Applied Mathematics in Biomedical Science

Applied Mathematics in Biomedical Science

Edited by Duncan Chambers

hayle medical

New York

Hayle Medical,
750 Third Avenue, 9th Floor,
New York, NY 10017, USA

Visit us on the World Wide Web at:
www.haylemedical.com

ISBN: 978-1-63241-844-9

Cataloging-in-Publication Data

Applied mathematics in biomedical science / edited by Duncan Chambers.
p. cm.
Includes bibliographical references and index.
ISBN 978-1-63241-844-9
1. Medical sciences--Mathematics. 2. Medical sciences--Mathematical models. 3. Biomedical engineering.
4. Applied mathematics. I. Chambers, Duncan.

R853.M3 A66 2020
610.151--dc23

Table of Contents

Preface

This book has been an outcome of determined endeavour from a group of educationists in the field. The primary objective was to involve a broad spectrum of professionals from diverse cultural background involved in the field for developing new researches. The book not only targets students but also scholars pursuing higher research for further enhancement of the theoretical and practical applications of the subject.

Biomedical science is the set of applied sciences that has applications in developing technology that can be of use in public health or healthcare. These applied sciences include clinical virology, medical microbiology, clinical epidemiology, biomedical engineering and genetic epidemiology, among others. An important branch of biomedical science is biomedical engineering, in which the concepts of engineering design and engineering principles are used to advance healthcare diagnosis, monitoring and therapy. Mathematical and theoretical biology applies mathematical models, theoretical analysis and abstractions to develop an insight into the structure, behavior and development of living systems. Mathematics is increasingly being applied to develop solutions to biomedical problems, particularly in toxicology, neurobiology and infectious diseases. The ever growing need of advanced technology is the reason that has fueled the research in the field of biomedical science in recent times. This book attempts to understand the use of mathematics in biomedical science and how such an integration has advanced the frontiers of medical science. It is a collective contribution of a renowned group of international experts.

It was an honour to edit such a profound book and also a challenging task to compile and examine all the relevant data for accuracy and originality. I wish to acknowledge the efforts of the contributors for submitting such brilliant and diverse chapters in the field and for endlessly working for the completion of the book. Last, but not the least; I thank my family for being a constant source of support in all my research endeavours.

Editor

1

Common Interferences Removal from Dense Multichannel EEG using Independent Component Decomposition

Weifeng Li, Yuxiaotong Shen, Jie Zhang, Xiaolin Huang, Ying Chen, and Yun Ge

School of Electronic Science and Engineering, Nanjing University, Nanjing 210023, China

Correspondence should be addressed to Xiaolin Huang; xlhuang@nju.edu.cn and Yun Ge; geyun@nju.edu.cn

Academic Editor: Fei Chen

To improve the spatial resolution, dense multichannel electroencephalogram with more than 32 leads has gained more and more applications. However, strong common interference will not only conceal the weak components generated from the specific isolated neural source, but also lead to severe spurious correlation between different brain regions, which results in great distortion on brain connectivity or brain network analysis. Starting from the fast independent component analysis algorithm, we first derive the mixing matrix of independent source components based on the baseline signals prior to tasks. Then, we identify the common interferences as those components whose mixing vectors span the minimum angles with respect to the unitary vector. By assuming that both the common interferences and their corresponding mixing vectors stay consistent during the entire experiment, we apply the demixing and mixing matrix to the task signals and remove the inferred common interferences. Subsequently, we validate the method using simulation. Finally, the index of global coherence is calculated for validation. It turns out that the proposed method can successfully remove the common interferences so that the prominent coherence of mu rhythms in motor imagery tasks is unmasked. The proposed method can gain wide applications because it reveals the true correlation between the local sources in spite of the low signal-to-noise ratio.

1. Introduction

Electroencephalogram (EEG) collected from the scalp is the integration of the electrical activities of amounts of cortex neurons blurred by the skull [1]. Although it is widely accepted that EEG has the advantage of high temporal resolution, the spatial resolution remains as a problem [2]. To improve the spatial resolution, dense multichannel EEG (with more than 32 channels) and high-density EEG (with more than 128 channels) have gained more and more applications. However, the more the channels are used, the more the redundant information is involved. It directly results in the fact that the weak components generated from the specific isolated neural source are deeply concealed by the common components from the surrounding sources [3]. Moreover, these redundancies can lead to a spurious correlation/coordination between different brain regions while in fact little or none is present. It will greatly distort the result of the brain connectivity or brain network analysis, which becomes more and more popular [4–15]. Therefore, it is of great importance to unmask the isolated source-corresponding component from the originally collected signals with too much redundant information or common interferences.

Among multichannel EEG redundancy-removal methods, one representative is surface Laplacian reference scheme [16, 17]. After subtracting the average potential in the local neighborhood, the original signals referencing to one or two common locations are converted to referencing to the respective local one. Typically, the signal amplitude will greatly decrease, with the expected return of redundancy removal. The surface Laplacian reference scheme is theoretically simple and easy to implement. However, using the arithmetical mean within the neighborhood as the local reference may be a little bit rough, regardless of the conduction differences among the neighbor leads. In addition, great attention should be paid to the selection of the neighborhood.

Another representative is independent component analysis (ICA) [18, 19]. In fact, ICA has long been applied to EEG preprocessing [20–27] including electrooculography artifacts removal. Recently, Whitmore and Lin have succeeded in removing distal electrical reference as well as volume-conducted noises from local field potentials using ICA [25]. It greatly motivates us to step further, trying a more general common interference removal.

In the presented manuscript, we do not identify the source or the frequency of the common interference. Instead, we only assume that the common interference will affect the different channel most evenly and the mixing vectors keep constant during the whole experiment, regardless of the mental activities. In addition, by regarding both the common interferences and their transfer vectors as identical in the entire experimental circumstance, we adopt the component extracted from the baseline data. We validate the proposed method on BCI competition dataset 1 [28, 29]. It turns out that the method can successfully unmask the coherence in mu rhythm during a motor imaginary task. Since high-density EEG and brain connectivity or brain network are the trends in neuroscience, the proposed method can gain wide applications.

In the manuscript, we first describe the method in Section 2, and then in Section 3 the method is validated using simulation series as well as experimental data provided in BCI Competition IV, and finally results are discussed in Section 4.

2. Methods

The method includes three steps in order: independent components decomposition, the common interference identification, and removal and inverse transformation.

2.1. Independent Component Decomposition. Mathematically, given the independent M sources as $\mathbf{S} = (s_{i,j})$, $i = 1, 2, \ldots, M$, $j = 1, 2, \ldots, L$, in which j represents the sampling time index, the N-channel ($N \geq M$) collected signal denoted as $\mathbf{X} = (x_{i,j})$, $i = 1, 2, \ldots, N$, $j = 1, 2, \ldots, L$, can be calculated as

$$\mathbf{X} = \mathbf{AS}, \tag{1}$$

in which $\mathbf{A}$ is the N-by-M mixing matrix. Theoretically, each row of $\mathbf{A}$ represents a set of combination weights of the M different sources on the specific channel, and each column of $\mathbf{A}$, denoted as $\overrightarrow{\mathbf{A}}_j$, reflects the relative impacts of the jth source on all the N different channels.

The independent component decomposition is to resolve (1) to obtain

$$\mathbf{S} = \mathbf{A}^{-1}\mathbf{X} = \mathbf{WX}, \tag{2}$$

where $\mathbf{W}$ is called demixing matrix. Because neither $\mathbf{W}$ nor $\mathbf{S}$ is known a priori, the maximization of non-Gaussianity or minimization of mutual information principle is conventionally employed to approximate the $\mathbf{W}$ as well as $\mathbf{S}$ through iteration [12].

Herein, we adopt FastICA algorithm proposed by Hyvärinen [13] for independent component decomposition. The fixed-point iteration scheme as well as the maximum-negative entropy principle is employed to find the orthogonal rotation matrix $\mathbf{W}$ with the maximal non-Gaussian measure of the prewhitened data. And then the mixing matrix $\mathbf{A}$ can be calculated as

$$\mathbf{A} = \mathbf{W}^{-1}. \tag{3}$$

2.2. Common Interference Identification and Removal. Subsequently, we try to identify and remove the common interference through analyzing the mixing matrix $\mathbf{A}$.

The putative common interference component is assumed as a distal signal that has approximately same effect on all electrodes. In order to obtain local brain activities more accurately, these distal common interference components should be removed. To do this, the vector angles are calculated between each $\overrightarrow{\mathbf{A}}_j$ and a unit vector, and the smaller the angle is, the more uniform the impacts of the corresponding source (independent component) across channels are and the more likely the corresponding source is a common interference. We delete this source through setting the corresponding kth independent source $s_{k,j}$, $j = 1, 2, \ldots, L$ as 0, obtain the processed $\widehat{\mathbf{S}}$, and finally derive the deabundancy signals as

$$\widehat{\mathbf{X}} = \mathbf{A}\widehat{\mathbf{S}} \tag{4}$$

3. Experiments

3.1. Simulation. To validate the proposed method, we first applied it to simulation series. We define the three collected channel signals which are determined by three independent components, i.e., $s_1 = \sin(2\pi \times 10t)$, $s_2 = \cos(2\pi t)$, and random Gaussian noises with $\mu = 0$, $\sigma = 10$, and the mixing matrix $\mathbf{A} = \begin{bmatrix} 1 & -0.5 & 0.19 \\ 0.2 & 1 & 0.21 \\ -0.4 & 0.4 & 0.2 \end{bmatrix}$. As described in Section 2, the collected signals are derived by $\mathbf{X} = \mathbf{AS}$. The Gaussian component is deliberately set with great amplitude and is treated as the common interference. Theoretically, we can obtain the pure signal without common interference via setting the 3rd column elements as 0 s. We plot the pure signal of Channels 1 and 2 in Figure 1(a), and the collected contaminated signals in Figure 1(b). Then, we apply the proposed method to X. After common interference removal, signals of Channels 1 and 2 are plotted in Figure 1(c). To quantitatively evaluate the signal quality, we also calculate the linear correlation coefficient between the collected signals and the pure signals, both before and after common interference removal.

Figure 1 shows that the proposed method nearly doubles the correlation coefficient with the pure signals, and wave form also indicates the signal quality is greatly improved, even in such low signal-to-noise ratios.

3.2. Application to Scalp EEG

3.2.1. Data Description. We apply the proposed method to the calibration data in dataset 1 of BCI Competition IV, provided by the Berlin BCI group [20, 21].

This dataset includes three artificial data (#c, #d, and #e) as well as four data pieces recorded from 4 healthy subjects (#a, #b, #f, and #g) in motor imagery experiments. Each data

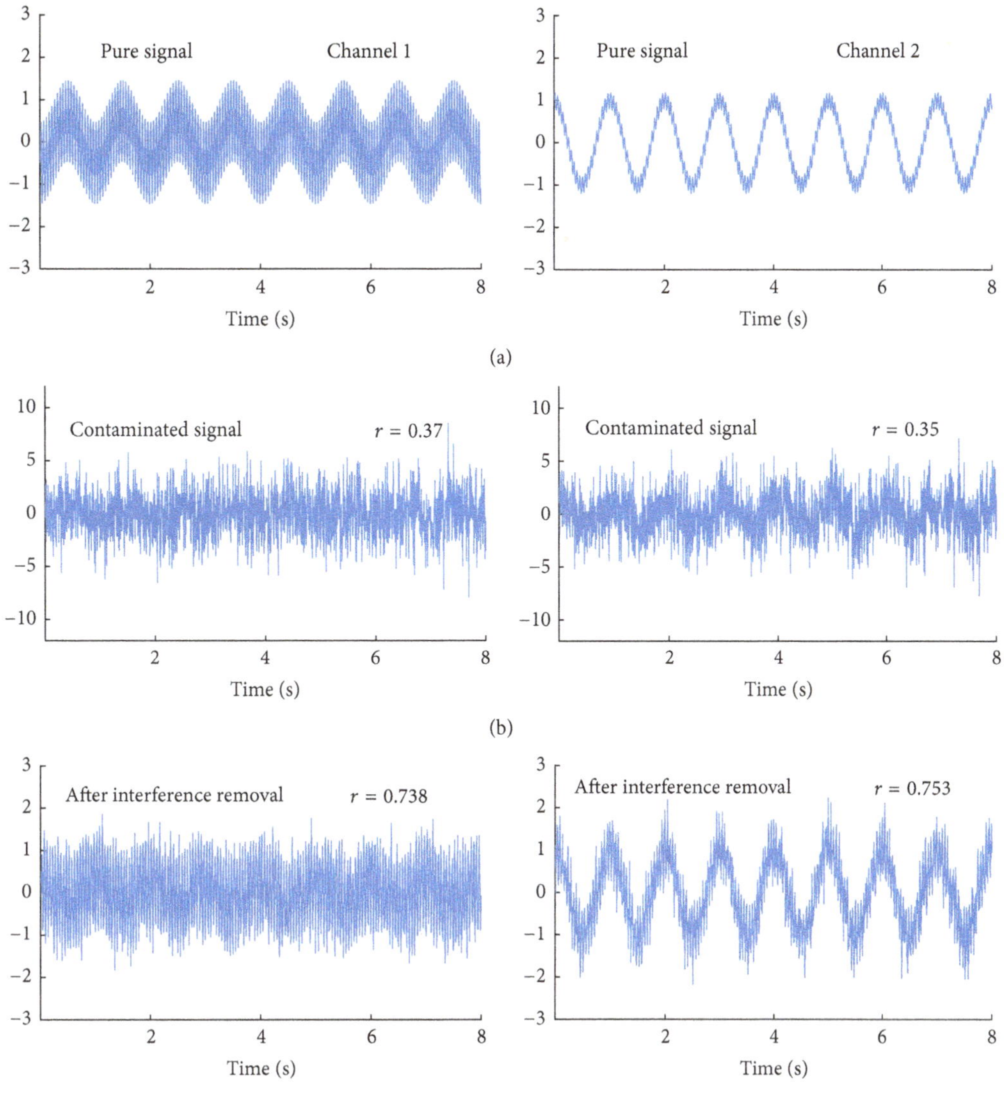

FIGURE 1: Simulation results ((a) is the pure signal, (b) is the contaminated signal, and (c) is the postprocessed signal. As we can see, although the noise is strong, the proposed method greatly improved the signal quality by doubling the correlation coefficient with the pure signal. Thus it validates the proposed method).

includes 59-channel continuous EEG or artificial simulated EEG, with a sampling rate of 1000 Hz and high cut-off frequency of 200 Hz. To compress the data size, the provider downsampled the data to 100 Hz after low-pass filtering them with stopband edge frequency 49 Hz [21]. According to the data information, we plot the lead locations in Figure 2.

In each experiment, before the first cue was given, the very first duration of 16 s can be considered the baseline signal, and then 200 trials of cue-response with 8 s duration were followed. Each trial consists of 4 s cue and motor imagery task, 2 s blank screen, and 2 s fixation. Motor imagery can be movement of left hand, right hand, or feet, and for each subject two classes of motor imagery were chosen. The first 2.56 s sections beginning with the cue are used for the following analysis.

3.2.2. Common Interference Removal. The baseline signals are firstly taken as original data to calculate the best orthogonal rotation matrix W and no more than 59 independent components S by FastICA [13]. The stopping criterion of FastICA is set as the minimum weight change of 10^{-5}.

Although the brain activities related independent sources might be different between the baseline and task trials, both the common interference signal itself and its corresponding transfer vector are assumed to be identical in the entire experiment. Therefore, the putative common interference components calculated by the baseline signals can be extended to the following task state of the EEG treatment. That is, $\mathbf{W}$ is applied to task trial signals:

$$\mathbf{S}^{\text{task}} = \mathbf{W}\mathbf{X}^{\text{task}} \quad (5)$$

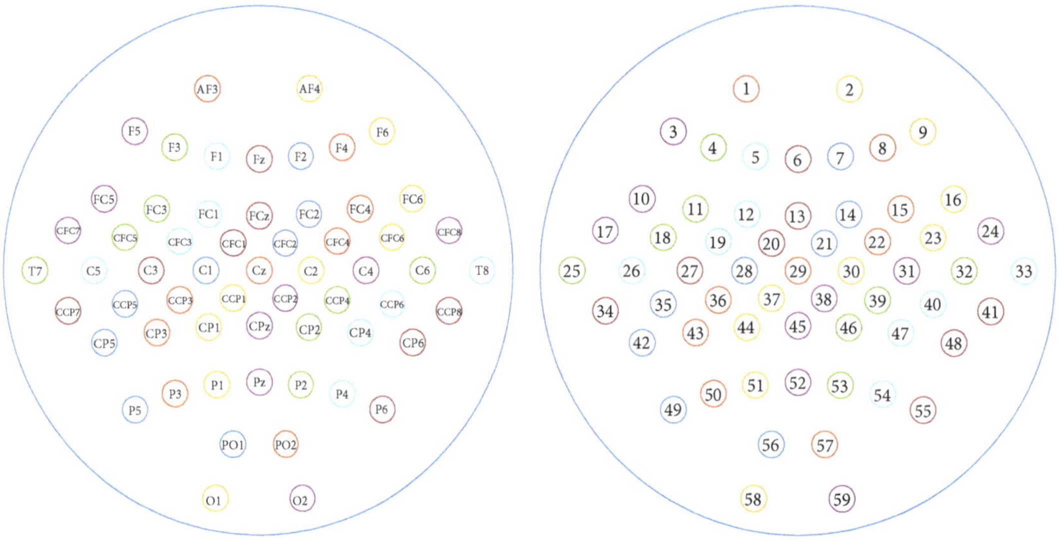

(a) (b)

FIGURE 2: Lead locations for signals in dataset 1 ((a) presents the lead label, and (b) presents the lead number, in case we would refer to it in the manuscript).

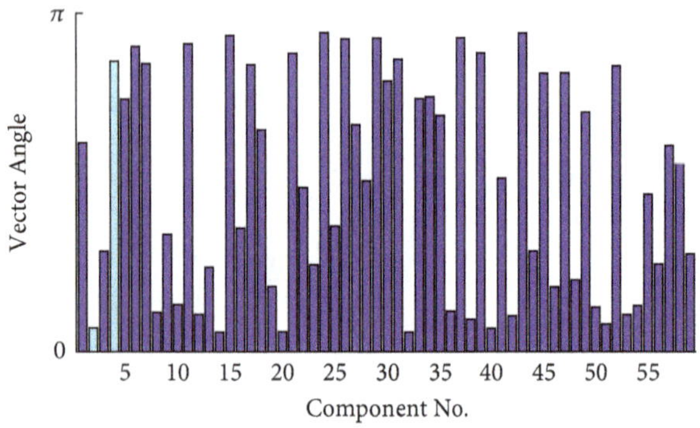

FIGURE 3: The vector angle of demixed independent component (the light blue marks the two components that are treated as common interference and removed).

After deleting the common interference, we obtain the processed signal as

$$\widehat{\mathbf{X}}^{\text{task}} = \mathbf{A}\widehat{\mathbf{S}}^{\text{task}} \tag{6}$$

3.2.3. EEG Results. We apply the proposed method to EEG. As a representative, we present the vector angle derived from #a in Figure 3, in which the light blue marks the two components treated as the common interference and then removed. As seen, these two components are not of the two smallest vector angles. However, we set an additional restriction that all elements in the mapping vector should be of the same sign. Therefore, in this case components 2 and 4 are determined as the common interference.

We also examined the EEG series before and after the processing. As a representative, we plot two leads of subject #a in Figure 4. As shown in Figure 4, the original signals collected from leads 5 (F1) and 7 (F2) are highly correlated. And the eye movement artifacts are obvious, occurring from

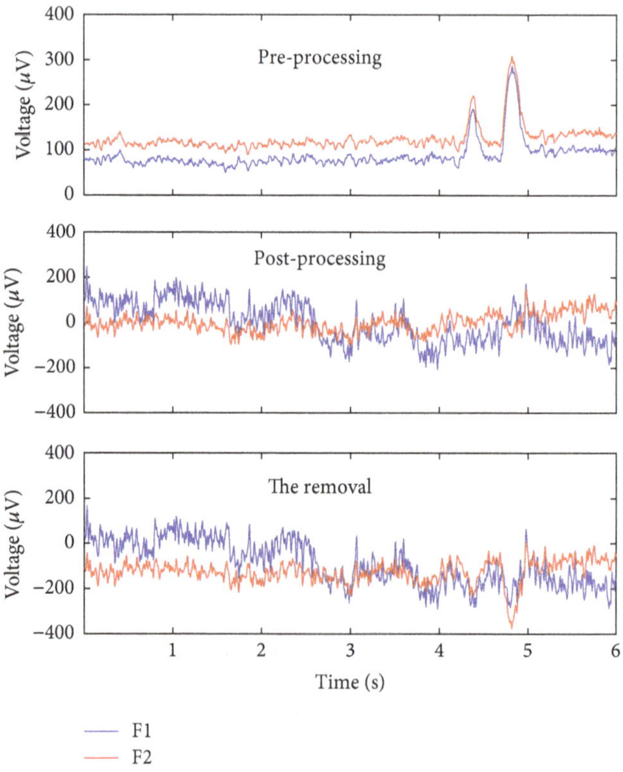

FIGURE 4: A representative EEG series result of subject #a. (Frontal EEG is usually contaminated by ocular and eye movement artifacts. This section includes two obvious ocular artifacts, occurring from 4.3 s to 5 s. After processing, the eye movement artifacts are successfully removed, and the correlation between F1 and F2 is alleviated)

4.3 s to 5 s. After processing, the correlation is alleviated, and the eye movement artifacts are removed.

It is difficult to provide an accurate signal quality evaluation, because we in fact do not know the "real" signal.

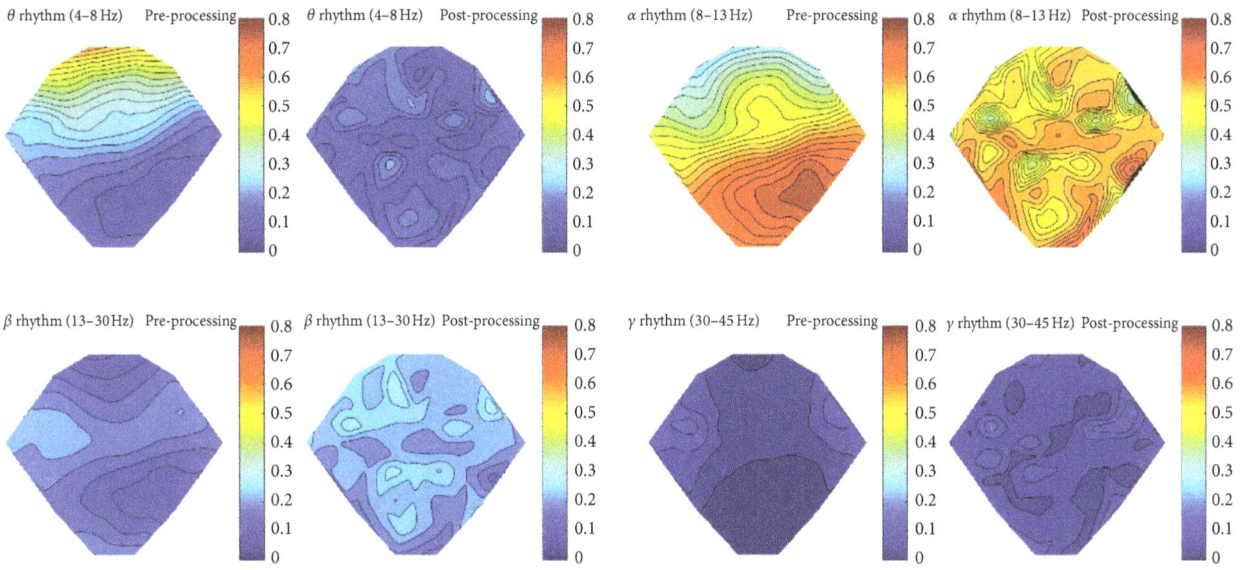

FIGURE 5: The relative power comparison between the original signal and the common interference removed signal. (Color represents the specific rhythm power relative to the power of the entire frequency band. As we see, after processing, the relative power reveals more distribution characteristics. It proves that we do uncover the intrinsic isolated neural activities, which were concealed by the strong common interference)

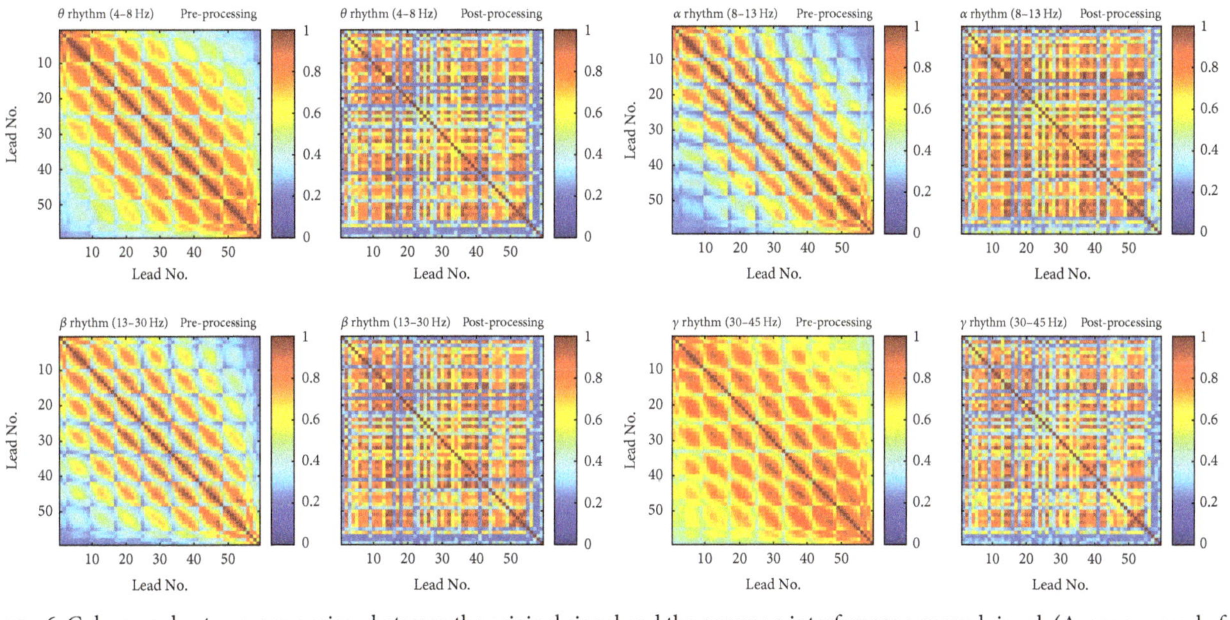

FIGURE 6: Coherence heatmap comparison between the original signal and the common interference removed signal. (As we can see, before processing, theta and gamma rhythm both present strong coherence for nearly all lead pairs. After processing, coherence differences among different pairs become obvious. In addition, the brighter lines parallel to the diagonal line diffuse to wider region after processing. It implies that after the common interference removal coherences between some far-away lead pairs become unconcealed and prominent)

However, we tried to calculate relative power as well as coherence and made comparison between the original signals (preprocessing) and processed signals with common interference removed (postprocessing). Taking the subject #a as an example, we present the relative power in Figure 5 and coherence heatmaps in Figure 6 for the commonly defined EEG rhythms.

As we can see from Figure 5, maps of the original signals have bigger connected regions, whereas after processing maps reveal more distribution characteristics. It proves that we do uncover the intrinsic isolated neural activities, which were concealed by strong common interference.

As we can see from Figure 6, for the original signal, the common interference imposes strong coherence on the

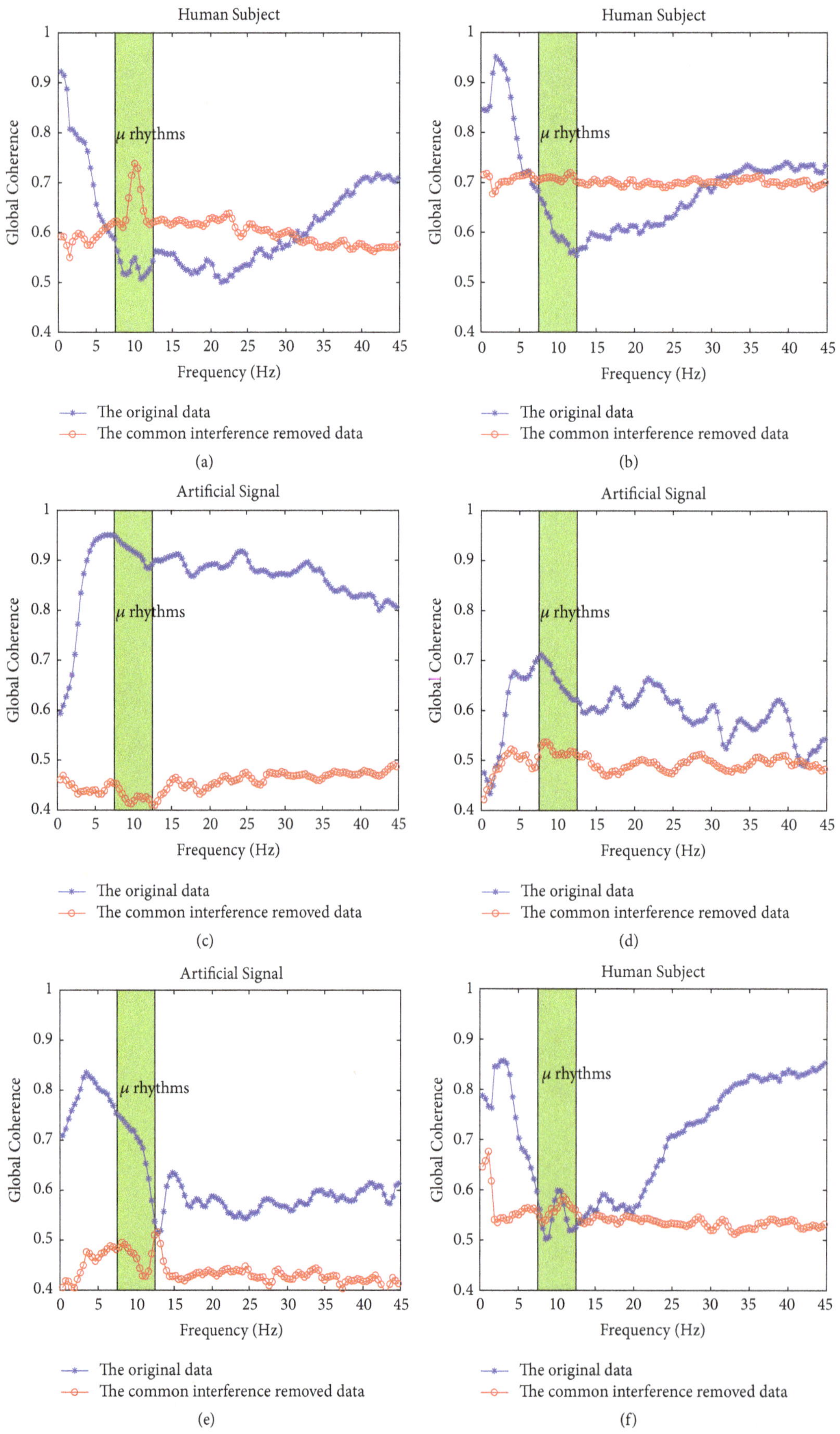

FIGURE 7: Continued.

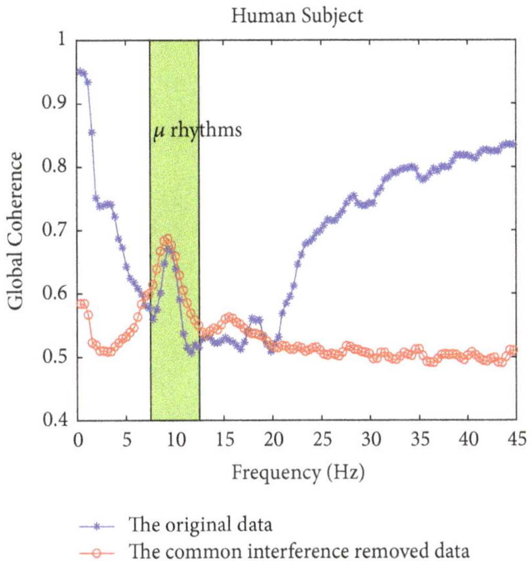

(g)

FIGURE 7: Comparison of the index of global coherence between the original and the processed signals. (The horizontal axis represents the frequency, and the vertical axis represents the index of global coherence. In the original data, all human subjects, i.e., (a), (b), (f), and (g), present high coherences in both low frequency band and high frequency band, which indicates a universal conductance induced consistency on scalp. However, as for the processed data, the high coherences in that two frequency bands are both suppressed while a coherence peak in mu rhythms (the green shade area) becomes prominent except for subject #b. It implies that although we did not mean to filter the specific frequency, the spurious high coherences caused by the common interferences are greatly alleviated. We cannot observe mu coherence in the artificial signals, i.e., (c), (d), and (e))

leads in the same neighborhood. That leads to the brighter lines parallel to the diagonal line in the heatmap, which may conceal coherence between leads that are not close in location. However, after being processed by the proposed method, the bright neighborhood diffused, and coherences between some far-away lead pairs become unconcealed and prominent.

We further calculated an interesting index, i.e., the global coherence [3, 22], and made comparison. All global coherence results for the data sets 1 are presented in Figure 7, in which the horizontal axis represents the frequency, and the vertical axis represents the index of global coherence.

As shown in Figures 7(a), 7(b), 7(f), and 7(g), in the original data, all human subjects present high coherences in both low frequency band and high frequency band, which indicates a universal conductance induced consistency on scalp. However, as for the processed data, the high coherences in that two frequency bands are both suppressed while a coherence peak in mu rhythms (the green shade area in Figure 7) becomes prominent except for subject #b. It implies that although we did not mean to filter the specific frequency, the spurious high coherences caused by the common interferences are greatly alleviated. Meanwhile, the coherence in mu rhythms, which are intrinsically related to the motor imaginary, is unmasked. And as to the artificial signals in Figures 7(c), 7(d), and 7(e), we cannot observe mu coherence. Since these signals are artificial, we consider it reasonable. Therefore, the above results demonstrate that the proposed method is successful.

4. Discussions and Conclusion

Coherence is the equivalence of correlation in frequency domain. In active brains, correlation analysis in time domain is difficult because the EEG amplitude is very weak for desynchronization. In these cases, coherence is the appropriate substitute. However, whether in time domain or in frequency domain, the spurious correlation brought by the common interference imposes a big problem on unmasking the true cooperation between the weak neural sources. In the presented work, we propose an independent component decomposition based method; the two most crucial innovations include the following: (1) the angle between the mixing vector and the unitary vector rather than the frequency or morphology is used to identify the common interference; and (2) the independent component source and the mixing vectors derived from the baseline signal are applied to the following task signals. As to (2), since most EEG experiments are implemented in stimulus-locking paradigm, the proposed method can gain wide applications. In brief, the proposed method presents successful application in the motor imaginary EEG of BCI Competition IV and reveals the coherence peak in motor related mu rhythms.

Appendix

The cross-spectral matrix $\mathbf{C}$ is calculated as

$$\mathbf{C}_{ij}^{X}(f) = \frac{1}{K}\sum_{k=1}^{K} X_i^k(f)\, X_j^k(f)^*, \qquad \text{(A.1)}$$

in which $X_i^k(f)$ and $X_j^k(f)$ are the spectrums calculated from channels i and j, respectively, at frequency f. Then the cross-spectral matrix is singular value decomposed as $\mathbf{C} = \mathbf{USV}$, where $\mathbf{S}$ is the diagonal matrix with each diagonal element, denoted as λ_i, being an eigenvalue, and $\lambda_1 \geq \lambda_2 \geq \cdots \geq \lambda_N$. Finally, the global coherence is calculated as

$$\mathrm{Coh}_{\mathrm{Global}} = \frac{\lambda_1}{\sum_{i=1}^{N} \lambda_i}. \quad \text{(A.2)}$$

Conflicts of Interest

The authors declare that they have no conflicts of interest.

Acknowledgments

This work is supported by Forward-Looking Project on the Integration of Industry, Education and Research of Jiangsu Province (Grant no. BY2015069-06) and Social Development Program of Primary Research & Development Plan in Jiangsu Province (Grant nos. BE2016733 and BE2017679).

References

[1] X. Ma, X. Huang, Y. Shen et al., "EEG based topography analysis in string recognition task," *Physica A: Statistical Mechanics and its Applications*, vol. 469, pp. 531–539, 2017.

[2] M. Gavaret, L. Maillard, and J. Jung, "High-resolution EEG (HR-EEG) and magnetoencephalography (MEG)," *Neurophysiologie Clinique / Clinical Neurophysiology*, vol. 45, no. 1, pp. 105–111, 2015.

[3] M. I. Franco, L. Turin, A. Mershin, and E. M. C. Skoulakis, "Molecular vibration-sensing component in *Drosophila melanogaster* olfaction," *Proceedings of the National Acadamy of Sciences of the United States of America*, vol. 108, no. 9, pp. 3797–3802, 2011.

[4] E. Bullmore and O. Sporns, "Complex brain networks: graph theoretical analysis of structural and functional systems," *Nature Reviews Neuroscience*, vol. 10, no. 3, pp. 186–198, 2009.

[5] M. Rubinov and O. Sporns, "Complex network measures of brain connectivity: Uses and interpretations," *NeuroImage*, vol. 52, no. 3, pp. 1059–1069, 2010.

[6] X. Ma, X. Huang, Y. Ge et al., "Brain Connectivity Variation Topography Associated with Working Memory," *PLoS ONE*, vol. 11, no. 12, p. e0165168, 2016.

[7] S. Palva and J. M. Palva, "Discovering oscillatory interaction networks with M/EEG: challenges and breakthroughs," *Trends in Cognitive Sciences*, vol. 16, no. 4, pp. 219–229, 2012.

[8] K. K. L. Liu, R. P. Bartsch, A. Lin, R. N. Mantegna, and P. C. Ivanov, "Plasticity of brain wave network interactions and evolution across physiologic states," *Frontiers in Neural Circuits*, vol. 9, no. OCTOBER, pp. 1–15, 2015.

[9] R. P. Bartsch, K. K. L. Liu, A. Bashan, and P. C. Ivanov, "Network physiology: How organ systems dynamically interact," *PLoS ONE*, vol. 10, no. 11, Article ID e0142143, 2015.

[10] P. C. H. Ivanov, K. K. L. Liu, and R. P. Bartsch, "Focus on the emerging new fields of network physiology and network medicine," *New Journal of Physics* , vol. 18, no. 10, Article ID 100201, 2016.

[11] A. Lin, K. K. L. Liu, R. P. Bartsch, and P. C. Ivanov, "Delay-correlation landscape reveals characteristic time delays of brain rhythms and heart interactions," *Philosophical Transactions of the Royal Society A: Mathematical, Physical & Engineering Sciences*, vol. 374, no. 2067, 2016.

[12] J. R. Moorman, D. E. Lake, and P. C. Ivanov, "Early detection of sepsis - A role for network physiology?" *Critical Care Medicine*, vol. 44, no. 5, pp. e312–e313, 2016.

[13] R. P. Bartsch and P. C. Ivanov, "Coexisting forms of coupling and Phase-Transitions in physiological networks," *Communications in Computer and Information Science*, vol. 438, pp. 270–287, 2014.

[14] P. C. H. Ivanov and et al., "Physiologic networks: topological and functional transitions across sleep stages," *Sleep*, vol. 35, 2012, Supplement S: A52-A53.

[15] A. Bashan, R. P. Bartsch, J. W. Kantelhardt, S. Havlin, and P. C. Ivanov, "Network physiology reveals relations between network topology and physiological function," *Nature Communications*, vol. 3, article no. 702, 2012.

[16] P. L. Nunez and R. Srinivasan, "Electric Fields of the Brain: The neurophysics of EEG," *Electric Fields of the Brain: The neurophysics of EEG*, pp. 1–611, 2009.

[17] G. Fein, J. Raz, F. F. Brown, and E. L. Merrin, "Common reference coherence data are confounded by power and phase effects," *Electroencephalography and Clinical Neurophysiology*, vol. 69, no. 6, pp. 581–584, 1988.

[18] P. Comon, "Independent component analysis, A new concept?" *Signal Processing*, vol. 36, no. 3, pp. 287–314, 1994.

[19] A. Hyvärinen, "Fast and robust fixed-point algorithms for independent component analysis," *IEEE Transactions on Neural Networks and Learning Systems*, vol. 10, no. 3, pp. 626–634, 1999.

[20] A. Delorme and S. Makeig, "EEGLAB: an open source toolbox for analysis of single-trial EEG dynamics including independent component analysis," *Journal of Neuroscience Methods*, vol. 134, no. 1, pp. 9–21, 2004.

[21] A. Delorme, T. Sejnowski, and S. Makeig, "Enhanced detection of artifacts in EEG data using higher-order statistics and independent component analysis," *NeuroImage*, vol. 34, no. 4, pp. 1443–1449, 2007.

[22] R. N. Vigário, "Extraction of ocular artefacts from EEG using independent component analysis," *Electroencephalography and Clinical Neurophysiology*, vol. 103, no. 3, pp. 395–404, 1997.

[23] J. Onton, M. Westerfield, J. Townsend, and S. Makeig, "Imaging human EEG dynamics using independent component analysis," *Neuroscience & Biobehavioral Reviews*, vol. 30, no. 6, pp. 808–822, 2006.

[24] G. G. Knyazev, J. Y. Slobodskoj-Plusnin, A. V. Bocharov, and L. V. Pylkova, "The default mode network and EEG alpha oscillations: An independent component analysis," *Brain Research*, vol. 1402, pp. 67–79, 2011.

[25] N. W. Whitmore and S.-C. Lin, "Unmasking local activity within local field potentials (LFPs) by removing distal electrical signals using independent component analysis," *NeuroImage*, vol. 132, pp. 79–92, 2016.

[26] B. Blankertz, G. Dornhege, M. Krauledat, K.-R. Müller, and G. Curio, "The non-invasive Berlin brain-computer interface: fast acquisition of effective performance in untrained subjects," *NeuroImage*, vol. 37, no. 2, pp. 539–550, 2007.

[27] K. K. Liu, R. P. Bartsch, Q. D. Ma, and P. C. Ivanov, "Major component analysis of dynamic networks of physiologic organ interactions," *Journal of Physics: Conference Series*, vol. 640, p. 012013, 2015.

2

A Novel Approach for Predicting Disease-lncRNA Associations Based on the Distance Correlation Set and Information of the miRNAs

Haochen Zhao,[1,2] Linai Kuang,[1,2] Lei Wang,[1,2] and Zhanwei Xuan[1,2]

[1]*College of Information Engineering, Xiangtan University, Xiangtan 411105, China*
[2]*Key Laboratory of Intelligent Computing & Information Processing, Xiangtan University, Xiangtan 411105, China*

Correspondence should be addressed to Lei Wang; wanglei@xtu.edu.cn

Academic Editor: Michele Migliore

Recently, accumulating laboratorial studies have indicated that plenty of long noncoding RNAs (lncRNAs) play important roles in various biological processes and are associated with many complex human diseases. Therefore, developing powerful computational models to predict correlation between lncRNAs and diseases based on heterogeneous biological datasets will be important. However, there are few approaches to calculating and analyzing lncRNA-disease associations on the basis of information about miRNAs. In this article, a new computational method based on distance correlation set is developed to predict lncRNA-disease associations (DCSLDA). Comparing with existing state-of-the-art methods, we found that the major novelty of DCSLDA lies in the introduction of lncRNA-miRNA-disease network and distance correlation set; thus DCSLDA can be applied to predict potential lncRNA-disease associations without requiring any known disease-lncRNA associations. Simulation results show that DCSLDA can significantly improve previous existing models with reliable AUC of 0.8517 in the leave-one-out cross-validation. Furthermore, while implementing DCSLDA to prioritize candidate lncRNAs for three important cancers, in the first 0.5% of forecast results, 17 predicted associations are verified by other independent studies and biological experimental studies. Hence, it is anticipated that DCSLDA could be a great addition to the biomedical research field.

1. Introduction

For long time, RNA was just considered to be transcriptional noise and intermediary between a DNA sequence and its encoded protein [1, 2]. However, sequence analyses point out that more than 98% of the human genome does not encode protein sequences [3]. Furthermore, increasing studies based on biological experiments have indicated that ncRNAs play important roles in numerous critical biological processes such as chromosome dosage compensation, epigenetic regulation, and cell growth [4]. In particular, the lncRNAs, as a class of important ncRNAs with a length more than 200 nucleotides [5], have been found to be associated with a wide range of human diseases, such as breast cancer [6], colorectal cancer [7], lung cancer [8], and cardiovascular diseases [9]. Hence, the study of finding novel disease-lncRNA associations has captured the attention of a lot of researchers and has been considered as one of the hottest topics in the research fields of diseases and lncRNAs. The identification of disease-lncRNA association can not only accelerate the understanding of human complex disease mechanism at the lncRNA level, but also serve as a biomarker identification for human disease diagnosis, treatment, and prevention [10]. So far, a lot of studies have generated a large amount of lncRNAs related biological data about sequence, expression, function, and so on [11–13]. However, compared with the rapidly increasing number of newly discovered lncRNAs, only few known lncRNA-disease associations have been reported. Hence, it is challenging and urgently needed to develop efficient and successful computational approaches to predict potential lncRNA-disease associations. In recent years, some computational methods have been proposed to predict novel lncRNA-disease associations, which can significantly decrease the time and cost of biological experiments by calculating the association probability of lncRNA-disease pairs. For example, Chen G et al. presented the first prediction method (genomic locus based) and constructed a lncRNA-disease association database as well [14]. Liang et al. proposed a genetic mediator and key regulator model to unveil the subtle relationships between lncRNAs and lung cancer. Liu et al. developed a computational framework to accomplish this by combining human lncRNA expression profiles, gene expression profiles, and human disease-associated gene data. Applying this framework to available human long intergenic noncoding RNAs (lincRNAs) expression data, Chen et al. developed a semi-supervised learning method based on framework of Laplacian Regularized Least Squares, LRL-SLDA, to infer potential lncRNA-disease associations which did not need negative samples and could obtain a reliable AUC of 0.7760 in the leave-one-out cross-validations [15]. In 2014, Sun et al. constructed a lncRNA functional similarity network and applied random walk with restart (RWR) to infer potential lncRNA-disease associations [16]. In the same year, Li et al. presented a bioinformatics method based on genomic location to predict the lncRNAs associated with vascular disease [17]. Then, Zhao et al. developed a computational method based on the naïve Bayesian classifier to identify cancer-related lncRNAs by integrating genome, regulome, and transcriptome data [18]. In 2015 Zhou et al. proposed a novel rank-based method named RWRHLDA to prioritize candidate lncRNA-disease associations by integrating miRNA-associated lncRNA-lncRNA crosstalk network, disease-disease similarity network, and known lncRNA-disease association network into a heterogeneous network and implemented a random walk with restart on the newly generated heterogeneous network [19].

Nowadays, with advent of many biological datasets, such as LncRNADisease [14], lncRNAdb [20], and NONCODE [13], the number of lncRNA-disease associations is still very limited. In 2015, Chen developed a method, named HGLDA, based on the information of miRNA [21], which predicted lncRNA-disease associations by integrating disease-miRNA associations with lncRNA-miRNA interactions and did not rely on known lncRNA-disease associations. Different from the method of HGLDA proposed by Chen et al., in this article, on the basis of experimentally reported lncRNA-disease associations collected from the HMDD database [22] and miRNA-lncRNA associations collected from the starBase database [23], a novel model based on distance correlation set is developed to predict potential lncRNA-disease associations by integrating known lncRNA-miRNA associations and known miRNA-disease associations. Compared with HGLDA, the advantage of DCSLDA lies in the introduction of the similarity of disease pairs and lncRNA pairs and distance correlation set. In addition, to optimize the prediction performance of DCSLDA, new methods to calculate the similarity of disease-disease pairs and lncRNA-lncRNA pairs are developed simultaneously. Finally, to evaluate the prediction performance of DCSLDA, LOOCV is implemented on the basis of the known lncRNA-disease associations and known lncRNA-cancer associations separately, and simulation results demonstrate that DCSLDA is superior to the state-of-the-art methods and can achieve a reliable AUC of 0.8517 in the LOOCV when the pregiven threshold parameter r is set at 6. Additionally, to further evaluate the prediction performance of DCSLDA, case studies of breast cancer, colorectal cancer, and lung cancer are implemented for DCSLDA; as a result, among the first 0.5% of predictive results, 9, 6, and 2 predicted potential associations are confirmed by recent experimental reports, respectively. Hence, considering the excellent prediction performance of DCSLDA, it is obvious that DSCLDA can become a useful and efficient computational tool for biomedical researches.

2. Materials and Methods

2.1. Disease-miRNA Associations. We downloaded known disease-miRNA associations from the Human MicroRNA Disease Database (HMDD) in July 2017 (see Supplementary file 1), which included 10381 experimentally verified disease-miRNA associations (including 572 miRNAs and 383 diseases). After merging miRNAs which produce the same mature miRNA and eliminating duplicate data, we obtained *dataset1* including 5430 disease-miRNA associations (including 383 human diseases and 495 lncRNAs). Let D be the number of different diseases and $M1$ be the number of different miRNAs collected from the *dataset1*, respectively, $S_D = \{d_1, d_2, \ldots, d_D\}$ represent the set of these D different diseases, and $S_{M1} = \{m1_{D+1}, m1_{D+2}, \ldots, m1_{D+M1}\}$ represent the set of these $M1$ different miRNAs; then for any given $d_i \in S_D$ and $m1_j \in S_{M1}$, we can define the *Association Strong Correlation* (*ASC1*) between d_i and $m1_j$ as follows:

$$\mathrm{ASC1}\left(d_i, m1_j\right) = \begin{cases} 1, & \textit{If } d_i \textit{ is related to } m1_j \textit{ in the dataset} 1 \\ 0, & \textit{otherwise}. \end{cases} \quad (1)$$

2.2. miRNA-lncRNA Associations. We downloaded known miRNA-lncRNA associations dataset from starBase v2.0 dataset in July 2017, which provided the most comprehensive experimentally confirmed lncRNA-miRNA interactions based on large scale CLIP-seq data. After data preprocessing (including elimination of duplicate values, erroneous data, disorganized data, and so on), *dataset2* (including 10195 lncRNA-miRNA associations, 275 miRNAs, and 1127 lncRNAs) was obtained from the starBase v2.0 (see Supplementary file 2). Let $M2$ be the number of different miRNAs and L be the number of different lncRNAs collected from the *dataset2*, $S_{M2} = \{m2_1, m2_2, \ldots, m2_{M2}\}$ represent the set of these $M2$ different miRNAs, and $S_L = \{l_{M2+1}, l_{M2+2}, \ldots, l_{M2+L}\}$ represent the set of these L different lncRNAs; then, for any given $m2_i \in S_{M2}$ and $l_j \in S_L$, we can define the *ASC2* between $m2_i$ and l_j as follows:

$$\mathrm{ASC2}\left(m2_i, l_j\right) = \begin{cases} 1, & \textit{If } m2_i \textit{ is related to } l_j \textit{ in the dataset2} \\ 0, & \textit{otherwise}. \end{cases} \quad (2)$$

2.3. lncRNA-Disease Associations. In order to evaluate the performance of DCSLDA, the newly lncRNA-disease associations were downloaded from LncRNADisease database, which integrated more than 1000 lncRNA-disease entries and 475 lncRNA interaction entries, including 321 lncRNAs and 221 diseases from ~500 publications. In this dataset, after duplicate associations and the lncRNA-disease associations involved in either diseases or lncRNAs which were not contained in the *dataset1* or *dataset2* were removed, 203 high-quality lncRNA-disease associations were obtained finally (see Supplementary file 3).

2.4. Disease Functional Similarity Based on miRNAs. For calculating the functional similarity between diseases, we introduced the concept of social network. In the social network, for any two nodes, we can calculate the similarities between them by comparing and integrating the similarities of nodes associated with these two nodes. In this section, based on the assumption that similar diseases tend to show a similar interaction and noninteraction pattern with the miRNAs, we calculated the disease similarity in the disease-miRNA interactive network. As illustrated in Figure 1, the calculation procedures of disease functional similarity based on miRNAs include 3 steps. First, we constructed miRNA-disease interactive network from known miRNA-disease associations (*dataset1*), whose topology can be abstracted as an undirected graph $G_1 = (V_1, E_1)$, where $V_1 = S_D \cup S_{M1} = \{d_1, d_2, \ldots, d_D, m1_{D+1}, m1_{D+2}, \ldots, m1_{D+M1}\}$ is the set of vertices, E_1 is the set of edges, and, for any two nodes a, $b \in V_1$, there is an edge between a and b in E_1, if and only if there are $a \in S_D, b \in S_{M1}$, and $ASC1(a,b) = 1$. However, since different miRNA terms in the *dataset1* may relate to different numbers of diseases, it is not suitable to assign the same contribution value to different miRNAs. Hence, we define the contribution value of each miRNA as follows:

$$C_D(m_i) = -\lg\left(\frac{\textit{the number of } m_i - \textit{related edges in } E_1}{\textit{the number of all edges in } E_1}\right). \quad (3)$$

Finally, we defined the functional similarity between diseases d_1 and d_J by integrating the miRNAs related to di, dj, or both of them as follows:

$$\mathrm{FSD}(d_i, d_j) = \frac{\exp \sum_{m_k \in (D(d_i) \cap D(d_j))} C_D(m_k)}{|D(d_i)| + |D(d_j)| - |D(d_i) \cap D(d_j)|} \quad (4)$$

where *FSD* is the disease functional similarity matrix calculated based on miRNA and $D(d_i)$ and $D(d_j)$ are the number of d_i related edges and d_j related edges in E_1, respectively. As an example, in Figure 1, there is $FSD(d_1, d_2) = \exp(C_D(m_1) + C_D(m_3) + C_D(m_4))/(4 + 5 - 3)$.

2.5. lncRNA Functional Similarity Based on miRNAs. Based on the assumption that similar lncRNAs tend to show a similar interaction and noninteraction pattern with the miRNAs, we can calculate the lncRNA similarity in the lncRNA-miRNA interactive network. Similar to the calculation procedures of disease functional similarity, first, we constructed lncRNA-miRNA interactive network from known lncRNA-miRNA associations (*dataset2*), whose topology can be abstracted as an undirected graph $G_2 = (V_2, E_2)$, where $V_2 = S_{M2} \cup S_L = \{m2_1, m2_2, \ldots, l_{M2+1}, l_{M2+2}, \ldots, l_{M2+L}\}$ is the set of vertices, E_2 is the set of edges, and, for any two nodes $a, b \in V_2$, there is an edge between a and b in E_2, if and only if there are $a \in S_{M2}$, $b \in S_L$, and $ASC2(a,b) = 1$. Then, considering the number of lncRNA-miRNA associations, we defined the contribution value of each miRNA as follows:

$$C_L(m_i) = -\log_2\left(\frac{\textit{the number of } m_i - \textit{related edges in } E_2}{\textit{the number of all edges in } E_2}\right). \quad (5)$$

Additionally, we defined the functional similarity between lncRNA l_i and l_j by integrating the miRNAs related to l_i, l_j, or both of them as follows:

$$\mathrm{FSL}(l_i, l_j) = \frac{\exp \sum_{m_k \in (D(l_i) \cap D(l_j))} C_L(m_k)}{|D(l_i)| + |D(l_j)| - |D(l_i) \cap D(l_j)|} \quad (6)$$

where *FSL* is the disease functional similarity matrix calculated based on miRNA and $D(l_i)$ and $D(l_j)$ are the number of l_i related edges and l_j related edges in E_2, respectively.

2.6. Method for Predicting Potential Association between lncRNAs and Diseases. Based on the assumptions that similar diseases tend to show a similar interaction and noninteraction pattern with the miRNAs and similar miRNAs tend to show a similar interaction and noninteraction pattern with the lncRNAs, we proposed a novel model, DCSLDA, based on miRNAs and distance correlation set to predict potential disease-lncRNA associations. As illustrated in Figure 2, the procedures of DCSLDA consist of the following 6 major steps.

Step 1 (construction of the disease-miRNA-lncRNA interaction network). On the basis of the above descriptions and letting $M = M1 \cap M2$, we can construct a disease-miRNA-lncRNA interaction network based on *dataset1* and *dataset2*, whose topology can be abstracted to an undirected graph $G_3 = (V_3, E_3)$, where $V_3 = S_D \cup S_M \cup S_L = \{d_1, d_2, \ldots, d_D, m_{D+1}, m_{D+2}, \ldots, m_{D+M}, l_{D+M+1}, l_{D+M+2}, \ldots, l_{D+M+L}\}$ is the set of vertices, E_3 is the edge set of G_3, and $\forall l_i \in L, m_j \in M, d_k \in D$. There is an edge between l_i and m_j in E_3, if and only if the lncRNA l_i relates to the miRNA m_j. Moreover, there is an edge between m_j and d_k in E_3, if and only if the miRNA m_j is related to the disease d_k. Then, for any given a, $b \in V_3$, we can define the *ASC3* between a and b as follows:

$$\mathrm{ASC3}(a,b) = \begin{cases} 1, & \textit{If there exists an edge between a and b in the } E_3 \\ 0, & \textit{otherwise.} \end{cases} \quad (7)$$

In addition, although we did not use any known disease-lncRNA associations, the diseases and lncRNAs can still be linked by integrating edges between diseases node and miRNAs node and edges between miRNAs nodes and lncRNAs nodes in the G_3.

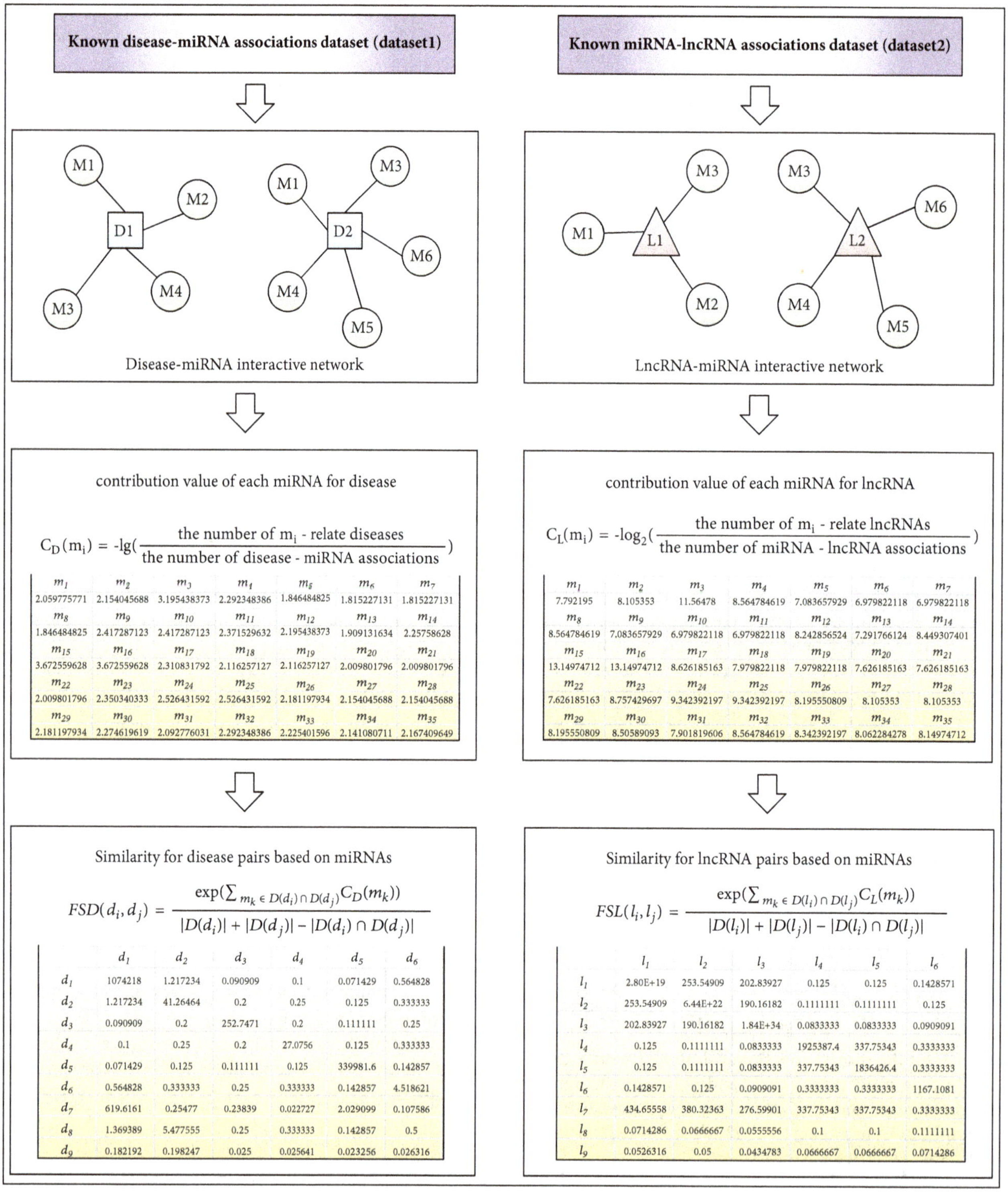

$$C_D(m_i) = -\lg\left(\frac{\text{the number of } m_i \text{ - relate diseases}}{\text{the number of disease - miRNA associations}}\right)$$

m_1	m_2	m_3	m_4	m_5	m_6	m_7
2.059775771	2.154045688	3.195438373	2.292348386	1.846484825	1.815227131	1.815227131
m_8	m_9	m_{10}	m_{11}	m_{12}	m_{13}	m_{14}
1.846484825	2.417287123	2.417287123	2.371529632	2.195438373	1.909131634	2.25758628
m_{15}	m_{16}	m_{17}	m_{18}	m_{19}	m_{20}	m_{21}
3.672559628	3.672559628	2.310831792	2.116257127	2.116257127	2.009801796	2.009801796
m_{22}	m_{23}	m_{24}	m_{25}	m_{26}	m_{27}	m_{28}
2.009801796	2.350340333	2.526431592	2.526431592	2.181197934	2.154045688	2.154045688
m_{29}	m_{30}	m_{31}	m_{32}	m_{33}	m_{34}	m_{35}
2.181197934	2.274619619	2.092776031	2.292348386	2.225401596	2.141080711	2.167409649

$$C_L(m_i) = -\log_2\left(\frac{\text{the number of } m_i \text{ - relate lncRNAs}}{\text{the number of miRNA - lncRNA associations}}\right)$$

m_1	m_2	m_3	m_4	m_5	m_6	m_7
7.792195	8.105353	11.56478	8.564784619	7.083657929	6.979822118	6.979822118
m_8	m_9	m_{10}	m_{11}	m_{12}	m_{13}	m_{14}
8.564784619	7.083657929	6.979822118	6.979822118	8.242856524	7.291766124	8.449307401
m_{15}	m_{16}	m_{17}	m_{18}	m_{19}	m_{20}	m_{21}
13.14974712	13.14974712	8.626185163	7.979822118	7.979822118	7.626185163	7.626185163
m_{22}	m_{23}	m_{24}	m_{25}	m_{26}	m_{27}	m_{28}
7.626185163	8.757429697	9.342392197	9.342392197	8.195550809	8.105353	8.105353
m_{29}	m_{30}	m_{31}	m_{32}	m_{33}	m_{34}	m_{35}
8.195550809	8.50589093	7.901819606	8.564784619	8.342392197	8.062284278	8.14974712

$$FSD(d_i, d_j) = \frac{\exp(\sum_{m_k \in D(d_i) \cap D(d_j)} C_D(m_k))}{|D(d_i)| + |D(d_j)| - |D(d_i) \cap D(d_j)|}$$

	d_1	d_2	d_3	d_4	d_5	d_6
d_1	1074218	1.217234	0.090909	0.1	0.071429	0.564828
d_2	1.217234	41.26464	0.2	0.25	0.125	0.333333
d_3	0.090909	0.2	252.7471	0.2	0.111111	0.25
d_4	0.1	0.25	0.2	27.0756	0.125	0.333333
d_5	0.071429	0.125	0.111111	0.125	339981.6	0.142857
d_6	0.564828	0.333333	0.25	0.333333	0.142857	4.518621
d_7	619.6161	0.25477	0.23839	0.022727	2.029099	0.107586
d_8	1.369389	5.477555	0.25	0.333333	0.142857	0.5
d_9	0.182192	0.198247	0.025	0.025641	0.023256	0.026316

$$FSL(l_i, l_j) = \frac{\exp(\sum_{m_k \in D(l_i) \cap D(l_j)} C_L(m_k))}{|D(l_i)| + |D(l_j)| - |D(l_i) \cap D(l_j)|}$$

	l_1	l_2	l_3	l_4	l_5	l_6
l_1	2.80E+19	253.54909	202.83927	0.125	0.125	0.1428571
l_2	253.54909	6.44E+22	190.16182	0.1111111	0.1111111	0.125
l_3	202.83927	190.16182	1.84E+34	0.0833333	0.0833333	0.0909091
l_4	0.125	0.1111111	0.0833333	1925387.4	337.75343	0.3333333
l_5	0.125	0.1111111	0.0833333	337.75343	1836426.4	0.3333333
l_6	0.1428571	0.125	0.0909091	0.3333333	0.3333333	1167.1081
l_7	434.65558	380.32363	276.59901	337.75343	337.75343	0.3333333
l_8	0.0714286	0.0666667	0.0555556	0.1	0.1	0.1111111
l_9	0.0526316	0.05	0.0434783	0.0666667	0.0666667	0.0714286

FIGURE 1: The flowchart of functional similarity calculation based on information of miRNA includes three steps: (1) constructing known disease-miRNA association and miRNA-lncRNA association network respectively; (2) obtaining contribution of each miRNA; (3) calculating functional similarity for diseases and lncRNAs, respectively.

Step 2 (construction of the *Adjacency Matrix* based on the disease-miRNA-lncRNA interactive network). We can construct a $(D + M + L) \times (D + M + L)$ dimensional *Adjacency Matrix* (*AM*) based on the disease-miRNA-lncRNA interactive network as follows:

$$AM(i,j)\begin{cases} ASC3(d_i,d_j), & if\ i \in [1,D],\ j \in [1,D]. \\ ASC3(d_i,m_j), & if\ i \in [1,D],\ j \in [D,D+M]. \\ ASC3(d_i,l_j), & if\ i \in [1,D],\ j \in [D+M,D+M+L]. \\ ASC3(m_i,d_j), & if\ i \in [D,D+M],\ j \in [1,D]. \\ ASC3(m_i,m_j), & if\ i \in [D,D+M],\ j \in [D,D+M]. \\ ASC3(m_i,l_j), & if\ i \in [D,D+M],\ j \in [D+M,D+M+L]. \\ ASC3(l_i,d_j), & if\ i \in [D+M,D+M+L],\ j \in [1,D]. \\ ASC3(l_i,m_j), & if\ i \in [D+M,D+M+L],\ j \in [D,D+M]. \\ ASC3(l_i,m_j), & if\ i \in [D+M,D+M+L],\ j \in [D+M,D+M+L] \end{cases} \tag{8}$$

where $i \in [1,D+M+L]$ and $j \in [1,D+M+L]$.

Step 3 (construction of the shortest distance matrix based on the disease-miRNA-lncRNA interactive network). Let r be a pregiven positive integer; then we can obtain r matrixes such as $AM^1, AM^2, \ldots, AM^r$ based on the *Adjacency Matrix*. Then, we can construct a $(D+M+L)\times(D+M+L)$ dimensional Shortest Path Matrix (*SPM*) as follows:

$$SPM(i,j) = \begin{cases} 0, & if\ AM^r(i,j) = 0 \\ 1, & if\ AM(i,j) = 1 \\ k, & otherwise \end{cases} \tag{9}$$

where $i \in [1,D+M+L]$, $j \in [1,D+M+L]$, $k \in [2,r]$, and k satisfies $AM^k(i,j) \neq 0$ while $AM^1(i,j) = AM^2(i,j) = \cdots = AM^{k-1}(i,j) = 0$.

Step 4 (collection of the *distance correlation sets* for nodes in the interactive network). In $G = (V,E)$, let $V = \{d_1,d_2,\ldots,d_D,m_{D+1},m_{D+2},\ldots,m_{D+M},l_{D+M+1},l_{D+M+2},\ldots,l_{D+M+L}\} = \{v_1,v_2,\ldots,v_D,v_{D+1},v_{D+2},\ldots,v_{D+M},v_{D+M+1},v_{D+M+2},\ldots,v_{D+M+L}\}$; then for each node $v_i \in V$, we can obtain its distance correlation set DCS_i according to the shortest distance matrix as follows:

$$DCS_i = \{v_j \mid r \geq SPM(i,j) > 0,\ i \neq j\}. \tag{10}$$

For instance, in the disease-miRNA-lncRNA interaction network illustrated in Figure 3, supposing that we hope to collect the DCS_{D1}, then according to the above description, we can easily know that the *distance correlation sets* of *D1* will be {M1, M2, M3, M4, L1, L2, L3, L4, L5} when $r = 2$.

And thereafter, for any given node $v_j \in DCS_i$, where $j \neq i$, we can compute the distance correlation coefficient $P(i,j)$ between the node v_i and v_j as follows:

$$P(i,j) = P(v_i,v_j) = \begin{cases} 1 - \dfrac{SPM(i,j)}{r+1}, & if\ SPM(i,j) \neq 0 \\ 0, & else. \end{cases} \tag{11}$$

Hence, based on (11), we can further obtain a $(D+M+L)\times(D+M+L)$ dimensional *Distance Correlation Coefficient Matrix* (*DCCM*) as follows:

$$DCCM(i,j) = \begin{cases} \dfrac{r}{r+1} & if\ node\ v_i = v_j \\ P(i,j), & if\ node\ v_j \in DCS_i \\ 0, & otherwise \end{cases} \tag{12}$$

where $i \in [1,D+M+L]$ and $j \in [1,D+M+L]$.

Step 5 (estimation of association degree between a pair of nodes in the disease-miRNA-lncRNA interactive network). Based on (12), we can obtain distance correlation coefficient of each nodes pair. For any given nodes pair (v_i,v_j) in $G = (V,E)$, where $V = \{d_1,d_2,\ldots,d_D,l_{D+1},l_{D+2},\ldots,l_{D+L}\} = \{v_1,v_2,\ldots,v_D,v_{D+1},v_{D+2},\ldots,v_{D+L}\}$ and $\{v_i,v_j\} \subseteq V$, we can obtain the association degree (AD) between them as follows:

$$AD(i,j) = \frac{\sum_{kD+M+L}^{k=1} DCCM(i,k) + \sum_{D+M+L}^{k=1} DCCM(k,j)}{D+M+L} \tag{13}$$

where $i \in [1,D+M+L]$ and $j \in [1,D+M+L]$.

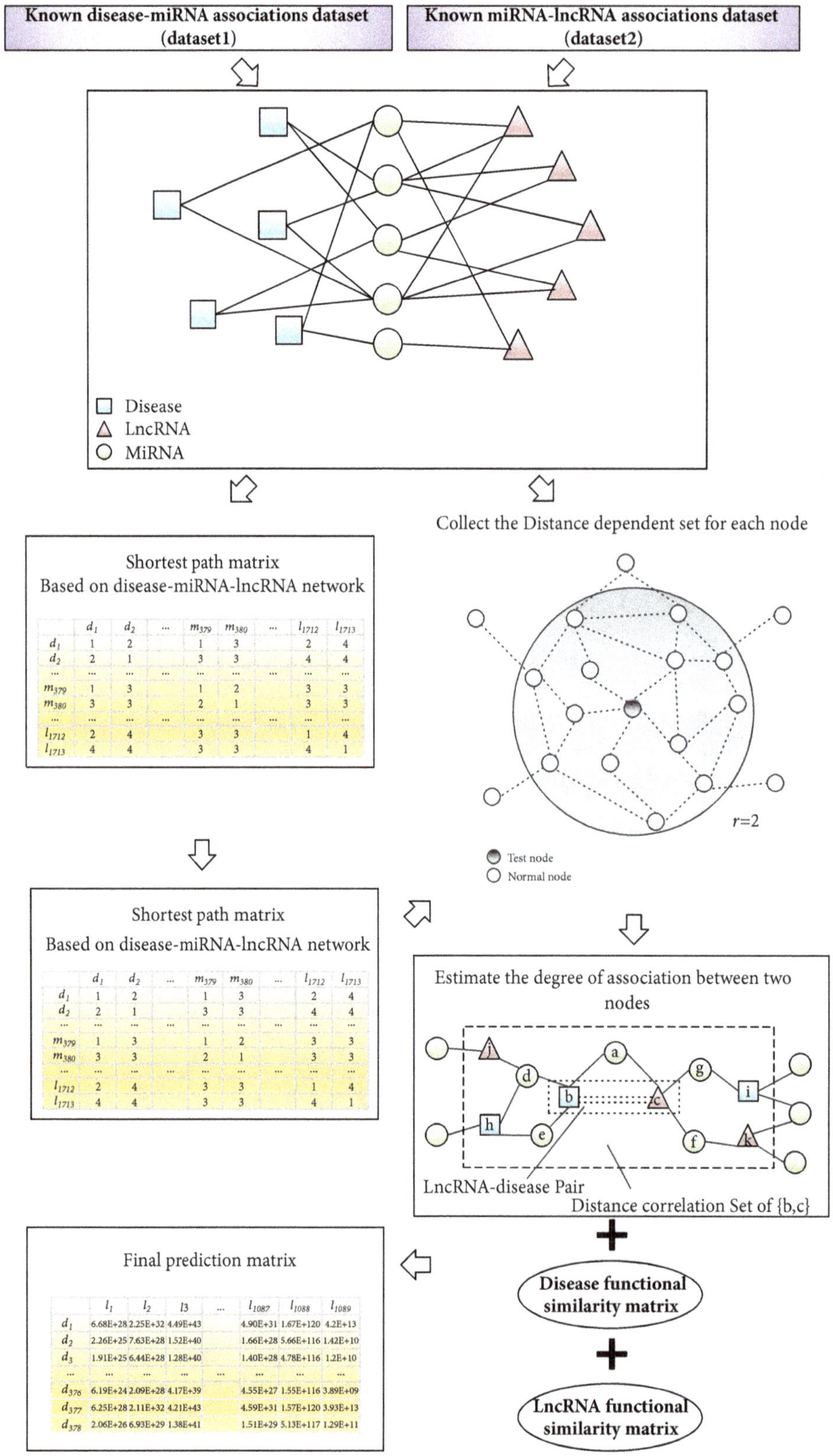

FIGURE 2: The procedures of DCSLDA.

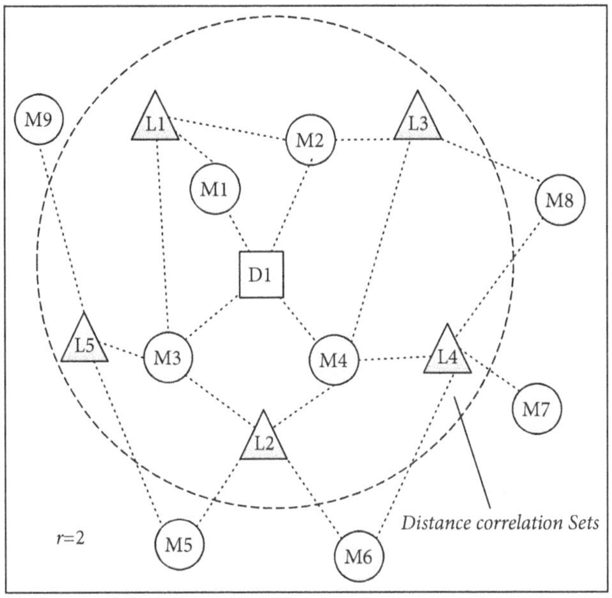

FIGURE 3: Distance correlation set of D1 with r=2.

Step 6 (construction of the *Final Prediction Result Matrix*). Based on (13), let $AD = \begin{bmatrix} C_{11} & C_{12} & C_{13} \\ C_{21} & C_{22} & C_{23} \\ C_{31} & C_{32} & C_{33} \end{bmatrix}$, where C_{11} is a $D \times D$ matrix, C_{12} is a $D \times M$ matrix, C_{13} is a $D \times L$ matrix, C_{21} is a $M \times D$ matrix, C_{22} is a $M \times M$ matrix, C_{23} is a $M \times L$ matrix, C_{31} is a $L \times D$ matrix, C_{32} is a $L \times M$ matrix, and C_{33} is a $L \times L$ matrix. It can be easily inferred that the matrix C_{13} will be our prediction results, which provided the association probability between each disease and lncRNA. Moreover, we can introduce disease functional similarity and lncRNA functional similarity for C_{13} as follows:

$$FAD = FSD \times C_{13} \times FSL \tag{14}$$

where the entity $FAD(i, j)$ in row i column j reflects the probability that the lncRNA $l(j)$ is related to the disease $d(i)$.

3. Results and Case Studies

To evaluate the prediction performance of DCSLDA, first of all, we implemented LOOCV (leave-one-out cross-validation) to compare DCSLDA with HGLDA [21] based on the lncRNA-disease association dataset downloaded from LncRNADisease database [14]. Next, LOOCV would be implemented to further evaluate the prediction performance of DCSLDA based on the known experimentally verified lncRNA-cancer associations. And then, the effects of the disease functional similarity and the lncRNA functional similarity to the prediction performance of DCSLDA would be analyzed also. Finally, experimental results about the prediction of associations between lncRNAs and three cancers were listed (see Table 1), and the performance comparisons between DCLSDA and HGLDA were implemented according to the rankings of these new disease-related lncRNAs in the case studies of three cancers (see Table 2).

TABLE 1: 17 predicted lncRNA-disease pairs with high predicted value while DCSLDA was applied to three important kinds of cancer (breast cancer, colorectal cancer, and lung cancer).

Cancer	LncRNA	PMID
Breast cancer	KCNQ1OT1	21304052; 26323944
Breast cancer	MALAT1	24525122; 19379481
Breast cancer	XIST	27248326
Breast cancer	NEAT1	25417700; 28034643
Breast cancer	LINC00657	26942882
Breast cancer	SNHG16	28232182
Breast cancer	CASP8AP2	28388918
Breast cancer	PPP1R9B	26387546
Breast cancer	TUG1	27791993
Colorectal cancer	KCNQ1OT1	16965397; 11340379
Colorectal cancer	MALAT1	25025966
Colorectal cancer	XIST	17143621
Colorectal cancer	NEAT1	26552600
Colorectal cancer	SNHG16	26823726
Colorectal cancer	CASP8AP2	22216762
Lung cancer	MALAT1	20937273; 24757675; 24667321
Lung cancer	XIST	27501756

TABLE 2: Performance comparisons between DCSLDA and HGLDA based on the rankings of ten lncRNA-disease associations related to three important kinds of cancer (breast cancer, colorectal cancer, and lung cancer).

Cancer	LncRNA	DCSLDA	HGLDA
Breast cancer	KCNQ1OT1	1	8
Breast cancer	MALAT1	4	30
Breast cancer	XIST	5	1
Breast cancer	NEAT1	8	12
Breast cancer	SNHG16	12	3
Colorectal cancer	KCNQ1OT1	1	5
Colorectal cancer	MALAT1	4	3
Colorectal cancer	XIST	5	1
Lung cancer	MALAT1	4	9
Lung cancer	XIST	5	1
Average ranks		4.9	7.3

3.1. Performance Evaluation of Potential Disease-lncRNA Association Prediction. According to the lncRNA-disease association datasets downloaded from LncRNADisease database, DCSLDA and HGLDA were applied in the framework of LOOCV, respectively. While the LOOCV was implemented for investigated diseases and lncRNAs, each known lncRNA-disease association would be left out in turn as test sample, and then we further evaluated how well this association ranked relatively to the candidate samples. Here, the candidate samples comprised all potential lncRNA-disease pairs without confirmed associations. Therefore, after the implementation of DCSLDA was completed, the rank of each left-out testing sample relative to the candidate samples

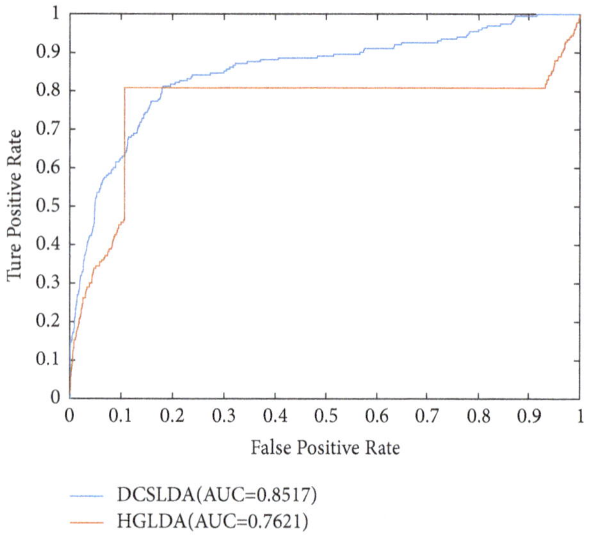

FIGURE 4: Performance comparisons between DCSLDA and HGDLA in terms of ROC curve and AUC based on LOOCV.

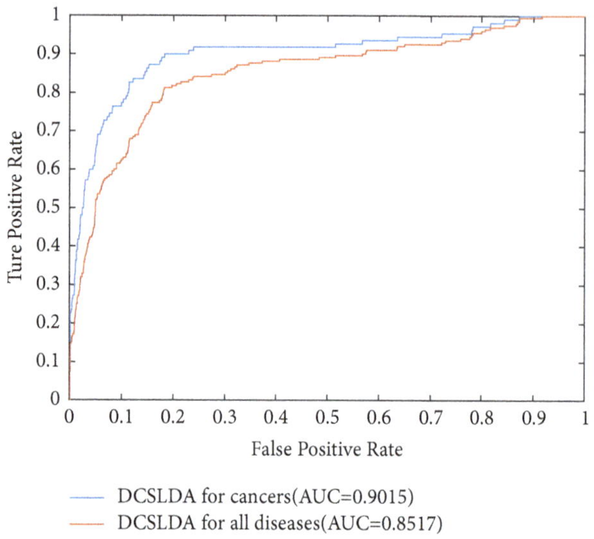

FIGURE 5: Performance evaluation of potential lncRNA-cancer association prediction in terms of ROC curve and AUC based on LOOCV.

could be further obtained. And then, the testing samples with a prediction rank higher than the given threshold were considered successfully predicted. Thus, we could further obtain the corresponding true positive rates (TPR, sensitivity) and false positive rates (FPR, 1-specificity) by setting different thresholds. Here, sensitivity refers to the percentage of test samples that were predicted with ranks higher than the given threshold, and the specificity was computed as the percentage of negative samples with ranks lower than the threshold. Therefore, the receiver-operating characteristics (ROC) curves could be drawn by plotting TPR versus FPR at different thresholds. And then, the areas under ROC curve (AUC) would be further calculated to evaluate the prediction performance of DCSLDA. An AUC value of 1 represented a perfect prediction while an AUC value of 0.5 indicated purely random performance.

The results of the performance comparison between DCSLDA and HGLDA were shown in Figure 4. Since the HGLDA method predicts lncRNA-disease associations without relying on the information of known disease-lncRNA association, it was selected for performance comparison with our method DCSLDA. As a result, it is clear that our newly proposed method DCSLDA achieved the AUC of 0.8517 in the framework of LOOCV, which is much higher than the AUC of 0.7621 achieved by HGLDA [21]. Simulation results indicate that DCSLDA significantly improved the performance of HGLDA by at least 0.0896 in the term of AUC values and fully demonstrate the performance superiority of HGLDA.

3.2. Performance Evaluation of Potential lncRNA-Cancer Association Prediction. Cancer has become one of the most dangerous killers for human beings [24, 25], and there is a high incidence of cancer in both developed countries and developing countries. Therefore, to further evaluate the prediction performance of DCSLDA, LOOCV was implemented on the basis of 117 lncRNA-cancer associations collected from the LncRNADisease dataset, and the simulation results were illustrated in Figure 5.

From Figure 5, it is easy to find that DCSLDA achieved the AUC of 0.9015 in the frameworks of LOOCV when r is set as 6, which indicates that our newly proposed method DCSLDA has a reliable predictive performance of cancers, and therefore it is a precise and high efficient method for the lncRNA-disease association prediction.

3.3. Effects of the Disease Functional Similarity and lncRNA Functional Similarity. In formula (14), we defined $FAD = FSD \times C_{13} \times FSL$. Then, in this section, we will analyze the effects of the disease similarity matrix *FSD* and the lncRNA similarity matrix *FSL* through comparing the prediction performances of DCSLDA in the framework of LOOCV while letting $FAD = C_{13}$ and $\mathrm{FAD} = \mathrm{FSD} \times C_{13} \times FSL$, respectively. The simulation results are illustrated in Figure 6. It is obvious that DCSLDA achieved the AUCs of 0.8517 while matrixes FSD and FSL were considered, but the AUC achieved by DCSLDA is 0.8352 only when letting $\mathrm{FAD} = C_{13}$. Simulation results indicated that the prediction performance of DCSLDA will be significantly improved by introducing the similarity matrixes FSD and FSC. Moreover, in Table 1, DCSLDA was applied to three important kinds of cancer (breast cancer, colorectal cancer, and lung cancer). As a result, 17 predicted lncRNA-disease pairs with high predicted value were publicly released to benefit the biological experimental validation.

3.4. Case Studies. Obviously, DCSLDA can predict all potential relationships between diseases and lncRNAs in *dataset1* and *dataset2* simultaneously. And of course, potential associations with high predicted value can be publicly released to benefit the biological experimental validation. It is anticipated that these potential disease-lncRNA associations that significantly share common miRNAs could be validated by

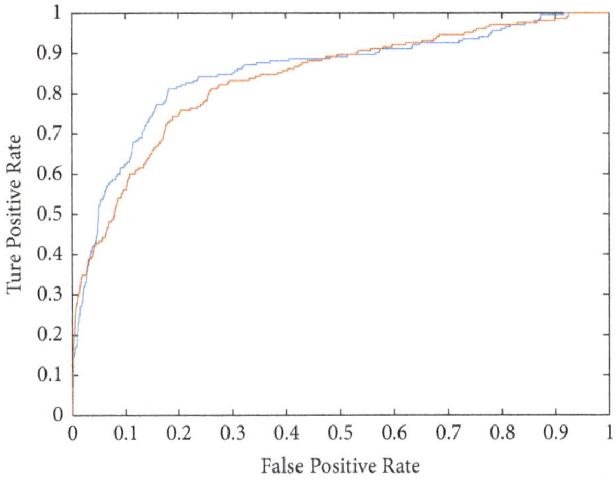

FIGURE 6: Comparison of effects of the disease functional similarity and lncRNA functional similarity to the prediction performance of PCSLDA in the framework of LOOCV with r =6.

biological experiments and provide important complement for experimental studies. Moreover, plentiful evidence has indicated that lncRNAs played important roles in various kinds of human cancers. The predicted results were sorted from best to worse, among which the first 0.5% results are selected to be analyzed (see Supplementary file 4). Case studies about three important kinds of cancers based on top 0.5% of predicted results were implemented to show the predictive performance of DCSLDA. Prediction results were verified based on the recent updates in the LncRNADisease dataset and recently published experimental literature (ranking results have been listed in Table 1).

In the world, breast cancer is the most prevalent cancer in women and a major public health problem. Several studies have focused on studying this disease, but more are needed, especially at the genetic and molecular levels [26, 27]. Therefore, it is necessary to predict breast cancer-related lncRNAs and identify lncRNA biomarkers. DCSLDA was implemented to prioritize candidate lncRNAs for breast cancer. Among the first 5% of predictive results, nine breast cancer-related lncRNAs have been confirmed based on recent experimental literature (see Table 1). For example, KCNQ1OT1, MALAT1, XIST, and NEAT1 are experimentally confirmed breast cancer-related lncRNAs, which have been ranked 2nd, 11th, 12th, and 19th in the predicted list based on the model of DCSLDA, respectively. KCNQ1OT1 had significantly higher expression levels in invasive breast carcinoma and was induced by estrogen in estrogen receptor-alpha expressing breast cancer cells [28]. 17β-Estradiol treatment affects breast tumor or nontumor cells proliferation, migration, and invasion in an ERα-independent, but a dose-dependent, way by decreasing the MALAT1 RNA level [29]. XIST expression is significantly reduced in breast cancer cell lines and breast cancer samples [30]. Breast cancer patients with high level of NEAT1 expression show low survival rate [31].

Colorectal cancer (CRC) is a leading cause of cancer deaths worldwide, one of the fundamental processes driving the initiation and progression of CRC is the accumulation of a variety of genetic and epigenetic changes in colon epithelial cells. Colorectal cancer is usually caused by the combination of various factors, such as genetic and epigenetic changes [32, 33]. Specially, lncRNAs have been demonstrated to play a critical role in the development and progression of colon cancer [34]. As a result, six colorectal cancer-related lncRNAs were listed in Table 1. For example, Tanaka K et al. proved that Loss of imprinting of KCNQ1OT1 is considered as a useful marker for diagnosis of colorectal cancer because of its frequent occurrences in colorectal cancer samples [35]. Ji Q et al. findings implied that MALAT1 might be a potential predictor for tumor metastasis and prognosis [36]. Furthermore, the interaction between MALAT1 and SFPQ could be a novel therapeutic target for CRC. Lassmann S et al. proved that expression level change of or DNA amplification of XIST is associated with colorectal cancer [37].

Over the past 30 years, the morbidity and mortality of lung cancer have been increasing and the cancer has the highest incidence and mortality across the world [38]. Due to the early diagnosis of lung cancer and the lack of effective treatment, its survival rate is around 10% within five years, which seriously endangers human health. More and more evidence has shown that lncRNAs play a critical role in treatment of lung cancers. Among the first 5% of predictive results, three predicted lncRNAs have been confirmed by published experimental literature [39]. According to this literature, MALAT1 has been shown to be highly associated with metastasis of lung cancer and promote lung cancer cell motility by regulating motility related gene expression [40, 41]. Long noncoding RNA XIST acts as an oncogene in non-small cell lung cancer by epigenetically repressing KLF2 expression [42].

In addition, performance comparisons between DCSLDA and HGLDA were implemented according to the rankings of these disease-related lncRNAs in the case studies of breast cancer, colorectal cancer, and lung cancer (see Table 2). By ranging the predicated results by HGLDA and our methods from good to bad, we selected the intersection of the underlying disease-lncRNA relationship predicated by HGLDA and the first 0.5 percent of the predicted results by our methods and listed the lncRNA items related to breast cancer, colorectal cancer, and lung cancer in this intersection in Table 2. As a result, DCSLDA significantly improved the prediction ability of HGLDA with higher ranks for these new disease-related lncRNAs.

4. Discussion and Conclusions

In recent years, plenty of studies have generated an enormous amount of biological data related to lncRNAs. Accumulating evidence shows that lncRNAs have played a very important role in the biological functions, and the study of lncRNA-disease association prediction is of great significance to human beings. However, there is a few computational models for predicting potential disease-lncRNA associations based on the information of miRNA. To utilize the wealth of disease-miRNA, miRNA-lncRNA, and disease-lncRNA associations data collected from three datasets and recently published in experimental literature, in this article, the novel model of DCSLDA was developed to predict potential disease-lncRNA associations. We calculated distance correlation set of each node based on disease-miRNA-lncRNA interactive network first and then further integrated disease functional similarity and lncRNA functional similarity for DCSLDA. The important difference from previous computational model is that DCSLDA does not rely on any known disease-lncRNA associations and it predicts disease-lncRNA associations only based on disease-miRNA-lncRNA interactive network. In order to evaluate the prediction performance of DCSLDA, the validation frameworks of LOOCV were implemented based on known disease-lncRNA and cancer-related-lncRNA associations downloaded from LncRNADisease database. And case studies were further implemented to three important cancers (breast cancer, colorectal cancer, and lung cancer) based on recently published experimental literature. The simulation results show that DCSLDA can achieve reliable and excellent prediction performance and is superior to the state-of-the-art methods. Hence, it is anticipated that DCSLDA could play an important role in the prospective biomedical researches.

Disease functional similarity plays an important role in disease-related molecular function research. Functional associations between disease-related genes are often used to identify pairs of similar diseases from different perspectives. Calculating lncRNA functional similarity could benefit lncRNA function inference and disease-related lncRNA prioritization. Therefore, based on the two assumptions that (1) similar diseases tend to show a similar interaction and noninteraction pattern with the miRNAs and (2) similar lncRNAs tend to show a similar interaction and noninteraction pattern with the miRNAs, DCSLDA was developed to predict potential disease-related lncRNA by integrating lncRNA functional similarity and disease functional similarity. Simulation results indicated that the prediction performance of DCSLDA will be significantly improved by disease similarity and lncRNA similarity.

However, there are also some limitations in our method. Firstly, DCSLDA measures the correlations between lncRNAs and investigated diseases by integrating walks with different lengths in a lncRNA-miRNA-disease network, which is constructed by combining the known disease-miRNA network, miRNA-lncRNA network, and disease similarity network. The value of distance threshold parameters r is an important factor in DCSLDA, and how to select this parameter is not yet solved well. Secondly, although DCSLDA does not rely on any known experimentally verified lncRNA-disease relationships, the performance of DCSLDA was not very satisfactory compared with that of several existing methods. In the future, we will further integrate data of diseases and lncRNAs that do not rely on the lncRNA-disease interactive network, disease-miRNA interactive network, or miRNA-lncRNA interactive network; then these above problems may be well solved. Finally, introducing more reliable measure of disease similarity and lncRNA similarity and developing more reliable similarity integration method would improve the performance of DCSLDA. In particular, disease similarity and lncRNA similarity in this model totally rely on known disease-miRNA and miRNA-lncRNA associations. The performance of DCSLDA would be further improved when sequence similarity of lncRNA and semantic similarity of disease are introduced.

Conflicts of Interest

The authors declare that there are no conflicts of interest regarding the publication of this paper.

Acknowledgments

The project is partly sponsored by the Natural Science Foundation of Hunan Province (No. 2018JJ4058, No. 2017JJ5036), the National Natural Science Foundation of China (No. 61640210, No. 61672447), and the CERNET Next Generation Internet Technology Innovation Project (No. NGII20160305).

Supplementary Materials

Supplementary file 1: the known miRNA-disease associations for constructing the ASC1. We list 5430 known miRNA-disease associations which were collected from HMDD dataset to construct the ASC1. Supplementary file 2: the known lncRNA-miRNA associations for constructing the ASC2. We list 10195 known lncRNA-miRNA associations which were collected from starBase v2.0 database to construct the ASC2. Supplementary file 3: the known lncRNA-disease associations. We list 203 high-quality lncRNA-disease associations which were collected from LncRNADisease database to validate the performance of our method. Supplementary file 4: the top 0.5% results were listed to validate the performance of our method. *(Supplementary Materials)*

References

[1] Y. Okazaki, M. Furuno, T. Kasukawa et al., "Analysis of the mouse transcriptome based on functional annotation of 60,770 full-length cDNAs," *Nature*, vol. 420, no. 6915, pp. 563–573, 2002.

[2] F. H. C. Crick, L. Barnett, S. Brenner, and R. J. Watts-Tobin, "General nature of the genetic code for proteins," *Nature*, vol. 192, no. 4809, pp. 1227–1232, 1961.

[3] T. E. P. Consortium, "Identification and analysis of functional elements in 1% of the human genome by the encode pilot project," *Nature*, vol. 447, no. 7146, pp. 799–816, 2007.

[4] F. F. Costa, "Non-coding RNAs: New players in eukaryotic biology," *Gene*, vol. 357, no. 2, pp. 83–94, 2005.

[5] T. R. Mercer, M. E. Dinger, and J. S. Mattick, "Long non-coding RNAs: insights into functions," *Nature Reviews Genetics*, vol. 10, no. 3, pp. 155–159, 2009.

[6] A. Katarzyna, M. C. Brian, E. F. Plow, and S. A. Khalid, "Mir-31 and its host gene lncrna loc554202 are regulated by promoter hypermethylation in triple-negative breast cancer," *Molecular Cancer*, vol. 11, no. 1, p. 5, 2012.

[7] X. He, X. Tan, X. Wang et al., "C-Myc-activated long noncoding RNA CCAT1 promotes colon cancer cell proliferation and invasion," *Tumor Biology*, vol. 35, no. 12, pp. 12181–12188, 2014.

[8] Y. Yang, H. Li, S. Hou, B. Hu, J. Liu, and J. Wang, " The noncoding RNA expression profile and the effect of lncRNA AK126698 on cisplatin resistance in non-small-cell lung cancer cell," *PLoS ONE*, vol. 8, no. 5, Article ID e65309, 2013.

[9] S. Uchida and S. Dimmeler, "Long noncoding RNAs in cardiovascular diseases," *Circulation Research*, vol. 116, no. 4, pp. 737–750, 2015.

[10] R. Spizzo, M. I. Almeida, A. Colombatti, and G. A. Calin, "Long non-coding RNAs and cancer: a new frontier of translational research," *Oncogene*, vol. 31, no. 43, pp. 4577–4587, 2012.

[11] J. Wang, R. Ma, W. Ma et al., "LncDisease: A sequence based bioinformatics tool for predicting lncRNA-disease associations," *Nucleic Acids Research*, vol. 44, no. 9, article no. e90, 2016.

[12] M. E. Dinger, K. C. Pang, T. R. Mercer, M. L. Crowe, S. M. Grimmond, and J. S. Mattick, "NRED: A database of long noncoding RNA expression," *Nucleic Acids Research*, vol. 37, no. 1, pp. D122–D126, 2009.

[13] D. Bu, K. Yu, S. Sun et al., "Noncode v3.0: integrative annotation of long noncoding rnas," *Nucleic Acids Research*, vol. 40, no. Database issue, pp. 210–215, 2012.

[14] G. Chen, Z. Wang, D. Wang et al., "LncRNADisease: a database for long-non-coding RNA-associated diseases," *Nucleic Acids Research*, vol. 41, no. 1, pp. D983–D986, 2013.

[15] X. Chen and G.-Y. Yan, "Novel human lncRNA-disease association inference based on lncRNA expression profiles," *Bioinformatics*, vol. 29, no. 20, pp. 2617–2624, 2013.

[16] J. Sun, H. Shi, Z. Wang et al., "Inferring novel lncRNA-disease associations based on a random walk model of a lncRNA functional similarity network," *Molecular BioSystems*, vol. 10, no. 8, pp. 2074–2081, 2014.

[17] J. W. Li, G. Cheng, Y. C. Wang, M. Wei, T. Jian, J. P. Wang et al., "A bioinformatics method for predicting long noncoding rnas associated with vascular disease," *Science China Life Sciences*, vol. 57, no. 8, pp. 852–857, 2014.

[18] T. Zhao, J. Xu, L. Liu et al., "Identification of cancer-related lncRNAs through integrating genome, regulome and transcriptome features," *Molecular BioSystems*, vol. 11, no. 1, pp. 126–136, 2015.

[19] M. Zhou, X. Wang, J. Li et al., "Prioritizing candidate disease-related long non-coding RNAs by walking on the heterogeneous lncRNA and disease network," *Molecular BioSystems*, vol. 11, no. 3, pp. 760–769, 2015.

[20] P. P. Amaral, M. B. Clark, D. K. Gascoigne, M. E. Dinger, and J. S. Mattick, "LncRNAdb: a reference database for long noncoding RNAs," *Nucleic Acids Research*, vol. 39, supplement 1, pp. D146–D151, 2011.

[21] X. Chen, "Predicting lncRNA-disease associations and constructing lncRNA functional similarity network based on the information of miRNA," *Scientific Reports*, vol. 5, Article ID 13186, 2015.

[22] Y. Li, C. Qiu, J. Tu et al., "HMDD v2.0: a database for experimentally supported human microRNA and disease associations," *Nucleic Acids Research*, vol. 42, pp. D1070–D1074, 2014.

[23] J. H. Li, S. Liu, H. Zhou, L. H. Qu, and J. H. Yang, "Starbase v2.0: decoding mirna-cerna, mirna-ncrna and protein-rna interaction networks from large-scale clip-seq data," *Nucleic Acids Research*, vol. 42, no. Database issue, p. D92, 2014.

[24] P. E. Spiess, J. Dhillon, A. S. Baumgarten, P. A. Johnstone, and A. R. Giuliano, "Pathophysiological basis of human papillomavirus in penile cancer: Key to prevention and delivery of more effective therapies," *CA: A Cancer Journal for Clinicians*, vol. 66, no. 6, pp. 481–495, 2016.

[25] M. K. Barton, "Local consolidative therapy may be beneficial in patients with oligometastatic non-small cell lung cancer," *CA: A Cancer Journal for Clinicians*, vol. 67, no. 2, pp. 89-90, 2017.

[26] M. Jin, P. Li, Q. Zhang, Z. Yang, and F. Shen, "A four-long non-coding rna signature in predicting breast cancer survival," *Journal of Experimental & Clinical Cancer Research*, vol. 33, no. 1, p. 84, 2014.

[27] N. Xu, F. Wang, M. Lv, and L. Cheng, "Microarray expression profile analysis of long non-coding rnas in human breast cancer: a study of chinese women," *Sichuan Building Materials*, vol. 69, no. 3, pp. 221–227, 2010.

[28] C. Lin, D. R. Crawford, S. Lin et al., "Inducible COX-2-dependent apoptosis in human ovarian cancer cells," *Carcinogenesis*, vol. 32, no. 1, pp. 19–26, 2011.

[29] Z. Zhao, C. Chen, Y. Liu, and C. Wu, "17β-Estradiol treatment inhibits breast cell proliferation, migration and invasion by decreasing MALAT-1 RNA level," *Biochemical and Biophysical Research Communications*, vol. 445, no. 2, pp. 388–393, 2014.

[30] Y.-S. Huang, C.-C. Chang, S.-S. Lee, Y.-S. Jou, and H.-M. Shih, "Xist reduction in breast cancer upregulates AKT phosphorylation via HDAC3-mediated repression of PHLPP1 expression," *Oncotarget* , vol. 7, no. 28, pp. 43256–43266, 2016.

[31] H. Choudhry, A. Albukhari, M. Morotti et al., "Tumor hypoxia induces nuclear paraspeckle formation through HIF-2α dependent transcriptional activation of NEAT1 leading to cancer cell survival," *Oncogene*, vol. 34, no. 34, pp. 4482–4490, 2015.

[32] D. C. Chung, "The genetic basis of colorectal cancer: Insights into critical pathways of tumorigenesis," *Gastroenterology*, vol. 119, no. 3, pp. 854–865, 2000.

[33] Y. Jia and M. Guo, "Epigenetic changes in colorectal cancer," *Chinese Journal of Cancer*, vol. 32, no. 1, pp. 21–30, 2013.

[34] Y. Yang, L. Zhao, L. Lei, W. B. Lau, B. Lau, Q. Yang et al., "Lncrnas, the bridge linking rna and colorectal cancer," *Oncotarget*, vol. 8, no. 7, 2016.

[35] K. Tanaka, G. Shiota, M. Meguro, K. Mitsuya, M. Oshimura, and H. Kawasaki, "Loss of imprinting of long QT intronic transcript 1 in colorectal cancer," *Oncology*, vol. 60, no. 3, pp. 268–273, 2001.

[36] Q. Ji, L. Zhang, X. Liu et al., "Long non-coding RNA MALAT1 promotes tumour growth and metastasis in colorectal cancer through binding to SFPQ and releasing oncogene PTBP2 from SFPQ/PTBP2 complex," *British Journal of Cancer*, vol. 111, no. 4, pp. 736–748, 2014.

[37] S. Lassmann, R. Weis, F. Makowiec et al., "Array CGH identifies distinct DNA copy number profiles of oncogenes and tumor suppressor genes in chromosomal- and microsatellite-unstable sporadic colorectal carcinomas," *Journal of Molecular Medicine*, vol. 85, no. 3, pp. 293–304, 2007.

[38] T. Hensing, A. Chawla, R. Batra, and R. Salgia, "A personalized treatment for lung cancer: molecular pathways, targeted therapies, and genomic characterization," in *Systems Analysis of Human Multigene Disorders*, Springer, New York, USA, 2014.

[39] W.-J. Gong, J.-Y. Yin, X.-P. Li et al., "Association of well-characterized lung cancer lncRNA polymorphisms with lung cancer susceptibility and platinum-based chemotherapy response," *Tumor Biology*, vol. 37, no. 6, pp. 8349–8358, 2016.

[40] K. Tano, R. Mizuno, T. Okada et al., "MALAT-1 enhances cell motility of lung adenocarcinoma cells by influencing the expression of motility-related genes," *FEBS Letters*, vol. 584, no. 22, pp. 4575–4580, 2010.

[41] G. Li, H. Zhang, X. Wan, X. Yang, C. Zhu, A. Wang et al., "Long noncoding rna plays a key role in metastasis and prognosis of hepatocellular carcinoma," *Biomed Research International*, vol. 5147, Article ID 780521, 2014.

[42] J. Fang, C.-C. Sun, and C. Gong, "Long noncoding RNA XIST acts as an oncogene in non-small cell lung cancer by epigenetically repressing KLF2 expression," *Biochemical and Biophysical Research Communications*, vol. 478, no. 2, pp. 811–817, 2016.

3

Modeling Inhibitory Effect on the Growth of Uninfected T Cells caused by Infected T Cells: Stability and Hopf Bifurcation

Yahui Ji, Wanbiao Ma, and Keying Song

Department of Applied Mathematics, School of Mathematics and Physics, University of Science and Technology Beijing, 100083, Beijing, China

Correspondence should be addressed to Wanbiao Ma; wanbiao_ma@ustb.edu.cn

Academic Editor: Ming-shi Yang

We consider a class of viral infection dynamic models with inhibitory effect on the growth of uninfected T cells caused by infected T cells and logistic target cell growth. The basic reproduction number R_0 is derived. It is shown that the infection-free equilibrium is globally asymptotically stable if $R_0 < 1$. Sufficient conditions for the existence of Hopf bifurcation at the infected equilibrium are investigated by analyzing the distribution of eigenvalues. Furthermore, the properties of Hopf bifurcation are determined by the normal form theory and the center manifold. Numerical simulations are carried out to support the theoretical analysis.

1. Introduction

The human immunodeficiency virus (HIV) is a lentivirus, which replicates by infecting and destroying primarily $CD4^+$ T cells. The end stage of HIV viral progression is acquired immune deficiency syndrome (AIDS) (see, for example, [1]), identified when the count of individual's $CD4^+$ cells count falls below 200. Since AIDS was found in America in 1981, it spread worldwide and became the public health and social problem which causes serious damage to human survival and development. In 2016, there exist about 38 million people living with human immunodeficiency virus (HIV) (see, for example, [2]). Thus, it is a challenge to study and control the virus.

It is widely known that mathematical models have made considerable contributions to understanding the HIV infection dynamics. Nowak et al. have proposed a class of classic mathematical model to describe HIV infection dynamics (see, for example, [3–6]),

$$\begin{aligned}\dot{x}(t) &= s - dx(t) - \beta x(t)v(t),\\ \dot{y}(t) &= \beta x(t)v(t) - py(t), \qquad (1)\\ \dot{v}(t) &= ky(t) - uv(t),\end{aligned}$$

where $x(t)$, $y(t)$, and $v(t)$ denote the concentrations of uninfected cells, infected cells, and free virus at time t, respectively. Uninfected cells are produced at the rate s ($s > 0$), die at the rate d ($d > 0$), and become infected at the rate β ($\beta > 0$). The constant p ($p > 0$) is the death rate of the infected cells due either to virus or to the immune system. The constant k ($k > 0$) is the rate of production of virus by infected cells and the constant u ($u > 0$) is the rate at which the virus is cleared.

Incorporating the life cycle of the virus in the cells, some researchers have considered that the HIV virus from HIV infection to produce new virus takes time. To make a better understanding for this phenomenon in mathematics, HIV models including time delay have been proposed (see, for example, [4, 7–9]). Several researchers have considered that when T cells stimulate by antigen or mitogen, this will differentiate and increase in the number. The HIV model with a full logistic mitosis term has been investigated (see, for example, [6, 10, 11]). Taking into account the growth of uninfected cells, they made a further investigation to add a full logistic term $rx(t)(1 - (x(t) + y(t))/T)$ (see, for example, [12, 13]).

In the above model, there are two factors that accelerate the reduction of uninfected cells: one is the natural death of uninfected cells and the other is that uninfected cells become infected cells. HIV gene expression products can be toxic and directly or indirectly induce apoptosis in uninfected cells. Some data show that viral proteins interact with uninfected cells and produce an apoptotic signals that accelerate the death of uninfected cells. Recently, Wang and Zhang proposed a spatial mathematical model to describe the predominance for driving CD4$^+$ T cells death, which is called caspase-1-mediated pyroptosis (see, for example, [14]).

Based on model (1), Guo and Ma have proposed a class of delay differential equations model of HIV infection dynamics with nonlinear transmissions and apoptosis induced by infected cells (see, for example, [15]). And then, Cheng et al. [16] have considered the following infection model with inhibitory effect on the growth of uninfected cells by infected cells:

$$\begin{aligned}\dot{x}(t) &= s - dx(t) - cx(t)y(t) - \beta x(t)v(t),\\ \dot{y}(t) &= \delta x(t-\tau)v(t-\tau) - py(t),\\ \dot{v}(t) &= ky(t) - uv(t),\end{aligned} \tag{2}$$

where the constant c ($c > 0$) represents the rate of apoptosis at which infected cells induce uninfected cells. δ ($\delta > 0$) denotes the surviving rate of infected cells before they become productively infected. The biological meanings of the other parameters in the model (2) are similar to that in the model (1).

Motivated by the above models, in this paper, we will study a delay differential equation model of HIV infection with a full logistic term of uninfected cells,

$$\begin{aligned}\dot{x}(t) &= s + rx\left(1 - \frac{x(t)+y(t)}{T}\right) - dx(t)\\ &\quad - cx(t)y(t) - \beta x(t)v(t),\\ \dot{y}(t) &= \delta x(t-\tau)v(t-\tau) - py(t),\\ \dot{v}(t) &= ky(t) - uv(t).\end{aligned} \tag{3}$$

In this model, the logistic growth of the healthy CD4$^+$ T cells is described by $rx(t)(1 - (x(t) + y(t))/T)$. The total concentration of CD4$^+$ T cells is $x(t) + y(t)$, where $x(t)$ denotes the concentration of uninfected cells, $y(t)$ is the concentration of infected cells, and T is the maximum level of CD4$^+$ T cells. δ ($\delta > 0$) is the infection rate of infected cells. The biological meanings of the other parameters in the model (3) are similar to that in the model (2).

The main purpose of this paper is to carry out a pretty theoretical analysis on the stability of the equilibria of the model (3) and to analyze the Hopf bifurcation by related theories of the differential equations. The organization of this paper is as follows. In Section 2, we investigate the existence and the ultimate boundedness of the solutions of the model (3). Then we consider the global stability of the infection-free equilibrium and the Hopf bifurcation at the infected equilibrium. In Section 3, some properties of Hopf bifurcation such as direction, stability, and period are determined. In Section 4, the brief conclusions are given and sets of numerical simulations are provided to illustrate the main results.

2. Local and Global Stability of the Equilibria

According to biological meanings, we assume that the initial condition of the model (3) is given as follows:

$$\begin{aligned}x(\theta) &= \phi_1(\theta),\\ y(\theta) &= \phi_2(\theta),\\ v(\theta) &= \phi_3(\theta)\\ &\qquad (\theta \in [-\tau, 0]),\end{aligned} \tag{4}$$

where $\phi = (\phi_1, \phi_2, \phi_3)^T \in C$ such that $\phi_i(\theta) \geq 0$ ($i = 1, 2, 3$). Here, $C = C([-\tau, 0]; R_+^3)$ denotes the Banach space of continuous functions mapping from the interval $[-\tau, 0]$ to R_+^3 equipped with the supnorm.

The existence and uniqueness, nonnegativity, and boundedness of the solutions of the model (3) with the initial condition (4) can be given as follows.

Theorem 1. *The solution $(x(t), y(t), v(t))$ of the model (3) with the initial condition (4) is existent, unique, and nonnegative on $[0, +\infty)$ and also has*

$$\begin{aligned}\limsup_{t\to+\infty} x(t) &\leq x_0,\\ \limsup_{t\to+\infty} (x(t) + y(t+\tau)) &\leq \frac{s + rx_0}{\tilde{d}},\\ \limsup_{t\to+\infty} v(t) &\leq \frac{k(s + rx_0)}{u\tilde{d}},\end{aligned} \tag{5}$$

where $\tilde{d} = \min\{d, p\}$ and $x_0 = (T/2r)(r - d + \sqrt{(r-d)^2 + 4sr/T})$.

In fact, by using standard theorems for existence and uniqueness of functional differential equations (see, for example, [17–19]), we can show that the solution $(x(t), y(t), v(t))$ of the model (3) with the initial condition (4) is existent, unique and nonnegative on $[0, +\infty)$, easily. And the proving of ultimately bounded of the solution $(x(t), y(t), v(t))$ is similar to [12, 16].

We can denote the basic reproduction number of the HIV virus for the model (3) as $R_0 = (k\delta/pu)x_0$, $x_0 = (T/2r)(r-d+\sqrt{(r-d)^2 + 4sr/T})$ (see, for example, [3]). For the existence of nonnegative equilibria of the model (3), we can obtain the following classifications:

(i) The model (3) always has the uninfected equilibrium $E_0 = (x_0, 0, 0)$.

(ii) If $R_0 = (k\delta/pu)x_0 > 1$, the model (3) has unique infected equilibrium $E^* = (x^*, y^*, v^*)$, where

$$\begin{aligned}x^* &= \frac{pu}{\delta k},\\ y^* &= \frac{u}{k}v^*,\\ v^* &= \frac{-rx^{*2}/T + (r-d)x^* + s}{rx^*u/kT + (cu/k)x^* + \beta x^*}.\end{aligned} \tag{6}$$

Theorem 2. *If $R_0 < 1$, the uninfected equilibrium E_0 of the model (3) is globally asymptotically stable.*

Proof. We consider linear system of the model (3) in E_0 near; we have

$$\begin{aligned}\dot{x}(t) &= \left(r - d - \frac{2r}{T}x_0\right)x(t) - \left(\frac{r}{T} + c\right)x_0 y(t) \\ &\quad - \beta x_0 v(t), \\ \dot{y}(t) &= \delta x_0 v(t-\tau) - p y(t), \\ \dot{v}(t) &= k y(t) - u v(t).\end{aligned} \quad (7)$$

The corresponding characteristic equation is given by

$$\left(\lambda - r + d + \frac{2r}{T}x_0\right)\left[(\lambda + p)(\lambda + u) - k\delta x_0 e^{-\lambda\tau}\right] = 0. \quad (8)$$

Clearly, one of the roots is $\lambda_1 = r - d - (2r/T)x_0 = -\sqrt{(r-d)^2 + 4rs/T} < 0$, so the local stability depends on the other two roots generated by

$$\lambda^2 + (p + u)\lambda + pu - k\delta x_0 e^{-\lambda\tau} = 0. \quad (9)$$

When $R_0 < 1$, $pu - k\delta x_0 \neq 0$. Therefore, $\lambda = 0$ is not root of (9). If (8) has pure imaginary root $\lambda = i\omega$ ($\omega > 0$) for some $\tau > 0$, substituting it into (8) and separating the real and imaginary parts, it has

$$\begin{aligned}pu - w^2 &= k\delta x_0 \cos w\tau, \\ (p + u) w &= -k\delta x_0 \sin w\tau.\end{aligned} \quad (10)$$

It follows that

$$f(\tilde{\omega}) \equiv \tilde{\omega}^2 + \left(p^2 + u^2\right)\tilde{\omega} + p^2u^2 - k^2\delta^2x_0^2 = 0, \quad (11)$$

where $\tilde{\omega} = \omega^2$. Since $p^2 + u^2 > 0$, $p^2u^2 - k^2\delta^2x_0^2 = p^2u^2(1 - R_0^2) > 0$, we have $f(\tilde{\omega}) > 0$, which contradicts $f(\tilde{\omega}) = 0$. This suggests that all the roots of (8) have negative real parts for any time delay $\tau \geq 0$. Therefore, the uninfected equilibrium E_0 of the model (3) is locally asymptotically stable.

Define

$$G = \{\phi = (\phi_1, \phi_2, \phi_3) \in C \mid 0 \leq \|\phi_1\| \leq x_0,\ \phi_2 \geq 0,\ \phi_3 \geq 0\}. \quad (12)$$

It is easy to show that G attracts all solutions of the model (3) and is also positively invariant with respect to the model (3).

Motivated by the methods in [20, 21], we choose the following Liapunov functional:

$$L(\phi) = \frac{1}{\delta}\phi_2(0) + \frac{p}{\delta k}\phi_3(0) + \int_{-\tau}^{0}\phi_1(\theta)\phi_3(\theta)\,d\theta \quad (13)$$

for any $\phi \in G$. The time derivative of L along the solutions of the model (3) is

$$\begin{aligned}\dot{L} &= \frac{1}{\delta}y'(t) + \frac{p}{\delta k}v'(t) + x(t)v(t) - x(t-\tau)v(t-\tau) \\ &= \left(x(t) - \frac{up}{k\delta}\right)v(t) \leq \left(x_0 - \frac{up}{k\delta}\right)v(t) \\ &= \left(1 - \frac{1}{R_0}\right)x_0 v(t) \leq 0,\end{aligned} \quad (14)$$

where $t \geq 0$. By using Liapunov-LaSalle invariance principle [18], the uninfected equilibrium E_0 of the model (3) is globally asymptotically stable.

Next, let us study the stability of the infected equilibrium E^*. The linearized system of the model (3) at E^* is

$$\begin{aligned}\frac{d}{dt}x(t) &= -\left(\frac{s}{x^*} + \frac{rx^*}{T}\right)x(t) - \frac{rx^*}{T}y(t) - \beta x^* v(t) \\ &\quad - cx^* y(t), \\ \frac{d}{dt}y(t) &= \delta\left[x^* v(t-\tau) + x(t-\tau)v^*\right] - py(t), \\ \frac{d}{dt}v(t) &= ky(t) - uv(t).\end{aligned} \quad (15)$$

Denote

$$\begin{aligned}B &= \frac{s}{x^*} + \frac{rx^*}{T}, \\ E &= \left(\frac{r}{T} + c\right)x^*, \\ F &= \beta x^*, \\ G &= \delta v^*, \\ H &= \delta x^*.\end{aligned} \quad (16)$$

The corresponding characteristic equation is

$$\begin{aligned}&\lambda^3 + (B + p + u)\lambda^2 + (Bp + uB + up)\lambda + uBp \\ &\quad + [(EG - kH)\lambda + (kGF + uEG - kBH)]e^{-\lambda\tau} \\ &= 0.\end{aligned} \quad (17)$$

Define

$$\begin{aligned}a_1 &= B + p + u > 0, \\ a_2 &= Bp + uB + up > 0, \\ a_3 &= uBp > 0, \\ b_2 &= EG - kH, \\ b_3 &= kGF + uEG - kBH,\end{aligned} \quad (18)$$

where $b_2 = pu(rv^*/kT - 1) + c\delta x^* v^*$ and $b_3 = pu(\beta v^* + ruv^*/kT - B) + c\delta ux^* v^*$.

Therefore, (17) becomes

$$\lambda^3 + a_1\lambda^2 + a_2\lambda + a_3 + [b_2\lambda + b_3]e^{-\lambda\tau} = 0. \quad (19)$$

When $\tau = 0$, (19) becomes $\lambda^3 + a_1\lambda^2 + (a_2 + b_2)\lambda + (a_3 + b_3) = 0$. Notice that $a_1 > 0$, $a_3 + b_3 = pu(\beta v^* + ruv^*/kT) + c\delta ux^* v^* > 0$. Thus, if $R_0 > 1$ and $\Delta_2 = a_1(a_2 + b_2) - (a_3 + b_3) > 0$ hold, by Routh-Hurwitz criterion, the infected equilibrium E^* is locally asymptotically stable when $\tau = 0$.

Now, let us investigate the stability of E^* when $\tau > 0$. Rewriting (19) as

$$P(\lambda) + Q(\lambda)e^{-\lambda\tau} = 0, \quad (20)$$

where

$$P(\lambda) = \lambda^3 + a_1\lambda^2 + a_2\lambda + a_3,$$
$$Q(\lambda) = b_2\lambda + b_3. \tag{21}$$

Since $a_3+b_3 = uBp+pu(\beta v^*+ruv^*/kT-B)+c\delta ux^*v^* > 0$, $\lambda = 0$ is not the root of (19). Assume that (19) has pure imaginary $\lambda = iw$ $(w > 0)$ for some $\tau > 0$; substituting it into (19), it has $-iw^3 - a_1w^2 + ia_2w + a_3 + (ib_2w + b_3)(\cos w\tau - i\sin w\tau) = 0$, and separating the real and imaginary parts, we have

$$w^3 - a_2w = b_2w\cos w\tau - b_3\sin w\tau,$$
$$a_1w^2 - a_3 = b_2w\sin w\tau + b_3\cos w\tau. \tag{22}$$

Therefore, it has

$$w^6 + c_1w^4 + c_2w^2 + c_3 = 0, \tag{23}$$

where $c_1 = a_1^2 - 2a_2$, $c_2 = a_2^2 - 2a_1a_3 - b_2^2$, $c_3 = a_3^2 - b_3^2$. Denote $v = w^2$; (23) becomes

$$v^3 + c_1v^2 + c_2v + c_3 = 0. \tag{24}$$

Define

$$h(v) = v^3 + c_1v^2 + c_2v + c_3, \tag{25}$$

hence $h'(v) = 3v^2 + 2c_1v + c_2$. Considering

$$3v^2 + 2c_1v + c_2 = 0. \tag{26}$$

It has two real roots, given as $v_1 = (-c_1 + \sqrt{\Delta})/3$ and $v_2 = (-c_1 - \sqrt{\Delta})/3$, where $\Delta = c_1^2 - 3c_2$.

Now, we will illustrate the following conclusions, and it has been proved in [22]. □

Lemma 3. *For the polynomial (24), the following conclusions are given:*

(i) *If $c_3 < 0$, (24) has at least one positive root.*

(ii) *If $c_3 \geq 0$ and $\Delta < 0$, (24) has no real root.*

(iii) *If $c_3 \geq 0$ and $\Delta > 0$, if and only if $v_1 = (-c_1+\sqrt{\Delta})/3 > 0$ and $h(v_1) \leq 0$, (24) has real roots.*

Assume that $h(v) = 0$ has positive real roots. Generally, we may suppose that (24) has k $(1 \leq k \leq 3)$ positive real roots, denoted as v_1, v_2, and v_3. Then, (23) has positive real roots $\omega_k = \sqrt{v_k}$. From (22), we attain

$$\cos\omega\tau = \frac{b_2w^4 + (a_1b_3 - a_2b_2)w^2 - a_3b_3}{b_2^2w^2 + b_3^2}. \tag{27}$$

Then, we get the corresponding $\tau_k^{(n)} > 0$ such that (23) has pure imaginary $\lambda = iw_k$, where

$$\tau_k^{(n)} = \frac{1}{w_k}\left\{\arccos\left(\frac{b_2w_k^4 + (a_1b_3 - a_2b_2)w_k^2 - a_3b_3}{b_2^2w_k^2 + b_3^2}\right) + 2n\pi\right\}, \quad k = 1,2,3, \; n = 0,1,2,\ldots. \tag{28}$$

Define

$$\tau^* = \min_{k\in[1,2,3]}\left\{\tau_k^{(0)}\right\}. \tag{29}$$

Differentiating the two sides of (19) with respect to τ, it follows that

$$\left(3\lambda^2 + 2a_1\lambda + a_2\right)\frac{d\lambda}{d\tau} + b_2e^{-\lambda\tau}\frac{d\lambda}{d\tau} - \tau\left(b_2\lambda + b_3\right)e^{-\lambda\tau}\frac{d\lambda}{d\tau} - \lambda\left(b_2\lambda + b_3\right)e^{-\lambda\tau} = 0. \tag{30}$$

Thus, we get

$$\left(\frac{d\lambda}{d\tau}\right)^{-1}_{\lambda=iw_k} = \frac{\left(a_2 - 3w_k^2\right) + 2a_1w_ki}{\left(a_2w_k^2 - w_k^4\right) - \left(a_3w_k - a_1w_k^3\right)i} + \frac{b_2}{-b_2w_k^2 + b_3w_ki}. \tag{31}$$

Then

$$\left[\frac{d(\operatorname{Res}(\lambda))}{d\tau}\right]^{-1}_{\lambda=iw_k} = \frac{\left(a_2 - 3w_k^2\right)\left(a_2w_k^2 - w_k^4\right) - 2a_1w_k\left(a_3w_k - a_1w_k^3\right)}{\left(a_2w_k^2 - w_k^4\right)^2 + \left(a_3w_k - a_1w_k^3\right)^2} + \frac{-b_2^2w_k^2}{-b_2^2w_k^4 + b_3^2w_k^2}. \tag{32}$$

From (19), we obtain $b_2w^2 + b_3^2 = (w^3 - a_2w)^2 + (a_1w^2 - a_3)^2$. Therefore,

$$\left[\frac{d(\operatorname{Res}(\lambda))}{d\tau}\right]^{-1}_{\lambda=iw_k} = \frac{3v_k^3 + 2c_1v_k^2 + c_2v_k}{w_k^2\left[b_2w_k^2 + b_3^2\right]} = \frac{h'(v_k)}{w_k^2\left[b_2w_k^2 + b_3^2\right]}. \tag{L}$$

Since $v_k > 0$, we get $\operatorname{Re}(d\lambda(\tau)/d\tau)|_{\tau=\tau_k^{(n)}}$ and $h'(v_k)$ have the same sign. Combining Lemma 3 with the above (L), we have the following conclusions.

Theorem 4. *$\tau_k^{(n)}$ and τ^* are defined by (28) and (29). If $R_0 > 1$, the following results hold:*

(i) *If $c_3 \geq 0$ and $\Delta \leq 0$, then infected equilibrium $E^*(x^*, y^*, v^*)$ is locally asymptotically stable.*

(ii) *If $c_3 < 0$ or $c_3 \geq 0$ and $\Delta > 0$, then infected equilibrium $E^*(x^*, y^*, v^*)$ is locally asymptotically stable when $\tau \in [0, \tau^*)$ and unstable when $\tau > \tau^*$.*

(iii) *If the conditions of (ii) are all satisfied and $h'(v_k) \neq 0$, then model (3) undergoes a Hopf bifurcation at E^* when $\tau = \tau_k^{(n)}$ $(n = 0, 1, 2, \ldots)$.*

3. Properties of Hopf Bifurcation

In the above section, we have given the sufficient condition where the model (3) undergoes a Hopf bifurcation at E^*. In this section, we will use the normal form method and the center manifold theory provided in [23, 24] to analysis direction, stability, and the period of the bifurcating periodic solution. By setting $\tau = \tau^* + \mu$, then $\mu = 0$ is a Hopf bifurcation value of the model (3). Let $\mu_1 = x - x^*$, $\mu_2 = y - y^*$, $\mu_3 = v - v^*$, and

$$u(t) = (\mu_1(t), \mu_2(t), \mu_3(t))^T \in R_+^3,$$
$$u_t(\theta) = u(t+\theta) \quad (\theta \in [-\tau, 0]). \tag{33}$$

Then, the model (3) is equivalent to the functional differential equations $\dot{u}_t = L_\mu(u_t) + f(\mu, u_t)$, defined in $C := C([-\tau, 0], R_+^3)$, where

$$f(\mu, \varphi) = \begin{pmatrix} -\frac{r}{T}\varphi_1^2(0) - \left(\frac{r}{T} + c\right)\varphi_1(0)\varphi_2(0) - \beta\varphi_1(0)\varphi_3(0) \\ \delta\varphi_1(-\tau)\varphi_3(-\tau) \\ 0 \end{pmatrix}. \tag{34}$$

For $\varphi = (\varphi_1, \varphi_2, \varphi_3)^T \in C$, define $L_\mu\varphi = A\varphi(0) + D\varphi(-\tau)$. Here,

$$A = \begin{pmatrix} -B & -E & -F \\ 0 & 0 & H \\ 0 & 0 & 0 \end{pmatrix},$$
$$D = \begin{pmatrix} 0 & 0 & 0 \\ G & -p & 0 \\ 0 & k & -u \end{pmatrix}. \tag{35}$$

Using the Riesz representation theorem, there is a 3×3 bounded variation matrix function $\eta(\theta, \mu)$, which exists for $\theta \in [-\tau, 0]$, such that $L_\mu\varphi = \int_{-\tau}^{0} d\eta(\theta, \mu)\varphi(\theta)$ holds for any $\varphi \in C$. We can choose $\eta(\theta, \mu) = A\rho(\theta) - D\rho(\theta + \tau)$, where

$$\rho(\theta) = \begin{cases} 1, & \theta = 0, \\ 0, & \theta \neq 0. \end{cases} \tag{36}$$

For $\varphi \in C([-\tau, 0], R^3)$, define

$$A(\mu)\varphi = \begin{cases} \frac{d\varphi(\theta)}{d\theta}, & \theta \in [-\tau, 0), \\ \int_{-\tau}^{0} d\eta(s, \mu)\varphi(s), & \theta = 0, \end{cases}$$
$$R\varphi = \begin{cases} 0, & \theta \in [-\tau, 0), \\ f(\mu, \varphi), & \theta = 0. \end{cases} \tag{37}$$

Then, the system is equivalent to the following operator equation:

$$\dot{u}_t = A(\mu)u_t + Ru_t. \tag{38}$$

Let $C^* = C([0, \tau], (R^3)^*)$, and adjoint operator A^* of A is defined by

$$A^*\psi(\xi) = \begin{cases} -\frac{d\psi(\xi)}{d\xi}, & \xi \in (0, \tau], \\ \int_{-\tau}^{0} d\eta(s, 0)\psi(-s), & \xi = 0. \end{cases} \tag{39}$$

Define the bilinear inner product of $\varphi \in C$ and $\psi \in C^*$ as

$$\langle\psi(\xi), \varphi(\theta)\rangle = \overline{\psi}(0)\varphi(0) - \int_{\theta=-\tau}^{0}\int_{s=0}^{\theta} \overline{\psi}(s-\theta)\, d\eta(\theta)\varphi(s)\, ds, \tag{40}$$

where $\eta(\theta) = \eta(\theta, 0)$.

Since $A(0)$ and $A^*(0)$ are adjoint operator and $\pm i\omega^*$ is the eigenvalue of $A(0)$, therefore $\pm i\omega^*$ also is the eigenvalue of A^*. Suppose that the eigenvector of $A(0)$ with respect to the eigenvalue $i\omega^*$ is $q(\theta)$; the eigenvector of A^* with respect to the eigenvalue $-i\omega^*$ is $q^*(\xi)$, and they all satisfy $\langle q^*(\xi), q(\theta)\rangle = 1$.

We choose $q(\theta) = (1, q_2, q_3)^T e^{i\omega^*\theta}$, $\theta \in [-\tau, 0]$, and $q^*(\xi) = \overline{R}(1, q_2^*, q_3^*)e^{i\omega^*\xi}$, $\xi \in [0, \tau]$. Since $A(0)q(\theta) = i\omega^* q(\theta)$, $A^* q^*(\xi) = -i\omega^* q^*(\xi)$, we get

$$q_2 = -\frac{(i\omega^* + u)(i\omega^* + B)}{E(i\omega^* + u) + kF},$$
$$q_3 = -\frac{k(i\omega^* + B)}{E(i\omega^* + u) + kF},$$
$$q_2^* = -\frac{i\omega^* - B}{Ge^{i\omega^*\tau^*}},$$
$$q_3^* = \frac{E}{k} + \frac{(i\omega^* - B)(i\omega^* - s)}{kGe^{i\omega^*\tau^*}}. \tag{41}$$

From $\langle q^*(\xi), q(\theta)\rangle = 1$ and the similar arguments as in [20–22], we attain the following formula:

$$R = \left[1 + \overline{q_2^*}q_2 + \overline{q_3^*}q_3 + \overline{q_2^*}\tau^*(G + q_3H)e^{-i\omega^*\tau^*}\right]^{-1}. \tag{42}$$

Following the algorithms given in [23] (see, also [13, 24–26]), it then follows that

$$g_{20} = 2R\left[-\frac{r}{T}(1 + q_2) - cq_2 - \beta q_3 + \overline{q_2^*}q_3\delta e^{-2i\omega^*\tau^*}\right],$$
$$g_{11} = R\left[-\frac{r}{T}(2 + q_2 + \overline{q_2}) - c(q_2 + \overline{q_2}) - \beta(q_3 + \overline{q_3}) + \overline{q_2^*}\delta(q_3 + \overline{q_3})\right],$$
$$g_{02} = 2R\left[-\frac{r}{T}(1 + \overline{q_2}) - c\overline{q_2} - \beta\overline{q_3} + \overline{q_2^*}\overline{q_3}\delta e^{2i\omega^*\tau^*}\right],$$

$$
\begin{aligned}
g_{21} = 2R\Bigg\{ & -\frac{r}{T}\Bigg[2\omega_{11}^{(1)}(0)+\omega_{20}^{(1)}(0)+\omega_{11}^{(2)}(0) \\
& +\frac{\omega_{20}^{(2)}(0)}{2}+q_2\frac{-\omega_{20}^{(1)}(0)}{2}+q_2\omega_{11}^{(1)}(0)\Bigg] \\
& -c\Bigg[\omega_{11}^{(2)}(0)+\frac{\omega_{20}^{(2)}(0)}{2}+q_2\frac{-\omega_{20}^{(1)}(0)}{2} \\
& +q_2\omega_{11}^{(1)}(0)\Bigg]-\beta\Bigg[\omega_{11}^{(3)}(0)+\frac{\omega_{20}^{(3)}(0)}{2} \\
& +q_3\frac{-\omega_{20}^{(1)}(0)}{2}+q_3\omega_{11}^{(1)}(0)\Bigg] \\
& +\overline{q_2^*}\delta\Bigg[\frac{\omega_{20}^{(3)}(-\tau^*)}{2}e^{i\omega^*\tau^*}+\omega_{20}^{(3)}(-\tau^*)e^{i\omega^*\tau^*} \\
& +\overline{q_3}\omega_{11}^{(1)}(-\tau^*)e^{i\omega^*\tau^*}\Bigg]\Bigg\},
\end{aligned}
\tag{43}
$$

where

$$
\begin{aligned}
\omega_{20}(\theta) &= \frac{ig_{20}}{\omega^*}q(0)e^{i\omega^*\theta}+\frac{i\overline{g_{02}}}{3\omega^*}\overline{q}(0)e^{-i\omega^*\theta}+E_1e^{2i\omega^*\theta}, \\
\omega_{11}(\theta) &= \frac{ig_{11}}{\omega^*}q(0)e^{i\omega^*\theta}+\frac{i\overline{g_{11}}}{\omega^*}\overline{q}(0)e^{-i\omega^*\theta}+E_2, \\
E_1 &= 2\begin{pmatrix} 2i\omega^*+B & E & F \\ -Ge^{-2i\omega^*\tau^*} & -2i\omega^*+p & -He^{-2i\omega^*\tau^*} \\ 0 & -k & 2i\omega^*+u \end{pmatrix}^{-1} \\
&\quad\times\begin{pmatrix} -\frac{r}{T}-\frac{r}{T}q_2-cq_2-\beta q_3 \\ \delta q_3e^{-2i\omega^*\tau^*} \\ 0 \end{pmatrix}, \\
E_2 &= \begin{pmatrix} B & E & F \\ -G & p & -H \\ 0 & -k & u \end{pmatrix}^{-1} \\
&\quad\times\begin{pmatrix} -\frac{2r}{T}-\frac{r}{T}(q_2+\overline{q_2})-c(q_2+\overline{q_2})-\beta(q_3+\overline{q_3}) \\ \delta(q_3+\overline{q_3}) \\ 0 \end{pmatrix}.
\end{aligned}
\tag{44}
$$

Then we can obtain the following quantities:

$$
\begin{aligned}
C_1(0) &= \frac{i}{2\omega^*}\left(g_{11}g_{20}-2|g_{11}|^2-\frac{|g_{02}|^2}{3}\right)+\frac{g_{21}}{2}, \\
\mu_2 &= -\frac{\operatorname{Re}(C_1(0))}{\operatorname{Re}(\lambda'(\tau^*))}, \\
\beta_2 &= 2\operatorname{Re}(C_1(0)), \\
T_2 &= -\frac{\operatorname{Im}(C_1(0))+\mu_2\operatorname{Im}(\lambda'(\tau^*))}{\omega^*}.
\end{aligned}
\tag{45}
$$

These quantities determine the properties of bifurcating periodic solutions. From the previous discussions, we have the following conclusions.

Theorem 5. *Suppose that the conditions in (iii) of Theorem 4 hold, then the infected equilibrium E^* undergoes a Hopf bifurcation at $\tau = \tau^*$, and μ_2, β_2, T_2 determine the direction, stability, and period of the Hopf bifurcation, respectively,*

(i) *If $\mu_2 > 0$, a bifurcating periodic solution exists in the sufficiently small τ^*-neighbourhood.*

(ii) *If $\beta_2 < 0$ ($\beta_2 > 0$), the bifurcating periodic solution is stable (unstable) when $t \longrightarrow +\infty$ ($t \longrightarrow -\infty$).*

(iii) *If $T_2 < 0$ ($T_2 > 0$), the period of the bifurcating periodic solution decreases (increases).*

4. Simulations and Conclusions

For the main results in Sections 2 and 3, we now give some numerical simulations.

Based on the numerical simulations in [16, 27–29], take the following data:

$$
\begin{aligned}
s &= 0.1, \\
r &= 0.01, \\
T &= 200, \\
d &= 0.02, \\
c &= 0.001, \\
\beta &= 0.0027, \\
\delta &= 0.002, \\
p &= 0.3, \\
k &= 0.1, \\
u &= 0.01.
\end{aligned}
\tag{46}
$$

We can get $R_0 = 0.6363 < 1$ and $E_0 = (9.5445, 0, 0)$ by direct calculations. The uninfected equilibrium E_0 is globally asymptotically stable by Theorem 2. Figure 1 gives the curves and orbits of the model (3) with appropriate initial condition.

Furthermore, we also simulate the occurrence of Hopf bifurcations as the time delay τ increases. Take the following data:

$$
\begin{aligned}
s &= 0.1, \\
r &= 1.01, \\
T &= 200, \\
d &= 0.02,
\end{aligned}
$$

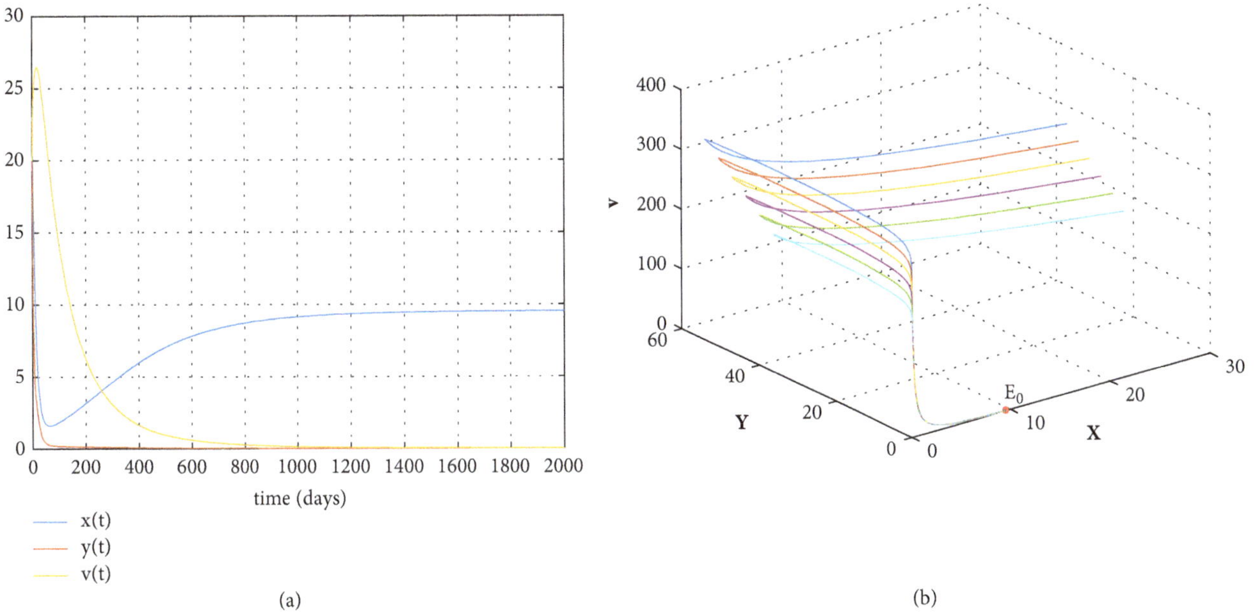

FIGURE 1: (a) The solution curves of the model (3) with $R_0 < 1$. (b) The orbits of the model (3) when $R_0 < 1$.

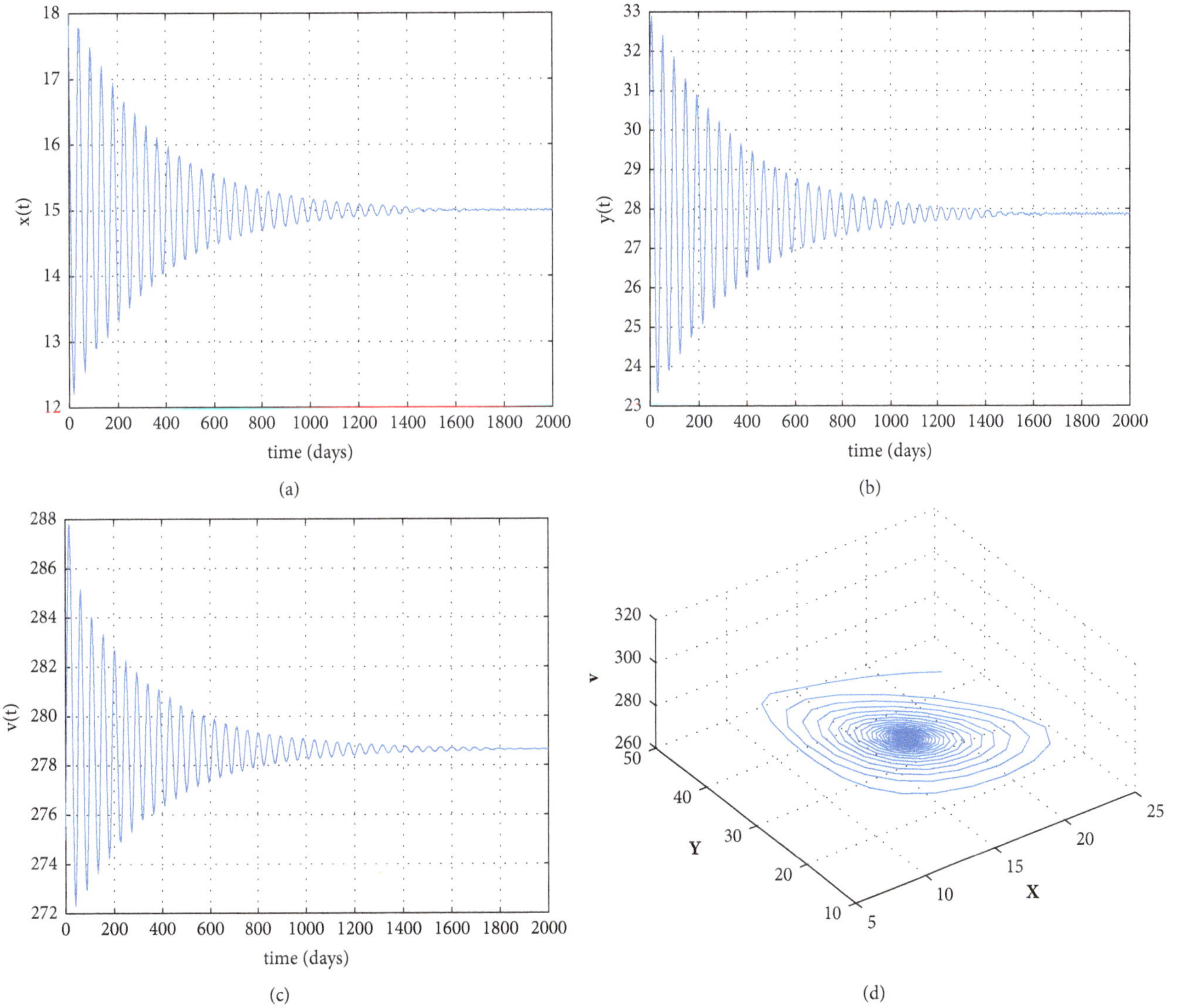

FIGURE 2: (a), (b), and (c) The solution curves of the model (3) with $R_0 > 1$, $\tau = 10 < \tau^*$. (d) The orbits of the model (3) when $R_0 > 1$, $\tau = 10 < \tau^*$.

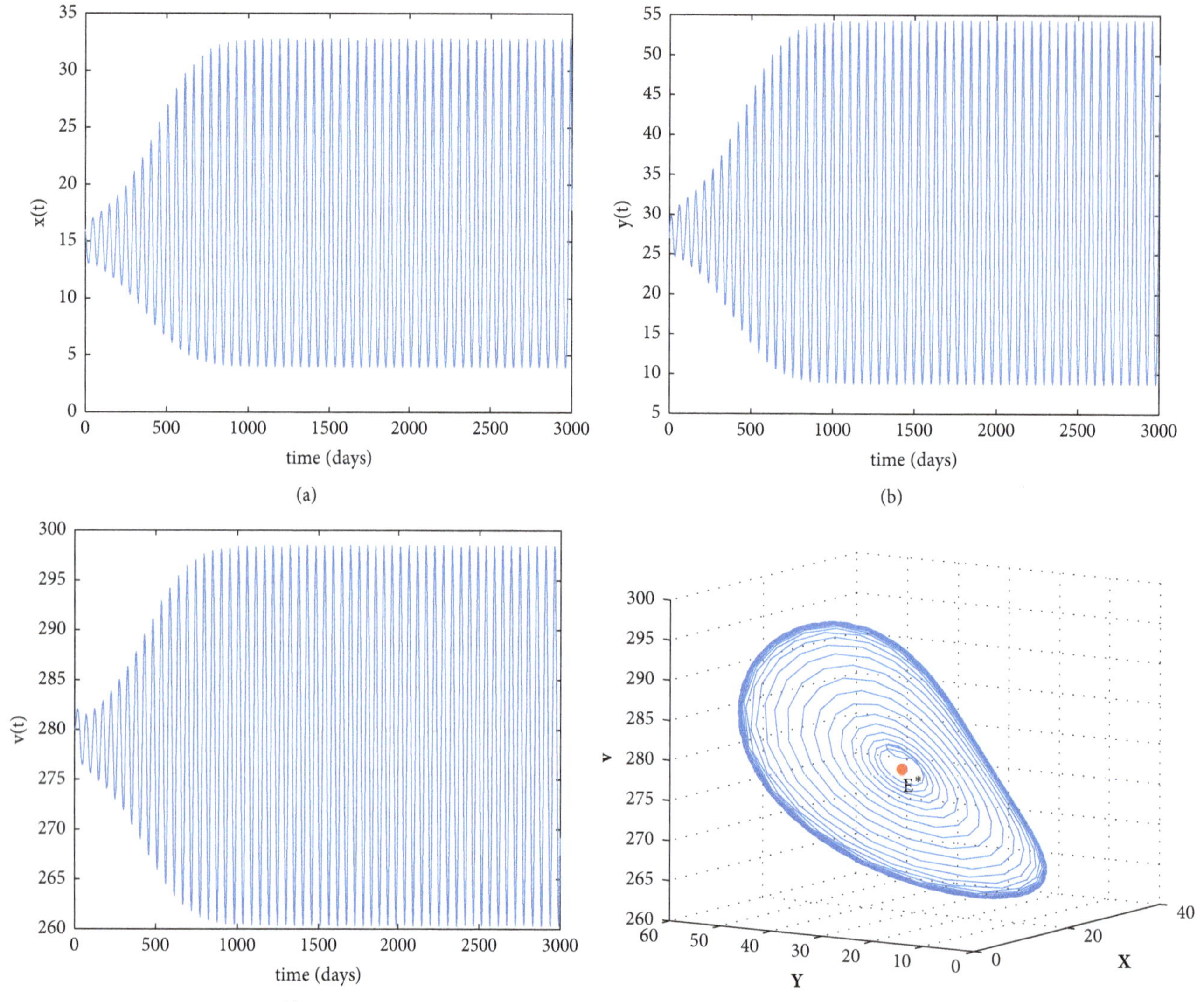

FIGURE 3: (a), (b), and (c) The solution curves of the model (3) with $R_0 > 1$, $\tau = 12 > \tau^*$. (d) The orbits of the model (3) when $R_0 > 1$, $\tau = 12 > \tau^*$.

$$
\begin{aligned}
c &= 0.001, \\
\beta &= 0.0027, \\
\delta &= 0.002, \\
p &= 0.3, \\
k &= 0.1, \\
u &= 0.01.
\end{aligned}
\tag{47}
$$

By direct calculations, we get that (19) has a positive root $v^* = 0.0175 > 0$, $R_0 = 13.0761 > 1$, and $E^* = (15, 27.8643, 278.6435)$. And by simple computations, we attain $\omega^* = 0.1322$, $\tau^* = 10.6528$, and $h'(v^*) = 0.0027 \neq 0$. From Theorem 4, the infected equilibrium E^* is locally asymptotically stable when $0 < \tau < \tau^*$ and unstable when $\tau > \tau^*$. Figure 2 gives the stable phase trajectories and orbits of the model (3) when $\tau = 10 < \tau^*$. Figure 3 gives the phase trajectories and orbits of model (3) when $\tau = 12 > \tau^*$ and it suggests that Hopf bifurcations occur. From (45), we obtain $\mathrm{Re}(C_1(0)) = -1.1035 \times 10^{-6} < 0$ for $\tau = 12$. Therefore, both bifurcating periodic solutions are stable.

In this paper, we has proposed a delay HIV infection model (3) with a full logistic term $rx(1-(x(t)+y(t))/T)$. Then, using the basic reproduction number $R_0 = (k\delta/pu)x_0$, we discuss the existence of the uninfected equilibrium E_0 and the infected equilibrium $E^* = (x^*, y^*, v^*)$. By Routh-Hurwitz criterion, Liapunov-LaSalle invariance principle, and Hopf bifurcation method, we prove the following results.

If $R_0 \leq 1$, the uninfected equilibrium E_0 is globally asymptotically stable when $\tau \geq 0$. That is to say, any solution $(x(t), y(t), v(t))$ trends to E_0. Biologically, this means that the virus cannot successfully invade uninfected cells and will soon be cleared of the immune system. And as the time t

increases, the virus will disappear. This suggests that we can control the disease by controlling the R_0.

If $R_0 > 1$, there exists a unique infected equilibrium E^*. The result of Theorem 4 implies that the time delay τ can destabilize the stability of the infected equilibrium E^* and leads to the occurrence of Hopf bifurcations. And if $\tau \in [0, \tau^*)$, the infected equilibrium E^* is locally asymptotically stable. Biologically, this means that the HIV infection may become chronic. The infected equilibrium E^* will be unstable and Hopf bifurcation occurs under some conditions when the time delay τ exceeds τ^*. In biology, this implies that the concentrations of uninfected cells, infected cells, and free virus will first tend to be constants and then oscillate as the time delay τ increases. In the immune response, this situation is very important for choosing the adequate drug treatment programs.

It can be found that the basic reproduction number R_0 for the model (3) is not the same as that for model (2). It is independent on the constant c, which represents inhibitory effect on the growth of uninfected cells by infected cells. But R_0 depends on the coefficient r of the full logistic term $rx(1 - (x(t) + y(t))/T)$. Furthermore, the value of x^* is independent on the coefficient r. And the values of y^* and v^* are the increasing functions with respect to r. And this paper shows that the time delay τ can produce richer dynamic behavior. As the time delay increases, the stability changes and periodic oscillations occur.

Conflicts of Interest

The authors declare that they have no conflicts of interest.

Acknowledgments

This work is partly supported by the National Natural Science Foundation of China for W. Ma (no. 11471034).

References

[1] D. C. Douek, M. Roederer, and R. A. Koup, "Emerging concepts in the immunopathogenesis of AIDS," *Annual Review of Medicine*, vol. 60, pp. 471–484, 2009.

[2] Y. Yan, P. Yan, L. Chen et al., "Research progress on AIDS treatment," *Chinese Journal of Zoonoses*, vol. 33, no. 5, pp. 383–388, 2017.

[3] M. A. Nowak and C. R. M. Bangham, "Population dynamics of immune responses to persistent viruses," *Science*, vol. 272, no. 5258, pp. 74–79, 1996.

[4] M. A. Nowak and R. M. May, *Virus Dynamics: Mathematics Principles of Immunology and Virology*, Oxford University Press, London, UK, 2000.

[5] A. S. Perelson, A. U. Neumann, M. Markowitz, J. M. Leonard, and D. D. Ho, "HIV-1 dynamics in vivo: virion clearance rate, infected cell life-span, and viral generation time," *Science*, vol. 271, no. 5255, pp. 1582–1586, 1996.

[6] A. S. Perelson and P. W. Nelson, "Mathematical analysis of HIV-1 dynamics in vivo," *SIAM Review*, vol. 41, no. 1, pp. 3–44, 1999.

[7] A. V. M. Herz, S. Bonhoeffer, R. M. Anderson, R. M. May, and M. A. Nowak, "Viral dynamics in vivo: limitations on estimates of intracellular delay and virus decay," *Proceedings of the National Acadamy of Sciences of the United States of America*, vol. 93, no. 14, pp. 7247–7251, 1996.

[8] J. Tam, "Delay effect in a model for virus replication," *Mathematical Medicine and Biology*, vol. 16, no. 1, pp. 29–37, 1999.

[9] W. Wang and W. Ma, "A diffusive HIV infection model with nonlocal delayed transmission," *Applied Mathematics Letters*, vol. 75, pp. 96–101, 2018.

[10] A. S. Perelson, D. E. Kirschner, and R. D. Boer, "Dynamics of HIV infection of CD4$^+$ T cells," *Mathematical Biosciences*, vol. 114, no. 1, pp. 81–125, 1993.

[11] R. V. Culshaw and S. Ruan, "A delay-differential equation model of HIV infection of CD4$^+$ T-cells," *Mathematical Biosciences*, vol. 165, no. 1, pp. 27–39, 2000.

[12] L. Wang and M. Y. Li, "Mathematical analysis of the global dynamics of a model for HIV infection of CD4$^+$ T cells," *Mathematical Biosciences*, vol. 200, no. 1, pp. 44–57, 2006.

[13] P. Hao, D. Fan, J. Wei, and Q. Liu, "Dynamic behaviors of a delayed HIV model with stage-structure," *Communications in Nonlinear Science and Numerical Simulation*, vol. 17, no. 12, pp. 4753–4766, 2012.

[14] W. Wang and T. Zhang, "Caspase-1-mediated pyroptosis of the predominance for driving CD4 + T cells death: a nonlocal spatial mathematical model," *Bulletin of Mathematical Biology*, vol. 80, no. 3, pp. 540–582, 2018.

[15] S. Guo and W. Ma, "Global behavior of delay differential equations model of HIV infection with apoptosis," *Discrete and Continuous Dynamical Systems - Series B*, vol. 21, no. 1, pp. 103–119, 2016.

[16] W. Cheng, W. Ma, and S. Guo, "A class of virus dynamic model with inhibitory effect on the growth of uninfected T Cells caused by infected T Cells and its stability analysis," *Communications on Pure and Applied Analysis*, vol. 15, no. 3, pp. 795–806, 2016.

[17] L. Chen, X. Meng, and J. Jiao, *Biodynamics*, Beijing Science Press, Beijing, China, 2009.

[18] J. K. Hale and S. M. Verduyn Lunel, *Introduction to Functional-Differential Equations*, Springer, Berlin, Germany, 1993.

[19] Y. Kuang, *Delay Differential Equations with Applications in Population Dynamics*, Academic Press, New York, NY, USA, 1993.

[20] Y. Wang, Y. Zhou, J. Wu, and J. Heffernan, "Oscillatory viral dynamics in a delayed HIV pathogenesis model," *Mathematical Biosciences*, vol. 219, no. 2, pp. 104–112, 2009.

[21] T. Zhang, X. Meng, and T. Zhang, "Global analysis for a delayed SIV model with direct and environmental transmissions," *Journal of Applied Analysis and Computation*, vol. 6, no. 2, pp. 479–491, 2016.

[22] S. Ruan and J. Wei, "On the zeros of a third degree exponential polynomial with applications to a delayed model for the control of testosterone secretion," *IMA Journal of Mathematics Applied in Medicine and Biology*, vol. 18, no. 1, pp. 41–52, 2001.

[23] B. D. Hassard, N. D. Kazarinoff, and Y.-H. Wan, *Theory and Applications of Hopf Bifurcation*, Cambridge University Press, 1981.

[24] J. Wei, H. Wang, and W. Jiang, *Bifurcation Theory And Application of Delay Differential Equation*, Science Press, Beijing, China, 2012.

[25] Z. Jiang and W. Ma, "Delayed feedback control and bifurcation analysis in a chaotic chemostat system," *International Journal of Bifurcation and Chaos*, vol. 25, no. 6, Article ID 1550087, 1550087, 13 pages, 2015.

[26] J. J. Wei and S. G. Ruan, "Stability and global Hopf bifurcation for neutral differential equations," *Acta Mathematica Sinica*, vol. 45, no. 1, pp. 93–104, 2002.

[27] F. Li, W. Ma, Z. Jiang, and D. Li, "Stability and Hopf bifurcation in a delayed HIV infection model with general incidence rate and immune impairment," *Computational and Mathematical Methods in Medicine*, Article ID 206205, Art. ID 206205, 14 pages, 2015.

[28] R. R. Regoes, D. Wodarz, and M. A. Nowak, "Virus dynamics: the effect of target cell limitation and immune responses on virus evolution," *Journal of Theoretical Biology*, vol. 191, no. 4, pp. 451–462, 1998.

[29] A. Miao, X. Wang, T. Zhang, W. Wang, and B. G. Sampath Aruna Pradeep, "Dynamical analysis of a stochastic SIS epidemic model with nonlinear incidence rate and double epidemic hypothesis," *Advances in Difference Equations*, Paper No. 226, 27 pages, 2017.

4

Validity and Reliability of the Newly Developed Surface Electromyography Device for Measuring Muscle Activity during Voluntary Isometric Contraction

Myung Hun Jang [1] Se Jin Ahn [2] Jun Woo Lee [3] Min-Hyung Rhee [4] Dasom Chae [5] Jinmi Kim [6] and Myung Jun Shin [1,5]

[1]*Department of Rehabilitation Medicine, Pusan National University Hospital, Pusan National University School of Medicine, Busan, Republic of Korea*
[2]*Division of Energy and Electric Engineering, Uiduk University, Gyeongju, Republic of Korea*
[3]*School of Mechanical Engineering, Pusan National University, Busan, Republic of Korea*
[4]*Department of Rehabilitation Medicine, Pusan National University Hospital, Busan, Republic of Korea*
[5]*Biomedical Research Institute, Pusan National University Hospital, Busan, Republic of Korea*
[6]*Department of Biostatistics, Clinical Trial Center, Biomedical Research Institute, Pusan National University Hospital, Busan, Republic of Korea*

Correspondence should be addressed to Myung Jun Shin; drshinmj@gmail.com

Academic Editor: Fumiharu Togo

Objective. The purpose of this study was to establish the validity and reliability of the newly developed surface electromyography (sEMG) device (PSL-EMG-Tr1) compared with a conventional sEMG device (BTS-FREEEMG1000). *Methods.* In total, 20 healthy participants (10 males, age 30.3 ± 2.9 years; 10 females, age 22.3 ± 2.7 years) were recruited. EMG signals were recorded simultaneously on two devices during three different isometric contractions (maximal voluntary isometric contraction (MVIC, 40% MVIC, 80% MVIC)). Two trials were performed, and the same session was repeated after 1 week. EMG amplitude recorded from the dominant biceps brachii (BB) and rectus femoris (RF) muscles was analyzed for reliability using intrasession intraclass correlation coefficient (ICC). Concurrent validity of the two devices was determined using Pearson's correlation coefficient. *Results.* Nonnormalized sEMG data showed moderate to very high reliability for all three contraction levels (ICC = 0.832–0.937 (BB); ICC = 0.814–0.957 (RF)). Normalized sEMG values showed no to high reliability (ICC = 0.030–0.831 (BB); ICC = 0.547–0.828 (RF)). sEMG signals recorded by the PSL-EMG-Tr1 showed good to excellent validity compared with the BTS-FREEEMG1000, at 40% MVIC ($r = 0.943$ (BB), $r = 0.940$ (RF)) and 80% MVIC ($r = 0.983$ (BB); $r = 0.763$ (RF)). *Conclusions.* The PSL-EMG-Tr1 was performed with acceptable validity. Furthermore, the high accessibility and portability of the device are useful in adjusting the type and intensity of exercise.

1. Introduction

Sarcopenia is defined as decreased skeletal muscle mass and muscle strength with age. Muscle mass and strength gradually decrease after reaching a peak in early adulthood, and the degree of decrease varies among individuals [1]. Elderly people with sarcopenia have a much higher fall risk and lower physical performance than do nonsarcopenic individuals [2]. Decreased muscle strength also reduces functional capacity and is a major cause of disability, mortality, and other adverse health outcomes [3, 4]. Because of individual differences, it is important to reduce the rate at which muscle mass declines to avoid premature sarcopenia. Sarcopenia can be evaluated by measuring skeletal muscle mass. It is common practice to examine the cross-sectional area, thickness, and weight of muscles using magnetic resonance imaging (MRI), computed tomography (CT), anthropometry, bioelectrical impedance analysis (BIA), and ultrasound. Muscle mass and strength are reduced in the third decade, and the prevalence of sarcopenia can be increased by the presence of obesity and the amount of physical activity. Therefore, managing the risk factors of sarcopenia through exercise is important in young and healthy adults [1, 5]. In addition, low physical performance can be assessed using functional measurements such as gait speed (e.g., 4 minute walking test) and grip strength [4, 6]. Muscle quality may be more important than muscle size in estimating the risk of falling, and monitoring muscle activity during daily activities can help in preventing sarcopenia and estimating the degree of frailty [7, 8]. It is also important to evaluate muscle quality in healthy elderly people before and after exercise and according to age [9, 10]. Muscle activity can be monitored and muscle quality can be evaluated, through surface electromyography (sEMG) [11, 12]. However, the sEMG devices developed so far are expensive and difficult to operate, which limits their use by nonspecialists. Therefore, a new sEMG device , that is, simple to use and highly accessible has been developed for people who are not familiar with EMG. The purpose of this study was to establish the validity and reliability of the new device.

2. Materials and Methods

2.1. Experimental Protocol. In total, 20 healthy participants (10 males, 10 females) between the ages of 21 and 34 years (males, age 30.3 ± 2.9 years, height 171.9 ± 3.8 cm, weight 74.1 ± 11.3 kg, body mass index (BMI) 25.4 ± 3.33 kg/m^2; females, age 22.3 ± 2.7 years, height 162.1 ± 5.0 cm, weight 56.4 ± 5.0 kg, BMI 21.5 ± 1.9 kg/m^2; mean ± SD) were recruited; all participants who provided informed consent prior to the study were recruited. Ethical approval was granted, and the informed consent form was approved by the Ethics Committee of Pusan National University Hospital, Busan, Korea (IRB number: 1703-018-052). Exclusion criteria included musculoskeletal disease, cardiopulmonary disease, and other diseases that could prevent exercise.

At each session, participants were first required to perform three maximal voluntary isometric contractions (MVIC) for 5 seconds each, with a 5-minute rest between contractions. Each session consisted of two trials. After three MVIC measurements, 15-second isometric contractions were performed at different intensity levels. In the pretest, it took at least 10–15 seconds to maintain the same intensity isometric contraction through visual feedback. First, 40% MVIC was performed, followed by 80% MVIC after 5 minutes of rest. In the second trial, the placement of the electrodes for the two devices (BTS-FREEEMG1000 and newly developed device) was interchanged, and contractions were again measured by the same method (Figure 1). During the test, participants received visual feedback about their performance from a monitor, which enabled them to maintain the muscle contraction at the target intensity. The same procedure was employed for the biceps brachii (BB) and rectus femoris (RF) muscles [13–15]. All tests were performed only with the dominant arm and leg. Participants were tested twice, with a week between sessions.

2.2. Mechanical Recording. The participants sat on a Biodex System 3 PRO dynamometer (Biodex Medical Systems, Shirley, NY, USA) with a visual torque feedback monitor. Each participant sat in an upright posture and was strapped firmly to the chair with adjustable belts across the arm, trunk, and thigh. To evaluate BB muscle contractions, the participant sat with the dominant arm flexed at 90° and the forearm flexed at 120° relative to the upper arm. To evaluate quadriceps (RF) contractions, the hips were flexed at 90° and the tested knee was flexed at 45°. The axis of the dynamometer was positioned at the center of the tested elbow or knee joint. The lever arm was fixed by the precalibrated force sensor [16].

2.3. EMG Recording. The EMG signal was recorded simultaneously using two different sEMG devices. The BTS-FREEEMG (BTS-FREEEMG1000; BTS Bioengineering, Milan, Italy) was set to a sampling rate of 1,000 Hz per channel, and the signals were band-pass filtered from 20 to 500 Hz. The newly developed sEMG device (PSL-EMG-Tr1; PhysioLab Co., Ltd., Busan, Korea) was set to a sampling rate of 30,000 Hz, and signals were amplified with a 3–2,000 Hz bandwidth (Figure 2(a)).

Adhesive hydrogel surface electrodes (35 mm teardrop-shaped Kendall™ 200 Foam Electrodes; Medtronic, Minneapolis, MN, USA) were used, and the interelectrode distance, electrode placement procedure, and skin preparation followed standard Surface Electromyography for the Non-Invasive Assessment of Muscles (SENIAM) guidelines [17]. Two pairs of surface electrodes were attached parallel to the muscle fibers at an interelectrode distance of 2.0 cm. The distance between the pairs of electrodes was also 2.0 cm. After the first trial, the second trial was performed by interchanging the positions of the two pairs of electrodes of the each EMG devices (Figure 2(b)). After the interchange of the electrodes, the average of the values was used to compare the concurrent validity of the two devices.

The root mean square (RMS) value was used to analyze and process the recorded electrical signals in the muscles. Based on the square root calculation, the RMS reflects the mean power of the signal and is the preferred recommendation for smoothing. The RMS value can be used as a parameter to reflect the physiological activities of the motor unit during muscle contraction [18].

2.4. Statistical Analysis. Sample size was calculated using G*Power software (ver. 3.1; Heinrich-Heine Universität, Düsseldorf, Germany). In this study, the number of subjects required for a null-correlation (R0) = 0, alternative correlation (R1) = 0.6, alpha = 5%, power = 80%, and two-tailed test value was 19. Statistical analysis was performed using SPSS software (ver. 18.0; SPSS Inc., Chicago, IL, USA). To determine concurrent validity between the two sEMG machines, Pearson's correlation coefficient (r) was used for the average of two trials in each device. Interpretation of the correlation coefficients was based on guidelines for Pearson's coefficients suggested by Portney and Watkins [19]: $r > 0.75$, good to excellent correlation; $r = 0.50$–0.75, moderate to good correlation; $r = 0.25$–0.50, fair correlation; and $r = 0.00$–0.25, little to no relationship [19]. The Bland–

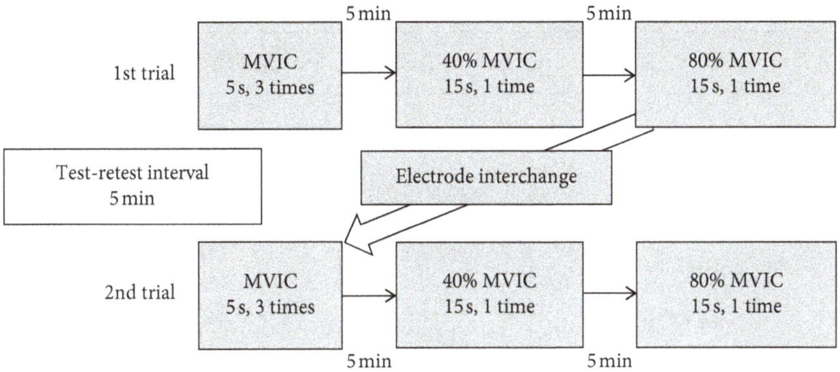

Figure 1: Scheme of the experimental protocol consisted of MVIC, 40%, and 80% MVIC. The same test was repeated after 1 week on the biceps brachii and rectus femoris muscles.

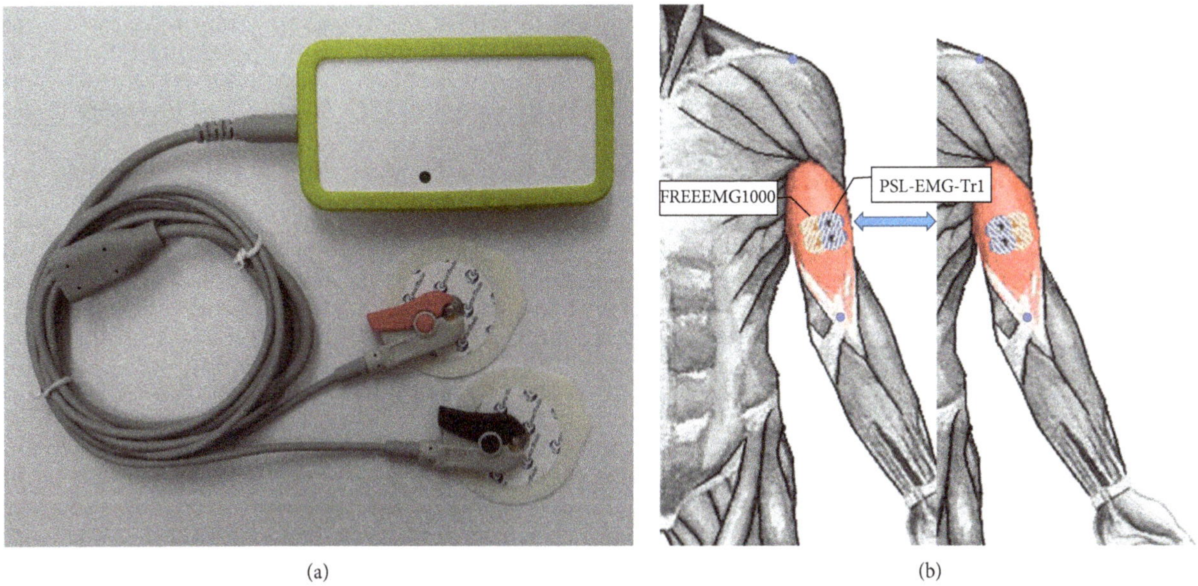

Figure 2: (a) The newly developed electromyography (EMG) machine (PSL-EMG-Tr1, PhysioLab Co., Ltd., Busan, Korea). (b) Placement of the two pairs of surface electrodes on the biceps brachii muscle.

Altman plot was used to visually compare the mean values of the two trials in each device. Mean differences were calculated by subtracting the % MVIC of the PSL-EMG-Tr1 from the % MVIC of the BTS-FREEEMG1000. Limits of agreements (LOA) were calculated by using 2 standard deviations around the mean difference.

The intraclass correlation coefficient (ICC) of two trials performed on each week was used to indicate the relative reliability of the measurements. For the test-retest reliability, ICC using a two-way mixed-effects model and absolute agreement definition is used [20]. Munro's descriptors for reliability coefficients were used to index the degree of reliability: very high correlation, 0.90–1.00; high correlation, 0.70–0.89; moderate correlation, 0.50–0.69; low correlation, 0.26–0.49; and little or no correlation, 0.00–0.25 [21]. The paired t-test was also conducted comparing the RMS (μV) and torque (N·m) between two trials of each week. Biodex is a device that has proved its reliability and validity. Therefore, Biodex was used only to evaluate the exact intensity during muscle contraction, and validity was compared between two sEMG devices [22].

3. Results

3.1. Torque Measurements. Twenty participants completed a total of four trials over 2 weeks. Table 1 shows the peak torque (N·m) values at three isometric contractions levels (MVIC, 40% MVIC, and 80% MVIC) for the first and second weeks. Very high relative reliability was found at all three isometric contraction levels for both muscles (ICC: 0.985–0.994 for BB; 0.948–0.981 for RF).

3.2. Amplitude of sEMG. Recorded sEMG data were processed for RMS analysis. The amplitudes (μV) of the non-normalized RMS values recorded by the PSL-EMG-Tr1 devices at the three contractions levels for the first and second weeks are shown in Table 1. Moderate to very high

Table 1: Reliability comparison of the Biodex System 3 PRO and BTS-FREEEMG, PSL-EMG-Tr1.

Device	Variable		Trial 1	Trial 2	ICC	Difference of means (95% CI)	p value
(a) Biceps brachii muscle							
MVIC	Biodex (N·m)	Week 1	36.65 ± 14.56	35.98 ± 13.78	0.985	0.68 (−0.9, 2.3)	0.387
		Week 2	38.60 ± 14.53	38.59 ± 14.27	0.986	0.01 (−1.6, 1.6)	0.990
	BTS-FREEEMG (μV)	Week 1	460.50 ± 257.49	395.52 ± 216.69	0.930	64.98 (14.4, 115.5)	0.014*
		Week 2	470.34 ± 243.38	413.91 ± 208.48	0.848	56.43 (−18.7, 131.5)	0.132
	PSL-EMG-Tr1 (μV)	Week 1	398.07 ± 231.36	435.05 ± 281.16	0.937	−36.98 (−96.3, 22.3)	0.207
		Week 2	392.39 ± 227.36	435.65 ± 268.89	0.875	−43.26 (−120.4, 33.9)	0.255
80% MVIC	Biodex (N·m)	Week 1	29.11 ± 11.65	28.52 ± 10.66	0.992	0.60 (−0.3, 1.5)	0.197
		Week 2	31.10 ± 11.18	30.95 ± 11.52	0.986	0.15 (−1.1, 1.4)	0.807
	BTS-FREEEMG (μV)	Week 1	364.27 ± 220.15	333.32±183.99	0.934	30.95 (−15.2, 77.1)	0.177
		Week 2	387.76 ± 220.15	356.38 ± 192.92	0.859	31.08 (−37.13, 99.3)	0.352
	PSL-EMG-Tr1 (μV)	Week 1	304.71 ± 198.40	354.03 ± 218.37	0.872	−49.32 (−115.1, 16.4)	0.132
		Week 2	324.07 ± 185.61	368.97 ± 233.94	0.916	−44.90 (−97.6, 7.8)	0.090
40% MVIC	Biodex (N·m)	Week 1	14.41±5.74	14.55 ± 5.09	0.986	−0.14 (−0.8, 0.5)	0.645
		Week 2	15.48 ± 5.72	15.75 ± 6.00	0.994	−0.28 (−0.7, 0.2)	0.199
	BTS-FREEEMG (μV)	Week 1	118.42 ± 81.22	101.81 ± 75.70	0.920	16.61 (−2.5, 35.7)	0.084
		Week 2	121.36 ± 75.72	115.91 ± 69.50	0.906	5.45 (−14.8, 25.7)	0.579
	PSL-EMG-Tr1 (μV)	Week 1	96.69 ± 67.98	94.32 ± 57.30	0.922	2.36 (−14.2, 19.0)	0.768
		Week 2	94.98 ± 53.06	116.68 ± 72.75	0.832	−21.81 (−43.1, −0.5)	0.045*
(b) Rectus femoris muscle							
MVIC	Biodex (N·m)	Week 1	147.80 ± 40.50	154.08 ± 36.38	0.948	−6.28 (−13.9, 1.4)	0.103
		Week 2	159.18 ± 46.04	160.05 ± 45.95	0.981	−0.88 (−6.8, 5.1)	0.762
	BTS-FREEEMG (μV)	Week 1	147.82 ± 65.95	144.25 ± 59.11	0.945	3.58 (−10.0, 17.2)	0.588
		Week 2	175.99 ± 59.53	156.78 ± 59.53	0.864	19.21 (−2.7, 41.1)	0.082
	PSL-EMG-Tr1 (μV)	Week 1	123.96±49.66	124.87 ± 55.45	0.899	−0.91 (−16.1, 14.3)	0.901
		Week 2	129.90 ± 52.05	138.30 ± 56.79	0.907	−8.40 (−23.2, 6.4)	0.249
80% MVIC	Biodex (N·m)	Week 1	115.58 ± 31.82	121.67 ± 30.34	0.964	−6.09 (−10.9, −1.3)	0.015*
		Week 2	127.06 ± 35.52	126.45 ± 35.75	0.977	0.61 (−4.5, 5.7)	0.805
	BTS-FREEEMG (μV)	Week 1	118.59 ± 80.28	115.13 ± 51.59	0.910	3.47 (−15.0, 21.9)	0.699
		Week 2	136.71 ± 67.52	123.54 ± 48.67	0.898	13.21 (−2.9, 29.3)	0.103
	PSL-EMG-Tr1 (μV)	Week 1	95.46 ± 57.58	101.13 ± 49.94	0.922	−5.66 (−19.3, 8.0)	0.396
		Week 2	100.46 ± 41.52	109.22 ± 45.45	0.943	−8.76 (−17.6, 0.1)	0.051
40% MVIC	Biodex (N·m)	Week 1	57.70 ± 15.90	61.50 ± 15.37	0.956	−3.80 (−6.3, −1.3)	0.005*
		Week 2	63.59 ± 18.34	63.81 ± 17.74	0.979	−0.23 (−2.7, 2.2)	0.851
	BTS-FREEEMG (μV)	Week 1	43.45 ± 17.65	44.53 ± 16.57	0.931	−1.08 (−5.2, 3.0)	0.590
		Week 2	50.89 ± 23.43	48.05 ± 21.21	0.883	2.84 (−4.0, 9.6)	0.393
	PSL-EMG-Tr1 (μV)	Week 1	36.15 ± 14.45	39.43 ± 18.16	0.814	−3.28 (−9.3, 2.8)	0.271
		Week 2	38.44 ± 15.68	41.24 ± 18.17	0.957	−2.80 (−5.8, 0.2)	0.070

Values are number or mean ± SD. MVIC, maximum voluntary isometric contraction; ICC, intraclass correlation coefficients; paired t-test, $^*p < 0.05$; CI, confidence interval.

relative reliability was found for all three contraction levels in both muscles (ICC: 0.832–0.937 for BB; 0.814–0.957 for RF). Overall, the reliability at various contraction levels was slightly lower for the PSL-EMG-Tr1 than for the Biodex device. This may be because the muscle group generating the torque includes other muscles in addition to the one measured by sEMG; this is discussed further below.

To compare EMG activity in the same muscle on different days or different individuals, or to compare EMG activity between muscles, the EMG must be normalized. Normalization of EMG signals (% MVIC) is shown in Table 2. Normalization of EMG signals is performed by dividing the EMG signals during the submaximal isometric contraction by a maximal EMG signal (MVIC). The normalized RMS values showed no to high relative reliability in BB and moderate to high relative reliability in RF (ICC: 0.030–0.831 for BB; 0.547–0.828 for RF). There were no statistical differences of normalized RMS values for two sEMG devices between the first and second trial ($p > 0.05$; Table 2).

3.3. Validity. Figure 3 shows the validity of the two sEMG devices. Pearson's r values were used to evaluate validity because all of the % MVIC values measured in the BB and RF muscles were normally distributed. The two sEMG devices were compared using averages of all four trials for two weeks of 40% MVIC and 80% MVIC. The 40% MVIC displayed excellent validity for BB ($r = 0.907$) and RF ($r = 0.965$), and the 80% MVIC showed good to excellent validity for BB ($r = 0.781$) and RF ($r = 0.757$). Figure 4 shows Bland–Altman plots which show the dispersion of the % MVIC of the two sEMG devices. The mean difference in % MVIC was small (0.0–1.1) with the majority of the data points within the 95% limits of agreement.

TABLE 2: Normalization of RMS and reliability of BTS-FREEEMG and PSL-EMG-Tr1.

Variable			Trial 1	Trial 2	ICC	Difference of means (95% CI)	p value
(a) Biceps brachii muscle							
80% MVIC (%)	BTS-FREEEMG	Week 1	78.92 ± 13.00	84.84 ± 18.92	0.321	−5.93 (−15.6, 3.7)	0.213
		Week 2	81.44 ± 16.97	84.09 ± 19.76	0.185	−2.65 (−14.2, 8.9)	0.637
	PSL-EMG-Tr1	Week 1	76.10 ± 14.83	82.08 ± 19.99	0.030	−5.98 (−17.8, 5.9)	0.306
		Week 2	83.14 ± 15.51	82.62 ± 17.93	0.246	0.53 (−11.1, 12.2)	0.925
40% MVCI (%)	BTS-FREEEMG	Week 1	27.52 ± 10.17	26.83 ± 10.89	0.862	0.69 (−2.8, 4.2)	0.683
		Week 2	26.86 ± 9.62	28.01 ± 11.22	0.662	−1.14 (−6.1, 3.8)	0.636
	PSL-EMG-Tr1	Week 1	26.07 ± 9.39	24.43 ± 10.10	0.831	1.63 (−1.9, 5.2)	0.350
		Week 2	26.07 ± 9.49	28.16 ± 11.58	0.307	−2.09 (−8.4, 4.3)	0.500
(b) Rectus femoris muscle							
80% MVIC (%)	BTS-FREEEMG	Week 1	76.46 ± 18.41	79.91 ± 12.59	0.509	−3.45 (−11.9, 5.0)	0.406
		Week 2	76.70 ± 12.19	78.22 ± 10.13	0.736	−1.53 (−6.4, 3.3)	0.517
	PSL-EMG-Tr1	Week 1	74.87 ± 19.24	80.50 ± 11.95	0.547	−5.63 (−13.9, 2.7)	0.171
		Week 2	77.56 ± 14.27	78.81 ± 10.54	0.580	−1.25 (−7.7, 5.2)	0.688
40% MVCI (%)	BTS-FREEEMG	Week 1	30.43 ± 7.32	32.11 ± 7.78	0.870	−1.68 (−4.0, 0.7)	0.152
		Week 2	30.07 ± 8.18	31.07 ± 8.06	0.752	−1.01 (−4.4, 2.4)	0.545
	PSL-EMG-Tr1	Week 1	29.93 ± 7.93	32.35 ± 8.23	0.765	−2.42 (−5.7, 0.8)	0.132
		Week 2	30.69 ± 7.89	30.84 ± 7.93	0.828	−0.15 (−3.0, 2.7)	0.912

Values are number or mean ± SD. MVIC, maximum voluntary isometric contraction; ICC, intraclass correlation coefficients; paired t-test, $^*p < 0.05$; CI, confidence interval.

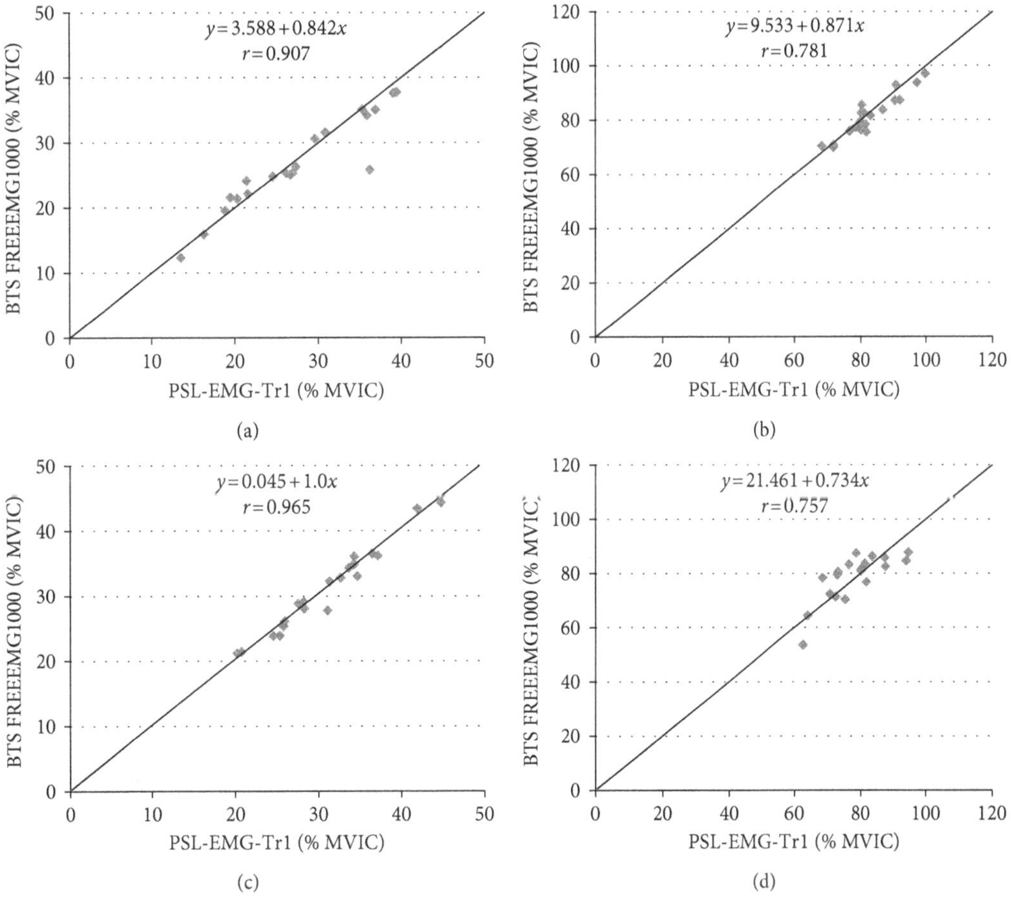

FIGURE 3: The relationship between BTS-FREEEMG1000 and PSL-EMG-Tr1 data. Data from 20 participants, for a total of 20 points in each plot. MVIC, maximum voluntary isometric contraction. (a) 40% MVIC (biceps brachii); (b) 80% MVIC (biceps brachii); (c) 40% MVIC (rectus femoris); (d) 80% MVIC (rectus femoris).

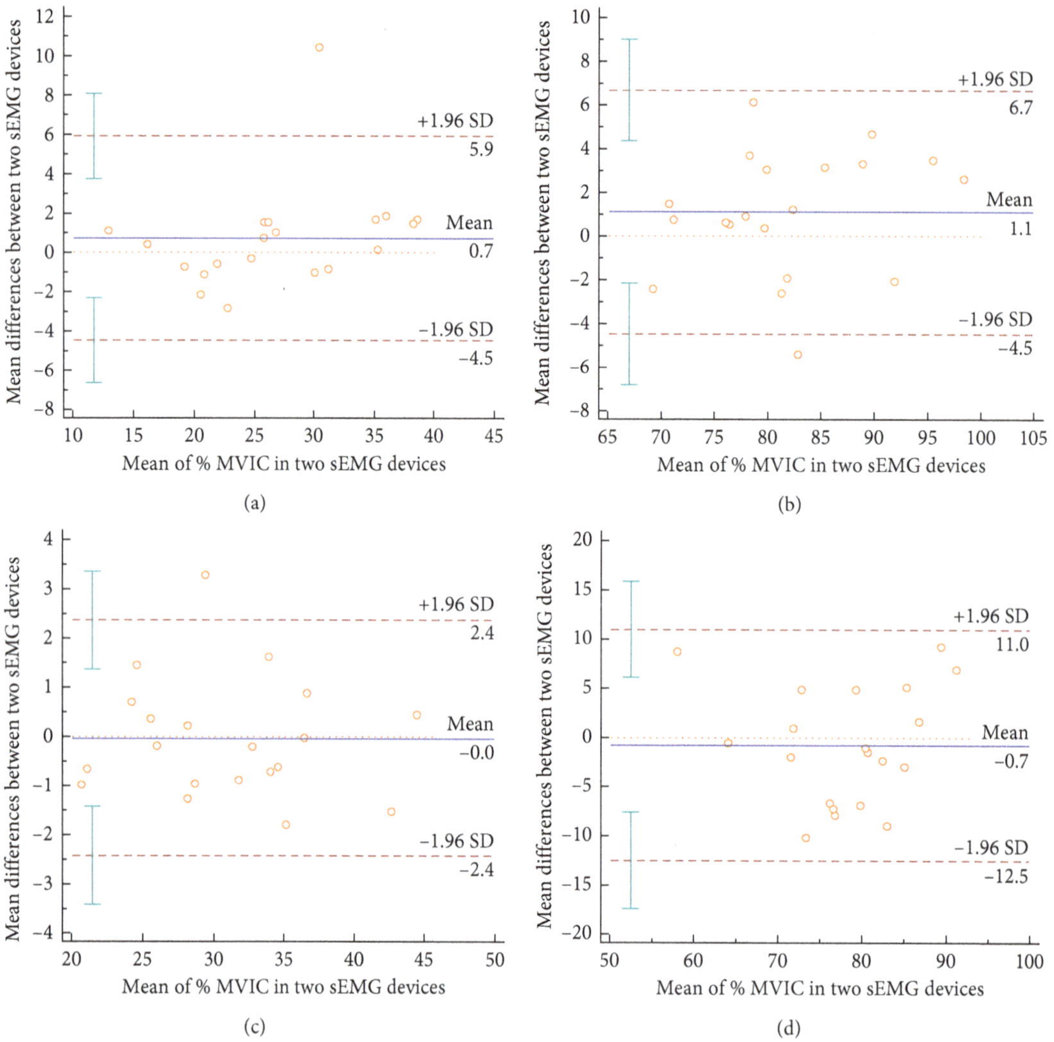

Figure 4: Agreement between BTS-FREEEMG1000 and PSL-EMG-Tr1. Means on the x-axis are the average of two sEMG devices for % MVIC; differences on the y-axis are the difference between the two devices. The 95% limits of agreement (LOA) are depicted (dashed lines). The error bars represent the 95% confidence interval for both the upper and lower limits of agreement. The 95% LOA include zero, indicating no systematic bias in performance between the two devices. (a) 40% MVIC (biceps brachii); (b) 80% MVIC (biceps brachii); (c) 40% MVIC (rectus femoris); (d) 80% MVIC (rectus femoris).

4. Discussion

In this study, we confirmed the reliability and validity of the newly developed sEMG device for monitoring muscle activity during exercise and in daily life. The nonnormalized RMS values measured on both devices showed high reliability (ICC: 0.832–0.937 for BB; 0.814–0.957 for RF). The normalized RMS values showed good to excellent validity ($r = 0.781$–0.907 for BB; $r = 0.757$–0.965 for RF) and showed nonsignificant results on the paired t-test ($p > 0.05$). Especially in the BB muscle, there was little reliability because of the low ICC of normalized RMS values.

Gaudet et al. reported the intersession reliability of maximal contraction of the elbow flexor group (BB, brachialis, and brachioradialis muscles) using sEMG. In this study, a relatively low ICC (range: 0.57–0.80) was seen in the BB in intersession single measurement. However, the average of repeated sEMG measurement was considered to obtain high reliability rather than single measurement [23]. Kollmitzer et al. evaluated the intersession reliability of measures of the knee extensor group (RF, vastus lateralis, and medialis muscles) and found that the overall reliability was good, especially for the RF muscle [16]. To improve reliability, testing in the lower limb can be a better choice than the upper limb and requires repeated measurements rather than a single measurement. Our study also confirmed higher ICC in RF than in BB. And our study compared the single measurements in each trial, which is one of the reasons for the low ICC. Based on previous studies and our results, it seems that EMG signal reproducibility has a great effect on the selection of certain muscles in upper and lower limbs.

In elderly populations, physical activity is reduced, with less than one-fifth of elderly individuals engaging in the recommended level of physical activity [24]. Commercially available computer-based physical activity monitors have

Table 3: Technical specifications of newly developed sEMG device (PSL-EMG-Tr1; PhysioLab Co., Ltd., Busan, Korea) and BTS-FREEEMG (BTS-FREEEMG1000; BTS Bioengineering, Milan, Italy).

	PSL-EMG-tr1	BTS-FREEEMG1000
	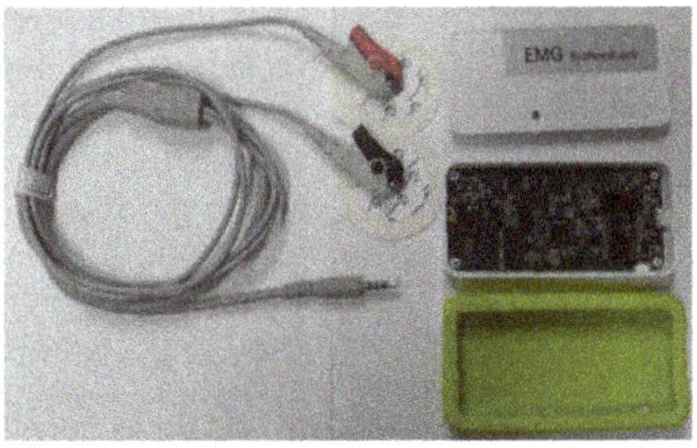	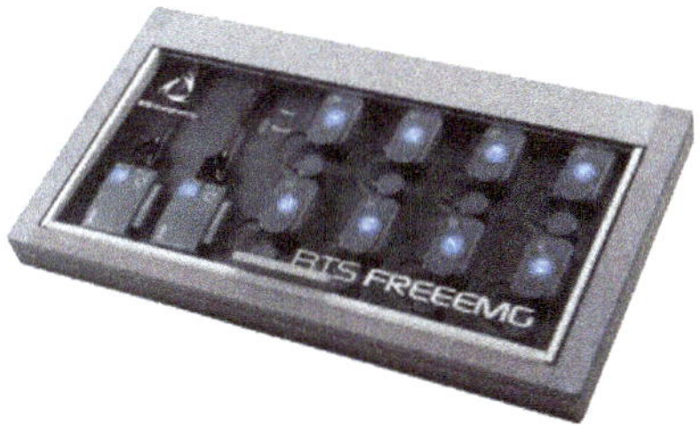
Price	~$500 USD	~$25,000 USD
Dimensions (mm)	48 L × 93 W × 15.5 H Lead wire length 1,100 mm (main 500 mm; branch 600 mm)	EMG probes: 41.5 L × 24.8 W × 14 H main electrode Ø 16 × 12 satellite electrode USB receiver: 82 L × 44 W × 22.5 H Charger: 350 L × 185 W × 20 H
Weight (g)	EMG device: 47 g Lead wire: 41 g	EMG probes: 10 g USB receiver: 80 g Charger: 1450 g
Channels	1 channel	Up to 10 wireless probes
Bandwidth (Hz)	3–2,000	25–500 Hz
Gain (V/V)	25	2,000
Sampling rate (Hz)	30,000	1,000
Common mode rejection (dB)	73	92

been developed in recent years; these devices can enhance motivation in elderly individuals, record physical activity, and support physical exercise [25, 26]. In frail elderly persons, single-repetition maximum resistance training (RT) at 30% MVIC or greater can significantly improve muscle strength, muscle power, and functional outcomes. Therefore, supervised and controlled RT can be an effective measure against frailty [27]. RT also has neuromuscular benefits, and changes in muscle quality can be monitored via sEMG [28]. Applying wearable devise to monitor physical activities is good for feasibility and effectiveness and can encourage exercise through self-monitoring and goal setting [29]. Developing sEMG devices with high accessibility will therefore be very useful in establishing therapeutic strategies and evaluating the muscle condition of elderly people. The newly developed sEMG device is small in size with low cost, and therefore has good portability (Table 3). These advantages can also increase the accessibility of muscle monitoring during various physical activities or exercise.

To evaluate the accuracy of the new device, we recruited young people free of disease and disability. However, elderly individuals may have chronic diseases that could cause peripheral neuropathy or myopathy due to disuse atrophy, so the quality of surface EMG data may vary. However, such difficulties would not indicate a problem with the accuracy of the device itself. In other words, it is possible to compare muscle activity within one individual, but caution is needed when comparing individuals with one another. Despite these limitations, it is very encouraging that there is a tool that allows easy and objective evaluation of muscle quality in elderly people. For the clinical application of the device, further studies will be necessary for healthy elderly or sacropenic patients. This study had the other limitation that should be addressed: the electrodes were attached according to the SENIAM guidelines, but it is considered that the 2.0 cm interelectrode distance was the main cause of the lower ICC in this study. However, this problem will not affect the clinical application of muscle monitoring over time for people undergoing monitoring or engaging in exercise, as only one device will be used. This is because ICC was also lower in clinically widely used sEMG device (BTS-FREEEMG1000), and good to excellent validity was found in normalized RMS values of the two sEMG devices.

The newly developed sEMG device is wired for a single channel, although a wireless model for two or more channels is under development. A high sampling rate was used for the sEMG device in this study. Since most signals from the human muscles have frequency characteristics that are valid at less than 400 Hz, we recommend that the signal analysis sample more than twice the major quard of interest frequency. While we do not need this sampling frequency for existing RMS and MDF analysis, we are interested in signal characteristics that we have not known before by increasing the maximum sampling frequency. This will be used for further study of the characteristics of EMG signals of damaged muscles. Therefore, the newly developed instrument is measuring at a sampling frequency much higher than the frequency of interest. However, since many burdens are expected in the signal processing during commercialization, the sampling rate will be reduced to 2,000 Hz; it will enable fast signal processing and long recording time. In addition, if the EMG signals from the patient's muscles are automatically stored and the system is programmed so that this information can be delivered to medical staff located elsewhere, the therapeutic value of the device will increase still further.

5. Conclusion

Signals from the BB and RF muscles, recorded by the newly developed PSL-EMG-Tr1 device, showed good to excellent validity and moderate to high ICC values with nonnormalized RMS values. However, low ICC values were seen with the normalized RMS values. Although the sEMG itself may have limitations, it can be overcome somewhat through repeated measurements and appropriate muscle selection. Since it has a high correlation compared to conventional sEMG devices, it can be used as an alternative to conventional sEMG devices. The newly developed device may be effective to evaluate and monitor the condition of individuals' muscles during repetitive daily activities or exercise, and it has higher accessibility and portability than do conventional sEMG devices.

Conflicts of Interest

The authors declare that they have no conflicts of interest.

Acknowledgments

This research was supported by the Bio & Medical Technology Development Program of the National Research Foundation, funded by the Korean government, Ministry of Science, ICT and Future Planning (2016M3A9E8942066).

References

[1] A. A. Sayer, H. Syddall, H. Martin, H. Patel, D. Baylis, and C. Cooper, "The developmental origins of sarcopenia," *Journal of Nutrition Health and Aging*, vol. 12, no. 7, pp. 427–432, 2008.

[2] F. Landi, R. Liperoti, A. Russo et al., "Sarcopenia as a risk factor for falls in elderly individuals: results from the ilSIRENTE study," *Clinical Nutrition*, vol. 31, no. 5, pp. 652–658, 2012.

[3] R. Roubenoff, "Origins and clinical relevance of sarcopenia," *Canadian Journal of Applied Physiology*, vol. 26, no. 1, pp. 78–89, 2001.

[4] R. J. Dhillon and S. Hasni, "Pathogenesis and management of sarcopenia," *Clinics in Geriatric Medicine*, vol. 33, no. 1, pp. 17–26, 2017.

[5] S. C. Shaw, E. M. Dennison, and C. Cooper, "Epidemiology of sarcopenia: determinants throughout the lifecourse," *Calcified Tissue International*, vol. 101, no. 3, pp. 229–247, 2017.

[6] T. Ikezoe, N. Mori, M. Nakamura, and N. Ichihashi, "Age-related muscle atrophy in the lower extremities and daily physical activity in elderly women," *Archives of Gerontology and Geriatrics*, vol. 53, no. 2, pp. e153–e157, 2011.

[7] D. E. Anderson, E. Quinn, E. Parker et al., "Associations of computed tomography-based trunk muscle size and density with balance and falls in older adults," *Journals of Gerontology Series: A Biological Sciences and Medical Sciences*, vol. 71, no. 6, pp. 811–816, 2016.

[8] O. Theou, G. R. Jones, A. A. Vandervoort, and J. M. Jakobi, "Daily muscle activity and quiescence in non-frail, pre-frail, and frail older women," *Experimental Gerontology*, vol. 45, no. 12, pp. 909–917, 2010.

[9] R. Radaelli, C. E. Botton, E. N. Wilhelm et al., "Low- and high-volume strength training induces similar neuromuscular improvements in muscle quality in elderly women," *Experimental Gerontology*, vol. 48, no. 8, pp. 710–716, 2013.

[10] E. Gaszynska, K. Kopacz, M. Fronczek-Wojciechowska, G. Padula, and F. Szatko, "Electromyographic activity of masticatory muscles in elderly women-a pilot study," *Clinical Interventions in Aging*, vol. 12, pp. 111–116, 2017.

[11] S. M. Ling, R. A. Conwit, L. Talbot et al., "Electromyographic patterns suggest changes in motor unit physiology associated with early osteoarthritis of the knee," *Osteoarthritis and Cartilage*, vol. 15, no. 10, pp. 1134–1140, 2007.

[12] R. J. Baggen, E. Van Roie, J. H. van Dieen, S. M. Verschueren, and C. Delecluse, "Weight bearing exercise can elicit similar peak muscle activation as medium-high intensity resistance exercise in elderly women," *European Journal of Applied Physiology*, vol. 118, no. 3, pp. 531–541, 2017.

[13] A. Rainoldi, G. Galardi, L. Maderna, G. Comi, L. Lo Conte, and R. Merletti, "Repeatability of surface EMG variables during voluntary isometric contractions of the biceps brachii muscle," *Journal of Electromyography and Kinesiology*, vol. 9, no. 2, pp. 105–119, 1999.

[14] S. Mathur, J. J. Eng, and D. L. MacIntyre, "Reliability of surface EMG during sustained contractions of the quadriceps," *Journal of Electromyography and Kinesiology*, vol. 15, no. 9, pp. 102–110, 2005.

[15] A. Rainoldi, J. E. Bullock-Saxton, F. Cavarretta, and N. Hogan, "Repeatability of maximal voluntary force and of surface EMG variables during voluntary isometric contraction of quadriceps muscles in healthy subjects," *Journal of Electromyography and Kinesiology*, vol. 11, no. 6, pp. 425–438, 2001.

[16] J. Kollmitzer, G. R. Ebenbichler, and A. Kopf, "Reliability of surface electromyographic measurements," *Clinical Neurophysiology*, vol. 110, no. 4, pp. 725–734, 1999.

[17] H. J. Hermens, B. Freriks, R. Merletti et al., *SENIAM: European Recommendations for Surface Electromyography: Results of the SENIAM Project*, Roessingh Research and Development, Enschede, Netherlands, 1999.

[18] T. Y. Fukuda, J. O. Echeimberg, J. E. Pompeu et al., "Root mean square value of the electromyographic signal in the isometric torque of the quadriceps, hamstrings and brachial biceps muscles in female subjects," *Journal of Applied Research*, vol. 10, pp. 32–39, 2010.

[19] L. G. Portney and M. P. Watkins, *Foundations of Clinical Research: Applications to Practice*, Davis Company, Upper Saddle River, NJ, USA, 3rd edition, 2009.

[20] T. K. Koo and M. Y. Li, "A guideline of selecting and reporting intraclass correlation coefficients for reliability research," *Journal of Chiropractic Medicine*, vol. 15, no. 2, pp. 155–163, 2016.

[21] S. B. Plichta and E. A. Kelvin, *MUNRO'S Statistical Methods for Health Care Research*, Lippincott Williams & Wilkins, Philadelphia, PA, USA, 6th edition, 2013.

[22] J. M. Drouin, T. C. Valovich-mcLeod, S. J. Shultz, B. M. Gansneder, and D. H. Perrin, "Reliability and validity of the Biodex system 3 pro isokinetic dynamometer velocity, torque and position measurements," *European Journal of Applied Physiology*, vol. 91, no. 1, pp. 22–29, 2004.
[23] G. Gaudet, M. Raison, F. D. Maso, S. Achiche, and M. Begon, "Intra-and intersession reliability of surface electromyography on muscles actuating the forearm during maximum voluntary contractions," *Journal of Applied Biomechanics*, vol. 32, no. 6, pp. 558–570, 2016.
[24] Department of Health and Human Services, Centers for Disease Control and Prevention (CDC), National Center for Chronic Disease Prevention and Health Promotion, and Division of Nutrition, Physical Activity, and Obesity, Atlanta, GA, USA, https://www.cdc.gov/physicalactivity/data/facts.htm.
[25] P. Silveira, E. van het Reve, F. Daniel, F. Casati, and E. D. de Bruin, "Motivating and assisting physical exercise in independently living older adults: a pilot study," *International Journal of Medical Informatics*, vol. 82, no. 5, pp. 325–334, 2013.
[26] S. K. McMahon, B. Lewis, M. Oakes, W. Guan, J. F. Wyman, and A. J. Rothman, "Older adults' experiences using a commercially available monitor to self-track their physical activity," *JMIR mHealth and uHealth*, vol. 4, no. 2, p. e35, 2016.
[27] P. Lopez, R. S. Pinto, R. Radaelli et al., "Benefits of resistance training in physically frail elderly: a systematic review," *Aging Clinical and Experimental Research*, vol. 30, no. 8, pp. 889–899, 2017.
[28] J. Cannon, D. Kay, K. M. Tarpenning, and F. E. Marino, "Comparative effects of resistance training on peak isometric torque, muscle hypertrophy, voluntary activation and surface EMG between young and elderly women," *Clinical Physiology and Functional Imaging*, vol. 27, no. 2, pp. 91–100, 2007.
[29] N. D. Ridgers, M. A. McNarry, and K. A. Mackintosh, "Feasibility and effectiveness of using wearable activity trackers in youth: a systematic review," *JMIR mHealth and uHealth*, vol. 4, no. 4, p. e129, 2016.

5

Mutual Information Better Quantifies Brain Network Architecture in Children with Epilepsy

Wei Zhang,[1,2] Viktoria Muravina,[3] Robert Azencott,[3] Zili D. Chu,[1,4] and Michael J. Paldino[1]

[1]*Department of Radiology, Texas Children's Hospital, 6701 Fannin St., Houston, TX, USA*
[2]*Outcomes and Impact Service, Texas Children's Hospital, 6701 Fannin St., Houston, TX, USA*
[3]*Department of Mathematics, University of Houston, 3507 Cullen Blvd, Houston, TX, USA*
[4]*Department of Radiology, Baylor College of Medicine, One Baylor Plaza-BCM360, Houston, TX, USA*

Correspondence should be addressed to Wei Zhang; wxzhang1@texaschildrens.org

Academic Editor: Giancarlo Ferrigno

Purpose. Metrics of the brain network architecture derived from resting-state fMRI have been shown to provide physiologically meaningful markers of IQ in children with epilepsy. However, traditional measures of functional connectivity (FC), specifically the Pearson correlation, assume a dominant linear relationship between BOLD time courses; this assumption may not be valid. Mutual information is an alternative measure of FC which has shown promise in the study of complex networks due to its ability to flexibly capture association of diverse forms. We aimed to compare network metrics derived from mutual information-defined FC to those derived from traditional correlation in terms of their capacity to predict patient-level IQ. *Materials and Methods.* Patients were retrospectively identified with the following: (1) focal epilepsy; (2) resting-state fMRI; and (3) full-scale IQ by a neuropsychologist. Brain network nodes were defined by anatomic parcellation. Parcellation was performed at the size threshold of 350 mm^2, resulting in networks containing 780 nodes. Whole-brain, weighted graphs were then constructed according to the pairwise connectivity between nodes. In the traditional condition, edges (connections) between each pair of nodes were defined as the absolute value of the Pearson correlation coefficient between their BOLD time courses. In the mutual information condition, edges were defined as the mutual information between time courses. The following metrics were then calculated for each weighted graph: clustering coefficient, modularity, characteristic path length, and global efficiency. A machine learning algorithm was used to predict the IQ of each individual based on their network metrics. Prediction accuracy was assessed as the fractional variation explained for each condition. *Results.* Twenty-four patients met the inclusion criteria (age: 8–18 years). All brain networks demonstrated expected small-world properties. Network metrics derived from mutual information-defined FC significantly outperformed the use of the Pearson correlation. Specifically, fractional variation explained was 49% (95% CI: 46%, 51%) for the mutual information method; the Pearson correlation demonstrated a variation of 17% (95% CI: 13%, 19%). *Conclusion.* Mutual information-defined functional connectivity captures physiologically relevant features of the brain network better than correlation. *Clinical Relevance.* Optimizing the capacity to predict cognitive phenotypes at the patient level is a necessary step toward the clinical utility of network-based biomarkers.

1. Introduction

Computational methods now have the capacity to model the cerebral network at the whole-brain scale [1]. In this context, the brain is represented as a collection of anatomical elements, or nodes; connections between pairs of nodes, referred to as edges, are then measured noninvasively. Once constructed, the organization of the resulting network can be quantified according to graph theoretical principles [2]. These techniques offer the potential to capture physiologically relevant architectural features of the cerebral network [3]. Resting-state functional MRI (rs-fMRI), a sequence that measures the blood oxygen level-dependent (BOLD) signal over time, is one method by which edges in the brain network can be quantified. Elements of the brain that interact to support a given function continue to exhibit similar BOLD fluctuations at rest [4]. Hence, the strength of a connection between each pair of nodes can be inferred from the similarity of their BOLD signal time courses. As this sequence is task free, it offers the potential to measure the functional status of children who are too young or too impaired to cooperate with traditional functional imaging. These attributes point to the potential for resting-state approaches to deliver new clinical tools, especially in disorders of the brain that emerge from reorganization of the cerebral network such as epilepsy [3]. Recent work has demonstrated the potential of network metrics derived from rs-fMRI to provide clinically meaningful markers of cognitive function in adults [5, 6], in healthy children [7], and in children with focal epilepsy [5–8]. Despite this promise, exactly how neuronal interaction across the cerebrum is reflected by these spontaneous fluctuations in the BOLD signal—and therefore how to best measure similarity in BOLD time courses—is yet to be determined.

The most commonly used measure of functional connectivity in resting-state studies is the Pearson correlation coefficient, defined as the linear covariance of two variables divided by the product of their standard deviations. The Pearson correlation coefficient is simple to calculate and facilitates communication among researchers of diverse disciplines. However, a critical assumption inherent to the use of correlation in the resting state—that the physiologically relevant information about interactions between two discrete brain regions is reflected by a linear relationship between the values of their respective BOLD signals at the same time—may not be valid. In particular, recent studies have shown that nonlinearities inherent to resting-state acquisitions, predominantly hemodynamic in origin, affect both the timing and the amplitude of the measured BOLD signal [9]. As a result, relationships between time series are influenced by the profile of temporal interactions rather than by zero-lag interactions alone [10, 11]. Furthermore, recent work has suggested that nonlinear relationships may play an even more prominent role in the connectivity of pathologic tissues [12]. Beyond issues of linearity, there is a great deal of uncertainty in terms of how the true neuronal interactions we hope to measure are represented by fluctuations in blood flow (BOLD); this challenge highlights the importance of generality [13]. Mutual information is an alternative measure of similarity that quantifies in a very general way how much one random variable tells us about another. It is a dimensionless quantity and can be thought of as the reduction in uncertainty about one variable given knowledge of another. Mutual information has been shown to outperform other methods for characterizing association between time series in simulated networks, in part for its generality and equitability [10, 13]. It has also been shown to provide a repeatable estimate of network connectivity in the brains of normal subjects [10]. Little data exist, however, regarding the importance of nonlinear association within resting-state networks with regard to the emergence of cognitive dysfunction. We therefore sought to compare brain networks constructed from mutual information to those based on correlation in terms of their capacity to support patient-level inferences on the relationship between brain network architecture and brain function.

2. Methods

2.1. Patients. The HIPAA-compliant study was approved by a local institutional review board. Informed consent was waived. Patient medical records were retrospectively reviewed to identify patients with the following inclusion criteria: (1) pediatric age group (21 years of age or younger); (2) a clinical diagnosis of focal epilepsy; (3) an available 3 tesla MR imaging of the brain, including an rs-fMRI sequence; and (4) full-scale intelligence quotient (IQ) using an age-appropriate Wechsler Intelligence Scale measured by a pediatric neuropsychologist within 3 months of the MR imaging. The above-defined cohort was refined by applying the following exclusion criteria: (1) any brain operations performed prior to the MR imaging or (2) having poor image quality due to either motion or other artifacts.

Imaging was performed from January 2013 to June 2015. Thirty-four patients met the inclusion criteria. Ten were excluded on the basis of prior brain surgery. Twenty-four patients (age range: 8–18 years; median: 13.4; 12 (46%) females) made up the final cohort. Of this cohort, 5 patients had structurally normal brains and 19 patients had demonstrable structural abnormalities at MRI, including focal cortical dysplasia ($n = 8$), mesial temporal sclerosis ($n = 5$), low-grade tumor ($n = 4$), and a single epileptogenic tuber in the setting of tuberous sclerosis ($n = 2$). An age-appropriate version of the Wechsler intelligence test was successfully administered in all patients; full-scale intelligence quotient in the cohort ranged from 52 to 129 (median: 91).

2.2. MR Imaging. All imaging procedures were performed on a 3 tesla Achieva system (Philips, Andover, Massachusetts) with a 32-channel phased array coil. The following sequences were obtained: (1) structural images: sagittal volumetric T1-weighted images (repetition time (TR)/echo time (TE): 7.2 ms/2.9 ms; 1 acquisition; flip angle: 7°, inversion time: 1100 ms; field of view (FOV): 22 cm; voxel size (mm): 1 × 1 × 1), and (2) resting-state fMRI: axial single-shot echo planar imaging (EPI) fMRI (TR/TE (ms): 2000/30; flip angle: 80°; 1 acquisition; FOV: 24 cm; voxel (mm): 3 × 3 × 3.75; 300 volumes (duration: 10 minutes)) performed in the resting state. Patients were instructed to lie quietly in the scanner with their eyes closed. All images were visually inspected for artifacts, including susceptibility and subject motion.

2.3. Image Processing and Analysis. The processing pipeline was implemented using MATLAB scripts (version 7.13; MathWorks, Inc.) in which adapter functions were embedded to execute FreeSurfer reconstruction (version 5.3.0; http://surfer.nmr.mgh.harvard.edu) and several FMRIB software library (FSL) suite tools [14]. Details regarding this pathway have been previously described [3, 8]. A brief summary is provided here.

2.3.1. Network Node Definition. The reference space was created from images of one patient in our database, who had no visible abnormality and with optimal registration to the MNI space [15]. Structural imaging data for each patient were aligned to a standard reference template (MNI152) using the FSL's nonlinear registration algorithm [14, 16]. Nodes in the network were defined on the template according to parcellation of whole-brain gray matter. First, FreeSurfer reconstruction of cerebral cortical surfaces was performed on the T1 structural image. This processing stream includes motion correction, skull stripping, intensity normalization, segmentation of white matter and gray matter structures, parcellation of the gray matter and white matter boundary, and surface deformation following intensity gradients which optimally place the gray matter/white matter and gray matter/cerebrospinal fluid borders [17, 18]. The pial and gray white surfaces were visually inspected using the Freeview software for accurate placement.

Next, a self-developed MATLAB program was applied to the FreeSurfer output to further subdivide the 75 standard gray matter parcels according to their surface area. During this process, each parcel was iteratively divided into two new parcels of equal size until the surface area of each parcel (as defined on the FreeSurfer gray-white surface mesh) was less than a predetermined threshold value. Networks were constructed with a size threshold of 350 mm^2. The final parcellation contained 780 nodes (Figure 1). Each surface parcel was then converted into a volume mask of gray matter at that region to form a node on the network. All nodes defined in the reference space were transformed into each individual patient's space by applying the nonlinear transformation matrix (12 degrees of freedom) obtained during registration.

2.3.2. FMRI Data Preprocessing. The first 5 volumes in each resting-state functional datum were removed to allow magnetization to reach equilibrium. Standard preprocessing and independent component analysis (ICA) of the functional datasets were performed using FSL MELODIC [14], consisting of motion correction, interleaved slice timing correction, brain extraction, spatial smoothing with a Gaussian kernel full width at half maximum of 5 mm, and high-pass temporal filtering equivalent to 100 seconds (0.01 Hz). Noise related to motion and other physiologic nuisance was addressed according to an independent component analysis technique [19]. Nonsignal components were removed manually by an expert operator with 6 years of experience using independent component analysis in this patient population. Although the optimal strategies for noise removal in fMRI are debatable [20, 21], an independent component analysis was selected because it has been shown to minimize the impact of motion on network metrics while, at the same time, decreasing the loss of temporal degree of freedom and preserving the signal of interest across a variety of resting-state datasets [21]. Affine boundary-based registration as implemented in FSL FLIRT was then used to align the preprocessed functional image volumes for each patient to that individual's structural T1 dataset using linear registration. The inverse transformation matrix was calculated in this step and subsequently used to transform all masks from structural to functional space. Mean BOLD signal time series were then computed for each node.

2.3.3. Network Edge Definition. The strength of an edge (connection) between 2 nodes was defined in two ways: (1) the absolute value of the Pearson correlation coefficient between their BOLD time series and (2) the mutual information calculated based on the following method.

For two discrete random variables X and Y, their mutual information takes the following form:

$$\mathrm{MI}(X,Y) = \sum_{x\in S_x}\sum_{y\in S_y} p(x,y)\log\left(\frac{p(x,y)}{p(x)p(y)}\right), \qquad (1)$$

where S_x and S_y are possible values of X and Y, $p(x,y)$ is the probability that the pair (X,Y) takes values x in S_x and y in S_y, and $p(x)$ and $p(y)$ are two marginal probabilities of X and Y. For a pair of time series taking small number of values, the probability functions $p(x)$, $p(y)$, and $p(x,y)$ are estimated by frequency counts of the values x and y appeared in the time series. Applying this formula to continuous time series seen in most studies requires a grid to discretize the continuous space into small boxes. The probability functions $p(x)$, $p(y)$, and $p(x,y)$ then are the frequency counts of values within the boundaries of a box centered at x and y. The boundaries and the resolution of the grid affect the value of mutual information. To avoid the ambiguity of choosing a grid, we take the largest mutual information of all possible grids of a predetermined resolution. This maximization applied in the mutual information calculation shares the same principal as the maximal information coefficient (MIC), where the maximization is taken over all grids up to a maximal resolution [13]. It is computationally impossible to search all grids for over 300 thousand pair time series of a single patient in our study however. Therefore, the resolution of the grids had to be predetermined. By testing data of several randomly selected patients, the 3-by-3 grids were chosen in the study as they provided similar mutual information compared to finer grids but required much shorter computation time. The boundaries of 3 bins on x- or y-axis of 3-by-3 grids were determined by 4 values. The two ends are min and max of a time series. The middle two values were determined by mean ± a multiple of standard deviation of the time series. We chose 5 values for the multiple, which yielded 25 possible choices for a pair of the middle two values, 25 choices for 3 bins on x- or y-axis, and 125 choices for 3-by-3 grids for a pair of time series.

2.4. Graph Construction and Network Metric Calculation. Two weighted, undirected connection matrices of each patient were constructed, named as "Pearson and mutual

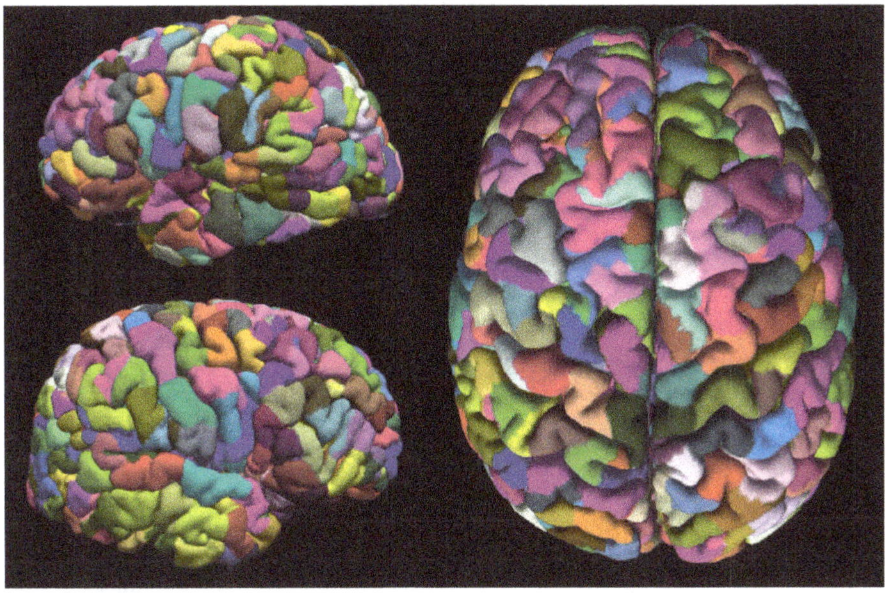

FIGURE 1: Final parcellation with a size threshold of 350 mm², resulting in 780 nodes.

information graphs," consisting, respectively, of the pairwise Pearson correlations and the mutual information between BOLD time series over all network nodes. The following topologic properties were calculated by using MATLAB scripts provided in the Brain Connectivity Toolbox (https://sites.google.com/site/bctnet/): clustering coefficient, modularity, characteristic path length, and global efficiency. A short description of each metric is provided in Table 1.

Clustering coefficient and modularity are metrics that measure the brain's tendency to segregate into relatively independent, local neighborhoods. In other words, these measures reflect the ability of the brain to process specialized functions within highly interconnected functional subnetworks. Characteristic path length and global efficiency measure the global integration of the brain. A short characteristic path length or a high global efficiency indicates that information can be integrated easily across the brain.

2.5. Statistical Analyses. Statistical testing was performed using SAS version 9.3 and R language version 3.4.0 (R Foundation for Statistical Computing, Vienna, Austria). The primary endpoint was the predictive value of the 4 output metrics of the brain network architecture (derived from either Pearson or mutual information graphs) with respect to individual intelligence. This multivariate analysis was accomplished using a random forest approach, which has been previously described in detail in [22]. In short, this ensemble learning method operates by constructing a multitude of decision trees during training and outputting the mean of predictions from individual trees. It is based on bootstrap aggregating, or bagging, in which numerous models are fitted during individual bootstrap sampling and then combined by averaging. During training, approximately one-third of the cohort is omitted at random from

TABLE 1: Metrics of the network architecture.

Metric	Description
Clustering coefficient	The fraction of the nodes of a given neighbor that are also neighbors of each other reflects segregation/subspecialization in the network
Modularity	The degree to which nodes tend to segregate into relatively independent modules reflects segregation/subspecialization within the network
Path length	The minimum number of edges required to traverse the distance between 2 nodes averaged over the network reflects the ease of information transfer across the network
Global efficiency	Inverse of the mean characteristic path length averaged over the network reflects integration in the network

Reproduced from Paldino MJ et al. (2016) [8] (under the Creative Commons Attribution License/public domain).

the training set—this omitted portion of the dataset is considered "out of bag." The IQ of each individual held out of bag is then predicted based on the "learned" model. Prediction accuracy for the out-of-bag cohort was quantified in two ways: (1) mean absolute error and (2) fractional variation explained [23]. To be specific, the random forest algorithm was given access to only the four network metrics and no other patient information during this analysis. The absolute errors of predictions from Pearson graphs were compared to those from mutual information graphs using the Wilcoxon signed rank test. All random forest models were run 500 times to obtain the 95% confidence interval (CI) for fractional variation explained.

The random forest algorithm was also used to measure the independent contribution of individual network metrics to the prediction of IQ. In other words, it measures the association of each variable after accounting for all other variables. This contribution is estimated for each variable by measuring the error for IQ prediction in the out-of-bag cohort compared with the error that results when that particular variable is negated during bagging.

Connections from a mutual information graph were compared to those from the corresponding Pearson graph through a scatter plot of each patient. Differences in network metrics computed on Pearson versus mutual information graphs were assessed using the Wilcoxon signed rank test. Relationships between Pearson-derived network metrics and mutual information-derived network metrics were also quantified using the Pearson correlation coefficient. The Pearson graph was chosen to measure this association since monotonic relationships were expected. Finally, the univariate association of each metric with IQ was measured in a univariate analysis by the Spearman correlation coefficient.

3. Results

3.1. Association between Pearson and Mutual Information Graphs. A representative example of a scatter plot of Pearson versus mutual information connections of one patient is provided in Figure 2. The reference line on the graph is $-1/2 \log(1-r^2)$, which is the relationship between mutual information and Pearson correlation if the joint distribution is Gaussian [24]. Deviation of our data from the reference line, reflecting nonlinear relationships between resting-state time series, was observed in all patients (data not shown).

Network metrics derived from Pearson graphs versus those from the mutual information graphs for each patient are presented in Figure 3. Although association between the Pearson and mutual information graph metrics was generally high-correlation coefficients ranging from 0.84 to 0.88, differences were apparent (Table 2). On average, clustering coefficient and global efficiency became smaller when computed on the mutual information graph. By contrast, path length tended toward higher values under the mutual information graph. Notably, modularity was not statistically different between the graphs (Table 2).

3.2. Network Architecture and Intelligence. Univariate correlation of the mutual information and Pearson-derived graph metrics with subject IQ is presented in Table 3. For most metrics, the association with patient IQ was greater when computed on the mutual information graph. Using a multivariate approach, mutual information graph metrics made the dominant contribution to subject IQ prediction by the random forest model (Figure 4).

Accuracy of the machine learning algorithm's prediction of IQ based on network metrics is presented in Table 4. Metrics derived from mutual information graphs demonstrated a significantly higher predictive value compared to that of the Pearson graph. The relationship between the magnitudes of prediction error for the two methods is demonstrated graphically in Figure 5.

4. Discussion

We evaluated two measures of association—the Pearson correlation and mutual information—that are commonly used to infer connectedness in brain networks constructed from resting-state functional MRI. We specifically assessed the impact of these measures on output metrics of the global brain architecture in terms of their capacity to support the prediction of global intelligence in children with focal epilepsy. We report that measuring brain network edges using mutual information significantly outperformed the use of the Pearson correlation in this setting.

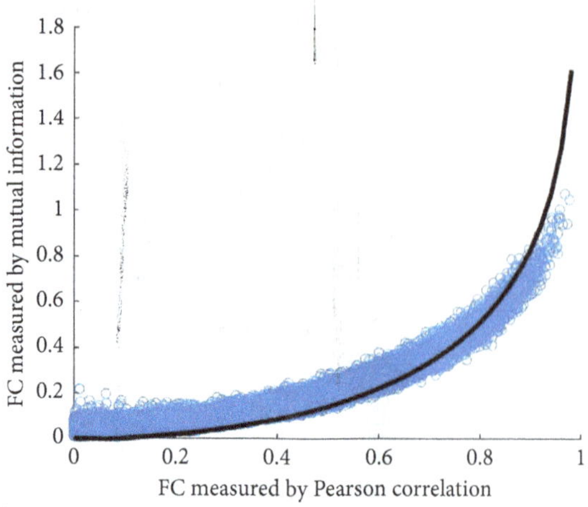

FIGURE 2: Scatter plot of Pearson and mutual information connections in a representative patient. Each blue dot corresponds to an edge between two nodes in the graph. The black reference line is the function $-1/2 \log(1-r^2)$, the relationship between mutual information and Pearson correlation when the data are jointly Gaussian.

Higher-order functions of the human brain are not accomplished by individual functional centers compartmentalized to a particular region of cortex. Rather, they emerge from parallel processing within subspecialized, but distributed, functional systems. The ability to decode these neuronal interactions, particularly as they relate to the emergence of brain function, has become a major focus in current neuroimaging research. Resting-state functional MRI is one modality that has been used extensively as a surrogate for connectedness in the human brain. A significant body of work now exists in support of its capacity to probe physiologically meaningful features of the human brain in a diversity of settings [4]. For example, studies have demonstrated an abnormal network architecture in a variety of disease states, including those with prominent cognitive dysfunction [25–30]; network reorganization has also been observed in adults [31–33] and children [29, 34] with focal epilepsies. Beyond group-level comparisons, a relationship of brain network features quantified by graph theory with intelligence has been demonstrated in many populations, including healthy adults [5, 6, 35], healthy children [7], normal aging [36], Alzheimer's disease [37, 38], autism [39], and epilepsy [8]. Given this capacity of resting-state networks to capture interindividual phenotypic variance in brain function, there is great interest in the development of subject-level markers that could be used to guide patient care [3, 8]. Despite this promise, exactly how neuronal interaction across the cerebrum is reflected by spontaneous

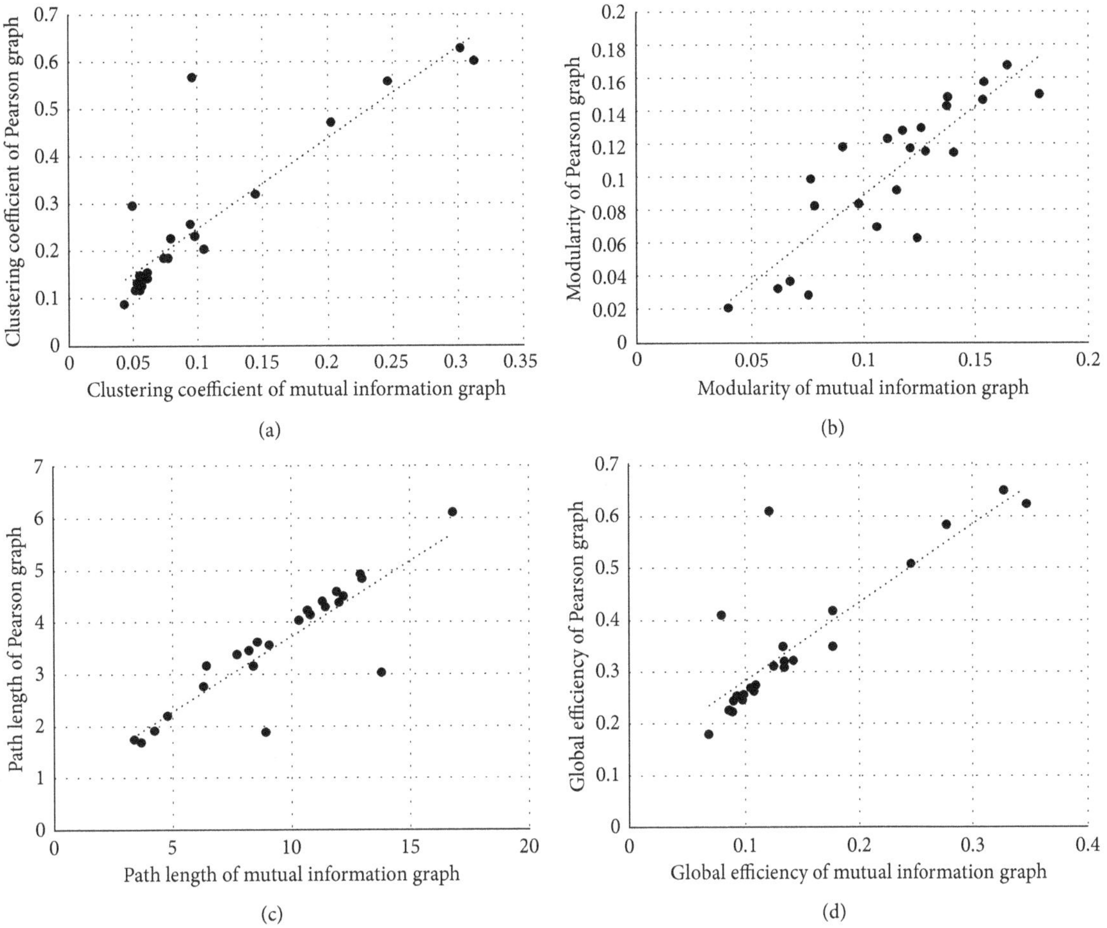

FIGURE 3: Network metrics derived from Pearson graphs versus those from mutual information graphs: (a) clustering coefficient ($r = 0.88$, $p < 0.001$); (b) modularity ($r = 0.86$, $p < 0.001$); (c) path length ($r = 0.88$, $p < 0.001$); (d) global efficiency ($r = 0.84$, $p < 0.001$).

TABLE 2: Comparison between Pearson and mutual information graph metrics.

	Pearson graph Mean ± SD	Mutual information graph Mean ± SD	p value	r (95% CI)
Clustering coefficient	0.26 ± 0.17	0.10 ± 0.08	<0.001	0.88 (0.74, 0.95)
Modularity	0.10 ± 0.04	0.11 ± 0.03	0.246	0.86 (0.68, 0.93)
Path length	3.57 ± 1.14	9.47 ± 3.45	<0.001	0.88 (0.73, 0.94)
Global efficiency	0.35 ± 0.14	0.15 ± 0.08	<0.001	0.84 (0.65, 0.93)

p values were adjusted for multiple comparison by the Bonferroni method. SD: standard deviation; r: correlation coefficient between Pearson and mutual information graph metrics; CI: confidence interval.

TABLE 3: Association between network metrics and patient IQ.

	Pearson graph		Mutual information graph	
	CC	p value	CC	p value
Clustering coefficient	−0.56	0.0320	−0.69	0.0016
Modularity	0.53	0.0656	0.52	0.0776
Path length	0.58	0.0232	0.64	0.0056
Global efficiency	−0.57	0.0272	−0.64	0.0064

p values were adjusted for multiple comparison by the Bonferroni method. CC: Spearman correlation coefficient between network metric and full-scale intelligence quotient.

fluctuations in the BOLD signal—and therefore how to best measure similarity in BOLD time courses—is yet to be determined. We observed that metrics of the network architecture computed on mutual information graphs outperformed network metrics based on the Pearson correlation in terms of the ability to predict subject-level intelligence in a cohort of children with epilepsy.

We observed that graph-based metrics from Pearson and mutual information graphs were relatively similar and demonstrated high linear correlation. Although this finding is consistent with prior work demonstrating only a small contribution of nonlinear associations to the rs-fMRI time

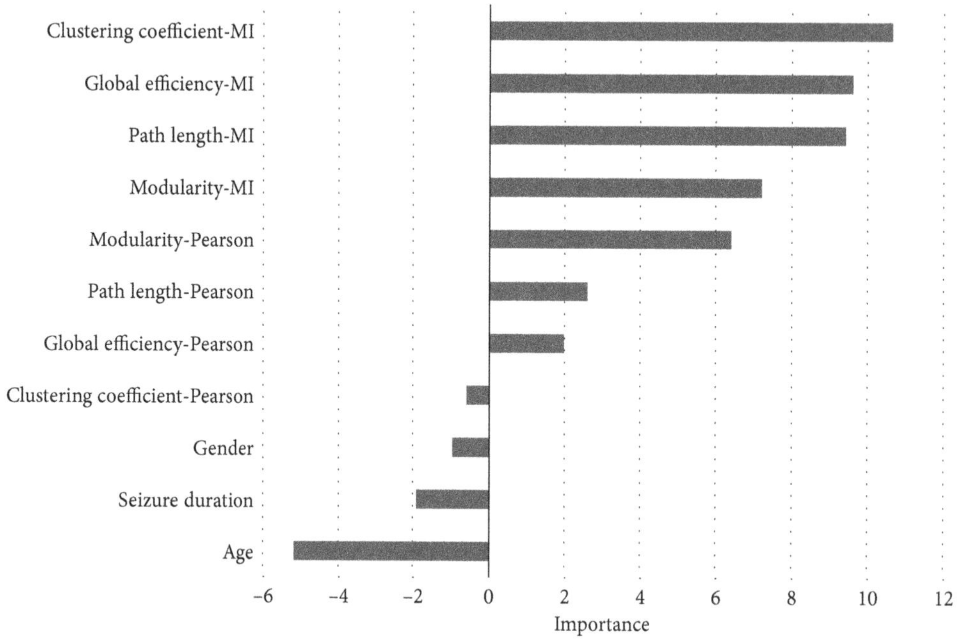

Figure 4: Independent contribution of individual network metrics to IQ prediction by the random forest model.

Table 4: Prediction accuracy for mutual information and Pearson graph metrics.

	Fractional variation explained (95% CI)	Absolute error (mean ± SD)	p value of absolute error comparison
Mutual information	49% (46%–51%)	9.1 ± 7.7	0.04
Pearson	17% (13%–19%)	13.0 ± 10.0	

CI: confidence interval; SD: standard deviation.

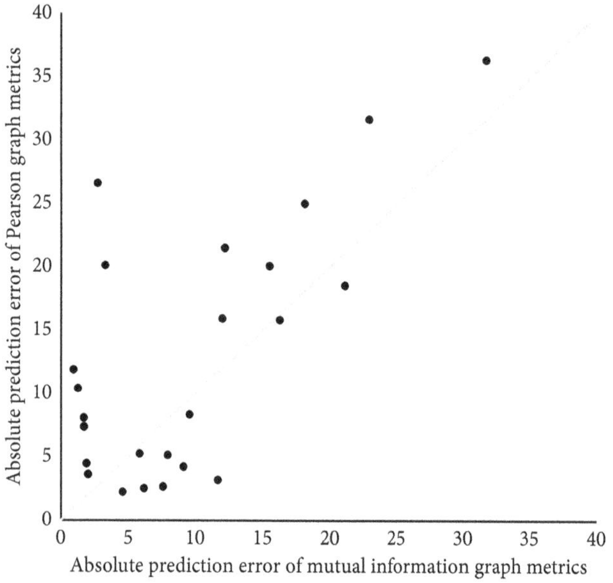

Figure 5: Comparison of absolute errors of "out-of-bag" IQ predictions based on metrics derived from Pearson and mutual information graphs. The gray dash reference line is where the two errors are equal.

series [24], we found that this "small amount" made a significant difference in terms of subject-level prediction in this population. Interestingly, we also observed larger non-Gaussian dependencies among the time series than what has been reported in a healthy adult population [24]. This idea is consistent with the work by Rummel et al. who used a uniform surrogate-based approach to study interrelations that significantly exceed linear correlation in EEG data of epilepsy patients [12]. They observed that nonlinearity occurred predominantly for epileptogenic tissue as well as during epileptic seizures [12]. Our results align with these studies, suggesting that the dynamics of the abnormal brain may be more complex than those of normal brains and that nonlinear associations may be more prevalent. Therefore, a general measure of brain interactions may be more important when analyzing a disease population.

Our results are in line with the previous work that has used mutual information to quantify network edges. Reshef et al. calculated the maximal information coefficient (MIC), based on the same concept as our calculation of mutual information; MIC was shown to be superior to linear association measures in terms of discovering important relationships [13]. It allows one to capture a wide range of interesting associations, not limited to specific function types, or even to all functional relationships. This generality is very crucial as many important relationships are not well modeled by a function. It was also shown that MIC was equitable in the sense of being able to retain the discovery of various types of associations even with increased noise in the simulation data [13]. These attributes may explain the superior prediction of subject intelligence using network metrics observed in our study. Along similar lines, a study in a cohort of patients with schizophrenia [28] demonstrated that nonlinear functional connectivity provided useful discriminative power toward making the diagnosis in each patient.

This study has several limitations. First, our cohort was a selected population of pediatric patients with focal epilepsy. The results may not be generalizable to other patient populations, or to normal subjects. Second, our sample size was small, which did not allow a study stratified by disease severity or a study on characteristics of patients who benefit more from using mutual information. Nevertheless, our goal was to show the general advantages of a nonlinear method used to quantify functional connections. Finally, the extensive computation time required to generate whole-brain networks under a range of nonlinear methods precludes comparison of an exhaustive list of available methods. Nevertheless, mutual information has been proven to be an effective measure in various disciplines for its generality and equitability.

5. Conclusion

Brain networks constructed using edges defined by mutual information significantly outperformed the use of the Pearson correlation for predicting global intelligence in a pediatric cohort with focal epilepsy. Network methodologies specifically optimized to make predictions about individuals will be critical to the development and implementation of clinical tools based on resting-state constructs.

Conflicts of Interest

The authors declare that there are no conflicts of interest regarding the publication of this paper.

References

[1] P. Hagmann, L. Cammoun, X. Gigandet et al., "Mapping the structural core of human cerebral cortex," *PLoS Biology*, vol. 6, no. 7, p. e159, 2008.

[2] M. Rubinov and O. Sporns, "Complex network measures of brain connectivity: uses and interpretations," *NeuroImage*, vol. 52, no. 3, pp. 1059–1069, 2010.

[3] M. J. Paldino, W. Zhang, Z. D. Chu, and F. Golriz, "Metrics of brain network architecture capture the impact of disease in children with epilepsy," *NeuroImage: Clinical*, vol. 13, pp. 201–208, 2017.

[4] B. B. Biswal, J. Van Kylen, and J. S. Hyde, "Simultaneous assessment of flow and BOLD signals in resting-state functional connectivity maps," *NMR in Biomedicine*, vol. 10, no. 4-5, pp. 165–170, 1997.

[5] Y. Li, Y. Liu, J. Li et al., "Brain anatomical network and intelligence," *PLoS Computational Biology*, vol. 5, no. 5, article e1000395, 2009.

[6] M. P. van den Heuvel, C. J. Stam, R. S. Kahn, and H. E. Hulshoff Pol, "Efficiency of functional brain networks and intellectual performance," *Journal of Neuroscience*, vol. 29, no. 23, pp. 7619–7624, 2009.

[7] D. J. Kim, E. P. Davis, C. A. Sandman et al., "Children's intellectual ability is associated with structural network integrity," *NeuroImage*, vol. 124, pp. 550–556, 2016.

[8] M. J. Paldino, F. Golriz, M. L. Chapieski, W. Zhang, and Z. D. Chu, "Brain network architecture and global intelligence in children with focal epilepsy," *American Journal of Neuroradiology*, vol. 38, no. 2, pp. 349–356, 2016.

[9] J. A. de Zwart, P. van Gelderen, J. M. Jansma, M. Fukunaga, M. Bianciardi, and J. H. Duyn, "Hemodynamic nonlinearities affect BOLD fMRI response timing and amplitude," *NeuroImage*, vol. 47, no. 4, pp. 1649–1658, 2009.

[10] B. Cassidy, C. Rae, and V. Solo, "Brain activity: connectivity, sparsity, and mutual information," *IEEE Transactions on Medical Imaging*, vol. 34, no. 4, pp. 846–860, 2015.

[11] P. J. Lahaye, J. B. Poline, G. Flandin, S. Dodel, and L. Garnero, "Functional connectivity: studying nonlinear, delayed interactions between BOLD signals," *NeuroImage*, vol. 20, no. 2, pp. 962–974, 2003.

[12] C. Rummel, E. Abela, M. Muller et al., "Uniform approach to linear and nonlinear interrelation patterns in multivariate time series," *Physical Review E*, vol. 83, no. 6, article 066215, 2011.

[13] D. N. Reshef, Y. A. Reshef, H. K. Finucane et al., "Detecting novel associations in large data sets," *Science*, vol. 334, no. 6062, pp. 1518–1524, 2011.

[14] S. M. Smith, M. Jenkinson, M. W. Woolrich et al., "Advances in functional and structural MR image analysis and implementation as FSL," *NeuroImage*, vol. 23, pp. S208–S219, 2004.

[15] V. Fonov, A. C. Evans, K. Botteron et al., "Unbiased average age-appropriate atlases for pediatric studies," *NeuroImage*, vol. 54, no. 1, pp. 313–327, 2011.

[16] I. J. Simpson, M. J. Cardoso, M. Modat et al., "Probabilistic non-linear registration with spatially adaptive regularisation," *Medical Image Analysis*, vol. 26, no. 1, pp. 203–216, 2015.

[17] B. Fischl, A. Liu, and A. M. Dale, "Automated manifold surgery: constructing geometrically accurate and topologically correct models of the human cerebral cortex," *IEEE Transactions on Medical Imaging*, vol. 20, no. 1, pp. 70–80, 2001.

[18] B. Fischl, D. H. Salat, A. J. van der Kouwe et al., "Sequence-independent segmentation of magnetic resonance images," *NeuroImage*, vol. 23, no. Suppl 1, pp. S69–S84, 2004.

[19] C. G. Thomas, R. A. Harshman, and R. S. Menon, "Noise reduction in BOLD-based fMRI using component analysis," *NeuroImage*, vol. 17, no. 3, pp. 1521–1537, 2002.

[20] M. G. Bright and K. Murphy, "Is fMRI "noise" really noise? Resting state nuisance regressors remove variance with network structure," *NeuroImage*, vol. 114, pp. 158–169, 2015.

[21] R. H. Pruim, M. Mennes, J. K. Buitelaar, and C. F. Beckmann, "Evaluation of ICA-AROMA and alternative strategies for motion artifact removal in resting state fMRI," *NeuroImage*, vol. 112, pp. 278–287, 2015.

[22] L. Breiman, "Random forests," *Machine Learning*, vol. 45, no. 1, pp. 5–32, 2001.

[23] H. Pang, A. Lin, M. Holford et al., "Pathway analysis using random forests classification and regression," *Bioinformatics*, vol. 22, no. 16, pp. 2028–2036, 2006.

[24] J. Hlinka, M. Palus, M. Vejmelka, D. Mantini, and M. Corbetta, "Functional connectivity in resting-state fMRI: is linear correlation sufficient?," *NeuroImage*, vol. 54, no. 3, pp. 2218–2225, 2011.
[25] M. Gottlich, T. F. Munte, M. Heldmann, M. Kasten, J. Hagenah, and U. M. Kramer, "Altered resting state brain networks in Parkinson's disease," *PloS One*, vol. 8, no. 10, Article ID e77336, 2013.
[26] H. He, J. Sui, Q. Yu et al., "Altered small-world brain networks in schizophrenia patients during working memory performance," *PloS One*, vol. 7, no. 6, Article ID e38195, 2012.
[27] E. J. Sanz-Arigita, M. M. Schoonheim, J. S. Damoiseaux et al., "Loss of 'small-world' networks in Alzheimer's disease: graph analysis of FMRI resting-state functional connectivity," *PloS One*, vol. 5, no. 11, Article ID e13788, 2010.
[28] L. Su, L. Wang, H. Shen, G. Feng, and D. Hu, "Discriminative analysis of non-linear brain connectivity in schizophrenia: an fMRI Study," *Frontiers in Human Neuroscience*, vol. 7, p. 702, 2013.
[29] E. Widjaja, M. Zamyadi, C. Raybaud, O. C. Snead, S. M. Doesburg, and M. L. Smith, "Disrupted global and regional structural networks and subnetworks in children with localization-related epilepsy," *American Journal of Neuroradiology*, vol. 36, no. 7, pp. 1362–1368, 2015.
[30] R. A. Yeo, S. G. Ryman, M. P. van den Heuvel et al., "Graph metrics of structural brain networks in individuals with schizophrenia and healthy controls: group differences, relationships with intelligence, and genetics," *Journal of the International Neuropsychological Society*, vol. 22, no. 2, pp. 240–249, 2016.
[31] M. N. DeSalvo, L. Douw, N. Tanaka, C. Reinsberger, and S. M. Stufflebeam, "Altered structural connectome in temporal lobe epilepsy," *Radiology*, vol. 270, no. 3, pp. 842–848, 2014.
[32] W. Liao, Z. Zhang, Z. Pan et al., "Altered functional connectivity and small-world in mesial temporal lobe epilepsy," *PloS One*, vol. 5, no. 1, Article ID e8525, 2010.
[33] M. C. Vlooswijk, M. J. Vaessen, J. F. Jansen et al., "Loss of network efficiency associated with cognitive decline in chronic epilepsy," *Neurology*, vol. 77, no. 10, pp. 938–944, 2011.
[34] M. J. Vaessen, H. M. Braakman, J. S. Heerink et al., "Abnormal modular organization of functional networks in cognitively impaired children with frontal lobe epilepsy," *Cerebral Cortex*, vol. 23, no. 8, pp. 1997–2006, 2013.
[35] N. Langer, A. Pedroni, L. R. Gianotti, J. Hanggi, D. Knoch, and L. Jancke, "Functional brain network efficiency predicts intelligence," *Human Brain Mapping*, vol. 33, no. 6, pp. 1393–1406, 2012.
[36] F. U. Fischer, D. Wolf, A. Scheurich, and A. Fellgiebel, "Association of structural global brain network properties with intelligence in normal aging," *PloS One*, vol. 9, no. 1, Article ID e86258, 2014.
[37] B. M. Tijms, H. M. Yeung, S. A. Sikkes et al., "Single-subject gray matter graph properties and their relationship with cognitive impairment in early- and late-onset Alzheimer's disease," *Brain Connectivity*, vol. 4, no. 5, pp. 337–346, 2014.
[38] J. Xiang, H. Guo, R. Cao, H. Liang, and J. Chen, "An abnormal resting-state functional brain network indicates progression towards Alzheimer's disease," *Neural Regeneration Research*, vol. 8, no. 30, pp. 2789–2799, 2013.
[39] Y. Zhou, F. Yu, and T. Duong, "Multiparametric MRI characterization and prediction in autism spectrum disorder using graph theory and machine learning," *PloS One*, vol. 9, no. 6, Article ID e90405, 2014.

6

Sample Entropy Analysis of Noisy Atrial Electrograms during Atrial Fibrillation

Eva María Cirugeda-Roldán,[1] Antonio Molina Picó,[1] Daniel Novák,[2] David Cuesta-Frau,[1] and Vaclav Kremen[3]

[1]Technological Institute of Informatics, Universitat Politècnica de València, Alcoi Campus, Plaza Ferrándiz y Carbonell 2, Alcoi, Spain
[2]Department of Cybernetics, Faculty of Electrical Engineering, Czech Technical University in Prague, Czech Republic
[3]Czech Institute of Informatics, Robotics and Cybernetics, Czech Technical University in Prague, Czech Republic

Correspondence should be addressed to David Cuesta-Frau; dcuesta@disca.upv.es

Academic Editor: Michele Migliore

Most cardiac arrhythmias can be classified as atrial flutter, focal atrial tachycardia, or atrial fibrillation. They have been usually treated using drugs, but catheter ablation has proven more effective. This is an invasive method devised to destroy the heart tissue that disturbs correct heart rhythm. In order to accurately localise the focus of this disturbance, the acquisition and processing of atrial electrograms form the usual mapping technique. They can be single potentials, double potentials, or complex fractionated atrial electrogram (CFAE) potentials, and last ones are the most effective targets for ablation. The electrophysiological substrate is then localised by a suitable signal processing method. Sample Entropy is a statistic scarcely applied to electrograms but can arguably become a powerful tool to analyse these time series, supported by its results in other similar biomedical applications. However, the lack of an analysis of its dependence on the perturbations usually found in electrogram data, such as missing samples or spikes, is even more marked. This paper applied SampEn to the segmentation between non-CFAE and CFAE records and assessed its class segmentation power loss at different levels of these perturbations. The results confirmed that SampEn was able to significantly distinguish between non-CFAE and CFAE records, even under very unfavourable conditions, such as 50% of missing data or 10% of spikes.

1. Introduction

Arrhythmia is an abnormal too fast, too slow, or irregular pattern heart rate. Most cardiac arrhythmias can be classified as atrial flutter, focal atrial tachycardia, or atrial fibrillation (AF) [1], the most prevalent arrhythmia. Causes of arrhythmia vary and are diverse: coronary heart disease, smoking, diabetes, obesity, age, some medications, hypertension, etc. They have been usually treated using drugs, but catheter ablation has proven more effective, especially in patients with persistent arrhythmia. This is an invasive method devised to cauterise the heart tissue that disturbs correct heart rhythm [2].

Radiofrequency or laser catheters have to be accurately guided by 3D anatomical navigation systems to this substrate. The acquisition and processing of atrial electrograms (AEGM) form the usual mapping technique [3], with a vast disparity of models and algorithms used in practice. Specifically, the assessment of AEGM complexity plays an increasingly important role in research as it can help physicians to minimise the inconvenience of Radiofrequency Ablation (RFA) procedures. Mapping complex fractionated AEGM (CFAE) as target sites for AF ablation is promising. CFAE areas represent critical sites for AF perpetuation and can serve as target sites for AF ablation [3].

The Dominant Frequency (DF) of AEGM signals is one of the most widely used common tools in this context. Algorithms to extract DF for AF ablation have been described in [4, 5]. A new strategy has also been reprogrammed and implemented in [6]. This strategy uses the complexity evaluation of CFAE, which was first introduced in [7] plus the semiautomatic implementation of the CARTO® (Biosense Webster, Diamond Bar, CA, US) CFAE algorithm [6]. The CARTO-XP® mapping system [8] has also been reimplemented in [6]. Two separate AEGM complexity measures have been extracted, the ICL (Interval Confidence Level) and SCI (Shortest Complex Interval) indices [9]. Both indices have also been described in [7] and used in [6, 8]. A measurement of intervals between the discrete peaks of AEGM signals has also been described. These methods contribute valuable information about the level of AEGM complexity which is extracted from CFAE by the unsupervised method [6], but it is still necessary to improve the level of the autonomous classification of AEGM complexity to further help the RFA of AF navigation procedures.

Since it is a highly invasive and complex technique, AEGM signal recording can be affected by many artifacts in the acquisition stage. For example, sensor failure or movement can introduce spikes during signal recording [10, 11], where spikes are sharp impulses of linearly rising and falling edges. Given the way experts classify CFAE signals, these artifacts can bias their interpretation by assigning CFAE records to an incorrect fractionation level. Although many signal processing techniques are available to reduce artifacts such as spikes [12], sometimes this is not possible because of their striking similarity to signal features [13], and the original signal cannot be completely reconstructed [14]. The influence of spikes on complexity measures has been previously characterised for electrocardiograph and electroencephalograph records [11, 15]. In [10], a comparative study of ApEn and SampEn robustness to spikes was carried out in stochastic processes and with simulated and real RR and ECG signals.

AEGM are also prone to having gaps in their time series. Unstable positioning, poor contact, or other problems related to catheters may lead to incomplete or incorrect data [16]. Previous studies have considered random and uniform sample loss in biomedical records and can be found in [17, 18]. These studies have assessed the influence of missing data on the complexity of electroencephalograph signals. In [19], a brief study about infant heart rate signals with random sample loss is presented. Similarly, in [20], Heart Rate Variability (HRV) signals have been considered but applied a uniform sample loss to beat to beat intervals (R-R intervals) from which HRV records were extracted. No study has analysed the influence of sample loss, or spikes, on AEGM records.

This work addresses the study of the influence of possible artifacts on the separability of AEGM records using entropy estimators. The metric SampEn [21] has proven successful in this task [22] using signals from different databases, but without the artifacts stated above. In this case, we included quantitative characterisation against spikes and sample loss to assess SampEn robustness against possible unfavourable real conditions for AEGM time series. Significant performance degradation would render SampEn unusable despite the good results obtained in [22]. SampEn performance and robustness have been evaluated in statistical test and correlation coefficient terms.

The remaining sections of the paper are arranged as follows: the next Section 2 describes the SampEn algorithm in detail, the experimental dataset, the synthetic artifacts to be included in the time series, and the employed statistical assessment. Section 3 presents the study results graphically and numerically. Discussion of these results takes place in Section 4. Finally, conclusions about the influence of perturbations on AEGM records in SampEn are drawn in Section 5.

2. Materials and Methods

2.1. Entropy Metrics. SampEn was first proposed by Richman et al. in [21]. It was devised as a solution to reduce the bias in ApEn and to, therefore, yield a more robust statistic. This new approach was based on avoiding template self-matches computing.

SampEn estimates the regularity of a time series by computing the negative logarithm of the conditional probability that two sequences, which are similar (template match[21]) for m points, remain similar for $m+1$ points at a dissimilarity level under a certain threshold r[19, 21]. It is largely independent of record length and exhibits relative consistency in circumstances in which ApEn does not. SampEn agrees much better than ApEn statistics with the theory for random numbers over wide-ranging operating conditions [21].

Given an input time series $\mathbf{x} = \{x_1, x_2, \ldots, x_N\}$ of size N, sequences to compare are obtained by splitting $\mathbf{x}$ into epochs of length m, $\mathbf{x}_i = \{x_i, x_{i+1}, \ldots, x_{i+m-1}\}$, $i = 1, \ldots, N - m + 1$. The dissimilarity measure between two of these sequences is defined as $d_{ij} = \max(|x_{i+k} - x_{j+k}|)$, $0 \le k \le m-1$, $j \ne i$. Two additional parameters are required to compute SampEn: the number of matches (number of sequences x_j so that $d_{ij} \le r$) for sequences of length m, $B_i(r)$, and the number of matches for sequences of length $m \leftarrow m+1$, $A_i(r)$. These parameters can then be averaged as

$$B_i^m(r) = \frac{1}{N-m-1} B_i(r)$$
$$A_i^m(r) = \frac{1}{N-m-1} A_i(r) \quad (1)$$

and expressed as probabilities:

$$B^m(r) = \frac{1}{N-m} \sum_{i=1}^{N-m} B_i^m(r)$$
$$A^m(r) = \frac{1}{N-m} \sum_{i=1}^{N-m} A_i^m(r) \quad (2)$$

SampEn can then be computed as the natural logarithm of the likelihood ratio:

$$\mathrm{SampEn}(m,r) = \lim_{N\to\infty} \left(-\ln\left[\frac{A^m(r)}{B^m(r)}\right]\right) \quad (3)$$

or for finite time series:

$$\mathrm{SampEn}(m,r,N) = -\ln\left[\frac{A^m(r)}{B^m(r)}\right] \quad (4)$$

The number of matches can be increased by decreasing m or increasing r, but it may impact the ability of SampEn to discern between classes [22]. Both parameters represent a trade-off criterion between accuracy and discrimination capability, and there are no guidelines to optimally choose them. In this case, and according to [21], m was set to 2 and $r = 0.2$.

2.2. Experimental Dataset. A final database containing 113 AEGM records from 12 different patients, nine of whom were males, was used in the experiments. AEGM were preselected by an expert from a larger database recorded in a single study in the Czech Republic [6, 22], after ruling out any noisy, unstable, or artifacted records. The selection criteria were as follows:

(i) Good endocardial contact.

(ii) Not close to the mitral annulus to avoid possible interferences from ventricular signals.

(iii) No visually apparent redundancies.

(iv) Featuring all forms: very organised, very fractionated, or intermediate.

AEGM signals were acquired in the AF mapping procedures performed on the patients indicated for RFA of AF [23]. Signals were sampled at 977 Hz and recorded by CardioLab 7000, Prucka Inc., and then resampled to 1 KHz. Each preselected AEGM signal in this dataset was 1,500 ms long. It would have been preferable to have longer records, but the expert signal selection was driven by the aim to achieve good stability and a high signal-to-noise ratio for later AEGM fractionation degree assessment by an expert. Relatively short records are a limitation of this study, but they guarantee more stability. Data were preprocessed for baseline wander and high frequency noise removal purposes.

According to [7, 24], AEGM were classified into two main classes: non-CFAE (NC) and CFAE (C). The first class, NC, included the AEGM recorded in regions where three independent experts (who perform AF ablation on a regular basis) would not recommend an ablative procedure to be performed (64 records, organised activity, or mild degree of fractionation). The C class contained the signals recorded in the areas where experts would ablate (49 records, intermediate or high degree of fractionation). The final classification corresponded to the average of the three experts' rankings [6]. This classification was based on the subjective perception of signals by the three experts, helped by a specific software tool that displays the AEGM grouped according to their aspect ratio [6]. Figure 1 shows a representative signal of each class considered in the database.

2.3. Synthetic Artifacts

2.3.1. Spikes. Spikes are considered nonstationarities which may arise from external conditions that have little to do with the intrinsic dynamics of the system [10], this being the fundamental basis of the spike generation algorithm.

The presence of a spike in a train is defined by a binomial random process: $\beta(N, p_s)$, where p_s is the probability of a

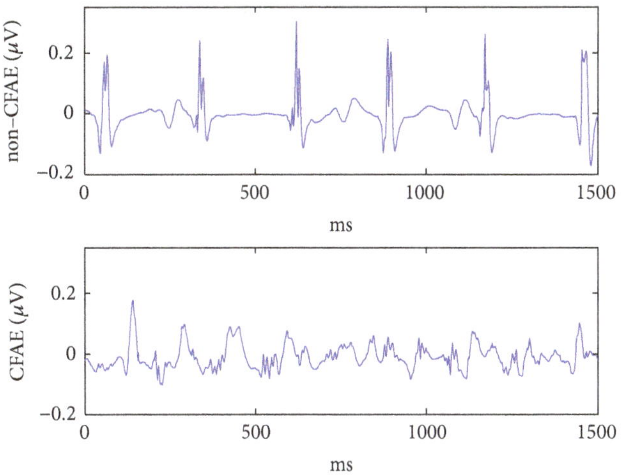

FIGURE 1: AEGM signals of each group of the database: noncomplex fractionated atrial electrogram (NC AEGM) and complex fractionated atrial electrogram (C AEGM).

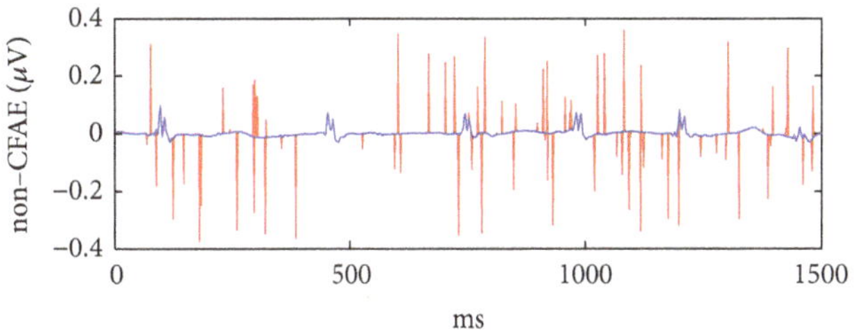

FIGURE 2: An NC signal in blue with a superimposed spike train ($p_s = 0.05$) in red.

spike occurring in a time series of length N. Spike amplitude was defined as a uniform random variable $\Omega(-3\lambda, 3\lambda)$, where λ accounts for the peak-to-peak amplitude of the original AEGM signal. All the spikes were considered to have a fixed length of one sample [15].

Mathematically speaking, spike train $s(t)$ is defined as

$$s(t) = \sum_i a_i \delta(t - t_i) \quad (5)$$

where a_i is the spike amplitude obtained from Ω and t_i is the spike temporal location, generated by means of β. Fifty realisations of independent random spike trains were added to the AEGM original signals in the experimental data set, with probabilities p_s = [0.01, 0.02, 0.03, 0.04, 0.05, 0.10, 0.15, 0.20, 0.30, 0.40, 0.50]. For illustrative purposes, Figure 2 shows one of these realisations, where a spike train was superimposed to an NC record.

2.3.2. Sample Loss. Two algorithms to generate sample losses were considered according to the realistic situations that can take place during catheter recording of the AEGM time series: distributed and consecutive sample losses. Once again, 50 realisations per signal were considered to preserve statistical properties. In both experiments, the number of samples to be removed from each signal was set at a percentage η of

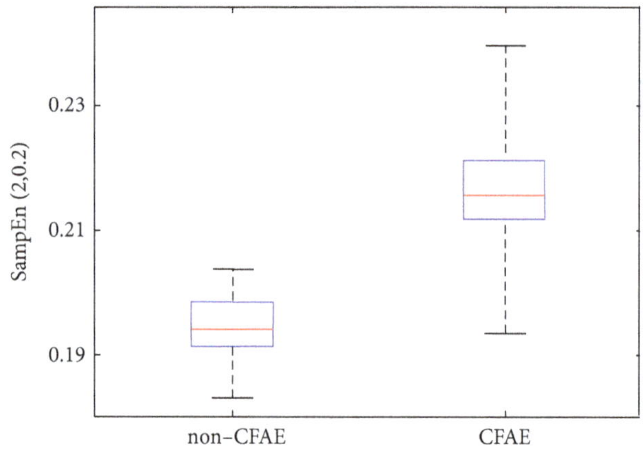

FIGURE 3: Boxplot distribution of C and NC AEGM SampEn values, with no artifact added to the experimental dataset.

total signal length N. Given the similarity to the previous spike experiment, the same percentages were considered, $\eta(\%) = [1, 2, 3, 4, 5, 10, 15, 20, 30, 40, 50]$. Due to this sample removal process, records were shortened by ηN samples. More specifically,

(i) distributed random sample loss was based on removing the isolated samples at the random locations given by β, until the total number of samples to be removed ηN was achieved.

(ii) consecutive random sample loss was based on removing a segment of ηN consecutive samples. Randomness was introduced into the initial sample that was removed. This sample was selected according to β to ensure that it would be different in all 50 realisations of each experiment.

2.4. Statistical Assessment. The segmentation results were assessed using a Mann–Whitney U test [25]. Specifically, this test was used to quantify the probability of the two groups, C and NC, having the same median value. The significance threshold was set at $\alpha = 0.01$. There was no need to check the normality of the results with this test. The performance deviation from the baseline case of no artifacts was quantified using a correlation coefficient ρ_{xy}.

3. Results

3.1. No Artifacts. By taking the value of SampEn(2, 0.2) as the distinguishing characteristic, it was possible to segment between the C and NC AEGM records significantly, with a p-value< 0.001. As shown in Figure 3, the interquartile ranges (featured by the blue box) do not overlap and the median values (red line) are far enough to be statistically different, according to the Mann–Whitney U test results.

Even though distributions were not statistically normal, the 95% confidence intervals given by $[\mu \pm 2\sigma]$, where μ is SampEn mean and σ is its standard deviation, do not overlap: [0.193, 0.199] for neither NC nor [0.216, 0.223] C AEGM.

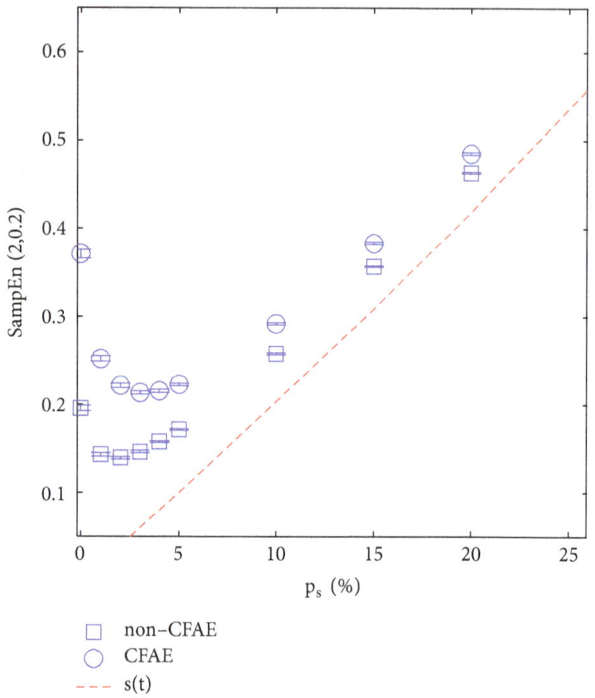

FIGURE 4: SampEn behaviour NC AEGM signals (box) and C AEGM signals (circle) when a spike train of probability p_s was superimposed to the signal. The red dashed line indicates the spike train entropy in terms of p_s. Boxplots fall inside the boxes or circles, respectively, due to the low variance of the SampEn values.

3.2. Spikes Influence on SampEn. Figure 4 depicts the influence that the inclusion of random spikes in AEGM signals had on SampEn values. When spikes were not present (p_s = 0) or found only in a small proportion ($p_s < 0.1$), both groups C and NC AEGM were statistically separated. Figure 5 shows the corresponding ROC curve for the case $p_s = 0.1$. For larger p_s, spikes masked the original AEGM signal entropy, and the ability to discern between AEGM fractionation was lost.

Table 1 shows, for different p_s, the numerical results related to the characterisation of the C and NC AEGM signals entropy at different spike perturbation levels. The metric SampEn can be considered robust enough to provide a good interpretation of the AEGM complexity in the presence of spikes for $p_s \leq 0.10$, with a correlation coefficient of $\rho_{xy} > 0.8$.

According to previous results, see Figure 4, the entropy of the spikes dominates the complexity of the artifacted signal for p_s above 0.10. The complexity of this signal exhibits the same behaviour as the regularity of the spike trains. Table 1 shows that, above this percentage, the measure should not be considered robust enough ($\rho_{xy}(15\%) < 0.8$) [26].

3.3. Sample Loss Influence on SampEn

3.3.1. Distributed Random Sample Loss. Figure 6 shows the behaviour of SampEn when AEGM undergo distributed random sample loss. It shows that AEGM complexity increases proportionally to the number of lost samples. Figure 7 depicts the corresponding ROC curve for η = 10%. The relationship

Table 1: SampEn statistical characteristics for both classes NC AEGM and C AEGM when a spike train of probability p_s is added. For each p_s, the statistical probability related to the separability between classes (p-value), the confidence intervals (CI) at 95% ($\mu \pm 2\sigma$), and the cross correlation coefficient ρ_{xy} between the SampEn values of the initial signal and the signal corrupted with spikes are given.

p_s	0.01	0.05	0.10	0.15
p-value	0.01	0.001	0.001	0.001
CI NC	0.196 ± 0.003	0.158 ± 0.001	0.171 ± 0.001	0.258 ± 0.001
CI C	0.371 ± 0.005	0.215 ± 0.002	0.223 ± 0.002	0.291 ± 0.001
ρ_{xy}	1	0.887	0.863	0.705

Table 2: SampEn statistical characteristics for both classes NC AEGM and C AEGM when distributed random sample loss occurs. For each η, the statistical probability related to the separability between classes (p-value), the confidence intervals (CI) at 95% ($\mu \pm 2\sigma$), and the cross correlation coefficient ρ_{xy} between the SampEn values of the initial signal and the signal with sample loss are given.

η(%)	0	10	30	50
p-value	0.001	0.001	0.001	0.001
CI NC	0.196 ± 0.003	0.211 ± 0.003	0.252 ± 0.004	0.315 ± 0.005
CI C	0.371 ± 0.005	0.402 ± 0.005	0.482 ± 0.006	0.602 ± 0.007
ρ_{xy}	1	0.999	0.996	0.987

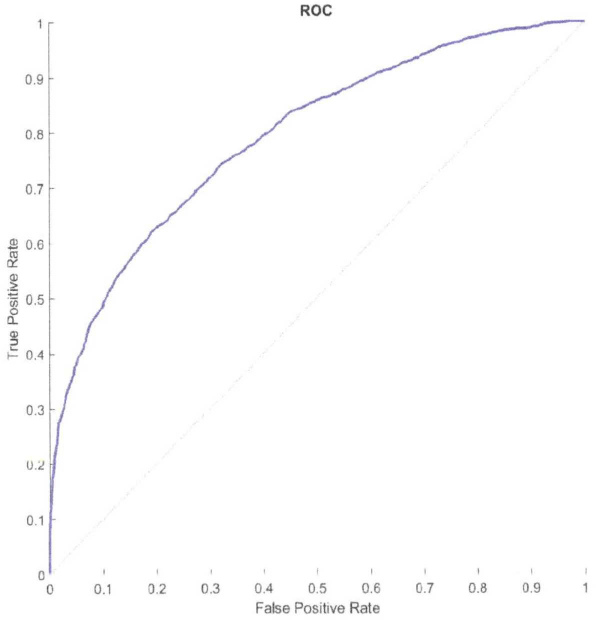

Figure 5: Influence of spikes on AEGM signals classification. ROC curve for $p_s = 0.1$.

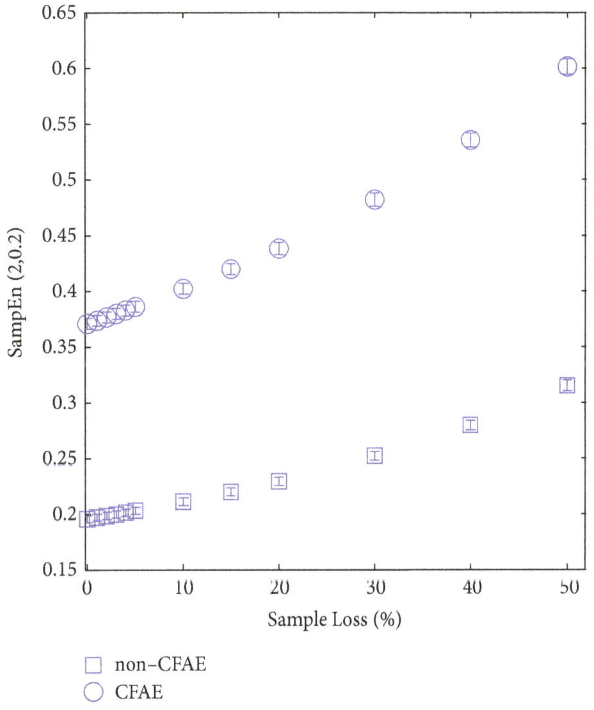

Figure 6: SampEn behaviour in terms of the percentage of random sample loss for NC (box) and C (circle) AEGM signals. Boxplots fall inside the boxes or circles respectively due to the narrow variance of the SampEn values.

between SampEn and the sample loss ratio can be accurately modelled linearly, $f(\eta) = 0.002\eta + 0.19$ for NC records, and $f(\eta) = 0.004\eta + 0.36$ for the C AEGM records, with an adjustment of 0.981 and 0.985, respectively, and a standard error less than 1% in both cases.

Finally, in Table 2, a statistical characterisation of each class for some considered sample loss ratios is given. Mean values are different enough to obtain a significant segmentation probability (p-value< 0.001) and the measure is robust enough to characterise these signals, even though half of the signal was removed ($\rho_{xy} > 0.80$, p-value< 0.001).

Table 2 shows, for the different η values, the numerical results related to the characterisation of the C and NC AEGM signals entropy at different distributed random loss levels. The metric SampEn can be considered robust enough to provide a good interpretation of the AEGM complexity, even with missing epochs for $\eta \leq 50\%$, at a correlation coefficient of $\rho_{xy} > 0.9$.

3.3.2. Consecutive Random Sample Loss. Figure 8 shows the evolution of SampEn values for NC and C AEGM

TABLE 3: SampEn statistical characteristics for both classes NC AEGM and C AEGM when consecutive sample loss was applied. For each η, the statistical probability related to the separability between classes (p-value), the confidence intervals (CI) at 95% ($\mu \pm 2\sigma$), and the cross correlation coefficient ρ_{xy} between the SampEn values of the initial signal and the signal with sample loss are given.

η(%)	0	10	30	50
p-value	0.001	0.001	0.001	0.001
CI NC	0.196 ± 0.003	0.197 ± 0.003	0.198 ± 0.003	0.200 ± 0.003
CI C	0.371 ± 0.005	0.371 ± 0.005	0.367 ± 0.005	0.359 ± 0.005
ρ_{xy}	1(0.001)	0.996(0.001)	0.981(0.001)	0.953(0.001)

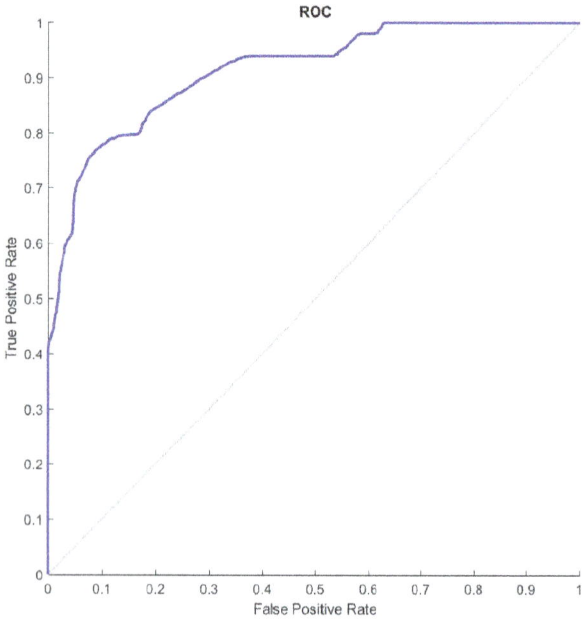

FIGURE 7: Influence of random sample loss on AEGM signals classification. ROC curve for η = 10%.

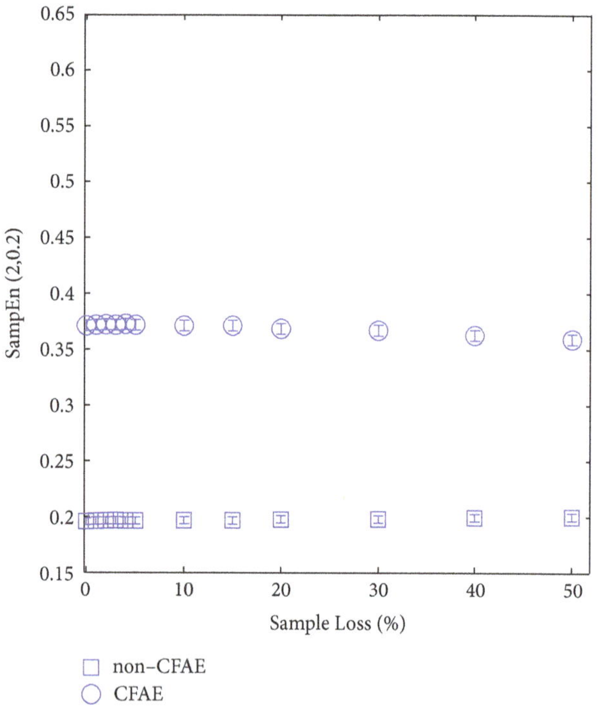

FIGURE 8: SampEn behaviour when consecutive sample loss occurs in the NC (square) and C (circle) AEGM signals. Boxplots fall inside the boxes or circles due to the narrow variance of the SampEn values.

when consecutive sample loss takes place. Unlike distributed random sample loss (Figure 6), this time SampEn remains more or less constant for a wide range of percentages. A slow and small SampEn decrease beyond 15% of sample loss is found in C signals, which is not observed for the NC signals. SampEn can be characterised as constant within a given range with consecutive random sample loss. Figure 9 depicts the corresponding ROC curve for η = 10%.

Table 3 provides the statistical characterisation of SampEn for some analysed percentages. Similar results to the distributed sample loss were found. Classes can be separated with statistical validity (p-value< 0.001). SampEn remained robust ($\rho_{xy} > 0.9$) and unchanged, even though samples were removed.

4. Discussion

All the experiments in this paper used a standard parameter configuration for SampEn, as suggested by [27] for ApEn. Other works have also used similar parameter configurations. In [28], the authors used $m = 2$ and $r = 0.25$ to compute SampEn complexity on paroxysmal AF. This work characterised both paroxysmal and persistent AF with no further consideration. In [29], the region inside $1 \le m \le 5$ and $0.1 \le r \le 0.6$ was considered appropriate for the same purpose. Therefore, it can be arguably reasonable to use the parameter configuration proposed herein.

In the baseline experiment, without external perturbations, SampEn was able to discern between classes. The results in Figure 3 show that the median values for C and NC clearly differ and can be statistically separated (p-value< 0.001). Thus SampEn is an appropriate measure to quantify the system complexity of AEGM signals, even with a short record length of 1.5s only. This length is a study limitation, and performance is arguably likely to improve with longer records, provided they are sufficiently stable.

The influence of spikes on the entropy of AEGM signals was characterised and quantified using synthetic spike trains added to the original signals. The results shown in Figure 4 and Table 1 account for SampEn performance under these conditions. For $p_s > 0.10$, it would be necessary to apply a signal processing technique to minimise the spike influence since its entropy supersedes that of the underlying record,

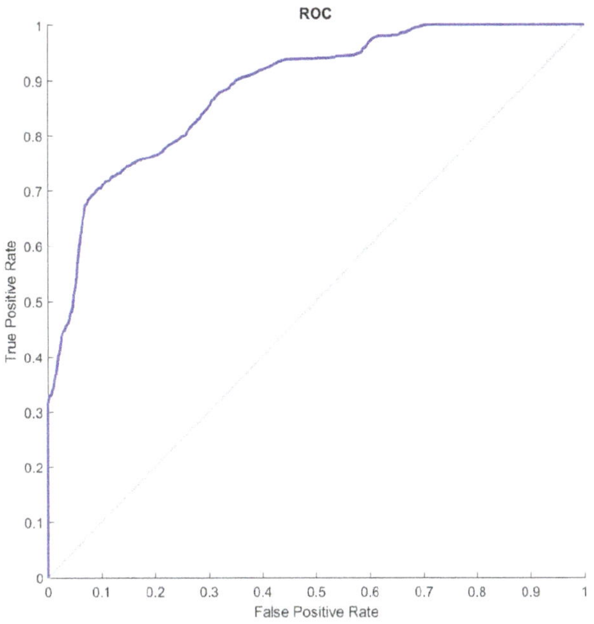

FIGURE 9: Influence of consecutive sample loss on AEGM signals classification. ROC curve for η = 10%.

and the measure loses its interpretability [26]. The results depicted in Figure 4 are similar to those obtained in [10] for the simulated ECG and RR signals. Firstly, SampEn abruptly drops to reach a minimum, from which it begins to increase. The drop is associated with an increase in the number of matches of length $m + 1$ because the randomness introduced by the spike tends to regularise the signal, but when spike probability increased, the number of matches of length $m + 1$ lowered. Thus complexity increased [19, 27]. In this case, SampEn did not measure the entropy of AEGM, but the entropy of the spike train.

Finally, the influence of distributed or contiguous sample loss was assessed. Previous works dealing with EEG signals have shown good performance for SampEn in this context [17]. The changes in performance observed for distributed sample loss are coherent with those presented in [17, 18, 20], where complexity increased due to a rise in randomness that removing samples introduced.

The expected behaviour in consecutive sample loss implied that complexity should be kept more or less constant as removing a segment of a signal implies removing approximately the same number of matches of length m and of length $m + 1$, so the ratio in (4) should be similar to the case before removal. However, this might render the record too short for an accurate SampEn estimation and, therefore, this prior assumption has to be validated. Figure 8 and Table 3 confirmed this expected behaviour, but with complexity of C signals slightly decreasing for the sample loss ratios higher than 15%, which is the same ratio as in [20], and with the same SampEn parameters, despite dealing with AEGM signals instead. In [20], signal epochs were removed from heart rate signals, and heart rate variability was analysed. This could be due to the bias that both ApEn and SampEn showed for short signal records [21] but could also be associated with the remaining correlation between the vectors that d_{ij} compared [30].

5. Conclusions

This study addressed the regularity characterisation of the AEGM signals recorded in RFA procedures of AF and their associated SampEn. It assessed the metric capability to distinguish between C and NC AEGM and provided insight into the influence of spikes or sample loss.

From the results, we conclude that

(i) SampEn is an appropriate regularity measure for AEGM signals as it enables the robust segmentation between C and NC regions. Hence this measure can be used in future clinical studies to prove that some RFA regions can be located by SampEn much more quickly and accurately. Furthermore, the method can be used in a real-time application as it provides reliable results, even on short records (1,500 ms) and exhibits a lower computational cost than other regularity measures such as ApEn or DFA;

(ii) when analysing the AEGM signals corrupted with spikes, if their frequency of occurrence is relatively low (10%), SampEn can be used without having to apply any prior processing as SampEn proved able to separate between classes NC and C. If more spikes are present, it is advisable to filter spikes out as much as possible because their influence may blur class separability;

(iii) SampEn is very robust to any type of sample loss and is able to separate between classes, even if the 50% of the samples are lost.

Conflicts of Interest

The authors declare that there are no conflicts of interest regarding the publication of this paper.

Acknowledgments

This research was supported by Research Center for Informatics (no. CZ.02.1.01/0.0/0.0/16-019/0000765).

References

[1] S. Ahmed, A. Claughton, and P. A. Gould, "Atrial flutter—diagnosis, management and treatment," in *Abnormal Heart Rhythms*, F. R. Breijo-Marquez, Ed., chapter 1, InTech, Rijeka, Croatia, 2015.

[2] P. Kirchhof and H. Calkins, "Catheter ablation in patients with persistent atrial fibrillation," *European Heart Journal*, vol. 38, no. 1, pp. 20–26, 2017.

[3] K. Nademanee, E. Lockwood, N. Oketani, and B. Gidney, "Catheter ablation of atrial fibrillation guided by complex fractionated atrial electrogram mapping of atrial fibrillation substrate," *Journal of Cardiology*, vol. 55, no. 1, pp. 1–12, 2009.

[4] J. Ng and J. J. Goldberger, "Understanding and interpreting dominant frequency analysis of AF electrograms," *Journal of Cardiovascular Electrophysiology*, vol. 18, no. 6, pp. 680–685, 2007.

[5] H. Kottkamp and G. Hindricks, "Complex fractionated atrial electrograms in atrial fibrillation: A promising target for ablation, but why, when, and how?" *Heart Rhythm*, vol. 4, no. 8, pp. 1021–1023, 2007.

[6] V. Křemen, L. Lhotská, M. Macaš et al., "A new approach to automated assessment of fractionation of endocardial electrograms during atrial fibrillation," *Physiological Measurement*, vol. 29, no. 12, pp. 1371–1381, 2008.

[7] K. Nademanee, J. McKenzie, E. Kosar et al., "A new approach for catheter ablation of atrial fibrillation: mapping of the electrophysiologic substrate," *Journal of the American College of Cardiology*, vol. 43, no. 11, pp. 2044–2053, 2004.

[8] D. Scherr, D. Dalal, A. Cheema et al., "Automated detection and characterization of complex fractionated atrial electrograms in human left atrium during atrial fibrillation," *Heart Rhythm*, vol. 4, no. 8, pp. 1013–1020, 2007.

[9] T. P. Almeida, G. S. Chu, J. L. Salinet et al., "Minimizing discordances in automated classification of fractionated electrograms in human persistent atrial fibrillation," *Medical & Biological Engineering & Computing*, vol. 54, no. 11, pp. 1695–1706, 2016.

[10] A. Molina-Picó, D. Cuesta-Frau, M. Aboy, C. Crespo, P. Miró-Martínez, and S. Oltra-Crespo, "Comparative study of approximate entropy and sample entropy robustness to spikes," *Artificial Intelligence in Medicine*, vol. 53, no. 2, pp. 97–106, 2011.

[11] D. Cuesta-Frau, P. Miró-Martínez, J. Jordán Núñez, S. Oltra-Crespo, and A. Molina Picó, "Noisy EEG signals classification based on entropy metrics. Performance assessment using first and second generation statistics," *Computers in Biology and Medicine*, vol. 87, pp. 141–151, 2017.

[12] N. S. Padhye, "Multiple timescale statistical filter for corrupt RR-series," in *Proceedings of the 25th Annual International Conference of the IEEE Engineering in Medicine and Biology Society (IEEE Cat. No.03CH37439)*, vol. 3, pp. 2432–2434, Cancun, Mexico, 2003.

[13] S. Demont-Guignard, P. Benquet, U. Gerber, and F. Wendling, "Analysis of intracerebral EEG recordings of epileptic spikes: Insights from a neural network model," *IEEE Transactions on Biomedical Engineering*, vol. 56, no. 12, pp. 2782–2795, 2009.

[14] G. Xu, J. Wang, Q. Zhang, and J. Zhu, "An automatic EEG spike detection algorithm using morphological filter," in *Proceedings of the IEEE International Conference on Automation Science and Engineering*, pp. 170–175, Shanghai, China, October 2006.

[15] A. Molina-Picó, D. Cuesta-Frau, P. Miró-Martínez, S. Oltra-Crespo, and M. Aboy, "Influence of QRS complex detection errors on entropy algorithms. Application to heart rate variability discrimination," *Computer Methods and Programs in Biomedicine*, vol. 110, no. 1, pp. 2–11, 2013.

[16] P. Ganesan, E. M. Cherry, A. M. Pertsov, and B. Ghoraani, "Characterization of Electrograms from Multipolar Diagnostic Catheters during Atrial Fibrillation," *BioMed Research International*, vol. 2015, Article ID 272954, 9 pages, 2015.

[17] E. M. Roldán, A. Molina-Picó, D. Cuesta-Frau, P. M. Martínez, and S. O. Crespo, "Characterization of entropy measures against data loss: application to EEG records," in *Proceedings of the 33rd Annual International Conference of the IEEE Engineering in Medicine and Biology Society*, pp. 6110–6113, Boston, Mass, USA, August 2011.

[18] E. M. Cirugeda-Roldán, A. Molina-Picó, D. Cuesta-Frau, S. Oltra-Crespo, and P. Miró-Martínez, "Comparative study between Sample Entropy and Detrended Fluctuation Analysis performance on EEG records under data loss," in *Proceedings of the 34th Annual International Conference of the IEEE Engineering in Medicine and Biology Society (EMBC)*, pp. 4233–4236, San Diego, Calif, USA, August 2012.

[19] D. E. Lake, J. S. Richman, M. P. Griffin, and J. R. Moorman, "Sample entropy analysis of neonatal heart rate variability," *American Journal of Physiology-Regulatory, Integrative and Comparative Physiology*, vol. 283, no. 3, pp. R789–R797, 2002.

[20] K. K. Kim, H. J. Baek, Y. G. Lim, and K. S. Park, "Effect of missing RR-interval data on nonlinear heart rate variability analysis," *Computer Methods and Programs in Biomedicine*, vol. 106, no. 3, pp. 210–218, 2012.

[21] J. S. Richman and J. R. Moorman, "Physiological time-series analysis using approximate entropy and sample entropy," *American Journal of Physiology—Heart and Circulatory Physiology*, vol. 278, no. 6, pp. H2039–H2049, 2000.

[22] E. Cirugeda-Roldán, D. Novak, V. Kremen et al., "Characterization of complex fractionated atrial electrograms by sample entropy: An international multi-center study," *Entropy*, vol. 17, no. 11, pp. 7493–7509, 2015.

[23] M. Porter, W. Spear, J. G. Akar et al., "Prospective study of atrial fibrillation termination during ablation guided by automated detection of fractionated electrograms," *Journal of Cardiovascular Electrophysiology*, vol. 19, no. 6, pp. 613–620, 2008.

[24] K. T. S. Konings, C. J. H. J. Kirchhof, J. R. L. M. Smeets, H. J. J. Wellens, O. C. Penn, and M. A. Allessie, "High-density mapping of electrically induced atrial fibrillation in humans," *Circulation*, vol. 89, no. 4, pp. 1665–1680, 1994.

[25] M. P. Fay and M. A. Proschan, "Wilcoxon-Mann-Whitney or t-test? On assumptions for hypothesis tests and multiple interpretations of decision rules," *Statistics Surveys*, vol. 4, pp. 1–39, 2010.

[26] J. S. Richman, "Sample entropy statistics and testing for order in complex physiological signals," *Communications in Statistics—Theory and Methods*, vol. 36, no. 5, pp. 1005–1019, 2007.

[27] S. M. Pincus, I. M. Gladstone, and R. A. Ehrenkranz, "A regularity statistic for medical data analysis," *Journal of Clinical Monitoring and Computing*, vol. 7, no. 4, pp. 335–345, 1991.

[28] R. Alcaraz and J. J. Rieta, "Non-invasive organization variation assessment in the onset and termination of paroxysmal atrial fibrillation," *Computer Methods and Programs in Biomedicine*, vol. 93, no. 2, pp. 148–154, 2009.

[29] R. Alcaraz, D. Abásolo, R. Hornero, and J. J. Rieta, "Optimal parameters study for sample entropy-based atrial fibrillation organization analysis," *Computer Methods and Programs in Biomedicine*, vol. 99, no. 1, pp. 124–132, 2010.

[30] M. Costa, A. L. Goldberger, and C.-K. Peng, "Multiscale entropy analysis of complex physiologic time series," *Physical Review Letters*, vol. 89, no. 6, Article ID 068102, 2002.

7

A Novel Model for Predicting Associations between Diseases and LncRNA-miRNA Pairs based on a Newly Constructed Bipartite Network

Shunxian Zhou,[1,2] Zhanwei Xuan,[2] Lei Wang,[2] Pengyao Ping,[2] and Tingrui Pei[2]

[1]*College of Software and Communication Engineering, Xiangnan University, Chenzhou 423000, China*
[2]*College of Information Engineering, Xiangtan University, Xiangtan 411105, China*

Correspondence should be addressed to Lei Wang; wanglei@xtu.edu.cn

Academic Editor: Yu Xue

Motivation. Increasing studies have demonstrated that many human complex diseases are associated with not only microRNAs, but also long-noncoding RNAs (lncRNAs). LncRNAs and microRNA play significant roles in various biological processes. Therefore, developing effective computational models for predicting novel associations between diseases and lncRNA-miRNA pairs (LMPairs) will be beneficial to not only the understanding of disease mechanisms at lncRNA-miRNA level and the detection of disease biomarkers for disease diagnosis, treatment, prognosis, and prevention, but also the understanding of interactions between diseases and LMPairs at disease level. *Results.* It is well known that genes with similar functions are often associated with similar diseases. In this article, a novel model named PADLMP for predicting associations between diseases and LMPairs is proposed. In this model, a Disease-LncRNA-miRNA (DLM) tripartite network was designed firstly by integrating the lncRNA-disease association network and miRNA-disease association network; then we constructed the disease-LMPairs bipartite association network based on the DLM network and lncRNA-miRNA association network; finally, we predicted potential associations between diseases and LMPairs based on the newly constructed disease-LMPair network. Simulation results show that PADLMP can achieve AUCs of 0.9318, 0.9090 $\pm$ 0.0264, and 0.8950 $\pm$ 0.0027 in the LOOCV, 2-fold, and 5-fold cross validation framework, respectively, which demonstrate the reliable prediction performance of PADLMP.

1. Introduction

MicroRNAs (miRNAs) are endogenous small and nonencoding RNA molecules, which can regulate gene expression at the posttranscriptional level by combining the $3'$ untranslated regions (UTRs) of target mRNAs (UTR) and lead the translation inhibited cleavage of the target mRNAs [1]. Moreover, long-noncoding RNAs (lncRNAs), as the biggest class of noncoding RNAs with length greater than 200 nt, can also regulate gene expression at different levels including transcriptional, posttranscriptional, and epigenetic regulation. Recently, increasing studies demonstrate that lncRNAs and miRNAs play a signification role in the cell proliferation and cell differentiation [2–5] and that the interactions between lncRNAs and microRNAs may have consequences for diseases, explain disease processes, and present opportunities for new therapies [6]. For example, Dey et al. proved that lncRNA H19 would give rise to microRNAs miR-675-3p and miR-675-5p to promote skeletal muscle differentiation and regeneration [7]. Yao et al. discovered that knockdown of lncRNA XIST could exert tumor-suppressive functions in human glioblastoma stem cells by upregulating miR-152 [8]. Wang et al. demonstrated that silencing of lncRNA MALAT1 by miR-101 and miR-217 would inhibit proliferation, migration, and invasion of esophageal squamous cell carcinoma cells [9]. Zhang et al. presented that lncRNA ANRIL indicated a poor prognosis of gastric cancer and promoted tumor growth by epigenetically silencing of miR-99a/miR-449a [10]. You et al. found that miR-449a inhibited cell growth in lung cancer and regulated lncRNA NEAT1 [11]. Emmrich et al. discovered that lncRNAs MONC and MIR100HG would act as oncogenes in AMKL blasts [12]. Leung et al. found that miR-222 and miR-221 upregulated by Ang II were transcribed from a large transcript and knockdown of Lnc-Ang362 would decrease expression of miR-221 and miR-222 and reduce cell proliferation [13]. Zhu et al. discovered that lncRNA H19 and H19-derived miRNA-675 were significantly downregulated in the metastatic prostate cancer cell line M12 compared with the non-meta-static prostate epithelial cell line [14]. Hirata et al. found that lncRNA MALAT1 was associated with miR-205 and promoted aggressive renal cell carcinoma [15]. Zhao and Ren demonstrated that TUG1 knockdown was significantly associated with decreased cell proliferation and promoted apoptosis of breast cancer cells through the regulation of miR-9 [16].

More and more researches have indicated that lncRNA-miRNA interactions are associated with the development of complex diseases, but until now, as far as we know, no prediction models have been proposed for large-scale forecasting of the associations between diseases and LMPairs. However, some prediction models have been reported to infer the associations between diseases and miRNA-miRNA pairs [17–21]. Moreover, there are researches showing that miRNA-miRNA pairs can work cooperatively to regulate an individual gene or cohort of genes that participate in similar processes [18, 22]. Inspired by these existing state-of-the-art methods and ideas for large-scale prediction of the associations between diseases and miRNA-miRNA pairs and based on the reasonable assumption that functionally similar LMPairs tend to be associated with similar diseases, in this paper, a new model named PADLMP is proposed to predict potential associations between diseases and LMPairs. To date, it is the first computational model used to predict disease-LMPairs associations. PADLMP can predict novel disease-LMPairs associations in a large scale by combining the known lncRNA-disease, miRNA-disease, and lncRNA-miRNA associations. To evaluate the prediction performance of the proposed model, evaluation frameworks of leave-one-out cross validation (LOOCV), 2-fold, and 5-fold cross validation were adopted based on the known disease-LMPairs. A series of comparison experiments were also implemented to evaluate the influence of the number of walks on prediction performance. As a result, PADLMP achieved its best performance when the number of walks was set as 2. Specifically, PADLMP achieved value of AUCs of 0.9318, 0.9090 ± 0.0264, and 0.8950 ± 0.0027 in the LOOCV, 2-fold, and 5-fold cross validation framework, respectively. The results of the prediction show that the PADLMP model is feasible and effective in predicting broad-scale disease-LMPairs associations by considering the topology information of the known disease-LMPairs dichotomous network.

2. Materials

2.1. LncRNA-Disease Associations. Known lncRNA-disease associations were downloaded from different databases such as the lncRNA-disease database lncRNADisease [23], MNDR [24], and Lnc2Cancer [25], respectively, and then, after preprocessing (getting rid of duplicate associations), 2048 distinct experimentally confirmed lncRNA-disease associations that including 1126 lncRNAs and 356 diseases were finally obtained (see Supplementary Table 1). Then we further constructed an adjacency matrix A1 of size 1126×356 as the information source.

2.2. miRNA-Disease Associations. We also downloaded known disease-miRNA associations from three different databases such as the miR2Disease [26], HMDD [27], and miRCancer [28], respectively. And then, after preprocessing (getting rid of duplicate associations) and mapping these newly obtained miRNAs and diseases to databases of miRBase v21 [29] and Disease Ontology (DO) [30] separately, we finally obtained 4041 disease-miRNA associations including 438 miRNAs and 263 diseases from HMDD, 1839 disease-miRNA associations including 83 cancers and 327 miRNAs from miRCancer, and 1487 disease-miRNA associations including 107 diseases and 276 miRNAs from miR2Disease (see Supplementary Table 2).

2.3. LncRNA-miRNA Associations. In this section, we downloaded two versions (2015 Version and 2017 Version) of lncRNA-miRNA association datasets from the starBasev2.0 database [31], which provided the most comprehensive experimentally confirmed lncRNA-miRNA interactions based on large-scale CLIP-Seq data. And then, after preprocessing (including elimination of duplicate values, erroneous data, and disorganized data), 20324 lncRNA-miRNA interactions including 494 miRNAs and 1127 lncRNAs were obtained finally (see Supplementary Table 3).

3. Methods

3.1. Methods Overview. In order to predict potential novel associations between diseases and LMPairs, a new model named PADLMP is proposed, which consists of three steps (Figure 1). First, the construction of association network and data integrate. Second, the similarities for lncRNAs, diseases, miRNAs, and lncRNA-miRNA pairs are calculated based on the association network. Finally, potential associations between disease and LMPairs are inferred.

3.2. Construct the Associated Network

3.2.1. LncRNA-Disease Network, Disease-miRNA Network, and LncRNA-miRNA Network. Based on these newly obtained known lncRNA-disease associations, we constructed the lncRNA-disease bipartite network $G_1 = (V_1, E_1)$ according to the following steps.

Step 1. Let V_{l1} be the set of newly collected 1126 lncRNAs, let V_{d1} be the set of newly collected 356 diseases, and $V_1 = V_{l1} \cup V_{d1}$, then we can obtain the vertex set V_1 of G_1.

Step 2. $\forall l_i \in V_{l1}$, if there is $d_j \in V_{d1}$ satisfying the fact that the association between l_i and d_j belongs to the set of newly collected 2048 lncRNA-disease associations, then we define that there is an edge between l_i and d_j in G_1, and by this way, we can obtain the edge set E_1 of G_1. Obviously, E_1 is composed of these newly collected 2048 lncRNA-disease associations.

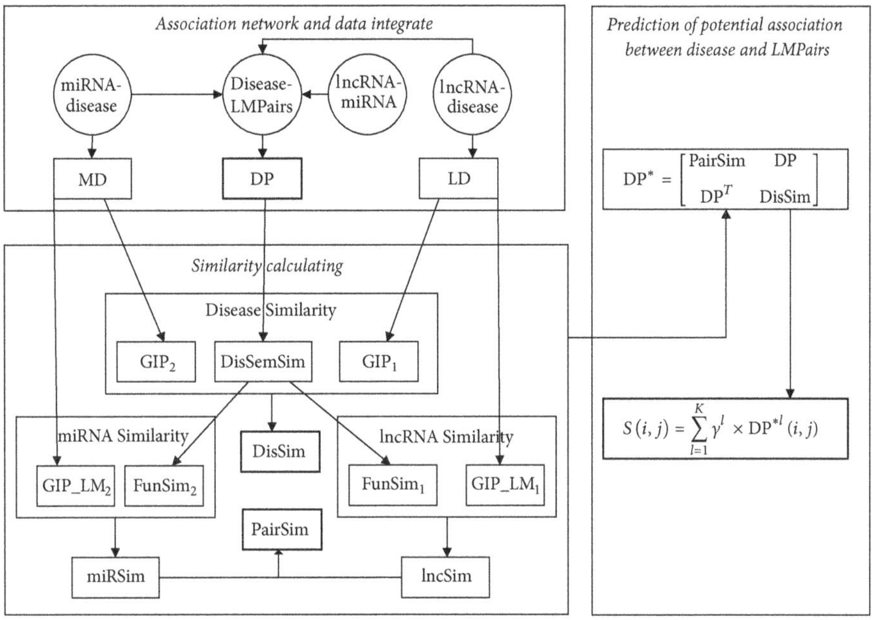

FIGURE 1: Flowchart of PADLMP based on known miRNA-disease, lncRNA-disease, and lncRNA-miRNA association network.

Similar to G_1, we constructed the disease-miRNA bipartite network $G_2 = (V_2, E_2)$ according to the following steps.

Step 1. Let V_{m1} be the set of all these newly collected miRNAs, let V_{d2} be the set of all these newly collected diseases, and $V_2 = V_{m1} \cup V_{d2}$, then we can obtain the vertex set V_2 of G_2.

Step 2. $\forall m_i \in V_{m1}$, if there is $d_j \in V_{d2}$ satisfying the fact that the association between m_i and d_j belongs to the set of all these newly collected disease-miRNA associations, then we define that there is an edge between m_i and d_j in G_2, and by this way, we can obtain the edge set E_2 of G_2. Obviously, E_2 is composed of all these newly collected disease-miRNA associations.

We also constructed the lncRNA-miRNA bipartite network $G_3 = (V_3, E_3)$ according to the following steps.

Step 1. Let V_{l2} be the set of newly collected 1127 lncRNAs, let V_{m2} be the set of newly collected 494 miRNAs, and $V_3 = V_{m2} \cup V_{l2}$, then we can obtain the vertex set V_3 of G_3.

Step 2. $\forall l_i \in V_{l2}$, if there is $m_j \in V_{m2}$ satisfying the fact that the association between l_i and m_j belongs to the set of newly collected 18286 lncRNA-miRNA associations, then we define that there is an edge between l_i and m_j in G_3, and by this way, we can obtain the edge set E_3 of G_3. Obviously, E_3 is composed of these newly collected 20324 lncRNA-miRNA associations.

3.2.2. Disease-LncRNA-miRNA Network. Based on above newly constructed bipartite networks such as G_1, G_2, and G_3, we constructed a new tripartite network $G_4 = (V_4, E_4)$ according to the following steps.

Step 1. Let $V_{l'} = V_{l1} \cap V_{l2}$, $V_{m'} = V_{m1} \cap V_{m2}$, and $V_{d3} = V_{d1} \cap V_{d2}$. $\forall d_i \in V_{d3}$, if there are $l_j \in V_{l'}$ and $m_k \in V_{m'}$ satisfying the fact that the association between d_i and l_j belongs to E_1, the association between d_i and m_k belongs to E_2, and the association between l_j and m_k belongs to E_3 simultaneously. Then we define that there are an edge between d_i and l_j, an edge between d_i and m_k, and an edge between l_j and m_k in G_4 separately, and by this way, we can obtain the edge set E_4 of G_4.

Step 2. Let $V_l \subseteq V_{l'}$ satisfying the fact that $\forall l_i \in V_l$ there is $d_j \in V_{d3}$ satisfying the fact that the association between d_j and l_i belongs to E_4. Let $V_m \subseteq V_{m'}$ satisfying the fact that $\forall m_i \in V_m$ there is $d_j \in V_{d3}$ satisfying that the association between d_j and m_i belongs to E_4. Let $V_4 = V_l \cup V_m \cup V_{d3}$, then we can obtain the vertex set V_4 of G_4.

3.2.3. Disease-LMPairs Network. Based on above newly obtained tripartite Disease-LncRNA-miRNA network G_4, we constructed a new bipartite disease-LMPairs network $G = (V, E)$ according to the following steps.

Step 1. $\forall l_i \in V_l$ and $m_j \in V_m$, let $p_{ij} = (l_i, m_j)$ and $V_p = \{p_{ij}\}$ where $i \in [1, |V_l|]$ and $j \in [1, |V_m|]$, then we define $V = V_{d3} \cup V_p$, and by this way, we can obtain the vertex set V of G.

Step 2. $\forall d_k \in V_{d3}$, there is $p_{ij} = (l_i, m_j) \in V_p$ satisfying the fact that the association between d_k and l_i belongs to E_1, the association between d_k and m_j belongs to E_2, and the association between l_i and m_j belongs to E_3 simultaneously. Then we define that there is an edge between d_k and p_{ij} in G, and by this way, we can obtain the edge set E of G.

To make it easier to understand the construction of the network, we list in "The Meaning of Vertex and Edges in the Networks" each of the vertices, edges, and their meanings that appear in Sections 3.2.1, 3.2.2, and 3.2.3.

3.3. Calculation the Similarity of Disease

3.3.1. Calculation of the Disease Semantic Similarity (DisSemSim). Firstly, we downloaded *MeSH* descriptors from the National Library of Medicine and curated the names of diseases using the standard *MeSH* disease terms. Next, we represented the relationship of different diseases by a structure of directed acyclic graph (DAG) such as $\mathrm{DAG}(D) = (T(D), E(D))$. Here, $T(D)$ represented the node set including node D and its ancestor nodes, and $E(D)$ denoted the edge set of corresponding direct links from a parent node to a child node, which represented the relationship between different diseases [32]. Then, based on the disease DAG, the contribution of an ancestor node d to the semantic value of disease D and the contribution of the semantic value of disease D itself can be calculated by the following two equations, respectively:

$$D_D(d) = 1 \quad \text{if } d = D$$

$$D_D(d) = \max\left\{\Delta * D_D\left(d'\right) \mid d' \in \text{children of } d\right\} \quad \text{if } d \neq D, \tag{1}$$

$$\mathrm{DV}(D) = \sum_{d \in T(D)} D_{D(d)}, \tag{2}$$

where $D_D(d)$ represents the contribution of an ancestor node d to the semantic value of disease D, $\mathrm{DV}(D)$ represents the contribution of the semantic value of disease D itself, and Δ is the semantic contribution decay factor with value between 0 and 1. The function of parameter Δ is to guarantee that, as the distances between disease D and its ancestor disease d increase, the contribution of d to D will progressively decrease. Moreover, from the above formula (1), it is easy to see that it is also reasonable to define the contribution of D to itself as 1. In addition, according to the experimental results of some previous state-of-the-art methods [33, 34], we will set the value of Δ as 0.5 in this paper.

In order to measure disease semantic similarity that two diseases with more common ancestor nodes in the DAG shall have higher semantic similarity, based on the assumption, we can define the semantic similarity between two diseases d_i and d_j as follows:

$$\mathrm{DisSemSim}\left(d_i, d_j\right) = \frac{\sum_{t \in T(d_i) \cap T(d_j)} \left(D_{d_i}(t) + D_{d_j}(t)\right)}{\mathrm{DV}(d_i) + \mathrm{DV}\left(d_j\right)}, \tag{3}$$

where $T(d_i)$ and $T(d_j)$ represented the node sets of the DAG of d_i and d_j, respectively.

3.3.2. Calculation of the Gaussian Interaction Profile Kernel Similarity for Diseases (GIPSim). According to the assumption that functionally similar genes tend to be associated with similar diseases, we can integrate the topologic information of known miRNA-disease association network and lncRNA-disease association network to measure the disease similarity. Moreover, in this section, we will adopt Gaussian Interaction Profile Kernel to calculate the similarity of diseases. Firstly, based on the networks such as G_1 and G_2 constructed above, we can obtain two adjacency matrices such as Y_1 (or Y_2) as follows. For any given lncRNA l_i (or miRNA m_i) and disease d_j, while k takes 1 or 2, we define that

$$Y_k(i, j) = \begin{cases} 1 & \text{exist an edge between } l_i\left(m_i\right) \text{ and disease } d_j \text{ in } G_1\left(G_2\right) \\ 0 & \text{otherwise.} \end{cases} \tag{4}$$

Hence, let $\mathrm{IP}_k(d_i)$ denote the ith column of matrix Y_k, then we can calculate the Gaussian Kernel Similarity between the diseases d_i and d_j based on their interaction profiles as follows:

$$\mathrm{GIP}_k\left(d_i, d_j\right) = \exp\left(-\gamma_k \left\|\mathrm{IP}_k(d_i) - \mathrm{IP}_k\left(d_j\right)\right\|^2\right)$$

$$\gamma_k = \frac{1}{(1/n_k)\sum_{i=1}^{n_k} \left\|\mathrm{IP}_k(d_i)\right\|^2}, \tag{5}$$

where the parameter n_k denotes the number of diseases in G_k $(k = 1, 2)$.

Based on formula (5), we can adopt squared root approach to calculate the Gaussian Interaction Profile Kernel Similarity for diseases as follows:

$$\mathrm{GIPSim}\left(d_i, d_j\right) = \left(\mathrm{GIP}_1\left(d_i, d_j\right) \times \mathrm{GIP}_2\left(d_i, d_j\right)\right)^{1/2}. \tag{6}$$

3.3.3. Calculation of the Integrated Similarity between Disease. Based on these formulas presented above, we can finally define the similarity measurement between diseases d_i and d_j as follows:

$$\mathrm{DisSim}\left(d_i, d_j\right) = \begin{cases} \mathrm{GIPSim}\left(d_i, d_j\right) & \text{if } \mathrm{DisSemSim}\left(d_i, d_j\right) = 0 \\ \dfrac{\mathrm{GIPSim}\left(d_i, d_j\right) + \mathrm{DisSemSim}\left(d_i, d_j\right)}{2} & \text{otherwise.} \end{cases} \tag{7}$$

3.4. Calculation of the Similarity between LncRNAs (miRNAs)

3.4.1. Calculation of the LncRNA (miRNA) Functional Similarity. For any given two lncRNAs (miRNAs) such as $l_i(m_i)$ and $l_j(m_j)$, let $DT_1 = \{dt_{11}, dt_{12}, \ldots, dt_{1m}\}$ be all diseases related to $l_i(m_i)$ in $G_1(G_2)$ and let $DT_2 = \{dt_{21}, dt_{22}, \ldots, dt_{2n}\}$ be all diseases related to $l_j(m_j)$ in $G_1(G_2)$, then we can define the functional similarity between $l_i(m_i)$ and $l_j(m_j)$ as follows ($k = 1$, $v = l$ or $k = 2$, $v = m$):

$$\operatorname{FunSim}_k(v_i, v_j) = \frac{\sum_{1\le p\le m} \operatorname{SemSims}(dt_{1p}, DT_2) + \sum_{1\le p\le n} \operatorname{SemSims}(dt_{2p}, DT_1)}{m+n}, \quad (8)$$

where

$$\operatorname{SemSims}(d_{t_{1p}}, DT_2) = \max_{1\le l\le n}\left(\operatorname{DisSemSim}(d_{t_{1p}}, d_{t_{21}})\right). \quad (9)$$

3.4.2. Calculation of the Gaussian Interaction Profile Kernel Similarity for lncRNAs (miRNA). For any given two lncRNAs (miRNAs) such as $l_i(m_i)$ and $l_j(m_j)$, in a similar way to the calculation of GIP_1, GIP_2 can be obtained as follows ($k = 1$, $v = l$ or $k = 2$, $v = m$):

$$\operatorname{GIP\_LM}_k(v_i, v_j) = \exp\left(-\gamma_k \left\|\operatorname{IP}_k(v_i) - \operatorname{IP}_k(v_j)\right\|^2\right)$$
$$\gamma_k = \frac{1}{(1/n_k)\sum_{i=1}^{n_k}\left\|\operatorname{IP}_k(v_i)\right\|^2}, \quad (10)$$

where $\operatorname{IP}_k(v_i)$ and $\operatorname{IP}_k(v_j)$ are the ith row and the jth row in matrix Y_k, respectively, and n_k is the number of lncRNAs (miRNA) in G_k.

3.4.3. Calculation of the Integrated Similarity between lncRNAs (miRNAs). Based on these formulas presented above, we can finally define the similarity measurement between lncRNAs l_i and l_j as follows:

$$\operatorname{lncSim}(l_i, l_j) = \frac{\operatorname{FunSim}_1(l_i, l_j) + \operatorname{GIP\_LM}_1(l_i, l_j)}{2}$$
$$\operatorname{miRSim}(m_i, m_j) = \frac{\operatorname{FunSim}_2(m_i, m_j) + \operatorname{GIP\_LM}_2(m_i, m_j)}{2}. \quad (11)$$

3.5. Similarity for LncRNA-miRNA Pairs (LMPairSim)

3.5. Similarity for LncRNA-miRNA Pairs (LMPairSim). Based on the bipartite disease-LMPairs network G constructed above, for any given two lncRNA-miRNA pairs $p_{ij} = (l_i, m_j)$ and $p_{ab} = (l_a, m_b)$, we can calculate the similarity between them according to the following three different ways:

(1) Average Approach

$$\operatorname{LMPairSim}(P_{ij}, P_{ab}) = \frac{\left(\operatorname{lncSim}(l_i, l_a) + \operatorname{miRSim}(m_j, m_b)\right)}{2}. \quad (12)$$

(2) Squared Root Approach

$$\operatorname{LMPairSim}(P_{ij}, P_{ab}) = \left(\operatorname{lncSim}(l_i, l_a) \times \operatorname{miRSim}(m_j, m_b)\right)^{1/2}. \quad (13)$$

(3) Centre Distance Approach

$$\operatorname{LMPairSim}(d_i, d_j) = \sqrt{\left(\operatorname{lncSim}(l_i, l_a) - \operatorname{AvglncSim}\right)^2 + \left(\operatorname{miRSim}(m_j, m_b) - \operatorname{AvgmiRSim}\right)^2}, \quad (14)$$

where

$$\operatorname{AvglncSim} = \frac{\sum_{i=1}^{n_l}\sum_{j=1}^{n_l}\operatorname{lncSim}(l_i, l_j)}{n_l^2},$$
$$\operatorname{AvgmiRSim} = \frac{\sum_{i=1}^{n_m}\sum_{j=1}^{n_m}\operatorname{miRSim}(m_j, m_i)}{n_m^2}. \quad (15)$$

3.6. Prediction of Potential Associations between Diseases and LMPairs. Inspired by the KATZ method in social networks [35], disease-gene correlation prediction [36], and lncRNA-association prediction of disease [37], we explored the PADLMP measure by developing a new computational model for predicting disease-LMPairs associations (see Figure 1). Obviously, based on the formulas (12), (13), (14), and (15), let N_d denote the number of diseases in G, N_p denote the number of LMPairs in G, N_l denote the number of lncRNAs in G, and N_m denote the number of miRNAs in G, respectively, then we can obtain a $N_d \times N_d$ dimensional matrix DisSim and $N_p \times N_p$ dimensional matrix PairSim. Moreover, we can construct $N_p \times N_p$ dimensional adjacency matrices DP as follows:

$$\operatorname{DP}(i, j) = \begin{cases} 1 & \text{exist an edge between } d_i \text{ and } p_j \text{ in } G \\ 0 & \text{otherwise,} \end{cases} \quad (16)$$

where d_i denotes the ith disease in G and p_j denotes the jth LMPair in G

Hence, inspired by the approach based on KATZHMDA [38] and KATZ [35], we can construct an integrated matrix

DP^* for further predicting the potential associations between diseases and LMPairs as follows:

$$DP^* = \begin{bmatrix} \text{PairSim} & DP \\ DP^T & \text{DisSim} \end{bmatrix}. \quad (17)$$

Based on the integrated matrix DP^* constructed above and letting $V_p = \{P_1, P_2, \ldots, P_{Np}\}$, then, for any given lncRNA-miRNA pair $p_i \in V_p$ and diseases node $d_j \in V_d$, the probability of potential association between p_i and d_k can be obtained as follows:

$$S(i,j) = \sum_{l=1}^{K} \gamma^l \times DP^{*l}(i,j), \quad (18)$$

where the parameter K is an integer bigger than 1 and the parameter γ satisfies $0 < \gamma < 1$.

Additionally, according to the above formula (18), it is obvious that the $(N_p + N_d) \times (N_p + N_d)$ dimensional matrix S depicts the possibilities of all associations between diseases and LMPairs in G, and it can be further modified into the following form:

$$S = \sum_{l \geq 1} \gamma^l \times DP^{*l} = (I - \gamma \times DP^*)^{-1} - I = \begin{bmatrix} S_{11} & S_{12} \\ S_{21} & S_{22} \end{bmatrix}, \quad (19)$$

where S_{11} is $N_p \times N_p$ dimensional matrix, S_{12} is $N_p \times N_d$ dimensional matrix, S_{21} is $N_d \times N_p$ dimensional matrix, and S_{22} is $N_d \times N_d$ dimensional matrix.

From formula (19), it is easily to know that S_{12} is exactly the *final prediction result matrix*, which includes all of the potential associations between diseases and LMPairs in G. In addition, considering that a long walker in a sparse network may be less meaningful, it will disrupt association prediction, so we set K to 2, 3, and 4 here. Then, final prediction result matrix could be represented by matrix DP, PairSim, and DisSim based on aforementioned equation (19).

While $K = 2$, there is

$$S_{122} = \gamma \times DP + \gamma^2 \times (\text{PairSim} \times DP + DP \times \text{DisSim}). \quad (20)$$

While $K = 3$, there is

$$S_{123} = S_{122} + \gamma^3 \times \left(DP \times DP^T \times DP + \text{PairSim}^2 \times DP + \text{PairSim} \times DP \times \text{DisSim} + DP \times \text{DisSim}^2\right). \quad (21)$$

While $K = 4$, there is

$$S_{124} = S_{123} + \gamma^4 \times \left(\text{PairSim}^3 \times DP + DP \times DP^T \times \text{PairSim} \times DP + \text{PairSim} \times DP \times DP^T \times DP + DP \times \text{DisSim} \times DP^T \times DP\right) + \gamma^4 \times \left(DP \times DP^T \times DP \times \text{DisSim} + \text{PairSim}^2 \times DP \times \text{DisSim} + \text{PairSim} \times DP \times \text{DisSim}^2 + DP \times \text{DisSim}^3\right). \quad (22)$$

4. Results

In order to estimate the prediction performance of our newly proposed model PADLMP, the leave-one-out cross validation (LOOCV) procedure was adopted based on the positive samples of disease-LMPair associations. In the LOOCV validation framework, each known disease-LMPair association is used as a test sample, and the remaining disease-LMPairs association is used as a training sample for model learning. In particular, all the disease-LMPairs without known relevance proofs will be considered as candidate samples. In the LOOCV, we can obtain the rank of each left-out testing sample relative to candidate samples, and if the test samples are with a prediction level higher than a given threshold, then it will be considered to be successfully predicted. The corresponding true positive rates (TPR, sensitivity) and false positive rates (FPR, 1 − specificity) could be obtained by setting different thresholds. Here, sensitivity measures the percentage of test samples which are predicted with a higher rank than given threshold, specificity is calculated as the percentage of negative samples ranked below a given threshold. The receiver operating characteristics (ROC) curves can be drawn by plotting TPR versus FPR by different thresholds. In order to evaluate the predictive performance of PADLMP, the areas under the ROC curve (AUC) were further calculated. 1 of the AUC value showed a perfect prediction, while 0.5 of the AUC value represented purely random performance.

From the above, we can find that there are some parameters such as K, γ adopted in our prediction model PADLMP. It is obvious that these parameters are critical to the prediction performance of our model. Moreover, in Section 3.5, three different ways have been proposed to calculate the similarity for lncRNA-miRNA pairs (LMPairSim), then we need to further evaluate the performances of these three different ways also. Hence, in this section, based on the validation framework of LOOCV, we implemented a series of comparison experiments to evaluate the influence of these parameters, and the simulation results were shown in Figure 2. As a result, from Figure 2, it is easy to see that PADLMP can achieve the best prediction performance while K was set to 2. Additionally, as for other parameters γ, during simulations, we will set γ as 0.01 based on the empirical values given by previous state-of-the-art works [37, 39–41]. Moreover, in the LOOCV, for the similarity calculation of LMPairSim, we use formulas (12), (13), and (14) in order and then select the formula that obtains the maximum AUC value. As a result, the AUC value of 0.9318, 0.9262, and 0.9247 were obtained when selecting formulas (12), (14), and (13), respectively.

Furthermore, we also compared the performance of our prediction model PADLMP with that of the RLSMDA [42], WBSMDA [39], and LRLSLDA [41] in LOOCV, since negative samples were not required in PADLMP, RLSMDA, WBSMDA, and LRLSLDA. The simulation results were shown in Figure 3. It is easy to see that PADLMP can achieve a reliable AUC of 0.9318, which is much higher than the AUC of 0.8104 and 0.9281 achieved by RLSMDA, WBSMDA, LRLSLDA, respectively, In addition, we can clearly see that the AUC value of the model LRSLDA is less than 0.5, which

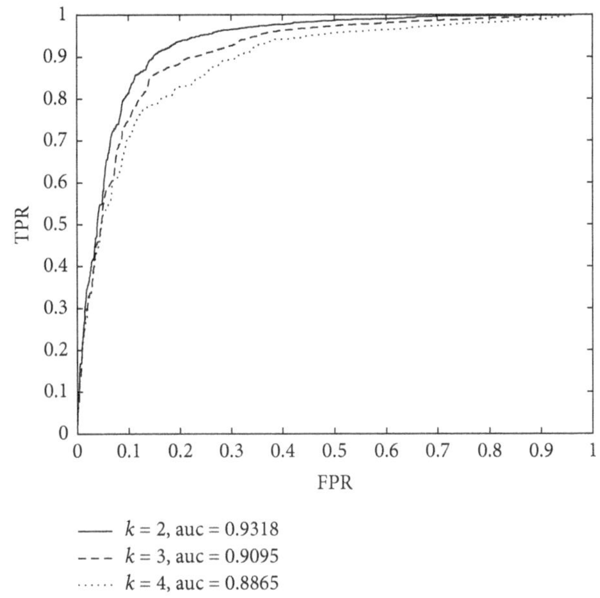

Figure 2: Prediction performance of PADLMP while K takes different values in LOOCV.

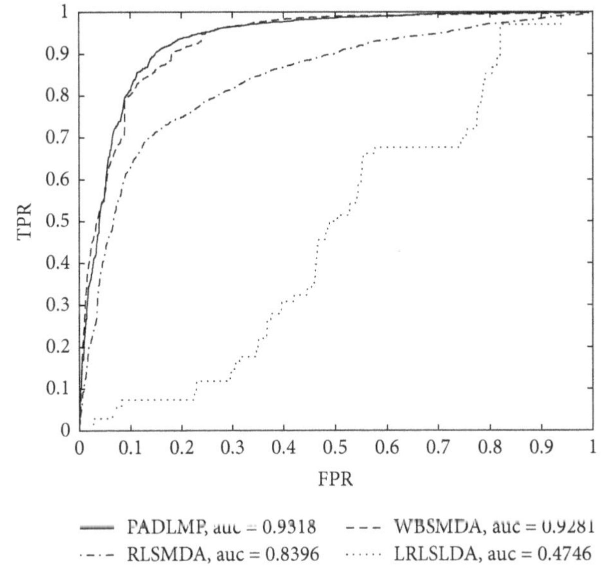

Figure 3: Comparison between PADLMP and RLSMDA, WBSMDA, and LRLSLDA in LOOCV.

is obviously unreasonable. So based on prior knowledge [43], we subtract this value less than 0.5 from 1 and then we get the AUC value of LRSLDA being 0.5254.

Moreover, in order to further evaluate the prediction performance of PADLMP, the k-fold cross validation was also implemented, in which all the known disease-LMPair association samples were randomly equally divided into k parts, and $k - 1$ parts were then used as training samples for model learning while the rest part was used as testing samples for model evaluation. Specifically, in this section, considering time complexity and costs, we would only implement 2-fold and 5-fold cross validation to evaluate the prediction

Table 1: Prediction performance of PADLMP while K was set to different values in the 2-fold and 5-fold cross validation, respectively.

5-fold	$K = 2$	$K = 3$	$K = 4$
AUC	0.8950	0.8367	0.7724
STD	0.0027	0.0050	0.0109
2-fold	$K = 2$	$K = 3$	$K = 4$
AUC	0.9090	0.8709	0.8518
STD	0.0264	0.0361	0.0441

performance of PADLMP. In a similar way to that of LOOCV, all the disease-LMPairs without known relevance evidences would be considered as candidate samples in the k-fold cross validation. Next, in case of the prediction performance bias caused by random division of the testing samples, we would repeat the random division of the testing samples and our simulations for 100 times, and then, the corresponding ROC curves and AUCs would be obtained in a similar way to that of LOOCV. Simulation results were shown in Table 1, and as a result, from the Table 1, it is easy to see that PADLMP can achieve the best prediction performance with average AUCs of 0.9090 and 0.8950 with Standard Deviation (STD) of 0.0264 and 0.0027 in the 2-fold and 5-fold cross validation, respectively, while setting $K = 2$.

From the above descriptions, it is obvious that the newly proposed model PADLMP can achieve a reliable and effective prediction performance in both LOOCV and k-fold cross validation. Therefore, we released the potential disease-LMPair associations with higher predicted relevance scores publicly (see Supplementary Table 4) and anticipated that these disease-LMPair associations may offer valuable information and clues for corresponding biological experiments and would be confirmed by experimental observations in the future.

5. Case Studies

Colon cancer is a malignant tumor that is usually found at the borders of rectum and sigmoid colon [44]. This is the third most common cancer and the third leading cause of cancer death in men and women in the United States [45]. However, patients with early colon tumors only suffer from subtle symptoms [46], which make the disease difficult to be detected. In addition, worse, it is reported that its incidence has an upward trend in recent years [47]. Therefore, there is an urgent need to predict potential miRNAs and lncRNAs associated with colon tumors. With the help of modern medicine, many miRNAs have been shown to be associated with colon tumors. For example, miRNA-145 targets the insulin receptor substrate-1 and thus inhibits the growth of colon cancer cells [48].

Moreover, as the second largest cause of cancer deaths in women, breast cancer accounts for the total number of cancers in women 22% [49, 50]. Breast cancer is caused by a variety of molecular changes, traditionally diagnosed by histopathological features such as tumor size, grading, and lymph node status [49]. Studies have shown that lncRNAs and

Table 2: PADLMP was applied to three kinds of important cancer.

Disease	LncRNA	miRNA	Evidence
Colon cancer	MALAT1	hsa-miR-145-5p	#, $, !
Colon cancer	MALAT1	hsa-miR-181a-5p	#, $, +
Colon cancer	MALAT1	hsa-miR-155-5p	#, $, !
Colon cancer	MALAT1	hsa-miR-101-3p	#, $, !
Colon cancer	MALAT1	hsa-miR-25-3p	#, $, +
Colon cancer	MALAT1	hsa-miR-143-3p	#, $, !
Colon cancer	MALAT1	hsa-miR-200c-3p	#, $, !
Colon cancer	MALAT1	hsa-miR-429	#, $, +
Colon cancer	MALAT1	hsa-miR-22-3p	#, $, !
Colon cancer	MALAT1	hsa-miR-320a	#, $, +
Breast cancer	XIST	hsa-let-7b-5p	#, $, !
Breast cancer	XIST	hsa-let-7a-5p	#, $, !
Breast cancer	XIST	hsa-miR-146a-5p	#, $, !
Breast cancer	XIST	hsa-miR-27a-3p	#, $, !
Breast cancer	XIST	hsa-let-7c-5p	#, $, !
Breast cancer	XIST	hsa-miR-181b-5p	#, $, !
Breast cancer	XIST	hsa-miR-181a-5p	#, $, !
Breast cancer	XIST	hsa-miR-34a-5p	#, $, !
Breast cancer	XIST	hsa-miR-25-3p	#, $, !
Breast cancer	XIST	hsa-miR-30a-5p	#, $, !
Prostate cancer	XIST	hsa-let-7b-5p	#, $, &
Prostate cancer	XIST	hsa-miR-146a-5p	*, $, &
Prostate cancer	XIST	hsa-miR-27a-3p	*, $, &
Prostate cancer	XIST	hsa-miR-7a-5p	*, $, &
Prostate cancer	XIST	hsa-miR-30a-5p	*, $, &
Prostate cancer	XIST	hsa-miR-34a-5p	*, $, &
Prostate cancer	XIST	hsa-miR-155-5p	*, $, +
Prostate cancer	XIST	hsa-miR-124-3p	*, $, +
Prostate cancer	XIST	hsa-miR-181b-5p	*, $, &
Prostate cancer	XIST	hsa-miR-25-3p	*, $, &

miRNAs play important role in many biological processes and are closely related to the formation of various cancers, including breast cancer [51, 52]. In order to better diagnose and treat breast cancer, it is necessary to predict breast cancer-related lncRNA or miRNAs and to identify lncRNA and miRNA biomarkers [52].

In addition, prostate cancer is a malignant tumor derived from prostate epithelial cells [53]. There are many factors, including age, family history of disease, and race, which may increase the risk of prostate neoplasms [54]. So far, many miRNAs and lncRNAs, such as miRNA has-let-7a-5p and lncRNA XIST in the prostate, have been found to be associated with prostate tumors.

As described previously, PADLMP has been demonstrated that it can achieve a reliable and effective prediction performance. Hence, in this section, case studies about above three kinds of important cancers based on top 5% of predicted results will be implemented to show the prediction performance of PADLMP. As illustrated in Table 2, the prediction results have been verified based on the recent updates in the databases such as lncRNADisease, MNDR v2.0, starBase v2.0, HMDD, miR2Disease, and miRCancer.

In Table 2, "#" and "*" stand for databases of lncRNA-disease and MNDR v2.0, respectively, which consist of known disease-lncRNA associations. "$" stands for starBase v2.0 database, which consists of known lncRNA-miRNA associations. "!,""&," and "+" stand for databases of HMDD, miR2Disease, and miRCancer, respectively, which consist of known disease-miRNA associations.

6. Discussion and Conclusion

Accumulating evidences show that the interaction of lncRNA-miRNAs is involved in the formation of many complex human diseases, such as breast cancer [16]; however, to our knowledge, there are no prediction models proposed for large scale forecasting the associations between diseases and LMPairs. Hence, based on the existing miRNA-disease associations, lncRNA-disease associations, lncRNA-miRNA interactions, and the assumption that genes with similar functions are often associated with similar diseases, we proposed a novel prediction model PADLMP to infer potential associations between diseases and LMPairs.

In this paper, we achieved the following contributions mainly: (1) we proposed the first computational model PADLMP for large-scale prediction of disease-LMPair associations, which can predict potential associations between diseases and lncRNA-miRNA pairs effectively. (2) We transformed the tripartite Disease-LncRNA-miRNA network into a bipartite disease-LMPair network, which greatly reduced the complexity of our prediction model. (3) Negative samples were not required in our prediction model.

However, although PADLMP is a powerful tool to infer novel associations between diseases and lncRNA-miRNA pairs, there are some limitations still existing in our method. For example, firstly, although we introduced semantic similarity for diseases and LMPairs, but the calculation of Gaussian Interaction Profile Kernel Similarity greatly relied on known disease-lncRNA associations, disease-miRNA associations, and disease-LMPairs associations. Therefore, it would cause inevitable bias towards those well-investigated diseases and LMPairs. Secondly, PADLMP could not be applied to unknown diseases and LMPairs, which were poorly investigated and had not any known associations. In the future, we will try to design new methods that do not rely on the topological information of disease-LMPair association network to solve these limitations.

The Meaning of Vertex and Edges in the Networks

G_1: LncRNA-disease bipartite network
G_2: Disease-miRNA bipartite network
G_3: LncRNA-miRNA bipartite network
G_4: Disease-LncRNA-miRNA tripartite network
G: Disease-LMPairs bipartite network
V_{l1}: LncRNA in lncRNA-disease association
V_{l2}: LncRNA in lncRNA-miRNA association
V_{d1}: Disease in lncRNA-disease association
V_{d2}: Disease in miRNA-disease association
V_{m1}: miRNA in miRNA-disease association
V_{m2}: Disease in lncRNA-miRNA association
$V_{l'}$: $V_{l'} = V_{l1} \cap V_{l2}$
$V_{m'}$: $V_{m'} = V_{m1} \cap V_{m2}$
V_{d3}: $V_{d3} = V_{d1} \cap V_{d2}$
V_l: $V_l \subseteq V_{l'}$
V_m: $V_m \subseteq V_{m'}$
p_{ij}: LncRNA-miRNA pair (l_i, m_j)
E_1: Edge of G_1, lncRNA l_i associated with disease d_j if edge $\langle l_i, d_j \rangle \in E_1$
E_2: Edge of G_2, miRNA m_i associated with disease d_j if edge $\langle m_i, d_j \rangle \in E_2$
E_3: Edge of G_3, lncRNA l_i associated with miRNA m_j if edge $\langle l_i, m_j \rangle \in E_3$
E_4: Edge of G_4, lncRNA l_i associated with disease d_j if edge $\langle l_i, d_j \rangle \in E_4$ or lncRNA l_i associated with miRNA m_k if edge $\langle l_i, m_k \rangle \in E_4$ or miRNA m_k associated with disease d_j if edge $\langle m_k, d_j \rangle \in E_4$
E_5: Edge of G_4, disease d_i associated with LMPair p_{jk} if edge $\langle d_i, p_{jk} \rangle \in E_5$.

Conflicts of Interest

The authors declare no conflicts of interest in this work.

Acknowledgments

The project is partly sponsored by the Natural Science Foundation of Hunan Province (no. 2018JJ4058 and no. 2017JJ5036), the National Natural Science Foundation of China (no. 61640210 and no. 61672447), and the CERNET Next Generation Internet Technology Innovation Project (no. NGII20160305).

Supplementary Materials

There are four supplementary tables in this manuscript. And among them, Supplementary Table 1 is a description of the lncRNA-disease associations, in which there are 2048 lncRNA-disease associations included, and the 1st column represents the lncRNAs and the 2nd column represents the diseases. Supplementary Table 2 is a description of the miRNA-disease associations, which contains the ID of diseases, the ID of miRNAs, and the associations between diseases and miRNAs. Supplementary Table 3 is a description of the lncRNA-miRNA associations, which contains 20343 lncRNA-miRNA associations and in which the first column represents the lncRNAs and the second column represents the miRNAs. Supplementary Table 4 is a description of the predictive results of associations between diseases and lncRNA-miRNA pairs while adopting PADLMP to execute prediction. *(Supplementary Materials)*

References

[1] E. Berezikov and E. Al, "Approaches to microrna discovery," *Nature Genetics*, vol. 38, p. 52, 2006.

[2] P. J. Batista and H. Y. Chang, "Long noncoding RNAs: cellular address codes in development and disease," *Cell*, vol. 152, no. 6, pp. 1298–1307, 2013.

[3] K. C. Wang and H. Y. Chang, "Molecular mechanisms of long noncoding RNAs," *Molecular Cell*, vol. 43, no. 6, pp. 904–914, 2011.

[4] C. P. Ponting, P. L. Oliver, and W. Reik, "Evolution and functions of long noncoding RNAs," *Cell*, vol. 136, no. 4, pp. 629–641, 2009.

[5] J. Zheng, H. Peng, and L. Wang, "Similarities/dissimilarities analysis of protein sequences based on recurrence quantification analysis," *Current Bioinformatics*, vol. 10, no. 1, pp. 112–119, 2015.

[6] L. Salmena, L. Poliseno, Y. Tay, L. Kats, and P. P. Pandolfi, "A *ceRNA* hypothesis: the rosetta stone of a hidden RNA language?" *Cell*, vol. 146, no. 3, pp. 353–358, 2011.

[7] B. K. Dey, K. Pfeifer, and A. Dutta, "The H19 long noncoding RNA gives rise to microRNAs miR-675-3p and miR-675-5p to promote skeletal muscle differentiation and regeneration," *Genes & Development*, vol. 28, no. 5, pp. 491–501, 2014.

[8] Y. Yao, J. Ma, Y. Xue et al., "Knockdown of long non-coding RNA XIST exerts tumor-suppressive functions in human glioblastoma stem cells by up-regulating miR-152," *Cancer Letters*, vol. 359, no. 1, pp. 75–86, 2015.

[9] X. Wang, M. Li, Z. Wang et al., "Silencing of long noncoding rna malat1 by mir-101 and mir-217 inhibits proliferation, migration, and invasion of esophageal squamous cell carcinoma cells," *The Journal of Biological Chemistry*, vol. 290, no. 7, pp. 3925–3935, 2015.

[10] E.-B. Zhang, R. Kong, D.-D. Yin et al., "Long noncoding RNA ANRIL indicates a poor prognosis of gastric cancer and promotes tumor growth by epigenetically silencing of miR-99a/miR-449a," *Oncotarget*, vol. 5, no. 8, pp. 2276–2292, 2014.

[11] J. You, Y. Zhang, B. Liu, Y. Li, N. Fang, L. Zu et al., "Microrna-449a inhibits cell growth in lung cancer and regulates long noncoding rna nuclear enriched abundant transcript 1," *Indian Journal of Cancer*, vol. 51, no. 7, p. e77, 2014.

[12] S. Emmrich, A. Streltsov, F. Schmidt, V. R. Thangapandi, D. Reinhardt, and J.-H. Klusmann, "LincRNAs MONC and MIR100HG act as oncogenes in acute megakaryoblastic leukemia," *Molecular Cancer*, vol. 13, no. 1, article 171, 2014.

[13] A. Leung, C. Trac, W. Jin et al., "Novel long noncoding RNAs are regulated by angiotensin II in vascular smooth muscle cells," *Circulation Research*, vol. 113, no. 3, pp. 266–278, 2013.

[14] M. Zhu, Q. Chen, X. Liu et al., "LncRNA H19/miR-675 axis represses prostate cancer metastasis by targeting TGFBI," *FEBS Journal*, vol. 281, no. 16, pp. 3766–3775, 2014.

[15] H. Hirata, Y. Hinoda, V. Shahryari et al., "Long noncoding RNA MALAT1 promotes aggressive renal cell carcinoma through Ezh2 and interacts with miR-205," *Cancer Research*, vol. 75, no. 7, pp. 1322–1331, 2015.

[16] X. B. Zhao and G. S. Ren, "Lncrna tug1 promotes breast cancer cell proliferation via inhibiting mir-9," *Cancer Biomarkers*, pp. 1–8, 2016.

[17] H. Peng, C. Lan, Y. Zheng, G. Hutvagner, D. Tao, and J. Li, "Cross disease analysis of co-functional microRNA pairs on a reconstructed network of disease-gene-microRNA tripartite," *BMC Bioinformatics*, vol. 18, no. 1, article 193, 2017.

[18] X. Li, J. Xu, Y. Li et al., "Dissection of the potential characteristic of miRNA-miRNA functional synergistic regulations," *Molecular BioSystems*, vol. 9, no. 2, pp. 217–224, 2013.

[19] X. Yun, C. Xu, J. Guan, Y. Ping, H. Fan, Y. Li et al., "Discovering dysfunction of multiple micrornas cooperation in disease by a conserved microrna co-expression network," *PLoS ONE*, vol. 7, no. 2, p. e32201, 2012.

[20] S. Yoon and G. D. Micheli, *Prediction of Regulatory Modules Comprising microRNAs and Target Genes*, Oxford University Press, Oxford, UK, 2005.

[21] B. Wu, C. Li, P. Zhang, Q. Yao, J. Wu, J. Han et al., "Dissection of mirna-mirna interaction in esophageal squamous cell carcinoma," *PLoS ONE*, vol. 8, no. 9, p. e73191, 2013.

[22] X. Lai, U. Schmitz, S. K. Gupta et al., "Computational analysis of target hub gene repression regulated by multiple and cooperative miRNAs," *Nucleic Acids Research*, vol. 40, no. 18, pp. 8818–8834, 2012.

[23] G. Chen, Z. Wang, D. Wang et al., "LncRNADisease: a database for long-non-coding RNA-associated diseases," *Nucleic Acids Research*, vol. 41, no. 1, pp. D983–D986, 2013.

[24] Y. Wang, L. Chen, B. Chen, X. Li, J. Kang, K. Fan et al., "Mammalian ncrna-disease repository: a global view of ncrna-mediated disease network," *Cell Death and Disease*, vol. 4, no. 8, p. e765, 2013.

[25] S. Ning, J. Zhang, P. Wang et al., "Lnc2Cancer: a manually curated database of experimentally supported lncRNAs associated with various human cancers," *Nucleic Acids Research*, vol. 44, no. 1, pp. D980–D985, 2016.

[26] Q. Jiang, Y. Wang, Y. Hao et al., "miR2Disease: a manually curated database for microRNA deregulation in human disease," *Nucleic Acids Research*, vol. 37, no. 1, pp. D98–D104, 2009.

[27] Y. Li, C. Qiu, J. Tu et al., "HMDD v2.0: a database for experimentally supported human microRNA and disease associations," *Nucleic Acids Research*, vol. 42, pp. D1070–D1074, 2014.

[28] B. Xie, Q. Ding, H. Han, and D. Wu, "miRCancer: a microRNA-cancer association database constructed by text mining on literature," *Bioinformatics*, vol. 29, no. 5, pp. 638–644, 2013.

[29] A. Kozomara and S. Griffiths-Jones, "miRBase: annotating high confidence microRNAs using deep sequencing data," *Nucleic Acids Research*, vol. 42, pp. D68–D73, 2014.

[30] L. M. Schriml, C. Arze, S. Nadendla et al., "Disease ontology: a backbone for disease semantic integration," *Nucleic Acids Research*, vol. 40, no. 1, pp. D940–D946, 2012.

[31] J. H. Li, S. Liu, H. Zhou, L. H. Qu, and J. H. Yang, "Starbase v2.0: decoding mirna-cerna, mirna-ncrna and protein–rna interaction networks from large-scale clip-seq data," *Nucleic Acids Research*, vol. 42, p. D92, 2014.

[32] D. Wang, J. Wang, M. Lu, F. Song, and Q. Cui, "Inferring the human microRNA functional similarity and functional network based on microRNA-associated diseases," *Bioinformatics*, vol. 26, no. 13, pp. 1644–1650, 2010.

[33] X. Chen, Z. You, G. Yan, and D. Gong, "IRWRLDA: improved random walk with restart for lncRNA-disease association prediction," *Oncotarget*, vol. 7, no. 36, pp. 57919–57931, 2016.

[34] Y. A. Huang, X. Chen, Z. H. You, D. S. Huang, and K. C. Chan, "ILNCSIM: improved lncRNA functional similarity calculation model," *Oncotarget*, vol. 7, no. 18, pp. 25902–25914, 2016.

[35] L. Katz, "A new status index derived from sociometric analysis," *Psychometrika*, vol. 18, no. 1, pp. 39–43, 1953.

[36] X. Yang, L. Gao, X. Guo, X. Shi, H. Wu, F. Song et al., "A network based method for analysis of lncrna-disease associations and prediction of lncrnas implicated in diseases," *PLoS ONE*, vol. 9, no. 1, p. e87797, 2014.

[37] X. Chen, "KATZLDA: KATZ measure for the lncRNA-disease association prediction," *Scientific Reports*, vol. 5, Article ID 16840, 2014.

[38] X. Chen, Y. A. Huang, Z. H. You, G. Y. Yan, and X. S. Wang, "A novel approach based on katz measure to predict associations of human microbiota with non-infectious diseases," *Bioinformatics*, vol. 33, no. 5, pp. 733–739, 2016.

[39] X. Chen, C. C. Yan, X. Zhang et al., "WBSMDA: within and between score for MiRNA-disease association prediction," *Scientific Reports*, vol. 6, Article ID 21106, 2016.

[40] X. Chen, Y. C. Clarence, X. Zhang, Z. H. You, Y. A. Huang, and G. Y. Yan, "HGIMDA: Heterogeneous graph inference for miRNA-disease association prediction," *Oncotarget*, vol. 7, no. 40, pp. 65257–65269, 2016.

[41] X. Chen and G.-Y. Yan, "Novel human lncRNA-disease association inference based on lncRNA expression profiles," *Bioinformatics*, vol. 29, no. 20, pp. 2617–2624, 2013.

[42] X. Chen and G. Y. Yan, "Semi-supervised learning for potential human microrna-disease associations inference," *Scientific Reports*, vol. 4, p. 5501, 2014.

[43] T. Fawcett, "An introduction to ROC analysis," *Pattern Recognition Letters*, vol. 27, no. 8, pp. 861–874, 2006.

[44] A. I. Phipps, N. M. Lindor, M. A. Jenkins et al., "Colon and rectal cancer survival by tumor location and microsatellite instability: The colon cancer family registry," *Diseases of the Colon & Rectum*, vol. 56, no. 8, pp. 937–944, 2013.

[45] F. Liu, D. Yuan, Y. Wei, W. Wang, L. Yan, T. Wen et al., "Systematic review and meta-analysis of the relationship between ephx1 polymorphisms and colorectal cancer risk," *PLoS ONE*, vol. 7, no. 8, p. e43821, 2012.

[46] S. Pita-Fernández, S. Pértega-Díaz, B. López-Calviño et al., "Diagnostic and treatment delay, quality of life and satisfaction with care in colorectal cancer patients: a study protocol," *Health and Quality of Life Outcomes*, vol. 11, no. 1, article 117, 2013.

[47] V. H. Chong, M. S. Abdullah, P. U. Telisinghe, and A. Jalihal, "Colorectal cancer: incidence and trend in Brunei Darussalam," *Singapore Medical Journal*, vol. 50, no. 11, pp. 1085–1089, 2009.

[48] B. Shi, L. Sepp-Lorenzino, M. Prisco, P. Linsley, T. Deangelis, and R. Baserga, "Micro RNA 145 targets the insulin receptor substrate-1 and inhibits the growth of colon cancer cells," *The Journal of Biological Chemistry*, vol. 282, no. 45, pp. 32582–32590, 2007.

[49] H. J. Donahue and D. C. Genetos, "Genomic approaches in breast cancer research," *Briefings in Functional Genomics*, vol. 12, no. 5, pp. 391–396, 2013.

[50] K. Karagoz, R. Sinha, and K. Y. Arga, "Triple negative breast cancer: a multi-omics network discovery strategy for candidate targets and driving pathways," *OMICS: A Journal of Integrative Biology*, vol. 19, no. 2, pp. 115–130, 2015.

[51] J. Meng, P. Li, Q. Zhang, Z. Yang, and S. Fu, "A four-long non-coding rna signature in predicting breast cancer survival," *Journal of Experimental and Clinical Cancer Research*, vol. 33, no. 1, article 84, 2014.

[52] N. Xu, F. Wang, M. Lv, and L. Cheng, "Microarray expression profile analysis of long non-coding rnas in human breast cancer: a study of chinese women," *Biomedicine Pharmacotherapy*, vol. 69, no. 3, pp. 221–227, 2015.

[53] G. A. Gmyrek, M. Walburg, C. P. Webb et al., "Normal and malignant prostate epithelial cells differ in their response to hepatocyte growth factor/scatter factor," *The American Journal of Pathology*, vol. 159, no. 2, pp. 579–590, 2001.

[54] P. C. Walsh and A. W. Partin, "Family history facilitates the early diagnosis of prostate carcinoma," *Cancer*, vol. 80, no. 9, pp. 1871–1874, 1997.

8

Computational Prediction of the Combined Effect of CRT and LVAD on Cardiac Electromechanical Delay in LBBB and RBBB

Aulia K. Heikhmakhtiar and Ki M. Lim

Department of IT Convergence Engineering, Kumoh National Institute of Technology, Gumi 39177, Republic of Korea

Correspondence should be addressed to Ki M. Lim; kmlim@kumoh.ac.kr

Guest Editor: Ka L. Man

Two case reports showed that the combination of CRT and LVAD benefits the end-stage heart failure patients with prolonged QRS interval significantly. In one of the reports, the patient had the LVAD removed due to the recovery of the heart function. However, the quantification of the combined devices has yet to be conducted. This study aimed at computationally predicting the effects of CRT-only or combined with LVAD on electromechanical behaviour in the failing ventricle with left bundle branch blocked (LBBB) and right bundle branch blocked (RBBB) conditions. The subjects are normal sinus rhythm, LBBB, RBBB, LBBB with CRT-only, RBBB with CRT-only, LBBB with CRT + LVAD, and RBBB with CRT + LVAD. The results showed that the CRT-only shortened the total electrical activation time (EAT) in the LBBB and RBBB conditions by 20.2% and 17.1%, respectively. The CRT-only reduced the total mechanical activation time (MAT) and electromechanical delay (EMD) of the ventricle under LBBB by 21.3% and 10.1%, respectively. Furthermore, the CRT-only reduced the contractile adenosine triphosphate (ATP) consumption by 5%, increased left ventricular (LV) pressure by 6%, and enhanced cardiac output (CO) by 0.2 L/min under LBBB condition. However, CRT-only barely affects the ventricle under RBBB condition. Under the LBBB condition, CRT + LVAD increased LV pressure and CO by 10.5% and by 0.9 L/min, respectively. CRT + LVAD reduced ATP consumption by 15%, shortened the MAT by 23.4%, and shortened the EMD by 15.2%. In conclusion, we computationally predicted and quantified that the CRT + LVAD implementation is superior to CRT-only implementation particularly in HF with LBBB condition.

1. Introduction

Heart failure (HF) plays a major role in the number of death worldwide [1]. Thus, the study of heart diseases including cardiac arrhythmia, which progressively leads to HF condition, is very important. Two types of cardiac therapy devices are commonly used to treat patients with cardiac disease: cardiac resynchronization therapy (CRT) and left ventricular assist device (LVAD). CRT is considered as a valuable treatment for patients with dyssynchrony HF with QRS interval >120 ms and left ventricular ejection fraction (EF) <35% [2, 3]. A number of studies showed significant benefits of using CRT. CRT synchronizes systolic function [4–6], restores heart structure [7, 8], and improves symptoms and the quality of life of the patients identified by the improvement of exercise endurance [3, 8–12]. However, 30% of patients with HF failed to benefit from the CRT [9]. Hu et al. [13] described that three major responses could be obtained from the CRT treatment: resynchronization of the intraventricular contraction, efficient ventricular preloading by a properly timed atrial contraction, and reduction of mitral regurgitation. One of the study findings was that resynchronization of the intraventricular contraction itself did not necessarily lead to stroke work improvement. However, the synchronization of the atrioventricular firing time was essential.

LVAD supports the ventricular pumping via mechanical unloading for weakened heart. LVAD was initially used as a bridge to transplantation for patients with end-stage disease [14, 15]. However, because the availability of heart donors is very limited, LVAD is now used as destination therapy as it lasts for years [16–18]. LVAD reverses the damaged ventricle and recovers myocardial functionalities by repairing left ventricular (LV) mass [19, 20], heart chamber size [20, 21], improves mitral filling [22], and induces cardiomyocyte hypertrophy regression [21, 22]. The use of LVAD also increased the quality of life of the patients [23–25]. Previously, we observed the effect of LVAD on the electromechanical delay (EMD) under mild and severe HF conditions [26]. The results showed that the LVAD not only increased the EF but also shortened the EMD under the mild HF and even better under severe HF conditions. The comparison study of the symptomatic relief of CRT and LVAD by Delgado et al. concluded that the use of both devices could synergistically improve cardiac functions for severe HF treatment [27].

In 2011, a case report article stated that the CRT supported the restoration of end-stage HF in a 15-year-old patient who underwent LVAD implantation [28]. The CRT shortened the septal to posterior wall motion delay from 146 ms to 104 ms, and overall, it backed up the hemodynamic improvements. After such improvement, the patient successfully had the LVAD removed. In another case report article, the CRT and LVAD cooperatively restored the cardiac functions of a 62-year-old patient who had cardiogenic shock and left bundle branch block (LBBB) [29]. The report stated that the combination of CRT and LVAD performed a profound treatment on the weakening heart under LBBB condition. It recovered the heart hypertrophy, and the EF was increased. Based on these reports, we conducted a computational modelling which combined the CRT and LVAD to the failing ventricle with LBBB and RBBB in order to understand the mechanism of the two devices combined to provide such improvement to the heart.

To the best of our knowledge, a computational study that quantifies the effect of combined CRT and LVAD has yet to be conducted. This study aims at predicting, computationally with an electromechanical failing ventricles model, the effects of CRT alone and the combination of CRT and LVAD treatment in patients with LBBB or right bundle branch block (RBBB). We used a well-developed electromechanical ventricular model which had been used to observe different heart conditions, including the prolonged EMD in the dyssynchrony HF condition [30], mechanoelectrical feedback on scroll wave stability [31], and spontaneous arrhythmia in acute regional ischemia [32]. Recently, by using similar electromechanical coupling model, our group revealed the effect of KCNQ1 S140G mutation on arrhythmogenesis and pumping performance [33]. We used computational methods to overcome the measurement limitations and risks of the experimental study. We analyzed seven HF diseases and therapies: (i) normal sinus rhythm, (ii) LBBB, (iii) LBBB with CRT alone (LBBB + CRT), (iv) LBBB with CRT and LVAD combination (LBBB + CRT + LVAD), (v) RBBB, (vi) RBBB with CRT alone (RBBB + CRT), and (vii) RBBB with combined CRT and LVAD (RBBB + CRT + LVAD) conditions.

2. Materials and Methods

We followed an existing well-developed electromechanical failing ventricle model with the fibers and laminar sheet structures based on diffusion tensor magnetic resonance imaging [34–37]. In this study, our electromechanical model was coupled with circulatory systems and LVAD models similarly as Lim et al. with additional Purkinje networks compartment to simulate LBBB and RBBB conditions [38]. The electromechanical model consisted of electrophysiological and myofilament dynamics model coupled by Ca^{2+} transient. The LVAD function included the circulatory systems, which connected to the 3D ventricular mechanics. Figure 1 shows a full schematic of the system we used in this study.

The electrical component was a failing ventricular mesh with 241,725 nodes and 1,298,751 tetrahedron elements. The electrical mesh has the characteristics of realistic heart compartment, which consists of endocardial, mid-myocardial, and epicardial cells following the ten Tusscher et al. human ventricular tissue model [39]. The line mesh type representing Purkinje networks was mapped onto a 3D ventricle chamber as well at the endocardial region (Figure 2(c)).

The Purkinje networks induced the electrical activation sequences of sinus rhythm (normal), LBBB, and RBBB (Figure 2(c)). The CRT pacing site of the LBBB was placed at the LV free-wall, while the CRT pacing site of the RBBB was placed at the RV endocardial apex as shown in Figure 2(b). The electrical stimulation was first induced at the root node of Purkinje fiber model, which propagates to the terminals, hence stimulating the ventricular tissue. The electrical propagation in the Purkinje can be described by solving a one-dimensional wave propagation equation and triggered the ventricular activation [40].

The electrical propagation signal represents an ion exchange across the myocyte as described by ten Tusscher et al. [39]. The electrophysiological phenomenon for the single cell can be described as follows:

$$\frac{dV}{dt} = \frac{-I_{\text{ion}} + I_{\text{stim}}}{C_{\text{m}}}, \tag{1}$$

where V represents the voltage difference of intracellular and extracellular, t represents time, I_{ion} represents the sum of all transmembrane ionic currents, I_{stim} represents the current if an external stimulus is applied, and C_{m} represents the cell capacitance per unit of surface area. I_{ion} consists of major ionic current as follows:

$$\begin{aligned} I_{\text{ion}} = {} & I_{\text{Na}} + I_{\text{K1}} + I_{\text{to}} + I_{\text{Kr}} + I_{\text{Ks}} + I_{\text{CaL}} + I_{\text{NaCa}} + I_{\text{NaK}} \\ & + I_{\text{pCa}} + I_{\text{pK}} + I_{\text{bCa}} + I_{\text{bNa}}, \end{aligned} \tag{2}$$

where I_{Na} is fast inward Na^+ current, I_{K1} is inward rectifier K1 current, I_{to} is transient outward K^+ current, I_{Kr} is rapid

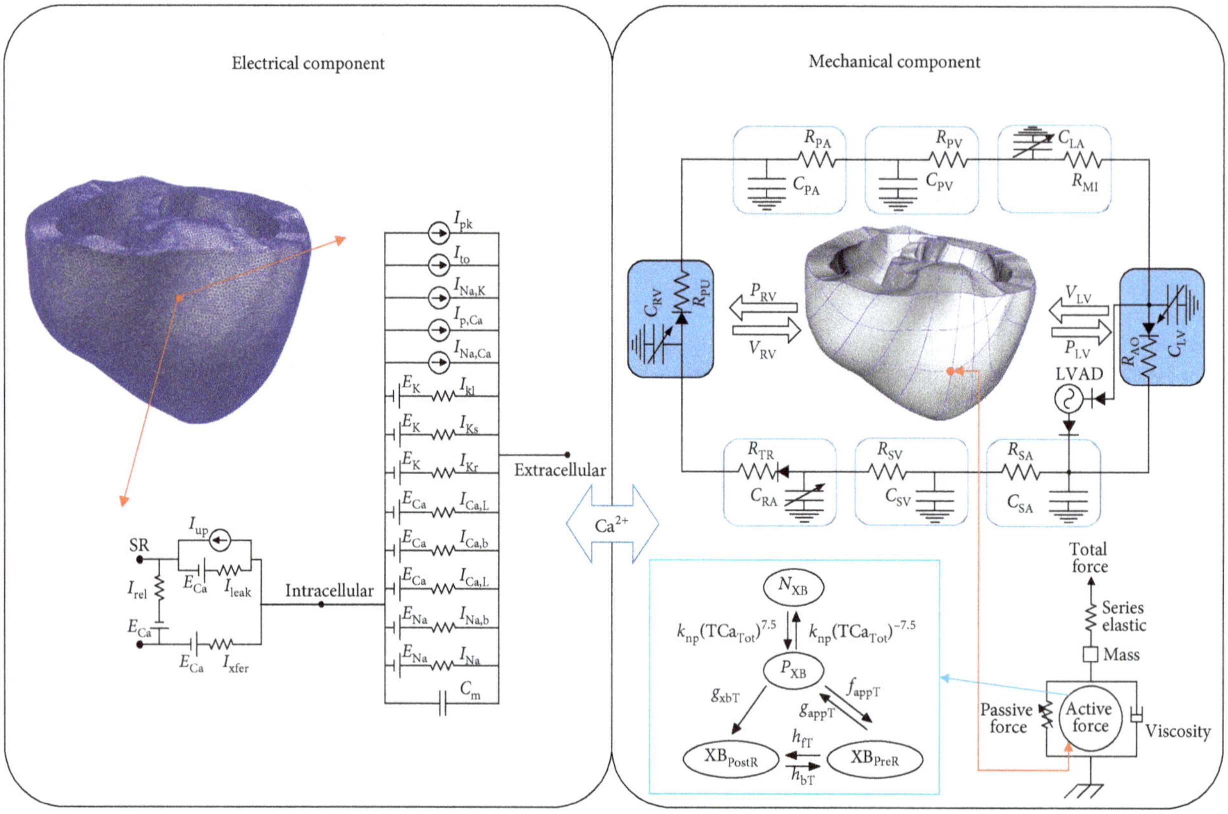

FIGURE 1: Schematics of the electrical and mechanical elements coupled with transient calcium. Electrical element: it represents the currents, pumps, and exchanger of the ten Tusscher ionic model as explained in equation (1). Mechanical element: a schematic diagram of the finite-element ventricular mechanical model coupled with the circulatory and LVAD models. P_{RV}, RV pressure; V_{RV}, RV volume; P_{LV}, LV pressure; V_{LV}, LV volume; R_{PA}, pulmonary artery resistance; C_{PA}, pulmonary artery compliance; R_{PV}, pulmonary vein resistance; C_{PV}, pulmonary vein compliance; R_{MI}, mitral valve resistance; C_{LA}, left atrium compliance; R_{AO}, aortic valve resistance; R_{SA}, systemic artery resistance; C_{SA}, systemic artery compliance; R_{SV}, systemic vein resistance; C_{SV}, systemic vein compliance; R_{TR} tricuspid valve resistance; C_{RA}, right atrium compliance; R_{PU}, pulmonary valve resistance.

delayed rectifier K^+ current, I_{Ks} is slow delayed rectifier K^+ current, I_{CaL} is L-type inward Ca^{2+} current, I_{NaCa} is Na^+/Ca^{2+} exchanger current, I_{NaK} is the Na^+/K^+ pump current, I_{pCa} and I_{pK} are sarcoplasmic plateau Ca^{2+} and K^+ currents, I_{bCa} is background Ca^{2+} current, and $I_{Na,b}$ is background Na^+ current.

To represent the electrical propagation through the conduction in 3D spatial, the cardiac tissue in this case could be described by the combination of the Equation (1) with the cellular resistivity (ρ) and surface-to-volume ratio (S) in x, y, and z directions, respectively. This phenomenon can be described by the following partial differential equation:

$$\frac{dV}{dt} = \frac{-I_{ion} + I_{stim}}{C_m} + \frac{1}{\rho_x S_x C_m}\frac{\partial^2 V}{\partial x^2} + \frac{1}{\rho_y S_y C_m}\frac{\partial^2 V}{\partial y^2} + \frac{1}{\rho_z S_z C_m}\frac{\partial^2 V}{\partial z^2}. \tag{3}$$

The mathematical equation for calcium dynamics for coupling the electromechanical simulation was also described by ten Tusscher et al. [39]:

$$I_{leak} = V_{leak}\left(Ca_{sr} - Ca_i\right),$$

$$I_{up} = \frac{V_{maxup}}{1 + K_{up}^2/Ca_i^2},$$

$$I_{rel} = \left(a_{rel}\frac{Ca_{sr}^2}{b_{rel}^2 + Ca_{sr}^2} + C_{rel}\right) dg,$$

$$Ca_{ibufc} = \frac{Ca_i \times Buf_c}{Ca_i + K_{bufc}},$$

$$\frac{dCa_{itotal}}{dt} = \frac{-I_{Cal} + I_{bCa} + I_{pCa} - 2I_{NaCa}}{2V_c F} + I_{leak} - I_{up} + I_{rel},$$

$$Ca_{srbufsr} = \frac{Ca_{sr} \times Buf_{sr}}{Ca_{sr} + K_{bufsr}},$$

$$\frac{dCa_{stotal}}{dt} = \frac{V_C}{V_{sr}}\left(-I_{leak} + I_{up} - I_{rel}\right), \tag{4}$$

where I_{leak} represents the calcium released from the sarcoplasmic reticulum (SR) into the cell. I_{up} represents the

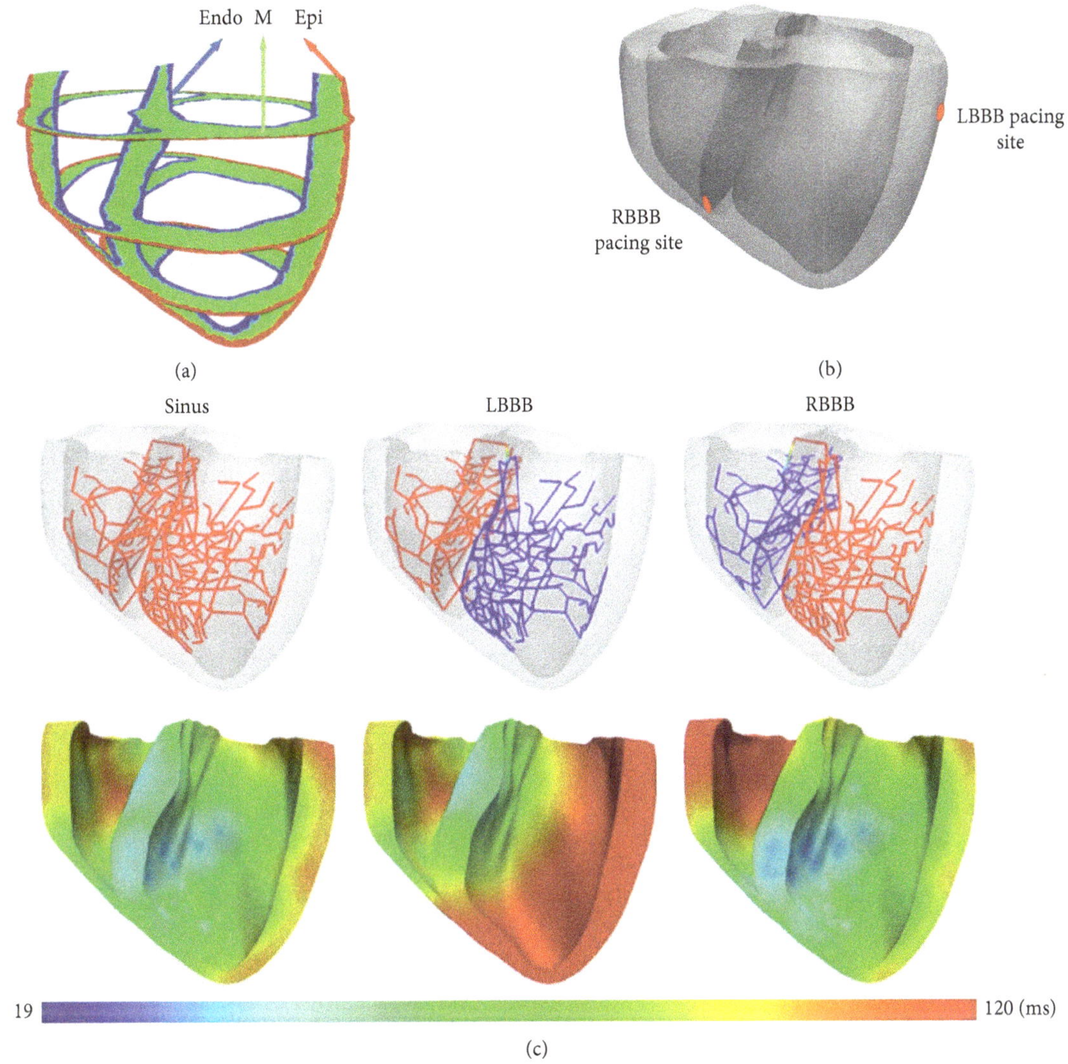

FIGURE 2: (a) The heterogeneous mesh that has the characteristics of endocardial, midmyocardial, and epicardial cells. (b) The CRT pacing site for the LBBB heart was placed on the LV free-wall, while that for the RBBB heart was placed inside the RV at the bottom of the septum. (c) The electrical propagation by the Purkinje network in the sinus, LBBB, and RBBB conditions. The electrical activation by the Purkinje networks is indicated in red. In sinus pacing, the Purkinje network delivers the electrical signal to its terminals. In the LBBB condition, the Purkinje network delivered the signal only to the right network in the RV area. In the RBBB condition, the Purkinje network delivered the signal only to the left network in the LV area. CRT, cardiac resynchronization therapy; LBBB, left bundle branch block; LV, left ventricular; RBBB, right bundle branch block; RV, right ventricular.

calcium pumping to restore the calcium again back to the SR. I_{rel} represents the calcium-induced calcium release current, d is the activation gate of I_{rel}, which was the same with I_{CaL}. Ca_{itotal} is the total calcium inside the cell, which consists of Ca_{ibufc}, the calcium buffer inside the cell, and Ca_i, the free calcium inside the cell. Accordingly, the $Ca_{srtotal}$ is the sum of calcium in the SR, which includes $Ca_{srbufsr}$, the calcium buffer, and Ca_{sr}, the free calcium inside the SR.

A Ca^{2+} transient serves as an input to the cell myofilament model representing the generation of active tension within each myocyte in which an ODE set and multiple algebraic equations describe Ca^{2+} binding to troponin C, cooperatively between regulatory proteins, and cross-bridge cycling. Ventricular contraction results from the active tension generation represented by the myofilament dynamics model described by Rice et al. [41]. Ventricular deformation is described by the equations of passive cardiac mechanics, with the myocardium being orthotropically hyperelastic, and nearly incompressible material with passive properties defined by an exponential strain-energy function. Simultaneous solutions of the myofilament model equations to those representing passive cardiac mechanics on the finite-element mesh constitute cardiac contraction. Considering the isometric contraction, we assumed that the sarcomere length (SL) is 0 at the initial value, $dSL/dt = 0$. To measure the isotonic contraction, the SL is solved using the following ordinary differential equation (ODE):

$$\frac{d}{dt}SL = \frac{\text{Integral}_{\text{Force}} + (\text{SL}_0 - \text{SL}) \times \text{viscosity}}{\text{mass}}, \tag{5}$$

the viscosity and mass are described in Figure 1 at the mechanical compartment, and $\text{Integral}_{\text{Force}}$ is the sum of the normalized force integrated toward time:

$$\text{Integral}_{\text{Force}} = \int_0^t (F_{\text{active}}(x) + F_{\text{passive}}(x) - F_{\text{preload}} - F_{\text{afterload}}(x))\, dt, \tag{6}$$

where the $F_{\text{active}}(x)$ is the active force and the $F_{\text{passive}}(x)$ is the passive force. F_{preload} is the constant force at the resting length of the initial sarcomere length, and $F_{\text{afterload}}$ is the force during the isotonic or isometric contraction. Thus, $F_{\text{afterload}}$ is expressed as follows:

$$F_{\text{afterload}}(x) = \text{KSE} \times (x - \text{SL}_0). \tag{7}$$

We calculated the ATP consumption by integrating the myofilament model in one cycle proposed by Rice et al. from each node [41]. In the myofilament model, the ATP consumption rate (E) is the outcome of cross-bridge detachment rate (g_{xbT}) and the single overlap fraction of thick filaments ($\text{SOVF}_{\text{Thick}}$):

$$E = g_{xbT} \times \text{SOVF}_{\text{Thick}}. \tag{8}$$

To construct an integrated model of an LVAD-implanted cardiovascular system, we added a compartment of LVAD function between LV and systemic arteries in the circulatory system based on Kerckhoffs et al. [42] as described previously by Lim et al. [38]. Briefly, the LVAD component was modelled as a flow generator with a specific mean flow rate of 3 L/min. Constant-flow conditions were used to simulate the continuous LVAD with the inlet at the LV apex and the outlet at the ascending aorta.

For the simulation protocol, first we simulated the electrical model with the Purkinje delivering the signal representing sinus rhythm, LBBB, or RBBB until the steady state was achieved. We set the conduction velocity by 60 cm/s and the basic cycle length by 600 ms. Here, we incorporated the dyssynchrony HF conditions (LBBB and RBBB) using CRT-alone or combined CRT and LVAD. We then used Gaussian point for the interpolation of transient Ca^{2+} from the electrical simulation as the input to the mechanical simulation. To model the HF condition, we multiplied the constant of passive scaling in the strain-energy function by 5 times to stiffen the myocardium. The mechanical model was simulated for 20 seconds to reach the steady state. We compared the ATP consumption rates and tension activation during end-systolic volume (ESV) and the strain during end-diastolic volume (EDV) by integrating the information of them from each node. EMD was defined as the time interval between mechanical activation time (MAT) and electrical activation time (EAT). MAT was identified when the local strain was shortened to 10% before its maximum, while EAT was identified when the myocyte started to depolarize, which in our case was −50 mV [30].

3. Results and Discussion

3.1. Electrophysiological Simulation Results. Figure 3 shows the membrane potential propagation in the normal sinus rhythm (sinus), LBBB, LBBB + CRT, LBBB + CRT + LVAD, RBBB, RBBB + CRT, and RBBB + CRT + LVAD conditions. The electrical wavelength almost covered the whole ventricle tissue at 100 ms in the sinus condition, and the EAT in the sinus condition was 120 ms (Table 1). The EAT in the LBBB condition was 173 ms, which was the longest among other cases. CRT shortened the EAT in the LBBB condition to 138 ms, which was close to that in the sinus condition. In the RBBB heart, the EAT was 164 ms. CRT shortened the EAT in the RBBB heart to 136 ms, which was close to the sinus condition as well.

Figure 4 shows the calcium activation sequences. The calcium activation sequence followed the electrical activation sequence for each case. Compared to the membrane potential, which deactivated after 450 ms, the Ca^{2+} deactivation occurred at 250 ms. CRT fastened the Ca^{2+} activation throughout the ventricle in the LBBB condition but insignificantly in the RBBB condition due to the CRT pacing site.

3.2. Cardiac Mechanics Simulation Results. Figure 5 shows the 3D ATP consumption rate, tension, and strain transmural distribution in the sinus, LBBB, LBBB + CRT, LBBB + CRT + LVAD, RBBB, RBBB + CRT, and RBBB + CRT + LVAD conditions. We pick one node at the LV free-wall as representative to compare the values of them. Overall, the ATP consumption rate and tension in the LBBB condition had the highest values, 3.3 and 3.5 times larger than those in the normal sinus condition, respectively. However, the CRT decreased the ATP consumption rate and tension in the LBBB condition to be 6% and 7% lower than those in the normal sinus condition. Furthermore, CRT and LVAD reduced the ATP consumption rate and tension in the LBBB condition to 10% and 12% lower than those in the normal sinus condition, respectively. The ATP consumption rate and tension in the RBBB condition were 8% and 9% higher than those in the control condition. The CRT reduced the ATP consumption rate and tension by 4% and 5%, respectively. CRT and LVAD reduced the ATP consumption rate and tension by 9% and 11% in the RBBB condition, respectively. The strain under the LBBB condition was 80 times larger than that in the normal condition (notified by major red region in the LV free-wall). The CRT reduced the strain in the LBBB 56 times lower than that in the normal sinus condition. CRT significantly restored the total strain under the LBBB condition with the pacing site at the LV free-wall. However, under LBBB + CRT + LVAD, the total strain was only eight times lower than that in the sinus condition. The continuous LVAD altered the overall strain in the ventricles. The total strain in the RBBB condition was 84 times larger than that in the normal condition. In the RBBB + CRT model, the strain activation was 122 times larger. In the RBBB + CRT + LVAD model, the strain

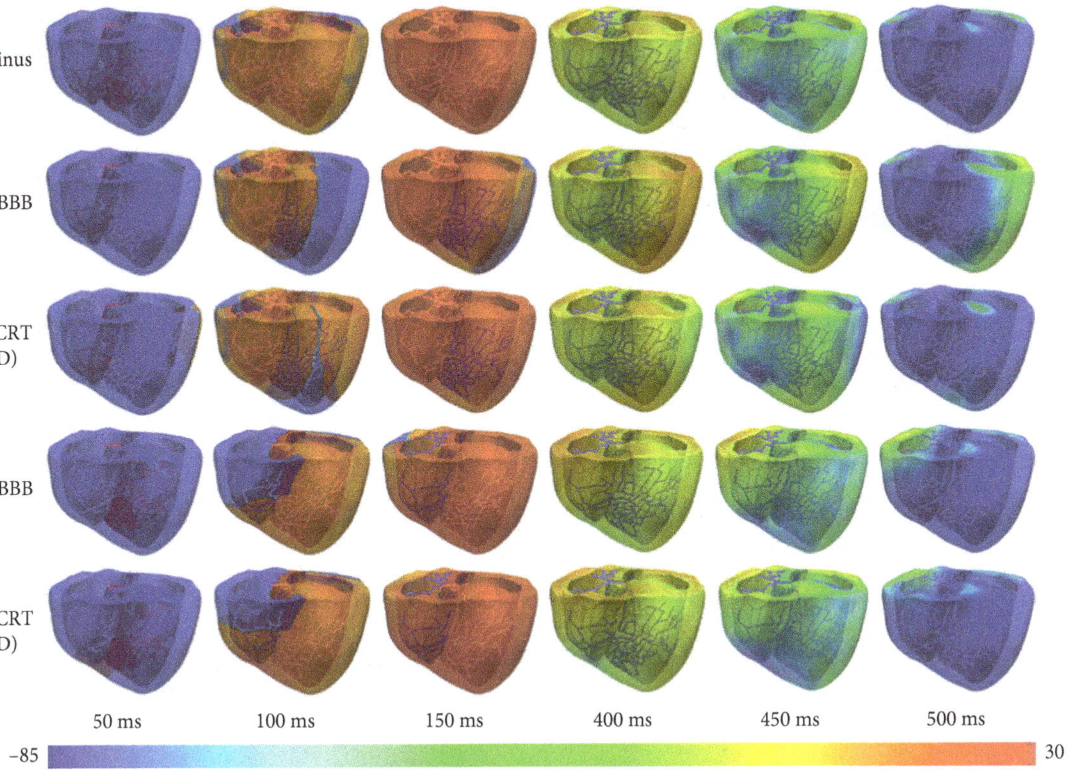

FIGURE 3: The membrane potential propagation of the sinus pacing, LBBB, LBBB + CRT, RBBB, and RBBB + CRT models. For the LBBB + CRT + LVAD and RBBB + CRT + LVAD models, we used the same electrical activation sequence as the LBBB + CRT and RBBB + CRT models, respectively, because the LVAD was incorporated into the mechanical computation. LBBB, left bundle branch block; CRT, cardiac resynchronization therapy; RBBB, right bundle branch block; LVAD, left ventricular assist device.

TABLE 1: Hemodynamic responses under normal, LBBB, LBBB + CRT, LBBB + CRT + LVAD, RBBB, RBBB + CRT, and RBBB + CRT + LVAD models.

Condition	EDV (mL)	ESV (mL)	CO (L/min)	EF (%)	Longest EAT (ms)	Average MAT (ms)	Average EMD (ms)
Normal sinus rhythm	88	55	3.4	38	120	157	78
LBBB	90	60	3	33.4	173	188	79
LBBB + CRT	89	57	3.2	36	138	148	71
LBBB + CRT + LVAD	—	—	3.9	—	138	144	67
RBBB	87	54	3.4	38	164	162	80
RBBB + CRT	88	55	3.4	38	136	157	81
RBBB + CRT + LVAD	—	—	4	—	136	155	79

activation was 23 times lower than that in the normal condition.

Figure 6(a) shows the LV pressure-volume (PV) loop diagram in the sinus, LBBB, LBBB + CRT, LBBB + CRT + LVAD, RBBB, RBBB + CRT, and RBBB + CRT + LVAD conditions. The LV PV-loop in the normal sinus rhythm condition was the same as those in the RBBB and RBBB + CRT conditions. The EDV in the three conditions was 88 mL, ESV was 54.5 mL, and EF was 38%. The LBBB condition had the highest EDV and ESV of 90 mL and 60 mL, respectively. The stroke volume (SV) and EF were 30 mL and 33.4%, respectively. CRT increased the EF up to 36% in the LBBB condition. The EDV, ESV, and SV in the LBBB + CRT condition were 89 mL, 57 mL, and 32 mL, respectively. We did not quantify the EF in models in which LVAD model was incorporated because the PV-loop of the LV was altered due to the LVAD implementation. However, the CO was presented to compare the effects of CRT-alone and combined CRT and LVAD. The complete EDV, ESV, CO, EF, MAT, and EMD data in all conditions are provided in Table 1.

Figure 6(b) shows the LV and systemic artery pressures coloured in black and red lines, respectively. In the normal sinus condition, the peak LV pressure was 148 mmHg. The LV pressure peaked at 358 ms, and the aortic valve was opened for 96 ms. In the LBBB condition, the LV peak pressure was 132.5 mmHg. The LV peak pressure time was prolonged to 407 ms, and the aortic valve was opened for 100 ms. The LV peak pressure in the LBBB + CRT condition

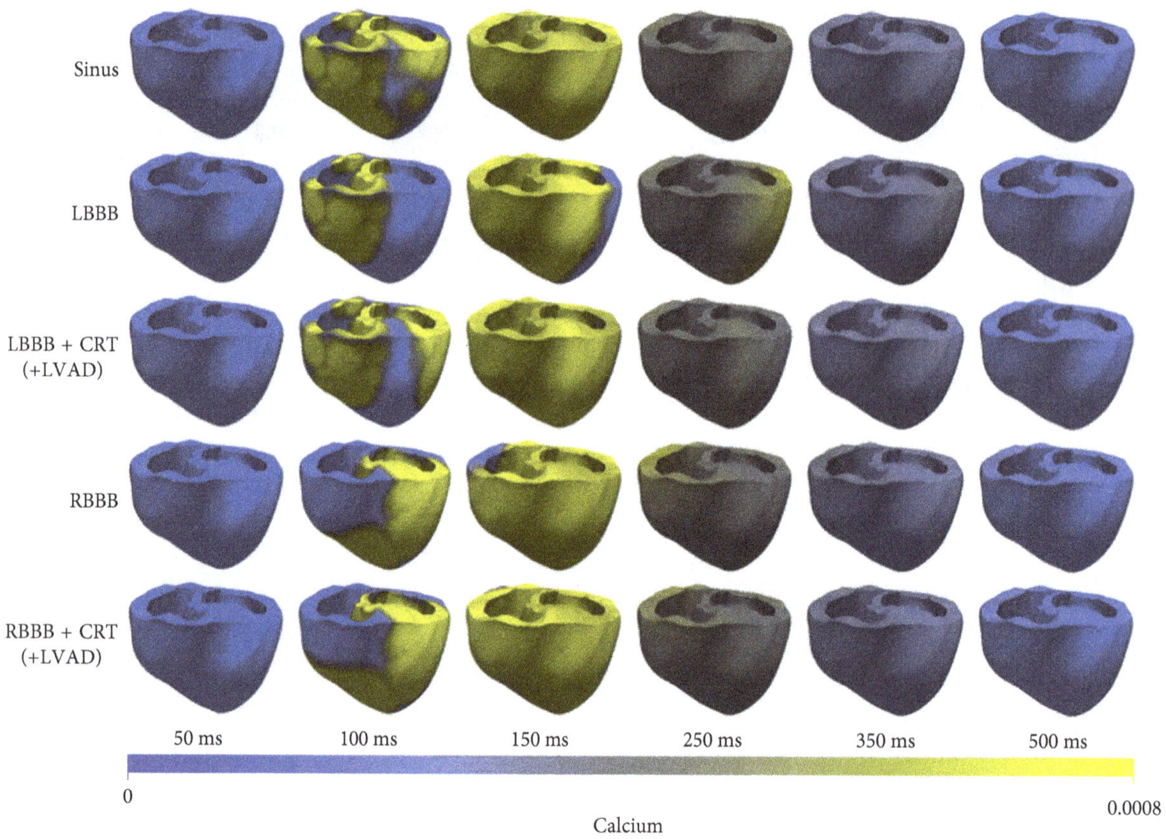

FIGURE 4: The Ca^{2+} propagation sequence following the membrane potential activation sequence in all cases. LBBB, left bundle branch block; CRT, cardiac resynchronization therapy; LVAD, left ventricular assist device; RBBB, right bundle branch block.

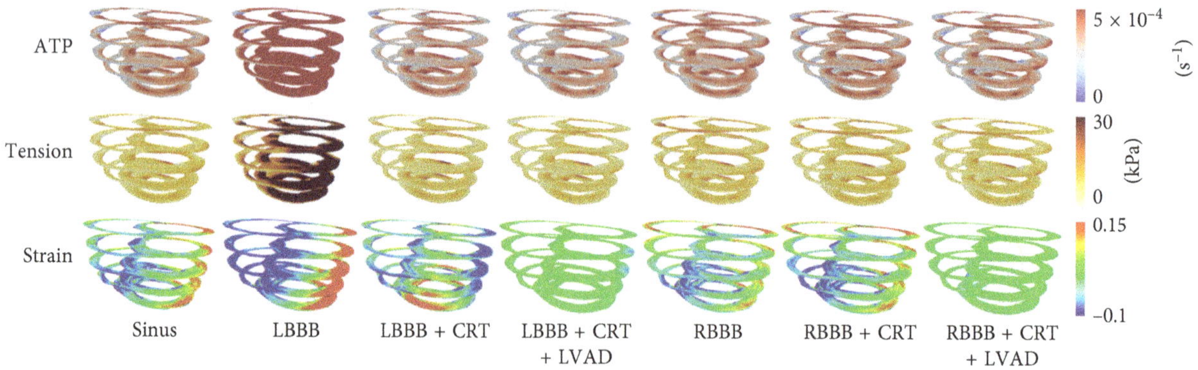

FIGURE 5: The 3D transmural distribution of ATP, tension, and strain in all cases. The snapshot for the ATP and tension was taken at the end-systolic volume, while the strain snapshot was taken at the end-diastolic volume time. ATP, adenosine triphosphate; LBBB, left bundle branch block; CRT, cardiac resynchronization therapy; LVAD, left ventricular assist device; RBBB, right bundle branch block.

was increased to 141 mmHg. The LV peak pressure time was shortened to 364 ms, and the aortic valve was opened for 96 ms. In the LBBB + CRT + LVAD condition, the peak LV pressure was 148 mmHg, the same as that in the normal condition, the LV peak pressure time was 363 ms, and the aortic valve was opened for 62 ms. The combination of CRT and LVAD restored the LV peak pressure and LV peak pressure time in the LBBB condition better than CRT alone. In the RBBB and RBBB + CRT conditions, the LV peak pressures and LV peak pressure time were the same at 148 mmHg and 353 ms, respectively, and the aortic valve was opened for 96 ms, the same as that in the normal condition. The reason was that the electrical activation of the LV was not altered in the RBBB condition. In the RBBB + CRT + LVAD condition, the peak LV pressure and LV peak pressure time were increased to 155 mmHg and 350 ms, respectively, and the aortic valve was opened for 63 ms. This finding shows that the combined CRT and LVAD increased the LV pressure and systemic artery more than the CRT-only implementation.

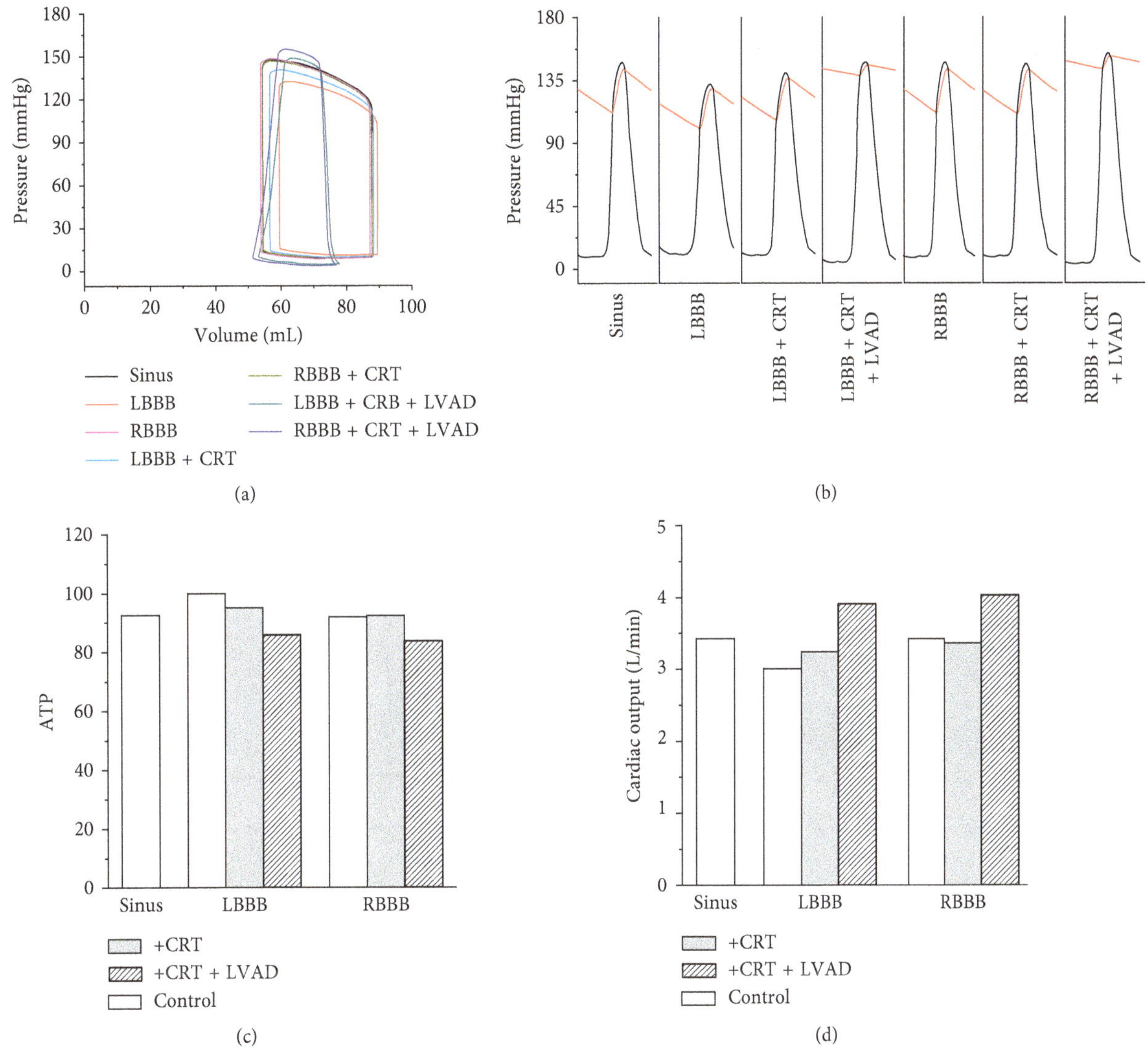

FIGURE 6: (a) LV pressure-volume loop, (b) LV pressure and aortic pressure, (c) ATP consumption rate, and (d) cardiac output of all cases. LV, left ventricular; LBBB, left bundle branch block; CRT, cardiac resynchronization therapy; LVAD, left ventricular assist device; RBBB, right bundle branch block; ATP, adenosine triphosphate.

Figure 6(c) shows the overall ATP consumption rate from one cycle of steady state. In the normal sinus condition, the ATP consumption rate was 93 s^{-1}. The ATP consumption rate in LBBB condition was the highest at 100 s^{-1}. CRT reduced the ATP consumption rate in the LBBB condition by 5%, while CRT and LVAD reduced the ATP consumption rate by 15%. In the RBBB and RBBB + CRT conditions, the ATP consumption rates were the same as that in the normal condition, 93 s^{-1}. However, with CRT and LVAD support, the ATP consumption rate in the RBBB condition was decreased by 16% to 84 s^{-1}.

Figure 6(d) shows the CO of the seven subjects. CRT increased the CO slightly in the LBBB condition but not in the RBBB condition. With the combination of CRT and LVAD, the CO of the LBBB and RBBB conditions was significantly increased (Table 1).

Figure 7(a) shows the 3D contour of EAT, MAT, and EMD, while Figure 7(b) shows the MAT and EMD of all cases. As shown in Figure 7(a), the activation sequence of MAT and EMD was identical to the EAT. The MAT and EMD values in the normal condition were 157 and 78 ms, respectively. In the LBBB condition, the MAT and EMD values were the greatest at 188 ms and 79 ms, respectively. CRT shortened the MAT and EMD to 148 ms and 71 ms in the LBBB condition. Furthermore, the MAT and EMD in the LBBB condition were further shortened with the combined CRT and LVAD to 144 and 67 ms, respectively. This finding showed that combination of CRT and LVAD performed better than CRT alone despite having the same EAT. In the RBBB condition, the MAT and EMD values were 162 and 80 ms, respectively. In the RBBB + CRT condition, the mean MAT and EMD values were reduced slightly to 157 and 81 ms, respectively. In the RBBB + CRT + LVAD condition, the mean MAT and EMD values were reduced to 155 and 79 ms (close to the control condition), respectively. In the RBBB condition, CRT alone only slightly affected the electrical and

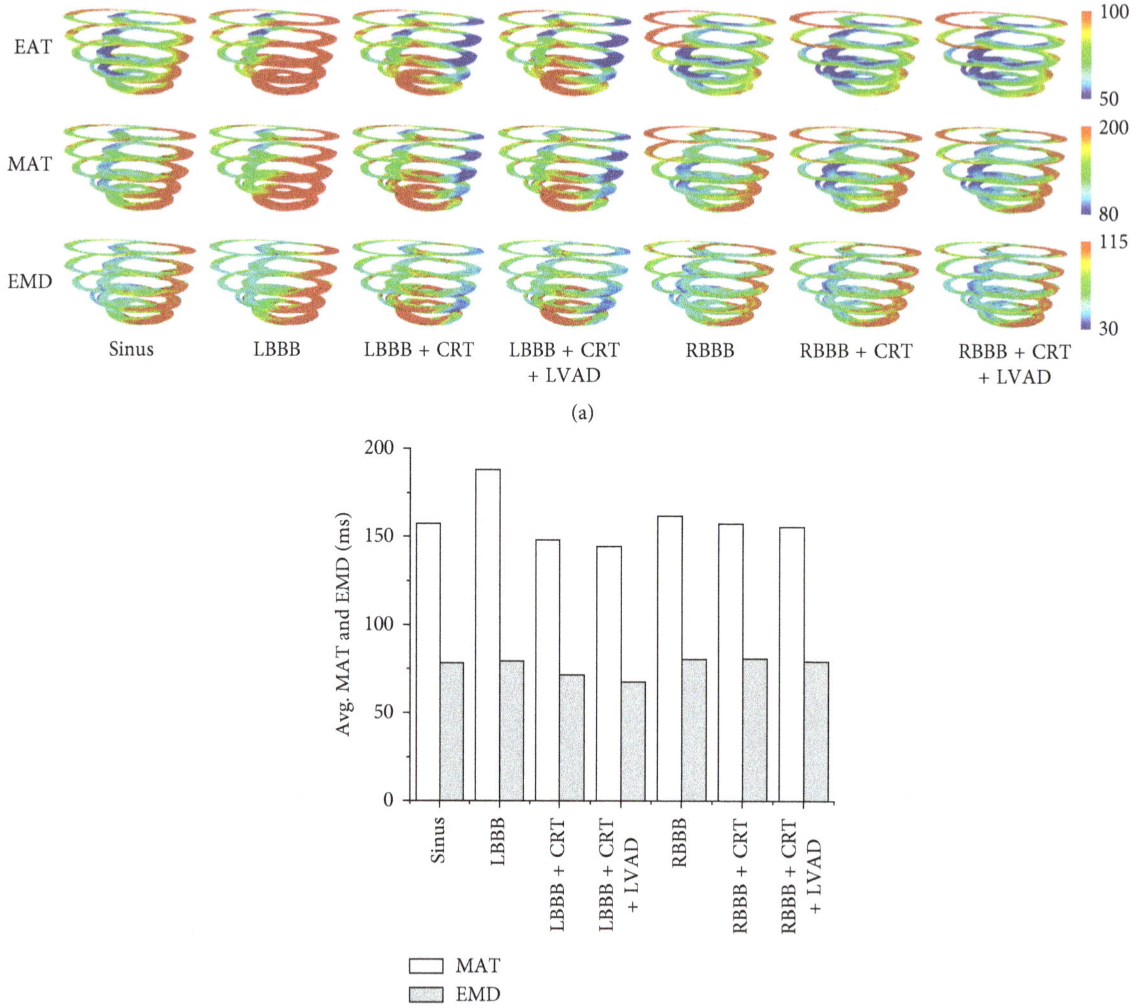

(a)

(b)

FIGURE 7: (a) Three-dimensional contour distribution of the EAT, MAT, and EMD and (b) the mean MAT and EMD values in all cases. EAT, electrical activation time; MAT, mechanical activation time; EMD, electromechanical delay; LBBB, left bundle branch block; CRT, cardiac resynchronization therapy; LVAD, left ventricular assist device; RBBB, right bundle branch block.

mechanical responses. However, CRT + LVAD increased CO in the RBBB condition significantly as expected.

In general, we performed a simulation and analyzed seven cardiac diseases and therapy conditions by using an electromechanical ventricular model incorporated with a circulatory systems, CRT, and LVAD models. The models including normal sinus rhythm, LBBB, LBBB + CRT, LBBB + CRT + LVAD, RBBB, RBBB + CRT, and RBBB + CRT + LVAD. The major findings of this study are as follows:

(1) CRT shortened the longest EAT by 20.2% in the LBBB condition and 17.1% in the RBBB condition. CRT shortened EMD by 10.1% in the LBBB condition but did not shorten EMD in the RBBB condition.

(2) Combination of CRT and LVAD treatment shortened EMD more than CRT alone in the LBBB condition (15.2%) and shortened EMD in the RBBB condition (1.3%).

(3) CRT reduced the ATP consumption by 5% as well as the tension and strain in the LBBB condition. CRT also slightly increased the LV peak pressure by 6% and increased the CO by 0.2 L/min in the LBBB condition. However, CRT-alone did not affect these mechanical responses in the RBBB condition.

(4) Combination of CRT and LVAD reduced the ATP consumption by 15% in the LBBB condition and by 16% in the RBBB condition. It also increased the LV pressure by 10.5% in the LBBB condition and 5.7% in the RBBB condition as well as the CO up to 4 L/min for both conditions, a degree greater than that in the control condition.

The pacing site at the tissue greatly affected synchronization. Placement at the LV free-wall showed faster activation throughout the chamber since the signal propagated evenly from the midway between the base and apex throughout the LV tissue. However, the pacing site at the RV endocardial apex showed a longer activation time for the electrical signal to propagate to the base.

In the RBBB condition, the electrical activation of the LV chamber was the same as normal sinus despite the electrical activation alteration in the RV. This is the major factor why the mechanical responses of the LV (LV PV-loop, LV pressure, and CO) were also the same as that in normal sinus rhythm. Even the CRT implementation in the RBBB condition did not affect the mechanical responses of the LV chamber. However, we observed significant improvement in CO in the RBBB + CRT + LVAD condition. CRT and LVAD also reduced the ATP consumption and tension and increased the LV and aortic pressure in the RBBB condition.

CRT-alone did not fully restore the mechanical responses under the LBBB condition to normal despite the resynchronization of the EAT, which shortened the MAT and EMD to back normal. On the contrary, the use of combined CRT and LVAD reduced the energy consumption (indicated by the ATP consumption rate), tension, increased the LV pressure, and produced CO by 18% more than that in the HF with sinus rhythm condition. In addition, the LVAD did not fully assist the blood distribution in the LBBB or RBBB condition.

The computational method allowed us to predict the electromechanical phenomenon in the dyssynchrony heart which underwent CRT and LVAD treatment. It is hardly possible to observe some parameters including ATP consumption, tension, MAT, and EMD from the patient's heart of that condition in experimental procedure. This study quantified the electrical activation and hemodynamic responses in several dyssynchrony HF combined with CRT-only, and CRT and LVAD, which has never been conducted previously. As for the clinical impact, the results of this study can be used as reference to generally predict the effect of the combination of CRT and LVAD devices to the HF patients with LBBB. Though, there are some parameters need to be consider deeply by the cardiologist expert.

This computational study has several limitations that need to be addressed. The study did not follow the standard biventricular pacing method [43]. Instead, we used only one CRT pacing site: the RV endocardial apex (for the RBBB condition) or the LV lateral wall (for the LBBB condition). The LV pacing site was not placed at the optimal position as described before [44]. We did not observe or describe the RV mechanical responses in the RBBB condition; instead, we showed the LV responses only. We used LVAD instead of a right ventricular assist device to support the RBBB condition. Because of our limitations, we did not validate the results of our simulation with experimental data. In addition, we did not describe long-term effects such as recovery of cardiac functions by the combined CRT and LVAD, as previously described [28, 29].

4. Conclusions

In conclusion, although CRT-alone shortened the MAT and EMD to more than normal in the LBBB condition, the mechanical responses in the LBBB condition were not restored to normal. The combined CRT and LVAD shortened the MAT and EMD more than CRT-alone, restored the hemodynamic, and produced a greater CO than normal in the LBBB and RBBB conditions. Using the combined system, LVAD contributed to the MAT reduction by mechanical unloading, shortened the EMD, reduced ATP consumption, and reduced tension, which contributes to the recovery of the heart shape and function. In short, we computationally predicted and quantified that the CRT + LVAD implementation is superior to CRT-only implementation particularly in HF with the LBBB condition.

Conflicts of Interest

The authors declare that they have no conflicts of interest.

Acknowledgments

This research was partially supported by the MSIT (Ministry of Science, ICT), under the ITRC support program (IITP-2018-2014-0-00639) and and Global IT Talent Support Program (IITP-2017-0-01811) supervised by the IITP, and NRF under basic engineering research project (2016R1D1A1B0101440) and the EDISON (NRF-2011-0020576) Programs.

References

[1] D. Lloyd-Jones, R. Adams, M. Carnethon et al., "Heart disease and stroke statistics—2009 update: a report from the American Heart Association Statistics Committee and Stroke Statistics Subcommittee," *Circulation*, vol. 119, no. 3, pp. e21–e181, 2009.

[2] C. Linde, C. Leclercq, S. Rex et al., "Long-term benefits of biventricular pacing in congestive heart failure: results from the MUltisite STimulation in cardiomyopathy (MUSTIC) study," *Journal of the American College of Cardiology*, vol. 40, no. 1, pp. 111–118, 2002.

[3] J. B. Young, W. T. Abraham, A. L. Smith et al., "Combined cardiac resynchronization and implantable cardioversion defibrillation in advanced chronic heart failure: the MIRACLE ICD Trial," *JAMA*, vol. 289, no. 20, pp. 2685–2694, 2003.

[4] M. Kawaguchi, T. Murabayashi, B. J. Fetics et al., "Quantitation of basal dyssynchrony and acute resynchronization from left or biventricular pacing by novel echo-contrast variability imaging," *Journal of the American College of Cardiology*, vol. 39, no. 12, pp. 2052–2058, 2002.

[5] G. S. Nelson, R. D. Berger, B. J. Fetics et al., "Left ventricular or biventricular pacing improves cardiac function at diminished energy cost in patients with dilated cardiomyopathy and left bundle-branch block," *Circulation*, vol. 102, no. 25, pp. 3053–3059, 2000.

[6] P. Søgaard, W. Y. Kim, H. K. Jensen et al., "Impact of acute biventricular pacing on left ventricular performance and volumes in patients with severe heart failure," *Cardiology*, vol. 95, no. 4, pp. 173–182, 2001.

[7] A. Auricchio, C. Stellbrink, S. Sack et al., "Long-term clinical effect of hemodynamically optimized cardiac

resynchronization therapy in patients with heart failure and ventricular conduction delay," *Journal of the American College of Cardiology*, vol. 39, no. 12, pp. 2026-2033, 2002.

[8] M. G. S. J. Sutton, T. Plappert, K. E. Hilpisch et al., "Sustained reverse left ventricular structural remodeling with cardiac resynchronization at one year is a function of etiology quantitative doppler echocardiographic evidence from the Multicenter InSync Randomized Clinical Evaluation (MIRACLE)," *Circulation*, vol. 113, no. 2, pp. 266–272, 2006.

[9] W. T. Abraham, W. G. Fisher, A. L. Smith et al., "Cardiac resynchronization in chronic heart failure," *New England Journal of Medicine*, vol. 346, no. 24, pp. 1845–1853, 2002.

[10] S. Cazeau, C. Leclercq, T. Lavergne et al., "Effects of multisite biventricular pacing in patients with heart failure and intraventricular conduction delay," *New England Journal of Medicine*, vol. 344, no. 12, pp. 873–880, 2001.

[11] J. G. Cleland, J.-C. Daubert, E. Erdmann et al., "The effect of cardiac resynchronization on morbidity and mortality in heart failure," *New England Journal of Medicine*, vol. 352, no. 15, pp. 1539–1549, 2005.

[12] A. J. Moss, W. J. Hall, D. S. Cannom et al., "Cardiac-resynchronization therapy for the prevention of heart-failure events," *New England Journal of Medicine*, vol. 361, no. 14, pp. 1329–1338, 2009.

[13] Y. Hu, V. Gurev, J. Constantino, and N. Trayanova, "Efficient preloading of the ventricles by a properly timed atrial contraction underlies stroke work improvement in the acute response to cardiac resynchronization therapy," *Heart Rhythm*, vol. 10, no. 12, pp. 1800–1806, 2013.

[14] R. John, F. Kamdar, K. Liao et al., "Improved survival and decreasing incidence of adverse events with the HeartMate II left ventricular assist device as bridge-to-transplant therapy," *Annals of Thoracic surgery*, vol. 86, no. 4, pp. 1227–1235, 2008.

[15] D. Casarotto, T. Bottio, A. Gambino, L. Testolin, and G. Gerosa, "The last to die is hope: prolonged mechanical circulatory support with a Novacor left ventricular assist device as a bridge to transplantation," *Journal of Thoracic and Cardiovascular Surgery*, vol. 125, no. 2, pp. 417-418, 2003.

[16] M. A. Daneshmand, K. Rajagopal, B. Lima et al., "Left ventricular assist device destination therapy versus extended criteria cardiac transplant," *Annals of Thoracic Surgery*, vol. 89, no. 4, pp. 1205–1210, 2010.

[17] E. J. Birks, "Left ventricular assist devices," *Heart*, vol. 96, no. 1, pp. 63–71, 2010.

[18] E. A. Rose, A. C. Gelijns, A. J. Moskowitz et al., "Long-term use of a left ventricular assist device for end-stage heart failure," *New England Journal of Medicine*, vol. 345, no. 20, pp. 1435–1443, 2001.

[19] G. T. Altemose, V. Gritsus, V. Jeevanandam, B. Goldman, and K. B. Margulies, "Altered myocardial phenotype after mechanical support in human beings with advanced cardiomyopathy," *Journal of heart and lung transplantation: The Official Publication of the International Society for Heart Transplantation*, vol. 16, no. 7, pp. 765–773, 1997.

[20] H. R. Levin, M. C. Oz, J. M. Chen et al., "Reversal of chronic ventricular dilation in patients with end-stage cardiomyopathy by prolonged mechanical unloading," *Circulation*, vol. 91, no. 11, pp. 2717–2720, 1995.

[21] A. Barbone, M. C. Oz, D. Burkhoff, and J. W. Holmes, "Normalized diastolic properties after left ventricular assist result from reverse remodeling of chamber geometry," *Circulation*, vol. 104, no. 1, pp. I-229–I-232, 2001.

[22] S. Nakatani, P. M. McCarthy, K. Kottke-Marchant et al., "Left ventricular echocardiographic and histologic changes: impact of chronic unloading by an implantable ventricular assist device," *Journal of the American College of Cardiology*, vol. 27, no. 4, pp. 894–901, 1996.

[23] K. L. Grady, P. Meyer, A. Mattea et al., "Improvement in quality of life outcomes 2 weeks after left ventricular assist device implantation," *Journal of Heart and Lung Transplantation*, vol. 20, no. 6, pp. 657–669, 2001.

[24] F. D. Pagani, L. W. Miller, S. D. Russell et al., "Extended mechanical circulatory support with a continuous-flow rotary left ventricular assist device," *Journal of the American College of Cardiology*, vol. 54, no. 4, pp. 312–321, 2009.

[25] M. S. Slaughter, J. G. Rogers, C. A. Milano et al., "Advanced heart failure treated with continuous-flow left ventricular assist device," *New England Journal of Medicine*, vol. 361, no. 23, pp. 2241–2251, 2009.

[26] A. K. Heikhmakhtiar, A. J. Ryu, E. B. Shim et al., "Influence of LVAD function on mechanical unloading and electromechanical delay: a simulation study," *Medical and Biological Engineering and Computing*, vol. 56, no. 5, pp. 911–921, 2017.

[27] R. M. Delgado and B. Radovancevic, "Symptomatic relief: left ventricular assist devices versus resynchronization therapy," *Heart Failure Clinics*, vol. 3, no. 3, pp. 259–265, 2007.

[28] J. Muratsu, M. Hara, I. Mizote et al., "The impact of cardiac resynchronization therapy in an end-stage heart failure patient with a left ventricular assist device as a bridge to recovery," *International Heart Journal*, vol. 52, no. 4, pp. 246-247, 2011.

[29] H. Keilegavlen, J. E. Nordrehaug, S. Faerestrand et al., "Treatment of cardiogenic shock with left ventricular assist device combined with cardiac resynchronization therapy: a case report," *Journal of Cardiothoracic Surgery*, vol. 5, no. 1, p. 1, 2010.

[30] J. Constantino, Y. Hu, A. C. Lardo, and N. A. Trayanova, "Mechanistic insight into prolonged electromechanical delay in dyssynchronous heart failure: a computational study," *American Journal of Physiology-Heart and Circulatory Physiology*, vol. 305, no. 8, pp. H1265–H1273, 2013.

[31] Y. Hu, V. Gurev, J. Constantino, J. D. Bayer, and N. A. Trayanova, "Effects of mechano-electric feedback on scroll wave stability in human ventricular fibrillation," *PLoS One*, vol. 8, no. 4, Article ID e60287, 2013.

[32] X. Jie, V. Gurev, and N. Trayanova, "Mechanisms of mechanically induced spontaneous arrhythmias in acute regional ischemia," *Circulation Research*, vol. 106, no. 1, pp. 185–192, 2010.

[33] K. M. Lim and D. U. Jeong, "Influence of the KCNQ1 S140G mutation on human ventricular arrhythmogenesis and pumping performance: simulation study," *Frontiers in Physiology*, vol. 9, p. 926, 2018.

[34] V. Gurev, T. Lee, J. Constantino, H. Arevalo, and N. A. Trayanova, "Models of cardiac electromechanics based on individual hearts imaging data," *Biomechanics and Modeling in Mechanobiology*, vol. 10, no. 3, pp. 295–306, 2011.

[35] J. Provost, V. Gurev, N. Trayanova, and E. E. Konofagou, "Mapping of cardiac electrical activation with electromechanical wave imaging: an in silico–in vivo reciprocity study," *Heart Rhythm*, vol. 8, no. 5, pp. 752–759, 2011.

[36] N. A. Trayanova, "Whole-heart modeling: applications to cardiac electrophysiology and electromechanics," *Circulation Research*, vol. 108, no. 1, pp. 113–128, 2011.

[37] N. A. Trayanova and J. J. Rice, "Cardiac electromechanical models: from cell to organ," *Frontiers in Physiology*, vol. 2, p. 43, 2011.

[38] K. M. Lim, J. Constantino, V. Gurev et al., "Comparison of the effects of continuous and pulsatile left ventricular-assist

devices on ventricular unloading using a cardiac electromechanics model," *Journal of Physiological Sciences*, vol. 62, no. 1, pp. 11–19, 2012.

[39] K. ten Tusscher, D. Noble, P. Noble, and A. Panfilov, "A model for human ventricular tissue," *American Journal of Physiology-Heart and Circulatory Physiology*, vol. 286, no. 4, pp. H1573–H1589, 2004.

[40] O. Berenfeld and J. Jalife, "Purkinje-muscle reentry as a mechanism of polymorphic ventricular arrhythmias in a 3-dimensional model of the ventricles," *Circulation Research*, vol. 82, no. 10, pp. 1063–1077, 1998.

[41] J. J. Rice, F. Wang, D. M. Bers, and P. P. De Tombe, "Approximate model of cooperative activation and crossbridge cycling in cardiac muscle using ordinary differential equations," *Biophysical Journal*, vol. 95, no. 5, pp. 2368–2390, 2008.

[42] R. C. Kerckhoffs, M. L. Neal, Q. Gu et al., "Coupling of a 3D finite element model of cardiac ventricular mechanics to lumped systems models of the systemic and pulmonic circulation," *Annals of Biomedical Engineering*, vol. 35, no. 1, pp. 1–18, 2007.

[43] J. B. Shea and M. O. Sweeney, "Cardiac resynchronization therapy a patient's guide," *Circulation*, vol. 108, no. 9, pp. e64–e66, 2003.

[44] Y. Hu, V. Gurev, J. Constantino, and N. Trayanova, "Optimizing cardiac resynchronization therapy to minimize ATP consumption heterogeneity throughout the left ventricle: a simulation analysis using a canine heart failure model," *Heart Rhythm*, vol. 11, no. 6, pp. 1063–1069, 2014.

9

An Improved FastICA Method for Fetal ECG Extraction

Li Yuan, Zhuhuang Zhou, Yanchao Yuan, and Shuicai Wu

College of Life Science and Bioengineering, Beijing University of Technology, Beijing, China

Correspondence should be addressed to Shuicai Wu; wushuicai@bjut.edu.cn

Academic Editor: Chuangyin Dang

Objective. The fast fixed-point algorithm for independent component analysis (FastICA) has been widely used in fetal electrocardiogram (ECG) extraction. However, the FastICA algorithm is sensitive to the initial weight vector, which affects the convergence of the algorithm. In order to solve this problem, an improved FastICA method was proposed to extract fetal ECG. *Methods.* First, the maternal abdominal mixed signal was centralized and whitened, and the overrelaxation factor was incorporated into Newton's iterative algorithm to process the initial weight vector randomly generated. The improved FastICA algorithm was used to separate the source components, selected the best maternal ECG from the separated source components, and detected the R-wave location of the maternal ECG. Finally, the maternal ECG component in each channel was removed by the singular value decomposition (SVD) method to obtain a clean fetal ECG signal. *Results.* An annotated clinical fetal ECG database was used to evaluate the improved algorithm and the conventional FastICA algorithm. The average number of iterations of the algorithm was reduced from 35 before the improvement to 13. Correspondingly, the average running time was reduced from 1.25 s to 1.04 s when using the improved algorithm. The signal-to-noise ratio (SNR) based on eigenvalues of the improved algorithm was 1.55, as compared to 0.99 of the conventional FastICA algorithm. The SNR based on cross-correlation coefficients of the conventional algorithm was also improved from 0.59 to 2.02. The sensitivity, positive predictive accuracy, and harmonic mean ($F1$) of the improved method were 99.37%, 99.00%, and 99.19%, respectively, while these metrics of the conventional FastICA method were 99.03%, 98.53%, and 98.78%, respectively. *Conclusions.* The proposed improved FastICA algorithm based on the overrelaxation factor, while maintaining the rate of convergence, relaxes the requirement of initial weight vector, avoids the unbalanced convergence, reduces the number of iterations, and improves the convergence performance.

1. Introduction

Electrocardiogram (ECG) is an important tool used by physicians for identifying abnormalities in the human heart activity [1]. Similarly, fetal ECG signal can also reflect electrophysiological activity of the fetal heart. Physicians can detect in time fetal abnormalities during fetal development through the fetal ECG waveform analysis, such as fetal distress and intrauterine hypoxia. In addition, a small number of abnormal fetal ECG waveforms are also a manifestation of congenital heart disease, for which early measures can be taken to reduce neonatal morbidity and mortality.

Currently, there are two ways for obtaining fetal ECG. One is the invasive scalp electrode method, which can directly measure the pure fetal ECG signal. However, it can only detect fetal ECG signal during the time of birth, and it is invasive so it may cause harm to the mother and the fetus. The other method is noninvasive, abdominal electrode method. The signals from the abdominal body surface are collected by placing an electrode patch in the abdomen of the mother, which allows for long-term monitoring during pregnancy without harming the mother or the fetus. However, the signals from maternal abdomen surface are very complex, which not only contain weak fetal ECG and maternal ECG but also include the mother's respiratory noise, frequency interference, and other signals [2]. In particular, the magnitude of the maternal ECG detected in the abdomen is about 2–10 times that of the fetal ECG [3], which makes the extraction of fetal ECG difficult. Therefore, it is necessary to develop a noninvasive method that can extract fetal ECG effectively.

At present, fetal ECG extraction algorithms mainly include adaptive filtering [4, 5], wavelet analysis [6], matched filtering [7], blind source separation [8], independent component analysis (ICA) [9], neural network [10, 11], and singular value decomposition (SVD) [12]. Among these methods,

ICA can separate the source signals from the mixed signals under the assumption that the source signals are statistically independent of each other, without needing any information regarding the source signals or the mixed matrix. Therefore, ICA is considered as a promising method for extracting fetal ECG. In recent years, researchers have proposed many improved ICA algorithms, which can separate non-Gaussian signals. Among them, because of its fast convergence, the fast fixed-point algorithm for independent component analysis (FastICA) [13] has been widely used in the extraction of fetal ECG. However, the FastICA algorithm is sensitive to the initial weight vector, and different initial weight vectors may lead to different convergence performances of the algorithm.

In this paper, an improved FastICA method was proposed to solve the above problem. By incorporating an overrelaxation factor into the iterative algorithm, the initial weight vector generated randomly can be relaxed. By choosing the appropriate overrelaxation factor, the iterative algorithm with slower convergence rate can converge, and the divergent iterative algorithm may become convergent.

2. Methods

2.1. FastICA Algorithm. FastICA is a fixed-point iterative algorithm, minimizing mutual information between estimated components [14]. Separation of independent components is accomplished when the maximum of non-Gaussianity is attained. There are different kinds of FastICA, including those based on kurtosis, based on the maximum likelihood, and based on the maximum negentropy (MNE), and so forth. In this paper, the MNE-based FastICA algorithm was used, which took the maximization of negentropy as a search direction and extracted each independent source signal in turn.

Before using the FastICA algorithm, the observed signal X was centralized and whitened. The mean removal process was conducted to subtract the mean vector of the signal from the observed signals so that the observed signal became zero mean, simplifying the FastICA algorithm. The observation signal was whitened using the principal component analysis (PCA) whitening algorithm so that the components after the whitening were uncorrelated. The purpose of the FastICA algorithm based on fixed-point iterative structure was to make $y = w^T x$ have the maximum non-Gaussianity, where w was a row of the separation matrix W. The objective function was set as

$$J(y) \approx \{E[G(y)] - E[G(v)]\}^2, \tag{1}$$

where $E[\cdot]$ was the expectation operator and v was a Gaussian random variable with zero mean and unit variance. It was assumed that y also had zero mean and unit variance. $G(\cdot)$ was a nonquadratic function.

According to the Kuhn-Tucker condition, the optimization of $E\{G(w^T x)\}$ could be obtained by (2) under the constraint of $E\{(w^T x)^2\} = \|w\|^2 = 1$:

$$E\left\{xg\left(w^T x\right)\right\} - \beta w = 0, \tag{2}$$

where β was a constant and could be obtained by $\beta = E\{{w_0}^T xg({w_0}^T x)\}$, where w_0 was the initial value of w and $g(\cdot)$ was a nonlinear function, which was the derivative of $G(\cdot)$. We chose the nonlinear function $g(y) = y^3$. The Newton iterative method was employed to solve (2). The left part of (2) was denoted as $F(w)$, and the Jacobian matrix $JF(w)$ was

$$JF(w) = E\left\{xx^T g'\left(w^T x\right)\right\} - \beta I \tag{3}$$

In order to simplify the computation of the inverse of the matrix, (3) was approximated. Because the data were whitened, (3) could be simplified as

$$\begin{aligned} E\left\{xx^T g'\left(w^T x\right)\right\} &\approx E\left\{xx^T\right\} E\left\{g'\left(w^T x\right)\right\} \\ &= E\left\{g'\left(w^T x\right)\right\} I \end{aligned} \tag{4}$$

The Jacobin matrix was a diagonal matrix, and its inverse matrix could be simply calculated. Similarly, replace the value of w_0 with the current value of w for the constant β. Therefore, we could obtain the approximated Newton iterative formula as follows:

$$w_{k+1} = w_k - \frac{\left[E\left\{xg\left(w_k^T x\right)\right\} - \beta w_k\right]}{\left[E\left\{g'\left(w_k^T x\right)\right\} - \beta\right]}, \tag{5}$$

where $\beta = E\{w^T xg(w^T x)\}$ and w_{k+1} represented the updated value of w_k. In order to improve the stability of the algorithm, w was normalized by $w_{k+1} = w_{k+1}/\|w_{k+1}\|$ after an iteration. To simplify (5), we obtained an iterative formula of simplified FastICA algorithm:

$$w_{k+1} = E\left\{xg\left(w_k^T x\right)\right\} - E\left\{g'\left(w_k^T x\right)\right\} w_k. \tag{6}$$

2.2. FastICA Algorithm Improvement

2.2.1. Selection of Overrelaxation Factor. In order to address the problem that FastICA is sensitive to the initial weight vector, we introduced an overrelaxation factor α_k into the iterative algorithm. If $F(w_k)$ is guaranteed to have a decreasing property for a given norm, (7) was satisfied:

$$\left\|E\left\{xg\left(w_{k+1}^T x\right)\right\} - \beta w_{k+1}\right\| < \left\|E\left\{xg\left(w_k^T x\right)\right\} - \beta w_k\right\| \quad k = 0, 1, \ldots, \tag{7}$$

that is,

$$\min_{\alpha_k} \left\|F\left(w_k - \frac{\alpha_k F(w_k)}{JF(w_k)}\right)\right\| \tag{8}$$

By introducing the overrelaxation factor α_k, it was guaranteed that $F(w_k)$ can enter the convergence area of the Newton iteration algorithm from a certain value of w_k, so as to ensure that the algorithm can achieve the convergence effect under any circumstance.

There are many methods for choosing the overrelaxation factors, such as the golden section method and step-by-step experimental method. In this paper, we used step-by-step experiment to obtain the optimal overrelaxation factor.

The value of α_k is $1 + 1/N, 1 + 2/N, \ldots, 1 + (N - 1)/N$, where $N = 100$. All the values of k that satisfied (9) were recorded. Among these values of k, the one that satisfied (8) was found and denoted as p. Then, α_p would be the optimal overrelaxation factor α.

$$\left\|F\left(w_k - \alpha_k \Delta w_k\right)\right\|^2 < \left\|F\left(w_k\right)\right\|^2, \tag{9}$$

where $\Delta w_k = F(w_k)/JF(w_k)$.

The selection of the overrelaxation factor α included the following steps.

Step 1. Set the initial value $N = 100$, $k = 1$, and create an empty vector v.

Step 2. $\alpha_k = 1 + k/N$.

Step 3. If the value of k satisfies (9), then k is used to calculate the target function TF, $\text{TF} = \|F(w_k - \alpha_k F(w_k)/JF(w_k))\|$, and the result of TF is added to v.

Step 4. $k = k + 1$.

Step 5. If $k < 100$, repeat Steps 2–4. Otherwise, the value of k corresponding to the smallest value of TF in the vector v is found and denoted as p. Then, α_p is the optimal overrelaxation factor α.

2.2.2. Improved FastICA. The convergence performance of the FastICA algorithm was affected by the initial weight vector. Since the initial weight vector of the FastICA algorithm was selected randomly, the efficiency of each iteration was different due to different initial weight vector. The obtained independent components would also be slightly different. Although it was also possible to select the principal component obtained during the whitening process as the initial weight vector, the algorithm easily converged to the initial value of the whitening. The FastICA algorithm should relax the initial weight vector requirements, that is, to achieve convergence in a wide range.

In order to improve the FastICA algorithm with respect to the initial weight vector w_0, Xu et al. [15] proposed the incorporation of relaxation factor α_k (low relaxation factor $0 < \alpha_k < 1$) into the FastICA iteration. Because the negative gradient direction was the fastest declining direction, the gradient value was chosen as the optimal relaxation factor α_k in [15]. However, the computational of the relaxation factor was of high complexity [15]. In this paper, the overrelaxation factor α_k $(1 < \alpha_k < 2)$ was introduced into the FastICA iteration to deal with the initial weight vector generated randomly, and the requirement of the initial weight vector of the FastICA algorithm was relaxed. Compared with the low relaxation iteration [15], the proposed overrelaxation iteration converged much faster and was of low computational complexity.

In this paper, we introduced the overrelaxation factor into the iteration of FastICA algorithm. The value of α was calculated according to Section 2.2.1. The iteration of w_{k+1} became as follows:

$$\begin{aligned} w'_{k+1} &= E\left\{xg\left(w_k^T x\right)\right\} + \alpha E\left\{g'\left(w_k^T x\right)\right\} w_k \\ w''_{k+1} &= E\left\{xg\left(w_k^T x\right)\right\} + E\left\{g'\left({w'}_{k+1}^{T} x\right)\right\} w_k \\ w_{k+1} &= \frac{w''_{k+1}}{\left\|w''_{k+1}\right\|} \end{aligned} \tag{10}$$

2.3. Fetal ECG Extraction by Improved FastICA. To achieve long-term monitoring of pregnant women during the perinatal period, noninvasive abdominal methods were preferred to collect mixed signals from the maternal abdomen. The collected mixed signals contained not only maternal ECG and fetal ECG, but also some noises. Before using the improved FastICA algorithm to extract fetal ECG, the observed signals were preprocessed. The third-order low-pass Butterworth filter was used to estimate the baseline signal of each channel, and the low-pass filter cut-off frequency was 5 Hz. The baseline drift removal signal was obtained by subtracting the baseline signal from the observed signal. Then, the processed signal was centralized and whitened to make the signal uncorrelated, thus reducing the complexity of the algorithm. The improved FastICA was used to separate each component of the source signal. As the amplitude of the maternal ECG signal is 2–10 times that of the fetal ECG signal, the extracted fetal ECG signal usually contained some maternal ECG interference. In order to remove the maternal ECG interference, the maternal ECG signal channel was selected from the separated signal components, and R-wave detection was conducted on the maternal ECG signal. Then, the SVD method was used to remove the maternal ECG components in each channel to obtain clean fetal ECG without maternal ECG interference [16].

Fetal ECG extraction steps were as follows.

Step 1. Remove baseline drift and centralize the observed signal X, $\overline{X} = X - E\{X\}$.

Step 2. $X = ED^{-1/2}E^T\overline{X}$.

Step 3. Initialize random vector w_0, and set the error of convergence $0 < \varepsilon < 1$.

Step 4. According to Section 2.2.1, calculate overrelaxation factor α.

Step 5. According to (10), adjust w_{k+1}.

Step 6. Calculate w_{k+1}, and normalize it.

Step 7. If $|w_{k+1} - w_k| > \varepsilon$, the algorithm does not converge; return to Step 5 until the algorithm converges.

Step 8. Using the resulting separation matrix w, all the estimates of the source signal y_i are obtained. The maternal ECG component is selected, and R-wave detection is performed.

Step 9. Use SVD to remove the maternal ECG components in each channel to get a clean fetal ECG signal.

3. Fetal ECG Extraction Algorithm Evaluation

The signal-to-noise ratio (SNR) and statistical evaluation were used to compare the performances of the proposed algorithm and the conventional FastICA algorithm in terms of fetal ECG extraction performance.

3.1. Signal-to-Noise Ratio Evaluation. The signal-to-noise ratio (SNR) based on eigenvalues and the SNR based on cross-correlation coefficients proposed by Outram [17] were used to evaluate the performance of the proposed algorithm and the conventional FastICA algorithm.

First, R-wave detection of the extracted fetal ECG was performed. Each R-wave was taken as a reference to cut off M signal segments whose length is N. Each signal segment contained a complete QRS wave. Then, the M signal segments were used to form a matrix U_{N*M}, and the normalization of each column of the matrix with zero mean and unit variance was performed. The SNR based on eigenvalues was defined as follows:

$$\mathrm{SNR}_{\mathrm{Eig}} = \sqrt{\frac{\lambda_{\max}}{\mathrm{sum}(\lambda) - \lambda_{\max}}}, \tag{11}$$

where λ was the M eigenvalues of the matrix $U^T U$ and $\lambda_{\max}$ was the maximum of the eigenvalues of the matrix $U^T U$.

(2) The SNR based on cross-correlation coefficients is defined in

$$\mathrm{SNR}_{\mathrm{RMS}} = \sqrt{\frac{\eta}{1-\eta}}, \tag{12}$$

where $\eta = (2/M(M-1)) \sum_{i=0}^{M-2} \sum_{k=i+1}^{M-1} f(i)^T f(k)$, where f is the fetal ECG signal that contains intact QRS waves.

3.2. Statistical Evaluation. The performance of the methods was evaluated on the total length of fetal QRS signals, using sensitivity (Sens), positive predictive accuracy (PPA) [18], and harmonic mean ($F1$) [19]:

$$\mathrm{Sens} = \frac{\mathrm{TP}}{\mathrm{TP}+\mathrm{FN}}$$
$$\mathrm{PPA} = \frac{\mathrm{TP}}{\mathrm{TP}+\mathrm{FP}} \tag{13}$$
$$F1 = 2\frac{\mathrm{PPA}\cdot\mathrm{Sens}}{\mathrm{PPA}+\mathrm{Sens}} = \frac{2\cdot\mathrm{TP}}{2\cdot\mathrm{TP}+\mathrm{FN}+\mathrm{FP}},$$

where TP, FP, and FN are the number of true positive (correct detection of fetal ECG QRS complexes), false positive (falsely detected absence of R-peak), and false-negative (false fetal ECG QRS complex detection), respectively. $F1$ is the overall probability that the fetal ECG QRS complex is correctly detected and can be used as a measure of the accuracy of the proposed method. The Pan and Tompkins algorithm [20] was used to detect the fetal QRS in this work.

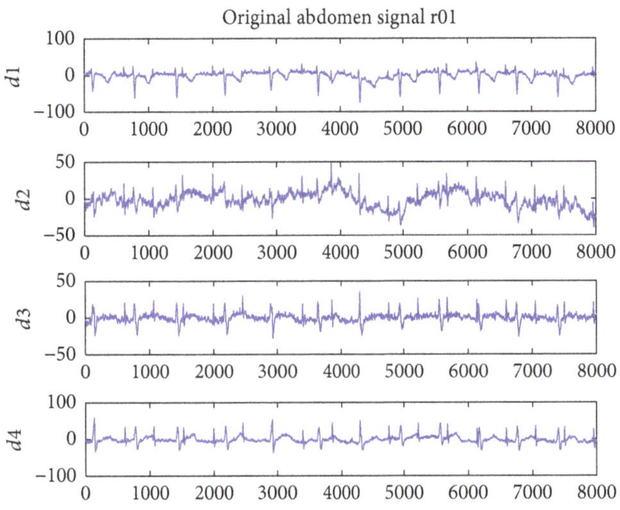

FIGURE 1: The original abdominal signal r01.

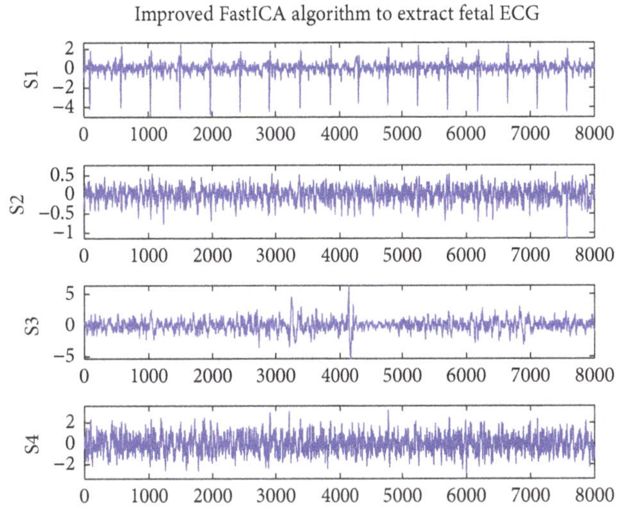

FIGURE 2: Improved FastICA algorithm to extract fetal ECG for r01.

4. Results

The improved FastICA algorithm was applied to fetal ECG signal extraction. The algorithm was validated using the clinical database Abdominal and Direct Fetal Electrocardiogram Database (ADFECGDB) [21]. The data were collected from five pregnant women of childbirth at 38–41 weeks of gestation. Each record contains four signals obtained from the maternal abdomen and one acquired directly from the fetal head at a sampling rate of 1 kHz and a collection time of 5 minutes.

Figure 1 shows the original record of the maternal abdomen signal database named r01. Figures 2 and 3 represent the residual signals after the cancelling of the maternal ECG component. Figure 2 shows the four ECG components of r01 extracted by the improved FastICA algorithm, where S1 is the extracted fetal ECG signal. Figure 3 shows the four ECG components of r01 extracted by the conventional FastICA algorithm, where S2 is the extracted fetal ECG signal.

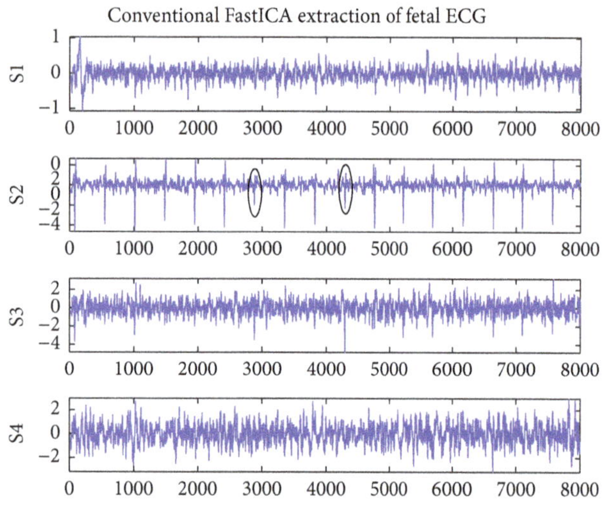

FIGURE 3: Conventional FastICA extraction of fetal ECG for r01.

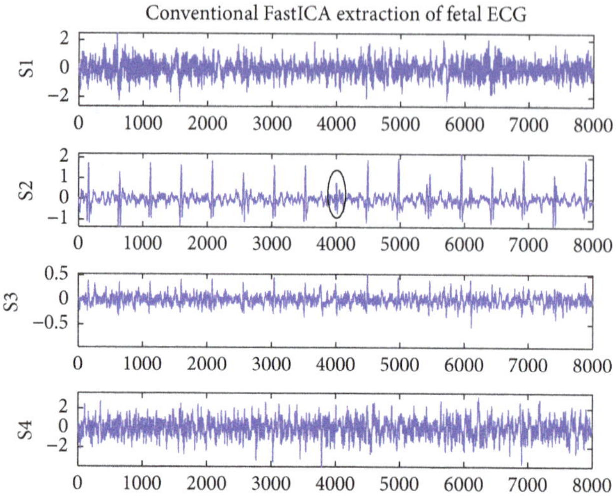

FIGURE 5: Conventional FastICA extraction of fetal ECG for r04.

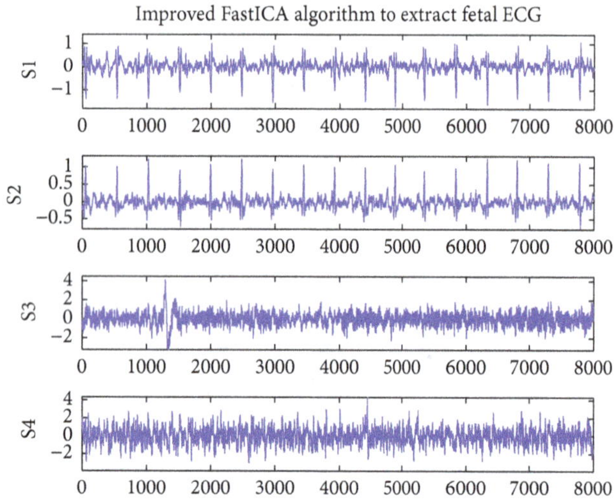

FIGURE 4: Improved FastICA algorithm to extract fetal ECG for r04.

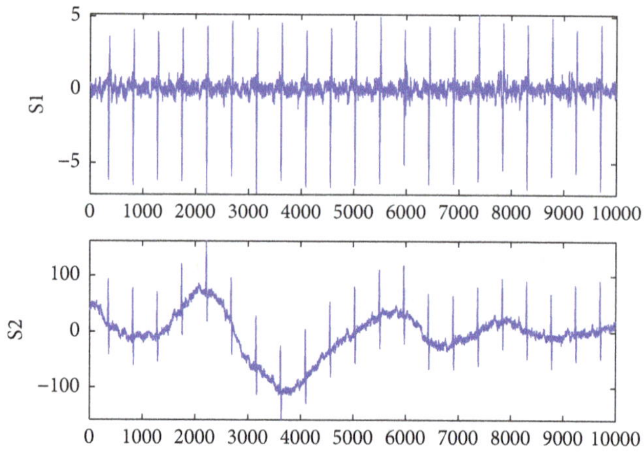

FIGURE 6: Improved FastICA algorithm for extraction of fetal ECG (S1) and golden standard (S2) for r01.

The amplitudes of R-waves (denoted by black circles in S2 of Figure 3) are small, which may render the R-waves undetected.

Figure 4 shows the four ECG components of r04 extracted by the improved FastICA algorithm, where both S1 and S2 contain fetal ECG signals. It can be seen that the proposed algorithm can extract clean fetal ECG from maternal abdominal mixed signals. Figure 5 shows the four ECG components of r04 extracted by the conventional FastICA algorithm, where S2 is the extracted fetal ECG signal. The amplitude of the 9th R-wave (denoted by black circles in S2 of Figure 5) is small, which may render the R-wave undetected.

In Figures 6 and 7, the S1 signals are the fetal ECG signal extracted from the abdomen signals of r01 and r08 using the proposed algorithm, respectively; the S2 signals are the fetal ECG signal provided the database as golden standard. It can be found that the proposed algorithm can extract a clean fetal ECG without loss of R-waves.

Table 1 shows the number of iterations and computational time of the conventional and improved FastICA algorithms for separating four source signal components. As the number of iterations of the two algorithms is related to the initial weight vector w_0, each algorithm ran 10 times. The average number of iterations of the conventional and proposed FastICA algorithms was 35 and 13, respectively, and the computational time was 1.25 s and 1.04 s, respectively. The number of iterations and computational time were decreased and the convergence rate was improved when using the improved FastICA algorithm.

Table 2 shows the SNR of the conventional and improved FastICA algorithms. Both the SNR based on eigenvalues and the SNR based on cross-correlation coefficients of the proposed algorithm were better than that of the conventional FastICA algorithm.

There was a one-channel annotated fetal ECG in ADFECGDB that can accurately provide the location of the fetal heart. As shown in Table 3, the proposed method correctly detected 3171 (TP) actual QRS complexes, falsely detected 32 (FP) extra QRS complexes, and missed 20 (FN) actual QRS complexes. The $F1$ of our proposed method was 99.19% while the $F1$ of the conventional FastICA method

Table 1: Number of iterations and running time of the improved and conventional FastICA algorithms.

No.	Improved FastICA		Conventional FastICA	
	Number of iterations	Running time (s)	Number of iterations	Running time (s)
1	16	1.03	34	1.73
2	14	1.06	36	1.20
3	12	1.03	28	1.21
4	12	1.03	32	1.18
5	14	1.02	36	1.23
6	12	1.02	34	1.18
7	14	1.06	34	1.19
8	13	1.05	38	1.20
9	12	1.06	42	1.17
10	12	1.01	36	1.18
Average	13	1.04	35	1.25

Table 2: Signal-to-noise ratio of the improved and conventional FastICA algorithms.

	Improved FastICA algorithm	Conventional FastICA algorithm
SNR_{Eig}	1.55	0.99
SNR_{RMS}	2.02	0.59

Table 3: Statistical evaluation of the improved and conventional FastICA algorithms.

Method	TP	FP	FN	Sens (%)	PPA (%)	*F*1 (%)
Improved FastICA	3171	32	20	99.37	99.00	99.19
Conventional FastICA	3160	47	31	99.03	98.53	98.78

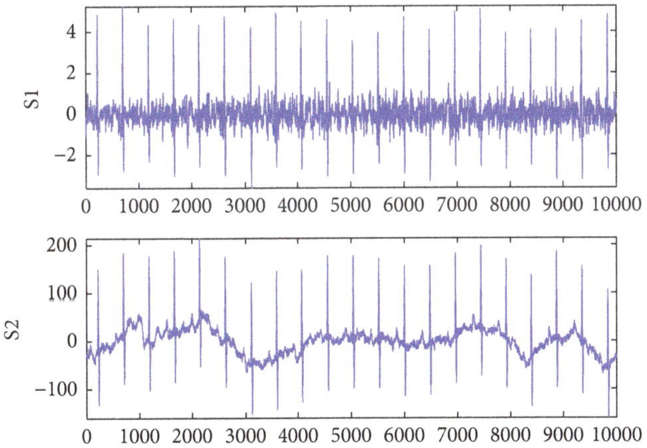

Figure 7: Improved FastICA algorithm for extraction of fetal ECG (S1) and golden standard (S2) for r08.

was 98.78%. It is demonstrated that the method proposed in this paper performs more favorably than the conventional FastICA method in statistical evaluation.

5. Discussion

The FastICA has been widely used in the extraction of fetal ECG because of its fast convergence rate. However, the FastICA algorithm is sensitive to the initial weight vector, and different initial weight vectors may lead to different convergence performances of the algorithm. So, in this paper, we introduced an overrelaxation factor, which can reduce the dependence of the FastICA algorithm on the initial weight vector and improve the convergence speed. The clinical database Abdominal and Direct Fetal Electrocardiogram Database (ADFECGDB) was selected to test the improved algorithm and the conventional FastICA algorithm. Figures 2 and 3 represent the residual signals obtained by maternal ECG component cancellation from the source components separated by the improved and conventional FastICA algorithms, respectively. It can be found that the proposed algorithm can extract a clean fetal ECG without loss of R-waves. We selected the four-channel AECG signal and compared the number of iterations and the computational time of the two algorithms. It can be seen from Table 1 that the average number of iterations of the improved algorithm is 13 and the average computational time is 1.04 s, significantly better than the conventional FastICA algorithm. As can be seen from Table 3, the improved algorithm only yielded 32 FP fetal heartbeat detections and 20 FN fetal heartbeat detections based on ADFECGDB, which contained a total of 3191 fetal heartbeats. The *F*1 of our improved method was 99.19% while the *F*1 of the conventional FastICA method was 98.78%. These results imply that the method improved in this paper is superior to the conventional FastICA method in statistical evaluation.

This study has a limitation. The improved algorithm and the conventional FastICA algorithm were only tested on the clinical database ADFECGDB. In future work, more clinical data may be used to further evaluate the performance of the improved FastICA algorithm.

6. Conclusions

In this paper, the FastICA algorithm based on the improved overrelaxation factor was proposed to extract fetal ECG. By incorporating an overrelaxation factor into the iterative algorithm, the initial weight vector generated randomly can be relaxed. ADFECGDB was used to assess the performance of the proposed algorithm and the conventional FastICA algorithm. Compared with the conventional FastICA algorithm, the proposed method not only had a fewer number of iterations but also performed better in SNR, Sens, PPA, and $F1$ metrics.

Conflicts of Interest

The authors declare that they have no conflicts of interest.

Acknowledgments

This work was supported by the National Natural Science Foundation of China under Grants 71661167001 and 71781260096, by China Postdoctoral Science Foundation under Grant 2017M620566, by Basic Research Fund of Beijing University of Technology, by Postdoctoral Research Fund of Chaoyang District, Beijing, under Grant 2017ZZ-01-03, and by Beijing Natural Science Foundation under Grant 4184081.

References

[1] R. Li, M. G. Frasch, and H.-T. Wu, "Efficient fetal-maternal ECG signal separation from two channel maternal abdominal ECG via diffusion-based channel selection," *Frontiers in Physiology*, vol. 8, no. MAY, article no. 277, 2017.

[2] M. Varanini, G. Tartarisco, R. Balocchi, A. Macerata, G. Pioggia, and L. Billeci, "A new method for QRS complex detection in multichannel ECG: Application to self-monitoring of fetal health," *Computers in Biology and Medicine*, vol. 85, pp. 125–134, 2017.

[3] G. M. Ungureanu, J. W. M. Bergmans, S. G. Oei, A. Ungureanu, and W. Wolf, "The event synchronous canceller algorithm removes maternal ECG from abdominal signals without affecting the fetal ECG," *Computers in Biology and Medicine*, vol. 39, no. 6, pp. 562–567, 2009.

[4] R. Martinek, R. Kahankova, H. Nazeran et al., "Non-invasive fetal monitoring: A maternal surface ECG electrode placement-based novel approach for optimization of adaptive filter control parameters using the LMS and RLS algorithms," *Sensors*, vol. 17, no. 5, article no. 1154, 2017.

[5] J. Behar, A. Johnson, G. D. Clifford, and J. Oster, "A comparison of single channel fetal ecg extraction methods," *Annals of Biomedical Engineering*, vol. 42, no. 6, pp. 1340–1353, 2014.

[6] S. Wu, Y. Shen, Z. Zhou, L. Lin, Y. Zeng, and X. Gao, "Research of fetal ECG extraction using wavelet analysis and adaptive filtering," *Computers in Biology and Medicine*, vol. 43, no. 10, pp. 1622–1627, 2013.

[7] A. Dessì, D. Pani, and L. Raffo, "An advanced algorithm for fetal heart rate estimation from non-invasive low electrode density recordings," *Physiological Measurement*, vol. 35, no. 8, pp. 1621–1636, 2014.

[8] A. Ghazdali, A. Hakim, A. Laghrib, N. Mamouni, and S. Raghay, "A new method for the extraction of fetal ECG from the dependent abdominal signals using blind source separation and adaptive noise cancellation techniques," *Theoretical Biology and Medical Modelling*, vol. 12, no. 1, article no. 25, 2015.

[9] G. Da Poian, R. Bernardini, and R. Rinaldo, "Separation and Analysis of Fetal-ECG Signals From Compressed Sensed Abdominal ECG Recordings," *IEEE Transactions on Biomedical Engineering*, vol. 63, no. 6, pp. 1269–1279, 2016.

[10] M. Lukoševičius and V. Marozas, "Noninvasive fetal QRS detection using an echo state network and dynamic programming," *Physiological Measurement*, vol. 35, no. 8, pp. 1685–1697, 2014.

[11] N. A. Sait, M. Thangarajan, and U. Snehalatha, "Neural network based on Verilog HDL for fetal ECG extraction," *International Journal of Biomedical Research*, vol. 7, no. 10, pp. 698–701, 2016.

[12] N. Zhang, J. Zhang, H. Li et al., "A novel technique for fetal ECG extraction using single-channel abdominal recording," *Sensors*, vol. 17, no. 3, article no. 457, 2017.

[13] A. Hyvärinen, "Fast and robust fixed-point algorithms for independent component analysis," *IEEE Transactions on Neural Networks and Learning Systems*, vol. 10, no. 3, pp. 626–634, 1999.

[14] Y. Jia and X. Yang, "A fetal electrocardiogram signal extraction algorithm based on fast one-unit independent component analysis with reference," *Computational and Mathematical Methods in Medicine*, Article ID 5127978, Art. ID 5127978, 10 pages, 2016.

[15] B. Xu, H. Jin, X. Tan et al., "Extracting fetal electrocardiogram based on a modified fast independent component analysis," in *9th International Conference on Fuzzy Systems and Knowledge Discovery*, pp. 1787–1791, IEEE, Chongqing, China, 2012.

[16] M. Varanini, G. Tartarisco, L. Billeci, A. Macerata, G. Pioggia, and R. Balocchi, "An efficient unsupervised fetal QRS complex detection from abdominal maternal ECG," *Physiological Measurement*, vol. 35, no. 8, pp. 1607–1619, 2014.

[17] N. J. Outram, *Intelligent pattern analysis of the fetal electrocardiogram*, University of Plymouth, Plymouth, England, 1998.

[18] AAMI, *ANSI/AAMI EC57:1998/(R)2008 - Testing and reporting performance results of cardiac rhythm and ST segment measurement algorithms*, American National Standards Institute, Arlington, VA, USA, 2008.

[19] L. Billeci and M. Varanini, "A combined independent source separation and quality index optimization method for fetal ECG extraction from abdominal maternal leads," *Sensors*, vol. 17, no. 5, article no. 1135, 2017.

[20] J. Pan and W. J. Tompkins, "A real-time QRS detection algorithm," *IEEE Transactions on Biomedical Engineering*, vol. 32, no. 3, pp. 230–236, 1985.

[21] "Abdominal and Direct FECG Database," Available online: https://physionet.org/physiobank/database/adfecgdb, 2018.

10

True Random Number Generation from Bioelectrical and Physical Signals

Seda Arslan Tuncer[1] **and Turgay Kaya**[2]

[1]*Department of Software Engineering, Faculty of Engineering, Fırat University, 23119 Elazig, Turkey*
[2]*Department of Electrical-Electronics Engineering, Faculty of Engineering, Fırat University, 23119 Elazig, Turkey*

Correspondence should be addressed to Seda Arslan Tuncer; satuncer@firat.edu.tr

Academic Editor: Yongqing Yang

It is possible to generate personally identifiable random numbers to be used in some particular applications, such as authentication and key generation. This study presents the true random number generation from bioelectrical signals like EEG, EMG, and EOG and physical signals, such as blood volume pulse, GSR (Galvanic Skin Response), and respiration. The signals used in the random number generation were taken from BNCIHORIZON2020 databases. Random number generation was performed from fifteen different signals (four from EEG, EMG, and EOG and one from respiration, GSR, and blood volume pulse datasets). For this purpose, each signal was first normalized and then sampled. The sampling was achieved by using a nonperiodic and chaotic logistic map. Then, XOR postprocessing was applied to improve the statistical properties of the sampled numbers. NIST SP 800-22 was used to observe the statistical properties of the numbers obtained, the scale index was used to determine the degree of nonperiodicity, and the autocorrelation tests were used to monitor the 0-1 variation of numbers. The numbers produced from bioelectrical and physical signals were successful in all tests. As a result, it has been shown that it is possible to generate personally identifiable real random numbers from both bioelectrical and physical signals.

1. Introduction

Random numbers are needed in some areas in computer science, such as authentication, secret key generation, game theory, and simulations. In these applications, particularly numbers should have good statistical properties and be unpredictable and nonreproducible. The number generation in the literature is performed in two different ways as deterministic and nondeterministic [1, 2]. PRNGs (Pseudo Random Number Generators), which are deterministic random number generators, generate numbers with fast, easy, inexpensive, and hardware independent solutions. The statistical qualities of these numbers produced are close to the ideal. PRNGs must meet the requirements specified in Table 1 to be used especially for authentication and key generation [3–5]. Therefore, nondeterministic functions are added to the output functions of PRNGs to guarantee these requirements.

TRNGs (True Random Number Generators), which are nondeterministic random number generators, present slower, more expensive, and hardware-dependent solutions compared to PRNGs. Contrary to PRNGs, there is no need to include extra components in the TRNG system designs for R2, R3, and R4 requirements. Because of the unpredictability of random numbers generated by the use of high noise sources with high entropy in TRNGs, it is assumed that the R2 requirement is met. If the R2 requirement is satisfied, then it is assumed that the R3 and R4 requirements are also satisfied. To meet the R1 requirement in TRNGs, postprocessing techniques are applied on the random numbers obtained by sampling from noise sources. This eliminates the statistical weaknesses of random numbers at the output of the TRNG. In addition, postprocessing techniques eliminate potential weaknesses and make TRNG designs strong and flexible [6, 7].

Recently, there have been studies performed on random number generation from human-based noise sources [8–12]. Elham et al. showed that two different people would produce different random numbers and that these numbers

TABLE 1: Requirements for random numbers.

Requirement	Explanation
R1	RNGs must generate random numbers having good statistical properties at the output to be used in cryptographic applications.
R2	In case of the attacker knows the sub-generators of random numbers, it must not be allowed to calculate or predict premise and consecutive random numbers with high accuracy.
R3	It must not be possible to predict or calculate previously generated random numbers with high accuracy by considering the known current internal state value of a RNG or without requiring its internal state information.
R4	It must not be possible to predict or calculate subsequent random numbers with high accuracy by considering the known current internal state value of a RNG or without requiring its internal state information.

could be used as biometric signatures [8]. Xingyuan et al. proposed a TRNG structure using a one-dimensional chaotic map based on mouse movements. The proposed structure showed that NIST tests were successful and could be used on personal PCs [9]. Hu et al. performed real random number generation by observing mouse movements of computer users. The statistical properties of the binary number generators generated from mouse movements of three different users were examined by the NIST test suite. Three chaos-based approaches were proposed to eliminate similar motions generated by the same user. Successful results were also achieved with these approaches [10]. Rahimi et al. used two different ECG signals for the cryptographic key generation and suggested two different approaches. The security analyses of keys obtained by both approaches were tested with distinctiveness, randomness, temporal variance, and NIST and successful results were obtained [11]. In the study performed by Chen et al. [12], random number generation was done from ECG signals and the analysis was tested by NIST test suite. It was revealed by the authors that the PRNG-based generated numbers had more successful results in classical PRNG structures. Dang et al. showed the possibility of random number generation from EEG signals. Four different EEG datasets were used to illustrate the use of obtained numbers in cryptography applications and their statistical properties were analyzed with the NIST test suite. In this PRNG-based approach, the samples consisting of EEG signals were transformed into 0 and 1 number generators. Mathematical definitions of the structure using modular arithmetic for the transformation of number generators were given. In the study, it was shown that EEG signals could be used for random number generation. The NIST test suite was used for this purpose and a success of higher than 99% was achieved [13]. In a study carried out by Chen et al. [14], the authors showed that EEG signals agreed with Gaussian distribution and also revealed whether random number could be generated from signals. They used the EEG signals obtained from both healthy and sick people for the PRNG number generation. They used NIST test suite for statistical analysis and they failed some tests. It was shown as a result of the study that the generated numbers could be used as a PRN. In a study done by Chen et al. [15], random number generation was performed by using white noise signals taken from MPEG-1, WEBCAM, and IPCAM video files and it was emphasized that successful results were obtained from statistical tests. Buhanuponp et al. proposed a new encoding method for random number generation using EEG signals. This number generator, which can be used in low cost and real applications, is based on TRNG. A success of 99.47% was obtained from statistical tests. It was revealed that it was possible to do simple and fast bit generation by encoding method [16]. The summary of the literature methods used for random number generation is shown in Table 2.

In this article, it was shown that it was possible to generate real random numbers from personally identifiable bioelectrical signals (EEG, EMG, and EOG) and physical information (blood volume pulse, GSR (Galvanic Skin Response), and respiration). The accuracy of random numbers obtained was analyzed by NIST SP 800-22, scale index, and autocorrelation tests that are commonly used in the literature and the results are given in tables. The contributions made to the literature in this article can be summarized as follows:

(1) It was shown that it was possible to generate personally identifiable random numbers.

(2) Random numbers were generated with the TRNG structure.

(3) It was revealed that random numbers can be generated by not only bioelectrical signals but also physical signals.

(4) The analyses of statistical properties were performed and successful results were obtained. Analyses were also performed by scale index and autocorrelation tests in addition to the NIST test.

The article is organized as follows to achieve the aim.

In the second section, the structures and properties of PRNG and TRNG are briefly explained. Moreover, the comparisons of these two structures are presented in tabular form. In the third section, bioelectrical and physical signals are briefly described and the properties of signals and the dataset used in the study are given. In the fourth section, the proposed TRNG structure, the normalization for number generation, and sampling and postprocessing operations are presented. The tests used for the statistical analysis of the numbers and the results obtained are tabulated in Section 5. In the last section of the article, the results are discussed and the suggestions are made about future works.

TABLE 2: Properties of random generation methods.

References	Implementation type	Noise Source	Tests	Performance
[2]	PRNG	MARC-bb Algorithm	TestU01	success
[3]	TRNG	jitter	NIST, scale index, Autocorrelation	success
[4]	PRNG	Chaos	NIST	success
[5, 17]	TRNG	jitter	NIST	success (for some test)
[7]	PRNG&TRNG	Chaos and jitter	NIST	success
[9]	TRNG	Chaotic signal	NIST	success
[10]	TRNG	Mouse movement	NIST	success
[11, 12]	PRNG	ECG	NIST	success
[13]	PRNG	EEG	NIST	success
[14]	PRNG	EEG	NIST	success (for some test)
[15]	TRNG (AVRNG)	Audio and Video	NIST	success
[16]	TRNG	EEG	NIST	success
[18]	TRNG&PRNG	Chaotic signal	NIST, FIPS	success
[19]	PRNG	Boolean function	NIST	success (for some test)
[20]	TRNG	Chaotic signal	NIST,TESTU01, scale index	success
[21, 22]	TRNG	jitter	NIST	success
[23]	PRNG	jitter	NIST	success
[24]	PRNG	chaotic maps	NIST, scale index	success
[25]	TRNG	chaotic maps	NIST, scale index	success
[26]	TRNG	Intel DRNG	TestU01, Autocorrelation	success
[27]	TRNG	Telegraph Noise	NIST, Autocorrelation	success

2. Random Number Generation Methods

Random numbers are widely used in areas such as cryptography and data transmission, luck games, secure communication, simulation, and game programming, where key generation is important. Random number generators can be divided into two classes: TRNG (True Random Number Generator) and PRNG (Pseudo Random Number Generator). Random numbers can be generated as hardware and software. The random numbers generated by the software can be defined by a specific mathematical model. On the other hand, it is possible to generate numbers by hardware with the help of noise source whose behavior cannot be predicted. Figure 1 shows the classification of random number generation.

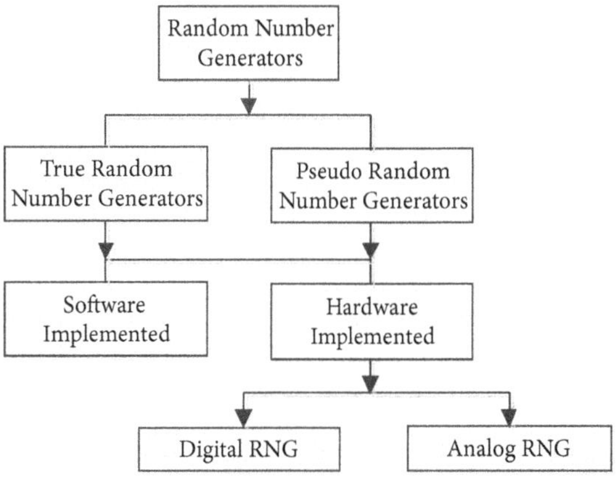

FIGURE 1: Random number generator classes.

2.1. PRNG. The general design architecture of PRNG is shown in Figure 2. $r_1, r_2, \ldots \ldots\ldots r_n \in R$ represents random number generator while $S_n \in S$ indicates the internal states of pure PRNG and P_s is defined as the probability distribution of random seed. PRNG generates r_n random number from the current S_n state provided that $\Psi : S \rightarrow R$ output function will be $r_n = \Psi(S_n)$. After that, using Φ transition function, S_n state is updated as $S_{n+1} = \Phi(S_n)$. S_0 represents the first internal state and S_1 value corresponds to the seed value of S_0 state and the equation $S_1 = \Phi(S_0)$ is generated [18]. In short, these generators need the starting parameters also known as seed. Random number generators with good quality statistics are generated by expanding these parameters with deterministic ways [19].

2.2. TRNG. The general design architecture of TRNG is shown in Figure 3. The values obtained by sampling noise

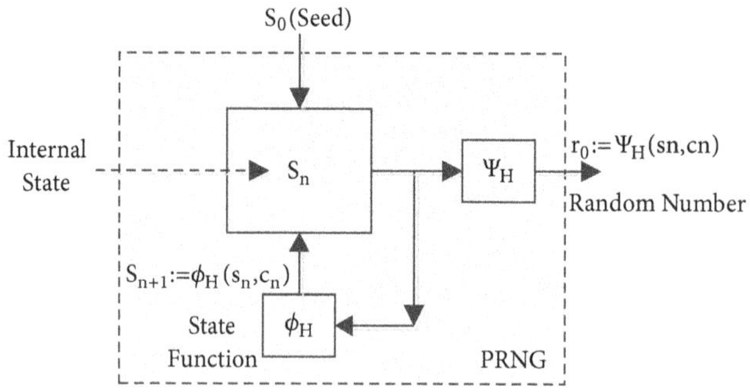

FIGURE 2: The general design architecture of PRNG.

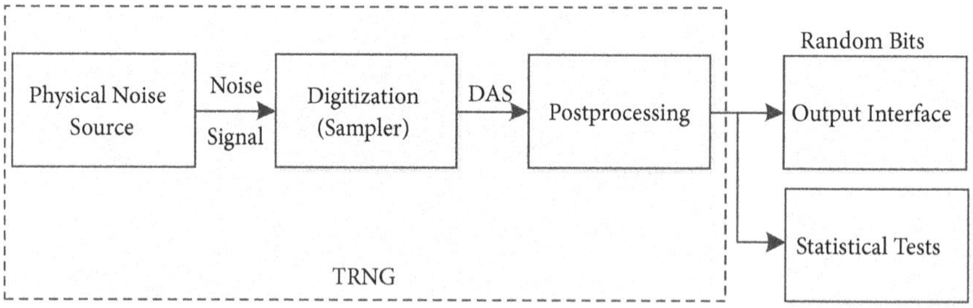

FIGURE 3: Block structure of TRNG.

TABLE 3: Comparison ofTRNG and PRNG.

	TRNG	PRNG
Realization type	Hardware required	Optional
Periodicity	Aperiodic	Periodic
Ease of application of design cycle	Complex	Easy because of standard structures
Efficiency	Weak	Perfect
Change of theoretical calculation limit	Constant (independent of time)	Dependent on time
Cryptographic security requirement	Rl, R2 requirement	Rl, R2, R3, and R4 requirements

sources are called digitalized analog signals (DAS). DAS random numbers correspond to a particular case of pure random numbers and they are subjected to algorithmic postprocessing to reduce their potential weaknesses. During this application, however, the output bit rate is reduced and the operating speed decreases.

The structural comparison of PRNG and TRNG number generators is shown in Table 3. According to Table 3, PRNGs generate fast, easily designable, and periodic numbers. On the other hand, TRNGs generate unpredictable, entropy dependent, and nonperiodic numbers. Beside these advantages, they are disadvantageous compared to PRNGs because they are hardware dependent and operate slowly.

3. Biolectrical and Physical Signals

Bioelectrical signals are low amplitude noises between 100 μV and 1 mV and are taken from the body through electrodes. The frequency spectra of such signals are in the low frequency range of 0.1 Hz ~ 2000 Hz. The amplitude and frequency characteristics of different bioelectrical signals taken from the body are shown in Table 4.

TABLE 4: Bioelectrical signals and their properties.

Signal Type	Amplitude	Frequency
EEG Electroencephalogram	2-100 μV	0.5-50 Hz
EMG Electromyogram	100 μV-1 mV	10- 500Hz
EOG Electrooculography	0.001-100 mV	0.1-10 Hz

During brain activity, continuous rhythmic electrical potentials are produced and also electrical signals are generated due to receptor activity. The recording of these electrical signals with the electrodes embedded in the skull is called electroencephalography (EEG). The amplitudes of EEG waves range from 5 to 400 μV and their frequencies change between 0.5 and 100 Hz. EEG signals are taken according to Extended International 10–20 system.

Electromyography (EMG) is a neurological examination method based on examining the electrical potentials of nerves and muscles. EMG is made in two ways by using surface electrodes and needle electrodes. In the tests using surface electrodes, electrodes are bonded to the skin surface.

TABLE 5: Bioelectrical signals and their properties.

Features	EEG	EMG	EOG	GSR	Blood Pressure	Respiration
Mean	-1.26×10^{4}	-1.825×10^{4}	3.104	150.11	-1.085×10^{5}	-1.397×10^{5}
Standard deviation	6.98×10^{3}	6.862×10^{3}	10.652	1.999	3.75×10^{3}	1.544×10^{4}

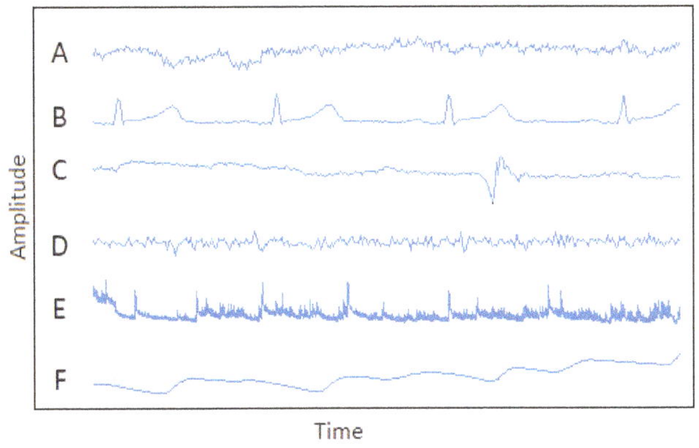

FIGURE 4: Bioelectrical and physical signals from database.

Superficial EMG can help monitor muscle and nerve disorders. In the tests using needle electrodes, needle electrodes are pricked into muscle tissue and electrical signals are recorded on muscle fibers. The amplitudes of EMG waves change between 100 μV and 1 mV and their frequencies range from 10 to 500 Hz.

Electrooculogram (EOG) signals are corneal-retinal signals between the cornea and retina formed by eye movements and caused by hyperpolarization and depolarization. EOG signals are taken with the help of electrodes placed around eyes. The EOG signals are in the frequency band of about 0.1–10 Hz and their amplitudes are about 0.001–100 mV. Horizontal and vertical EOG signals vary with eye movement. One degree of movement causes a variation of 16 μV in horizontal amplitude and 14 μV in vertical amplitude.

Among physical signals, the blood volume pulse (BVP) is used to measure heart rate. BVP measurement is obtained using a photoplethysmography (PPG) sensor. This sensor measures changes in blood volume corresponding to changes in heart rate in arteries and capillaries and blood flow. The GSR signal is one of the most sensitive indicators of emotional stimulation to show whether individuals are under stress. It gives information about the conductivity of the skin. Another physical signal, respiration, is caused by the difference between breathing air and exhaling air. With the temperature converter, the heat exchange during respiration is converted into electrical activity.

Figure 4 shows the samples bioelectrical and physical signals in the BNCIHORIZON2020 database. In this figure, the six rows of signals from top to bottom are samples EEG, EOG, EMG, GSR, and blood pressure respiration signals from the datasets A, B, C, D, E, and F, respectively. Table 5 shows mean and standard deviation of bioelectrical and physical signals.

4. Personally Identifiable Number Generation from Bioelectrical and Physical Signals

In this study, to generate TRNG-based random numbers, bioelectrical and physical signals obtained from BNCIHORIZON2020 database were used. The overall number of the databases used is fifteen. These data are four EEG, four EMG, four EOG, one blood volume pulse, one GSR (Galvanic Skin Response), and one respiration. For EEG data, the signals in the database were recorded using thirty-two Ag/AgCl active electrodes with a sampling frequency of 512 Hz according to Extended International 10–20 system. EOG and EMG signals were recorded over the left and right flexor digitorum profundus. GSR, blood volume pulse, and respiration data were recorded simultaneously with bioelectrical signals.

Real random number generation from these data includes three steps, as shown in Figure 5. These steps are normalization, digitization (sampler), and postprocessing.

In normalization, all data obtained from noise sources (raw signals) first should be transformed into binary number system. To achieve this, the operations given with their mathematical explanations below are applied. Let each signal obtained from individuals be $x=(x_1,x_2,\ldots x_n)^T$. Each sample is expressed as 5 bits by using modular arithmetic as shown in

$$y_i = x_i \bmod 32 \quad for\ i \in [1, n]. \tag{1}$$

To produce 0 and 1 from 5-bit y_i generators, z_i generator is obtained according to (2). Each element of z_i generator is in a range of [0–5].

$$z_i = \sum_{k=1}^{5} y_{i_k}. \tag{2}$$

Lastly, b_i random binary generator is obtained by using z_i generator with the help of (3). The algorithm of normalization is given below.

$$b_i = z_i \bmod 2 \quad for\ i \in [1, n]. \tag{3}$$

After this step, sampling is applied to b_i generator obtained from bioelectrical and physical signals that are used as the noise source. Periodic and nonperiodic signals are used in the literature for sampling [17, 20]. In this article, logistic map presenting nonperiodic behavior was used for sampling. Logistic map presenting chaotic behavior is defined as

$$a_{i+1} = r * a_i * (1 - a_i) \quad i = 0, 1, 2, \ldots \tag{4}$$

where r is the system parameter, a_1 is the seed or initial value, and i is the number of iterations. The numbers produced by logistic map and in a range of [0, 1] are real. Let these numbers

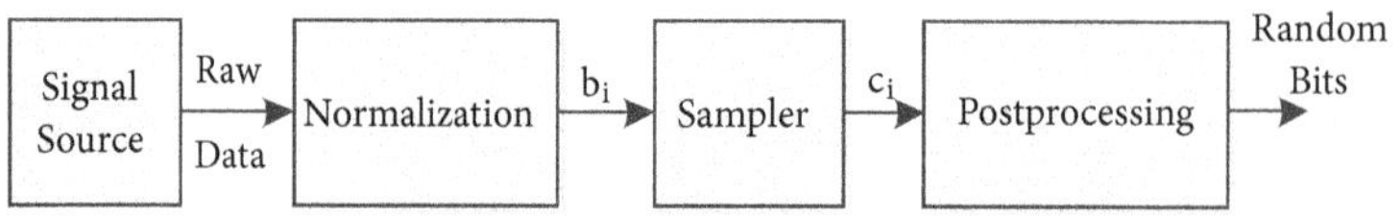

FIGURE 5: The steps of number generation.

TABLE 6: Obtaining the sampled signal.

Signals	Obtained Bits
b_i (Normalized signals)	0,1,1,1,0,1,0,1,0,0,1,0,1,0
c_i (Sampled signal obtained from Logistic map)	0,1,1,0,1,1,1,0,1,1,0,0,1,1,1
d_j (Sampled signal)	1,1, 1,0,1 1,0 0,1,0

be $_{a1}, _{a2}, _{a3} \ldots$. The expression "$a_i$ >=0.5" produced at the ith iteration indicates that the output of logistic map is assumed to be 1; otherwise it is 0. For r=3.91 and a_1=0.2, first fifteen values are 0.2, 0.625, 0.916, 0.301, 0.823, 0.568, 0.959, 0.153, 0.508, 0.977, 0.087, 0.311, 0.837, 0.533, and 0.973. The produced sampling signal will be as follows: 0,1,1,0,1,1,1,0,1,1,0,0,1,1,1. When the sampling signal becomes 1, then d_j=b_i is satisfied. When it is 0, b_i signal is neglected. This phenomenon is illustrated in Table 6. Sampling operation is given in Algorithm 2.

Postprocessing is applied to improve statistical properties of sampled random number generators. XOR, Von Neumann, LFSR, and Hash function structures are commonly used in the literature for postprocessing [21, 28]. In this study, XOR postprocessing was used. When sequential numbers are 0,1 and 1,0 with XOR in the random number generator, real random number is assumed to be 1 and otherwise 0. When XOR postprocessing is applied to the sampled 1110110010 number generator obtained in Table 5, the number generator obtained will be 01001.The algorithm for postprocessing is given in Algorithm 3.

5. Statistical Analysis of Random Numbers

NIST SP 800-22, scale index, and autocorrelation tests—commonly used in the literature—were used for the statistical analysis of generated random numbers.

5.1. NIST SP 800-22 Statistical Test Suite. NIST SP 800-22 is a test commonly used for statistical analysis of the numbers obtained from TRNG, PRNG, Physical Unclonable Function (PUF), and their hybrid generators [21–23]. NIST test suite includes fifteen tests and the parameters of each test are given in the related study [29]. The α value known as the level of significance is one of the most important parameters in the test. The selection of α as 0 indicates that the randomness of numbers to be tested has a confidence value of 99%. Another parameter is p value and it is known as the measure of randomness. If this value is equal to 1, numbers are said to have perfect randomness. If p value becomes 0, numbers are not random. The α value of personally identifiable random numbers to be used for key and verification applications should be appropriately selected. For each test, if p value is greater than or equal to α value, then the test is successful. Otherwise the test becomes unsuccessful; i.e., the numbers generated are not random. Generally, α is selected from [0.001, 0.01] range.

NIST test suite analysis results of personally identifiable random numbers obtained from bioelectrical and physical signals in the dataset are shown in Tables 7 and 8, respectively. As can be seen from tables, all data used was successful in the NIST test because their p value was higher than 0.01.

5.2. Scale Index Test. The scale index test was applied for statistical analysis of numbers. The scale index technique was proposed by Benitez [30]. This technique was used to determine the information about the degree of nonperiodicity of a signal or generated number series. In literature, for determining the periodicity of TRNG and PRNG, the scale index test was used [24, 25]. The scale index was based on the continuous wavelet transform and wavelet multiresolution analyses. The scales s and f at time u in the continuous wavelet transform (CWT) and scalogram were shown as given in equations (5) and (6) [22]. One has

$$Wf(u,s) := \langle f, \psi_{u,s} \rangle = \int_{-\infty}^{+\infty} f(t)\, \psi^*_{u,s}(t)\, dt \quad (5)$$

$$(s) := \|Wf(u,s)\| = \left(\int_{-\infty}^{+\infty} |Wf(u,s)|^2 du \right) \quad (6)$$

The continuous wavelet transform's energy of f at a scale s was illustrated as $S(s)$. Equation (7) shows the inner scalogram of f at a scale s.

$$\mathrm{S^{in}}(s) := \|\mathrm{Wf}(u,s)\|_{j(s)} = \left(\int_{c(s)}^{d(s)} |\mathrm{Wf}(u,s)|^2 \mathrm{du} \right)^2 \quad (7)$$

where $J(s) = [c(s), d(s)] \subseteq I$ is the maximal subinterval in I for which the support of $\psi_{u,s}$ is included in I for all $u \in j(s)$. Considering that the length of $J(s)$ depends on the scale s, the values of the inner scalogram at different scales cannot be compared. The normalized s^{in} is defined as shown in

$$\overline{S}^{in}(s) = \frac{S^{in}(s)}{(d(s) - c(s))^{1/2}}. \quad (8)$$

TABLE 7: NIST test results obtained from bioelectrical signals.

Test Type	EEG1	EEG2	EEG3	EEG4	EMG1	EMG2	EMG3	EMG4	EOG1	EOG2	EOG3	EOG4
Frequency Monobit	*0.4564*	0.016	0.539	0.784	0.324	0.523	0.663	0.961	0.701	0.406	0.047	0.737
Frequency Test within a Block	0.492	0.184	0.252	0.744	0.253	0.594	0.294	0.058	0.805	0.916	0.725	0.264
Runs	0.445	0.221	0.358	0.734	0.676	0.453	0.506	0.258	0.440	0.246	0.842	0.388
Longest Run of Ones in a Block	0.277	0.428	0.295	0.131	0.853	0.046	0.094	0.221	0.087	0.871	0.616	0.973
Binary Matrix Rank	0.774	0.648	0.980	0.458	0.579	0.402	0.795	0.354	0.481	0.481	0.636	0.448
Discrete Fourier Transform	0.212	0.295	0.798	0.784	0.996	0.964	0.408	0.108	0.032	0.773	0.531	0.348
Non Overlapping Template Matching	*0.234*	0.451	0.553	0.947	0.880	0.925	0.218	0.431	0.477	0.397	0.568	0.843
Overlapping Template Matching	0.510	0.310	0.712	0.119	0.631	0.615	0.348	0.028	0.633	0.838	0.363	0.715
Universal	0.436	0.235	0.533	0.661	0.748	0.117	0.659	0.527	0.219	0.371	0.567	0.512
Linear Complexity	0.745	0.874	0.236	0.225	0.318	0.374	0.453	0.178	0.959	0.985	0.406	0.210
Serial	0.560 /0.437	0.026 /0.211	0.540 /0.357	0.909 /0.734	0.565 /0.679	0.616 /0454	0.723 /0.498	0.526 /0.257	0.714 /0.468	0338 /0.224	0.138 /0.826	0.651 /0.388
Approximate Entropy	0.254	0.330	0.690	0.532	0.840	0.305	0.026	0.757	0.345	0.324	0.176	0.710
Cumulative Sums	0.469	0.014	0.171	0.875	0.503	0.802	0.410	0.405	0.894	0.416	0.042	0736
Random excursions test*	0.712	0.337	0.501	0.287	0.746	0.253	0.413	0.682	0.485	0.226	0.711	0.603
Random excursions variant test*	0.519	0.483	0.645	0.831	0.452	0.846	0.445	0.577	0.186	0.705	0.694	0.279

*More than one p value was obtained and it was found that p value > 0.01. The values given for these tests are average.

TABLE 8: NIST test results obtained from physical signals.

Test Type	GSR	Blood Pressure	Respiration
Frequency Monobit	0.715	0.079	0.951
Frequency Test within a Block	0.125	0.213	0.412
Runs	0.445	0.490	0.290
Longest Run of Ones in a Block	0.230	0.762	0.639
Binary Matrix Rank	0.490	0.232	0.208
Discrete Fourier Transform	0.916	0.469	0.826
Non Overlapping Template Matching	0.817	0.734	0.140
Overlapping Template Matching	0.415	0.040	0.962
Universal	0.043	0.115	0.636
Linear Complexity	0.388	0.560	0.680
Serial	0.698 /0.444	0.166 /0.473	0.578 /0.295
Approximate Entropy	0.422	0.0.485	0.092
Cumulative Sums	0.773	0.055	0.345
Random excursions test*	0.252	0.289	0.601
Random excursions variant test*	0.333	0.427	0.397

*More than one p value was obtained and it was found that p value > 0.01. The values given for these tests are average.

TABLE 9: Scale index test results of datasets.

	1. Dataset	2. Dataset	3. Dataset	4. Dataset
EEG	0.924	0.936	0.973	0.951
EMG	0.944	0.955	0.957	0.924
EOG	0.756	0.763	0.861	0.804
Blood Pressure	0.936			
GSR	0.964			
Respiration	0.879			

Equation (9) shows the scale index of f in the scale interval $[s_0, s_1]$.

$$i_{scale} := \frac{S(s_{min})}{S(s_{max})}. \tag{9}$$

The degree of nonperiodicity of bioelectrical and physical magnitudes was determined by the scale index test whose details were explained above. Table 9 shows obtained scale index values.

The scale index value i_{scale} should be in the range of $0 \leq i_{scale} \leq 1$. If the scale value obtained from the generated system is 0 or near 0, then the system is defined as periodic and if 1 or near to 1, then it is defined as nonperiodic. According to Table 8, it was observed that the results obtained from both bioelectrical and physical signals were successful in scale index test and they were close to 1.

5.3. Autocorrelation Test. Finally, to observe the variations of 0 and 1 s in the generated random numbers the autocorrelation test was used [26, 27].

Equation (10) shows the mathematical definitions of the test [31].

$$A(d) = \sum_{i=0}^{n-d-1} b_i \oplus b_{i+d} \tag{10}$$

where $\oplus$ is the XOR operator, n is the length of the generated number sequences, and b_i represents the number sequence. The d value is the constant integer and between $[1,(n/2)]$. Equation (11) shows the relationship between 0 and 1s.

$$X5 = \frac{2\left[A(d) - (n-d)/2\right]}{\sqrt{n-d}}. \tag{11}$$

For $\alpha = 0.05$, if $|X5| < 1.6449$, then the test is successful.

Autocorrelation test was used to determine 0-1 change in the random numbers obtained from both bioelectrical and physical magnitudes. Table 10 shows autocorrelation test results. As seen in Table 9, for each dataset, $|X5|$ value is in the specified interval. Thus, random numbers obtained from both bioelectrical and physical signals were successful in autocorrelation test.

TABLE 10: Autocorrelation test results of datasets.

d		8	10	13
EEG datasets	1	0.205	0.445	0.302
	2	1.289	0.159	0.896
	3	0.216	0.285	1.169
	4	0.627	0.776	0.599
EMG datasets	1	1.175	0.593	0.633
	2	0.253	1.08	0.382
	3	1.261	0.688	0.991
	4	0.836	1.498	1.137
EOG datasets	1	1.068	0.812	0.107
	2	1.089	1.431	0.727
	3	1.497	0.927	1.182
	4	0.896	0.346	0.111
Blood Pres.	1	1.381	0.468	0.359
GSR	1	0.833	0.890	0.188
Respiration	1	0.730	0.993	1.030

```
x = (x_1, x_2, ... x_n)^T            //Data set
for i=1 to n
    y_i=x_i mod (32)                 // y_i between [0-31]
    convert y_i to binary format
    z_i=0
    for k=1 to 5
        z_i= z_i+ y_{i,k}
    end
    b_i= z_i mod (2)                 //normalized 0-1 data
end
```

ALGORITHM 1: Normalization procedure.

```
Set the initial value: a_1=0.2, r=3.91, c_1=0
for i=1 to n
    a_{i+1}=a_i*r*(1- a_i)           // a_i between [0-1]
    if a_i ≥ 0.5 then
        c_i=1
    else
        c_i=0
    end if
end
j=1
for i=1 to n
    if c_i==1 then
        d_j= b_i                     //d_j: sampled number
        j=j+1
    end if
end
```

ALGORITHM 2: Sampler procedure.

```
Set the initial value: k=1
for i=1 to j-1, update i=i+2
    number_k=d_i XOR d_{i+1}
    k=k+1
end
```

ALGORITHM 3: Postprocessing procedure.

6. Discussion and Conclusion

Random numbers have been generated in the literature from bioelectrical signals such as EEG. These numbers have the PRNG structure. However, the statistical properties of the numbers generated from EEG signals are not good. In this article, the TRNG structure using bioelectrical and physical signals as a source of randomness was proposed. Although the taken signals are periodic, the level of noise that would emerge from any source on the signal causes the signal to be nonperiodic. In this case, the random numbers to be generated are unpredictable. Personally identifiable random numbers were generated from the obtained raw signals using normalization (see Algorithm 1), sampling, and postprocessing operations. The process is faster than the TRNG structures in the literature because of the simple structure of normalization, sampling, and postprocessing. NIST SP 800-22 test was used to show that the statistical properties of the generated numbers were improved; scale index test was used to reveal the level of nonperiodicity and autocorrelation tests were used to observe 0 and 1 change of numbers. All test results were presented in tabular form and all results were found to be successful. The results indicate that TRN generation from bioelectrical and physical signals obtained from the human body is possible.

Thus, the obtained random numbers are suitable for use in different areas, such as key generation, authentication, games of chance, simulation, and game programming. It is possible to carry out various studies on random number generation using these bioelectrical and physical signals as well as different types of signals like EGG and ECG. The present study will be the basis for random number generation using such signals.

Conflicts of Interest

The authors declare that there are no conflicts of interest regarding the publication of this paper.

References

[1] M. Bakiri, C. Guyeux, J.-F. Couchot, and A. K. Oudjida, "Survey on hardware implementation of random number generators on FPGA: theory and experimental analyses," *Computer Science Review*, vol. 27, pp. 135–153, 2018.

[2] J. Li, J. Zheng, and P. Whitlock, "Efficient deterministic and non-deterministic pseudorandom number generation," *Mathematics and Computers in Simulation*, vol. 143, pp. 114–124, 2018.

[3] T. Tuncer, "The implementation of chaos-based PUF designs in field programmable gate array," *Nonlinear Dynamics*, vol. 86, no. 2, pp. 975–986, 2016.

[4] F. Özkaynak, "Cryptographically secure random number generator with chaotic additional input," *Nonlinear Dynamics*, vol. 78, no. 3, pp. 2015–2020, 2014.

[5] T. Tuncer, "Implementation of duplicate TRNG on FPGA by using two different randomness source," *Elektronika ir Elektrotechnika*, vol. 21, no. 4, pp. 35–39, 2015.

[6] M. Dichtl, *Bad and Good Ways of Post-processing Biased Physical Random Numbers*, vol. 4593 of *Lecture Notes in Computer Science*, Springer, Berlin, Germany, 2007.

[7] E. Avaroglu, T. Tuncer, A. B. Özer, and M. Türk, "A new method for hybrid pseudo random number generator," *Journal of Microelectronics, Electronic Components and Materials*, vol. 4, no. 4, pp. 303–311, 2014.

[8] E. Jokar and M. Mikaili, "Assessment of Human Random Number Generation for Biometric Verification," *Journal of Medical Signals and Sensors*, vol. 2, no. 2, pp. 82–87, 2012.

[9] W. Xingyuan, Q. Xue, and T. Lin, "A novel true random number generator based on mouse movement and a one-dimensional chaotic map," *Mathematical Problems in Engineering*, vol. 2012, Article ID 931802, 9 pages, 2012.

[10] Y. Hu, X. Liao, K.-W. Wong, and Q. Zhou, "A true random number generator based on mouse movement and chaotic cryptography," *Chaos, Solitons & Fractals*, vol. 40, no. 5, pp. 2286–2293, 2009.

[11] S. R. Moosavi, E. Nigussie, S. Virtanen, and J. Isoaho, "Cryptographic key generation using ECG signal," in *Proceedings of the 14th IEEE Annual Consumer Communications and Networking Conference, CCNC 2017*, pp. 1024–1031, usa, January 2017.

[12] X. Chen, Y. Zhang, G. Zhang, and Y. Zhang, "Evaluation of ECG random number generator for wireless body sensor networks security," in *Proceedings of the 2012 5th International Conference on Biomedical Engineering and Informatics, BMEI 2012*, pp. 1308–1311, October 2012.

[13] D. Nguyen, D. Tran, W. Ma, and K. Nguyen, "EEG-Based random number generators," *Lecture Notes in Computer Science (including subseries Lecture Notes in Artificial Intelligence and Lecture Notes in Bioinformatics): Preface*, vol. 10394, pp. 248–256, 2017.

[14] G. Chen, "Are electroencephalogram (EEG) signals pseudo-random number generators?" *Journal of Computational and Applied Mathematics*, vol. 268, pp. 1–4, 2014.

[15] I.-T. Chen, "Random numbers generated from audio and video sources," *Mathematical Problems in Engineering*, vol. 2013, Article ID 285373, 7 pages, 2013.

[16] B. Petchlert and H. Hasegawa, "Using a low-cost electroencephalogram (EEG) directly as random number generator," in *Proceedings of the 3rd IIAI International Conference on Advanced Applied Informatics, IIAI-AAI 2014*, pp. 470–474, September 2014.

[17] T. Tuncer, E. Avaroglu, M. Türk, and A. B. Ozer, "Implementation of non-periodic sampling true random number generator on fpga," *Informacije Midem*, vol. 44, no. 4, pp. 296–302, 2014.

[18] E. Avaroglu, İ. Koyuncu, A. B. Özer et al., "Hybrid pseudo-random number generator for cryptographic systems," *Nonlinear Dynamics*, vol. 82, no. 1-2, pp. 239–248, 2015.

[19] A. A. Maaita and H. A. A. Al_Sewadi, "Deterministic Random Number Generator Algorithm for Cryptosystem Keys," *World Academy of Science, Engineering and Technology International Journal of Computer and Information Engineering*, vol. 9, no. 4, 2015.

[20] E. Avaroğlu, T. Tuncer, A. B. Özer, B. Ergen, and M. Türk, "A novel chaos-based post-processing for TRNG," *Nonlinear Dynamics*, vol. 81, no. 1-2, pp. 189–199, 2015.

[21] S. Buchovecká, R. Lórencz, F. Kodýtek, and J. Buček, "True random number generator based on ring oscillator PUF circuit," *Microprocessors and Microsystems*, vol. 53, pp. 33–41, 2017.

[22] I. Cicek, A. E. Pusane, and G. Dundar, "A novel design method for discrete time chaos based true random number generators," *Integration, the VLSI Journal*, vol. 47, no. 1, pp. 38–47, 2014.

[23] S. Chen, B. Li, and C. Zhou, "FPGA implementation of SRAM PUFs based cryptographically secure pseudo-random number generator," *Microprocessors and Microsystems*, vol. 59, pp. 57–68, 2018.

[24] Y. Yang and Q. Zhao, "Novel pseudo-random number generator based on quantum random walks," *Scientific Reports*, vol. 6, no. 1, 2016.

[25] B. Karakaya, V. Çelik, and A. Gülten, "Chaotic cellular neural network-based true random number generator," *International Journal of Circuit Theory and Applications*, vol. 45, no. 11, pp. 1885–1897, 2017.

[26] J. J. Chan, P. Thulasiraman, G. Thomas, and R. Thulasiram, "Ensuring Quality of Random Numbers from TRNG: Design and Evaluation of Post-Processing Using Genetic Algorithm," *Journal of Computer and Communications*, vol. 04, no. 04, pp. 73–92, 2016.

[27] X. Chen, L. Wang, B. Li et al., "Modeling Random Telegraph Noise as a Randomness Source and its Application in True Random Number Generation," *IEEE Transactions on Computer-Aided Design of Integrated Circuits and Systems*, vol. 35, no. 9, pp. 1435–1448, 2016.

[28] V. Rozic, B. Yang, W. Dehaene, and I. Verbauwhede, "Iterating von Neumann's post-processing under hardware constraints," in *Proceedings of the 2016 IEEE International Symposium on Hardware Oriented Security and Trust, HOST 2016*, pp. 37–42, May 2016.

[29] NIST Special Publication 800-22, 2001. http://csrc.nist.gov/rng/rng2.html.

[30] R. Benìtez, V. J. Bolos, and M. E. Ramìrez, "A wavelet-based tool for studying non-periodicity," *Computers & Mathematics with Applications. An International Journal*, vol. 60, no. 3, pp. 634–641, 2010.

[31] A. J. Menezes, P. C. van Oorschot, and S. A. Vanstone, *Handbook of Applied Cryptography*, CRC Press, New York, NY, USA, 1996.

11

The Application of Dynamic Models to the Exploration of β_1-AR Overactivation as a Cause of Heart Failure

Xiaoyun Wang,[1,2] Min Zhao,[1] Xiaoqiang Wang,[2] Shuping Li,[3] Ning Cao,[4,5] and Huirong Liu[4,5]

[1]*College of Mathematics, Taiyuan University of Technology, Taiyuan, Shanxi, China*
[2]*Department of Scientific Computing, Florida State University, Tallahassee, FL, USA*
[3]*Department of Mathematics, North University of China, Taiyuan, Shanxi, China*
[4]*Department of Physiology and Pathophysiology, School of Basic Medical Sciences, Capital Medical University, Beijing, China*
[5]*Beijing Key Laboratory of Metabolic Disorders Related Cardiovascular Diseases, Capital Medical University, Beijing, China*

Correspondence should be addressed to Xiaoyun Wang; xywang0708@126.com, Xiaoqiang Wang; wwang3@fsu.edu, and Huirong Liu; liuhr2000@126.com

Academic Editor: Jesús Poza

High titer of β_1-adrenoreceptor autoantibodies (β_1-AA) has been reported to appear in heart failure patients. It induces sustained β_1-adrenergic receptor (β_1-AR) activation which leads to heart failure (HF), but the mechanism is as yet unclear. In order to investigate the mechanisms causing β_1-AR non-desensitization, we studied the beating frequency of the neonatal rat cardiomyocytes (NRCMs) under different conditions (an injection of isoprenaline (ISO) for one group and β_1-AA for the other) and established three dynamic models in order to best describe the true relationships shown in medical experiments; one model used a control group of healthy rats; then in HF rats one focused on conformation changes in β_1-AR; the other examined interaction between β_1-AR and β_2-adrenergic receptors (β_2-AR). Comparing the experimental data and corresponding Akaike information criterion (AIC) values, we concluded that the interaction model was the most likely mechanism. We used mathematical methods to explore the mechanism for the development of heart failure and to find potential targets for prevention and treatment. The aim of the paper was to provide a strong theoretical basis for the clinical development of personalized treatment programs. We also carried out sensitivity analysis of the initial concentration β_1-AA and found that they had a noticeable effect on the fitting results.

1. Introduction

The incidence of heart failure (HF) is increasing year by year throughout the world, as is the cost of treating it [1]. Accurately recognising the cardiac signals associated with HF not only would prevent the progress of chronic HF, but also can guide individual treatment and positively influence the normal progression of the disease [2]. A variety of mechanisms are involved in HF progression, including nervous system inhibition. Heart failure itself causes cardiovascular irregularity due to material imbalance and cell damage [3]. Studies have shown that sustained activation of the sympathetic nervous system (SNS) is the core mechanism trigger of heart failure [4]. The main way in which the overactivation of the SNS occurs is the overactivation of the cardiomyocytes at the β_1-adrenergic receptor (β_1-AR) [5]. β_1-adrenergic receptor autoantibodies (β_1-AA) were found in the serum of patients with dilated cardiomyopathy in a study [6]. As β_1-AA can bind with and activate β_1-AR, it has a β_1-AR agonist-like effect [7]. Excessive activation of β_1-AR leads to impaired cardiac function [8]. A study found that, in addition to catecholamine β_1-AR agonist ISO, β_1-adrenoceptor (β_1-AA) autoantibodies that could cause continuous activation of β_1-AR [9] were detected in 40%–60% of HF patients [8]. β_1-AR and β_2-AR (β_1-adrenergic receptors) link through the C-terminal, which are within cardiac cells, and belong to the G protein-coupled receptor family [10]. β_1-AR and β_2-AR can form heterodimers [11], where β_2-AR downstream couples with stimulatory G protein (G_s) and inhibitory G protein (G_i) [12]. Another study [13] found that, in the early stages of heart failure, when β_1-AR is activated, it can cause the β_2-AR downstream signal to be converted from G_s to G_i, and G_i is activated by the activity of G protein-coupled receptor kinase 2 (GRK2), which then causes β_1-AR phosphorylation, as well as β-arrestin binding to form endocytosis, after which β_1-AR endocytosis [13] inhibits the overactivation of β_1-AA. There are two main mechanisms involved in the continuous activation of β_1-AR: β_1-AR conformation changes and interaction between β_1-AR and β_2-AR. However, the mechanisms for how β_1-AA induces continuous activation of β_1-AR are not entirely clear.

To identify the core molecular mechanism of β_1-AR non-desensitization, we adopted a novel approach by establishing differential dynamic models. We used C_{++} to estimate the parameters, obtained modified 60-minute snapshots highlighting the experimental data, and made predictions on how the images would progress over the next 60 minutes. Then we took advantage of AIC to select the optimal model of β_1-AR non-desensitization induced by β_1-AA, and the corresponding mechanism. β_2-AR plays an important role in the activation of β_1-AR, which can be used to estimate cardiac function, prevent deterioration of cardiac function, and improve the quality of life of the patients with HF.

This paper is organized as follows. In Section 2, we established the models and listed the differential equations separately. Section 3 focused on the analysis of the models and determination of the parameters. We select the optimal model to identify the key molecular mechanism, by applying the Akaike information criterion (AIC). Results on the sensitivity analysis of parameters are given in Section 4. Section 5 is the conclusion.

Figure 1 shows the interrelationships between the various substances. It reflects the receptor desensitization when the β_1-AR is combined with ISO and non-desensitization when the β_1-AR is combined with β_1-AA, causing conformational changes and interaction between the β_1-AR and the β_2-AR, eventually leading to HF.

2. Methods

2.1. Extraction and Detection of Neonatal Rat Cardiomyocytes. Laboratory animal medicine of Capital Medical University provided 20 male newborn rats born 0–3 days as raw materials for extracting neonatal rat cardiomyocytes. According to previous method [14], the details of myocardial cell isolation and culture of neonatal rats are as follows: (1) open the sternum, expose the heart, clip it with tweezers, and wash in cold phosphate-buffered saline (PBS); (2) remove excess connective tissue from the washed heart and cut with ophthalmic scissors; (3) the heart fragments were aspirated into a centrifuge tube, and cold PBS was added and then centrifuged at 1000 *rpm* for 5 *mins*; (4) remove the centrifuge tube and vacuum suction PBS; (5) add 1 *ml* of 0.25 % trypsin and 1 *ml* of 0.25 % collagenase, blow vigorously, set in a 37°*C* water bath, and shake for 20 *mins*; (6) add 1 *ml* fetal bovine serum to stop digestion; (7) digestion was collected by adding 2 *ml* of DMEM containing 10% fetal bovine serum (FBS), 1000 *rpm*, and after centrifugation for 10 *mins*, the supernatant was discarded and fresh medium was added for differential adherence; (8) after adherence for 1 *h*, the culture medium was transferred to a new centrifuge tube and centrifuged at 1000 *rpm* for 5 *mins*. Cells were collected and the supernatant was discarded. Fresh medium was added and transferred to a 6-well plate for cell culture and 2 *ml* of DMEM low-glucose medium was added to each well. Detection of the beating frequency of NRCMs [15] was as follows: the culture medium was replaced on the day of the experiment and stably incubating in a 37°*C* cell culture incubator for 30 minutes, the 6-well plate was placed on a constant-temperature table of inverted microscopy, and a total of 10 fields of view of 3 six-well plates were randomly observed. Each field was measured for 30 seconds at a time, and the number of synchronized contractions of an isolated single cell or a group of cardiomyocytes in the untreated group was measured.

Table 1: Data on frequency of beats of measured NRCMs added to ISO.

Time (*min*)	Mean values (*bmp*) n=3	Standard Deviation (*bmp*)
0.0	0	3.055
1.0	24.667	5.292
3.0	36.667	3.464
5.0	33.46	7.211
7.0	37.837	4.163
9.0	22.0	4.163
10.0	15.333	5.774
20.0	10.0	1.155
30.0	9.333	3.055
60.0	2.667	4.0

Then, we used 0.1μM of ISO, β_1-AA, and IgG (immunoglobulin G) (eliminating the effects of β_1-AA itself) to stimulate, respectively. After that, the beating frequency of NRCMs was measured by Live Cell Imaging System offered by Medical Sciences Center Lab of Capital Medical University. Specifically, we measured the frequency in beat per minute of the cardiomyocytes after stimulation by live cell workstation and visualization at 63-fold magnification. Before being exposed to drugs, the cells had been stabilized for 10 *mins* in the system. The present study complies with the recommendations in the Guide for the Care and Use of Laboratory Animals protocol, NIH guidelines (Guide for the Care and Use of Laboratory Animals), and conformed to AVMA Guidelines on Euthanasia.

Tables 1 and 2 showed the measured data of beating frequency of NRCMs added to ISO and β_1-AA. We used the beat frequency of NRCMs at time 0 as the base value, which was recorded as 0. When the standard deviation was greater than or equal to 4, the data was appropriately adjusted within the scope of standard deviation.

Figure 2 reflects the positive correlation between concentration and beating frequency of NRCMs. Also, Martinsson et al. [16] studied the relationship between ISO and heart rate in their experiment results.

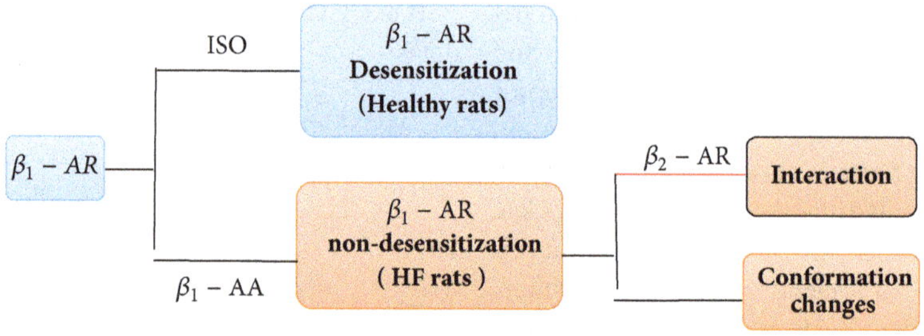

FIGURE 1: Relation diagram among the ISO, β_1-AA, β_1-AR, and β_2-AR.

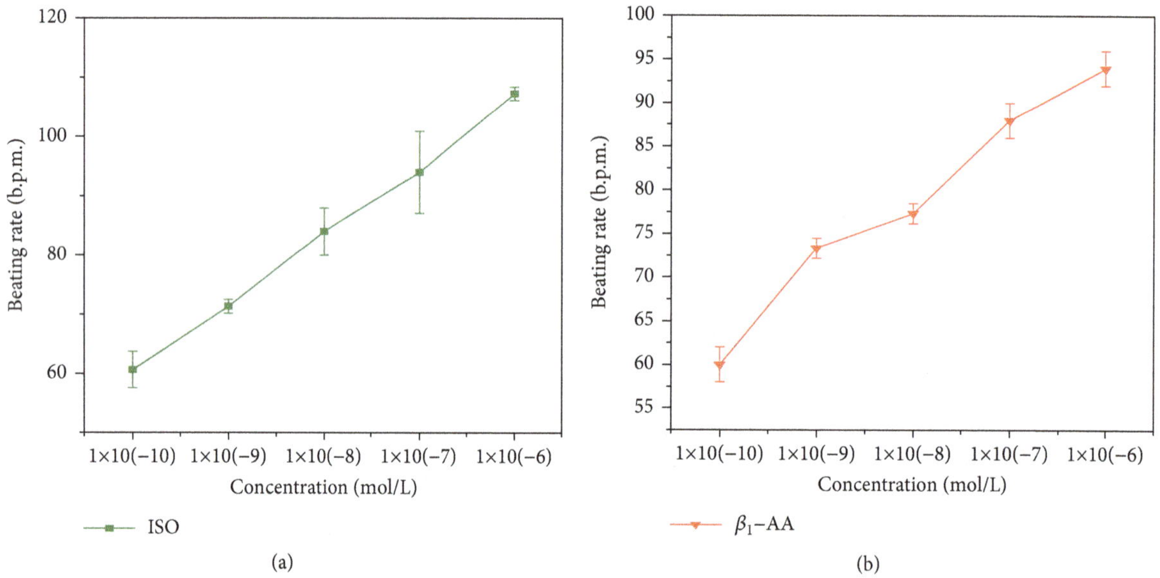

FIGURE 2: Relationship between different reactant concentrations and beating frequency of NRCMs. **(a)** Control model in three minutes. **(b)** Experiment model in three minutes. Multiple sets of experiments were performed using the previously mentioned method for detecting NRCMs, and the beating frequency of NRCMs at a concentration of 0.1 nM to 1 μM was measured.

TABLE 2: Data on frequency of beats of measured NRCMs added to $\beta_1 - AA$.

Time (min)	Mean values (bmp) n=3	Standard Deviation (bmp)
0.0	0.0	2.0
1.0	22.0	2.0
3.0	26.0	2.0
5.0	30.0	3.464
7.0	31.5	7.024
9.0	32.2	5.774
10.0	32.33	4.619
20.0	32.5	7.211
30.0	33.0	5.292
60.0	33.0	6.0

2.2. The Models. There are many molecular mechanisms causing β_1-AR non-desensitization, among which conformation changes and interaction are the most likely ones. In order to clarify the most likely molecular mechanism, we established dynamical models including control model and experiment models to study the specific molecular mechanisms.

2.2.1. Explanation of Interaction

Definition 1 (a protein-to-protein interaction (*PPI*) [17]). Proteins rarely act alone as their functions tend to be regulated. Many molecular processes within a cell are carried out by molecular machines that are built from a large number of protein components organized by their *PPIs* (protein-protein interactions). In the experimental groups, β_1-AR and β_2-AR belong to the G protein-coupled receptor family that are connected through the C-terminus [10] which belongs to PPI. Although β_1-AA does not directly bind to β_2-AR, β_1-AA will indirectly affect the conformation of β_2-AR by activating β_1-AR based on the studies of laboratory animal medicine of Capital Medical University. Therefore, β_1-AA can interfere with their dimerization which reflects the fact that β_2-AR can affect the persistence of β_1-AR activation.

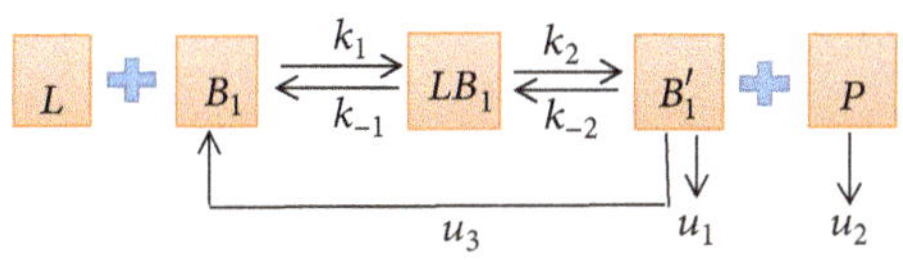

FIGURE 3: The block diagram of control model. ISO (L) activates β_1-AR (B_1) receptor generating intermediate complexes LB_1 causing endocytosis of β_1-AR, so that it can no longer come into contact with the protected ligand; then the complexes LB produce a new substance P and structurally changed receptor β_1-AR (B_1') that returns to the cell surface to terminate the signal.

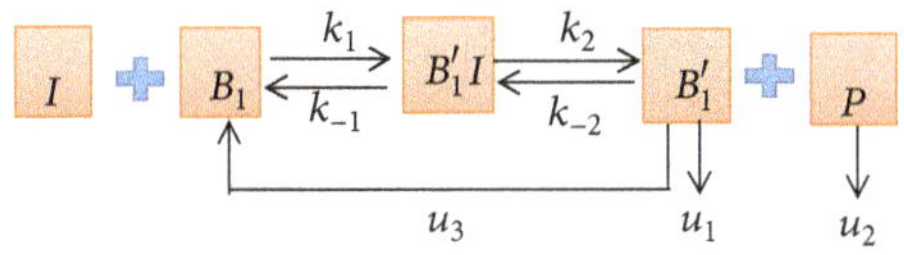

FIGURE 4: The block diagram of conformation changes model. β_1-AA (I) activates β_1-AR (B_1) receptor generating intermediate complexes $B_1'I$ with conformation changes. The production of $B_1'I$ continues to activate the signal, and then it produces a new substance P and structurally changed receptor β_1-AR (B_1').

2.2.2. The Establishment of the Model Block Diagrams. The possible molecular mechanisms about β_1-AR overactivation are conformation changes and interaction. To determine a more specific molecular mechanism, we propose the dynamical models including control model and experiment models, where experiment models are composed of conformation changes model and interaction model. In order to facilitate the study and simplify the reaction diagram, we use corresponding letters instead of reactants and the definition of the corresponding parameters in dynamical models; see Table 3.

(1) The Block Diagram of Control Model (See Figure 3). In Figure 3, k_1 represents the combined velocity of L and B_1, k_{-1} represents the reverse reaction velocity, k_2 represents the velocity of LB_1 decomposition, k_{-2} is the reverse reaction velocity, and u_1 and u_2 represent the degradation velocity of B_1' and P, respectively. u_3 represents the velocity at which undegraded B_1' returns to the cell surface and participates in the reaction again.

(2) The Block Diagram of Conformation Changes Model (See Figure 4). In Figure 4, k_1 represents the combined velocity of I and B_1, k_{-1} represents the reverse reaction velocity, k_2 represents the velocity of $B_1'I$ decomposition, k_{-2} is the reverse reaction velocity, and u_1 and u_2 represent the degradation velocity of B_1' and P, respectively. u_3 represents the velocity at which undegraded B_1' returns to the cell surface and participates in the reaction again.

(3) The Block Diagram of Interaction Model (See Figure 5). In Figure 5, k_1 represents the combined velocity of I and B_1B_2, k_{-1} represents the reverse reaction velocity, k_2 represents the velocity of B_1IB_2 decomposition, k_3 represents the velocity of $(B_1I)'$ decomposition, and u_1 and u_2 represent the degradation velocity of B_1' and P, respectively. u_3 represents the velocity at which undegraded B_1' returns to the cell surface and participates in the reaction again. Also, β_1-AR and β_2-AR

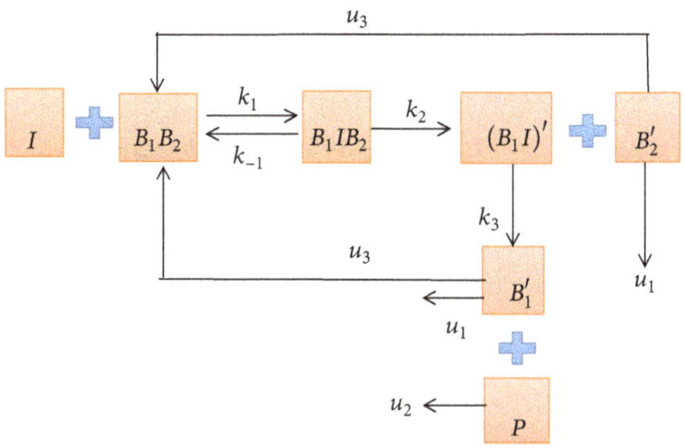

FIGURE 5: The block diagram of interaction model. We also take β_2-AR (B_2) into consideration in the reaction based on medical experiments. According to the studies of laboratory animal medicine of Capital Medical University, they found that β_1-AA had a unique characteristic that can inhibit heterodimerization of β_1/β_2-AR and thus lead to decompose of β_1-AR and β_2-AR that are originally connected, resulting in endocytosis inhibition and sustained activation of the signal. Therefore, there is no conjugation of β_1-AR and β_2-AR (B_1B_2) in the products. Besides, β_1-AA (I) cannot directly bind to β_2-AR (B_2), so there is no IB_2 in the products. Thus, we consider that B_1IB_2 (I and B_2 are combined to B_1) are intermediate complexes and $B_1'I$, B_2' are the products with structure change.

belong to the G protein-coupled receptor family [10], and thus we assume that they have the same degradation velocity u_1.

Next, we established three mathematical models as shown in Figures 3, 4, and 5 and established the corresponding ordinary differential equations based on the relevant theoretical knowledge of biochemical reaction models in cell and molecular biology [18, 19].

2.2.3. Corresponding Differential Equations

(1) The Control Model. we propose a control model for healthy rats based on Figure 3. The time evolution of control model is described by five coupled differential equations.

$$\begin{aligned}
\frac{d[L]}{dt} &= -k_1[L][B_1] + k_{-1}[LB_1], \\
\frac{d[B_1]}{dt} &= -k_1[L][B_1] + k_{-1}[LB_1] + u_3[B_1'], \\
\frac{d[LB_1]}{dt} &= k_1[L][B_1] - k_{-1}[LB_1] - k_2[LB_1] \\
&\quad + k_{-2}[B_1'][P], \\
\frac{d[B_1']}{dt} &= k_2[LB_1] - u_1[B_1'] - u_3[B_1'] \\
&\quad - k_{-2}[B_1'][P], \\
\frac{d[P]}{dt} &= k_2[LB_1] - k_{-2}[B_1'][P] - u_2[P],
\end{aligned} \tag{1}$$

TABLE 3: Nonstandard abbreviations.

L	ISO	P	product
B_1	β_1-AR	LB_1	intermediate complexes
B_1'	β_1-AR with structure changes	$B_1'I$	intermediate complexes
B_2	β_2-AR	B_1B_2	conjugation of β_1-AR andβ_2-AR
B_2'	β_2-AR with structure changes	$(B_1I)'$	the product with structure change
I	β_1-AA	B_1IB_2	intermediate complexes

where the initial conditions of the control model are $[L](0) = [L_0] = 1 \times 10^{-7} mol/L$, $[B_1](0) = [B_{10}] = 3 \times 10^{-8} mol/L$, $[LB_1](0) = 0$, $[B_1'](0) = 0$, and $[P](0) = 0$.

(2) The Conformation Changes Model. We have known that β_1-AA and ISO compete for different binding sites of β_1-AR, which belongs to the competitive inhibition in different positions of β_1-AR [10]. Assuming that there is no reaction between β_1-AA and β_2-AR, the time evolution of conformation changes model based on Figure 4 is described by five coupled differential equations.

$$\begin{aligned}
\frac{d[I]}{dt} &= -k_1[I][B_1] + k_{-1}[B_1'I], \\
\frac{d[B_1]}{dt} &= -k_1[I][B_1] + k_{-1}[B_1'I] + u_3[B_1'], \\
\frac{d[B_1'I]}{dt} &= k_1[I][B_1] - k_{-1}[B_1'I] - k_2[B_1'I] \\
&\quad + k_{-2}[B_1'][P], \\
\frac{d[B_1']}{dt} &= k_2[B_1'I] - k_{-2}[B_1'][P] - u_1[B_1'] \\
&\quad - u_3[B_1'], \\
\frac{d[P]}{dt} &= k_2[B_1'I] - k_{-2}[B_1'][P] - u_2[P],
\end{aligned} \tag{2}$$

where the initial conditions of the conformation changes model are $[I](0) = [I_0] = 1 \times 10^{-7} mol/L$, $[B_1](0) = [B_{10}] = 2.3 \times 10^{-9} mol/L$, $[B_1'I](0) = 0$, $[B_1'](0) = 0$, and $[P](0) = 0$.

(3) The Interaction Model. In the preliminary study, β_1-AR and β_2-AR form heterodimer through the C-terminal [10], while β_1-AA can be combined with β_1-AR but not directly with β_2-AR [15]. Thus, we consider the effect of β_2-AR on the experimental group to establish interaction model, while the other conditions of the experiment group remain unchanged.

$$\begin{aligned}
\frac{d[I]}{dt} &= -k_1[I][B_1B_2] + k_{-1}[B_1IB_2], \\
\frac{d[B_1B_2]}{dt} &= -k_1[I][B_1B_2] + k_{-1}[B_1IB_2] + u_3[B_1'] \\
&\quad + u_3[B_2'], \\
\frac{d[B_1IB_2]}{dt} &= k_1[I][B_1B_2] - k_{-1}[B_1IB_2] \\
&\quad - k_2[B_1IB_2], \\
\frac{d[(B_1I)']}{dt} &= k_2[B_1IB_2] - k_3[(B_1I)'], \\
\frac{d[B_1']}{dt} &= k_3[(B_1I)'] - u_1[B_2'] - u_3[B_1'], \\
\frac{d[B_2']}{dt} &= k_2[B_1IB_2] - u_1[B_2'] - u_3[B_2'], \\
\frac{d[P]}{dt} &= k_3[(B_1I)'] - u_2[P],
\end{aligned} \tag{3}$$

where the initial conditions of the interaction model are $[I](0) = [I_0] = 1 \times 10^{-7} mol/L$, $[B_1B_2](0) = 1.8 \times 10^{-9} mol/L$, $[B_1IB_2](0) = 0$, $[(B_1I)'](0) = 0$, $[B_1'](0) = 0$, $[B_2'](0) = 0$, and $[P](0) = 0$.

Next, we will use second order Runge-Kutta method to estimate the parameters of systems (1), (2), and (3) and then select the optimal model of β_1-AR non-desensitization.

3. Model Analysis and Results

3.1. Parameter Fitting and Graphs Analysis. Second order Runge-Kutta method is used to solve the ODE systems obtained in our models. Our parameter fitting is an optimization process, which minimizes the squared summation of $[AB]_{pred} - [AB]_{data}$ at all time $[AB]_{data}$ got measured, where for simplicity we use $[AB]$ to denote the concentrations of the intermediate products LB_1, $B_1'I$, and B_1IB_2 in the three models, respectively (i.e., $[LB_1]$, $[B_1'I]$, and $[B_1IB_2]$). We also denote the total squared summation by S. Obviously S is a function of all the parameters that require fitting. Given a set of parameters, second order Runge-Kutta method gives the value of $[AB]_{pred}$ and thus S. We use steepest descent method to find the minimum of S. In this process, the gradient of S over all parameters is calculated numerically. For example, for positive parameter k_i,

$$\frac{\partial S}{\partial k_i} = \frac{S(k_i(1+\Delta)) - S(k_i)}{k_i \Delta}. \tag{4}$$

In our program $\Delta = 1.0e - 6$, and the time step in the Runge-Kutta method is chosen to be 0.01 min.

We use the measured values in Table 1 to do the parameter fitting for the control model and the values in Table 2 for the experiment models. Note that the measured data in the tables is not the exact concentration of $[AB]$. Instead, we assumed that the measured data is proportional to the concentration of $[AB]$. In other words, we introduce an extra parameter λ, and $[AB]_{data} = \lambda T_{data}$, where T_{data} is the measured data in the tables. In the optimization process, we trait λ in the same way we trait other parameters. And λ is also get fitted. Combining Figure 2 and parameter fitting method, we determined that the concentration is directly proportional to the heart rate of NRCMs and the proportionality factor is 0.0025.

Next, we analyze the fitting of the graphs and the prediction of the different time points, as shown in Figures 6–8.

Figure 6(a) shows the fitting results of control group model from 0 *min* to 60 *mins*, in which the points are experimentally measured and the curve is the solution of dynamical control group model of $[LB_1]$. And the fitting curve finally declined which reflects the fact that β_1-AR desensitizes when reacting with ISO in healthy rats. However, the situation was quite different with HF rats.

Figure 6(b) displays the prediction result from 60 *mins* to 120 *mins*. It predicts that $[LB_1]$ continues to decrease, eventually tends to zero, and becomes stable, which clearly showed the mechanism of β_1-AR desensitization.

Figure 7(a) presents the fitting results of the conformation changes model from 0 *min* to 60 *mins*, in which the points are experimentally measured and the curve is the solution of dynamical conformation changes model of $[B_1'I]$.

Figure 7(b) is the prediction results from 60 *mins* to 120 *mins*. The $[B_1'I]$ curve eventually stabilized in (b), which clearly showed the mechanism of β_1-AR non-desensitization.

Figure 8(a) presents the fitting results of the interaction model from 0 *min* to 60 *mins*, in which the points are experimentally measured, the curve is the solution of dynamical interaction model of $[B_1IB_2]$, and the fitting curve finally stabilized.

Figure 8(b) is the prediction results from 60 *mins* to 120 *mins*. The upward trend of the $[B_1IB_2]$ curve reflects the effects of β_1-AA and β_2-AR on the non-desensitization of the β_1-AR.

Then, we analyze the reaction speeds and Table 4 lists the reaction velocities of three models. Since the units of positive reaction velocities and reverse reaction velocities are different, they cannot be directly compared. Therefore, we simulated the reaction speeds figures of the control group and the experimental groups, and the reaction speed is the product of the reaction velocity and concentration. See Figure 9.

As can be seen from Figure 9, the positive and negative reaction speeds of the control model and experimental models are greater than those of the reverse reaction, and the positive reaction speeds decrease rapidly. In the course of the decrease of the positive reaction speeds, the speed of reversed reaction continues to rise. Finally, their tendency gradually slows down.

3.2. Model Selection. **Akaike's information criterion** [20–22] (AIC) is a measure of the goodness of fit of an estimated statistical model and a tool for model selection. Given a data set, several competing models can be ranked according to their AIC, with the one with the lowest AIC being the best. The AIC is defined as follows:

$$AIC = nInR_e + 2k, \qquad R_e = \frac{RSS}{n}, \tag{5}$$

where RSS is the residual sum of squares, n is the amount of the real data, and k is the total amount of estimated parameters in the model. AIC_c is AIC with a second order correction for small sample sizes ($n/k < 40$), to start with

$$AIC_c = AIC + \frac{2k(k+1)}{n-k-1}. \tag{6}$$

Moreover, AIC difference is defined as $\Delta_i = AIC_i - AIC_{min}$, where AIC_i is the AIC or AIC_c of the ith model, and AIC_{min} is the AIC or AIC_c of the model with minimal AIC. If $0 \le \Delta_i \le 2$, the ith model has substantial data support. If $4 \le \Delta_i \le 7$, the ith model has considerable less data support. If $\Delta_i \ge 10$, the ith model has essentially no data support.

Since the $n/k = 10/4 < 40$, we use AIC_c to select the model, which determines the mechanism of the β_1-AR non-desensitization. In order to verify the validity of the models, we apply AIC to view the residuals between theoretic and real data under three models. We calculated the AIC_c values of the conformation model and interaction model which are, respectively, $AIC_{c1} \approx -7.287$, $AIC_{c2} \approx -8.494$. By comparing the AIC_c values calculated in the two models above, we conclude easily that $AIC_{c1} > AIC_{c2}$, $AIC_{cmin} \approx -8.494$. It is obvious that the possibility of interaction is the largest, which conforms to the analysis of graphs and parameter.

4. Sensitivity Analysis

We determined that the interaction model between β_1-AR and β_2-AR is the optimal model for heart failure through the AIC criterion. Next, when the initial concentration of β_1-AA is different, we analyzed the figures and data (measured by Capital Medical University) fitting of the interaction model between β_1-AR and β_2-AR. From Figure 10, we can see that the initial concentration of β_1-AA has a certain effect on the fitting result. Table 5 shows the reaction velocity for the interaction model at different concentrations.

Figure 10, respectively, showed the graphs of $[B_1IB_2]$ when the initial concentrations of β_1-AA are $1 \times 10^{-9} mol/L$, $1 \times 10^{-8} mol/L$, and $1 \times 10^{-6} mol/L$ in 10 minutes, while the concentration of B_1B_2 remains unchanged at $1.8 \times 10^{-9} mol/L$. And we can see that when the concentration of β_1-AA is $1 \times 10^{-9} mol/L$, the fitting result is the worst, followed by $1 \times 10^{-6} mol/L$ and $1 \times 10^{-8} mol/L$. As can be seen from Figure 8, when concentration of β_1-AA is $1 \times 10^{-7} mol/L$, the fitting result is the best. Therefore, the optimum concentration of mice monoclonal β_1-AA leading to the NRCMs beating frequency was 0.1 μM (detected from 1 nM to 1 μM).

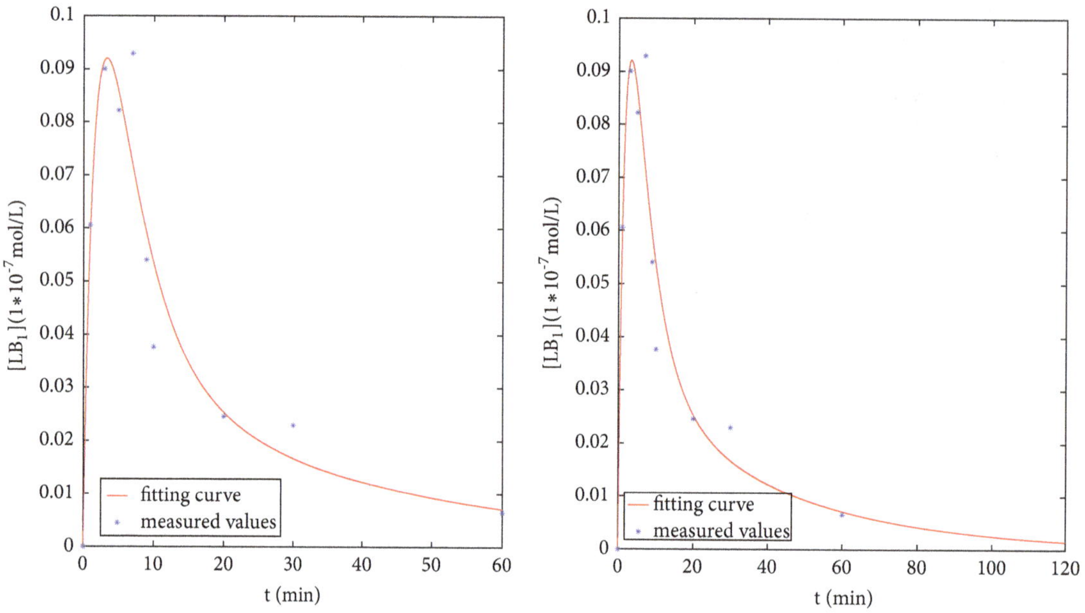

(a) (b)

FIGURE 6: The fitting and prediction graphs of control model. **(a)** Fitting graph. **(b)** Prediction graph at 120 mins.

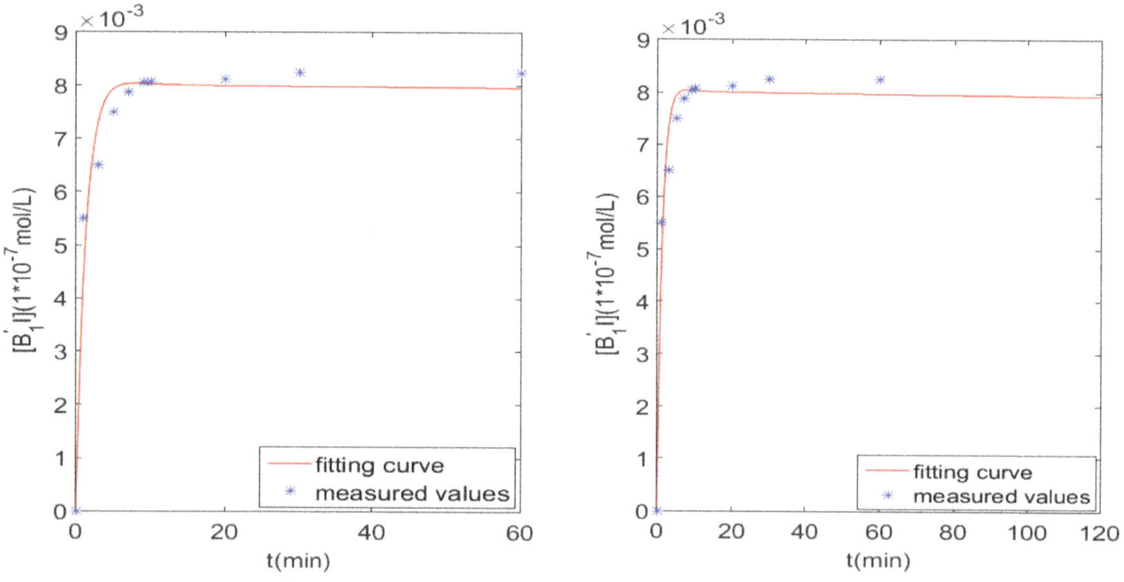

(a) (b)

FIGURE 7: The fitting and prediction graphs of conformation changes model. **(a)** Fitting graph. **(b)** Prediction graph at 120 mins.

TABLE 4: Velocities in three models.

models	k_1 $M^{-1}min^{-1}$	k_{-1} min^{-1}	k_2 min^{-1}	k_{-2} $M^{-1}min^{-1}$	k_3 min^{-1}	u_1 min^{-1}	u_2 min^{-1}	u_3 min^{-1}
control model	0.279	0.107	0.273	$1*10^{-6}$	–	0.039	0.011	0.028
conformation changes model	0.275	0.474	0.018	0.021	–	$1*10^{-6}$	0.100	0.271
interaction model	0.361	0.422	0.014	–	0.153	0.122	0.100	0.191

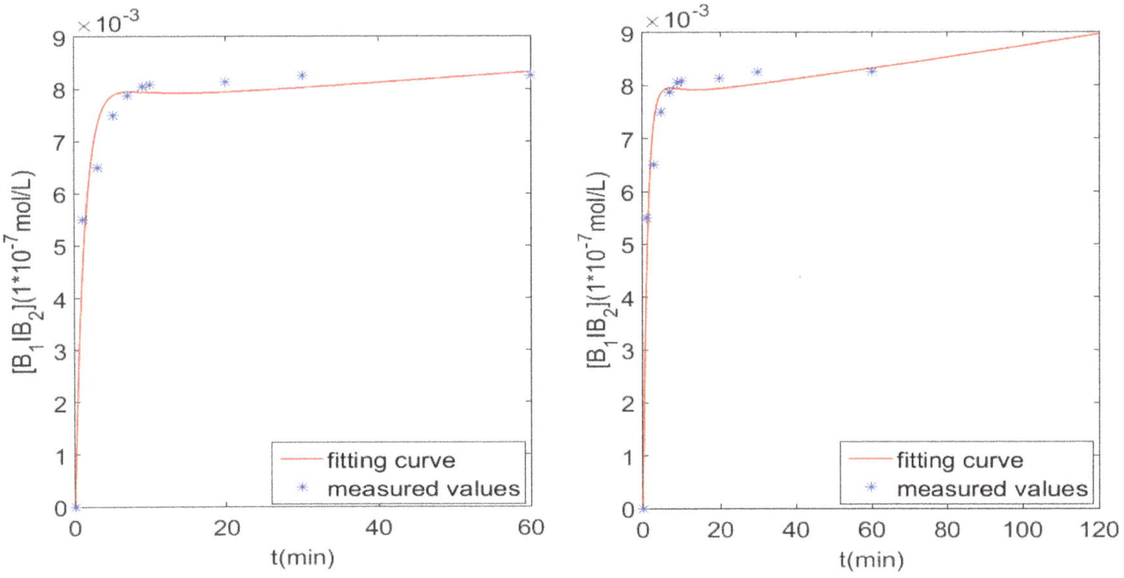

(a) (b)

FIGURE 8: The fitting and prediction graphs of interaction model. **(a)** Fitting graph. **(b)** Prediction graph at 120 mins.

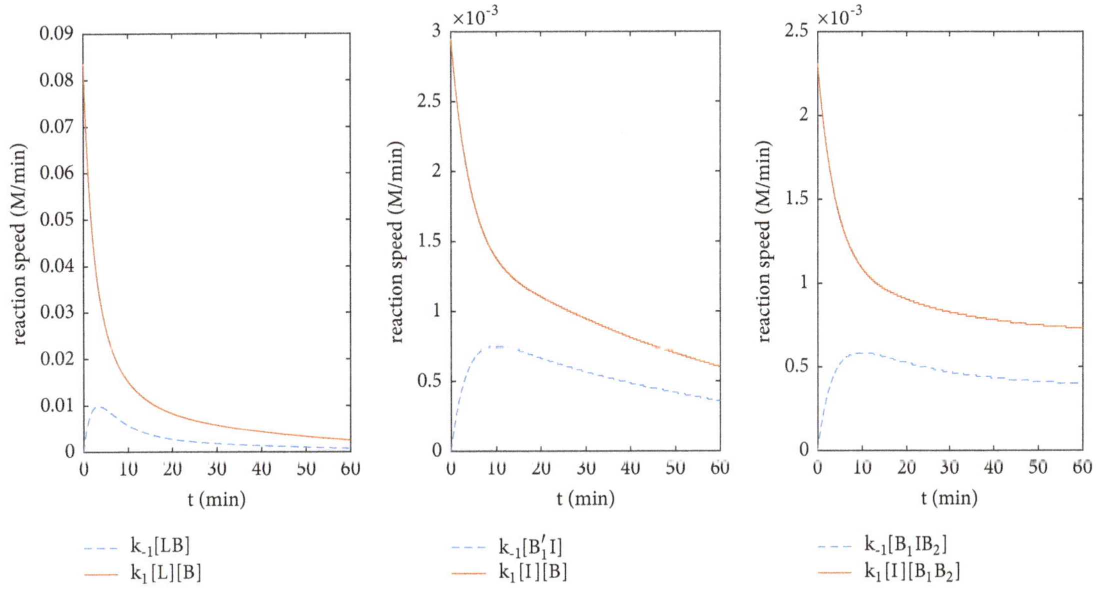

(a) (b) (c)

FIGURE 9: Comparison of speeds of positive and negative reactions between experimental models and control model. **(a)** Control model. **(b)** Conformation changes model. **(c)** Interaction model.

TABLE 5: Velocity values in interaction model.

Concentration of β_1-AA (mol/L)	k_1 $(M^{-1}min^{-1})$	k_{-1} (min^{-1})	k_2 (min^{-1})	k_3 (min^{-1})
1×10^{-9}	11.173	0.000001	0.067	0.000001
1×10^{-8}	3.201	0.753	0.059	0.408
1×10^{-6}	0.035	0.362	0.343	0.238

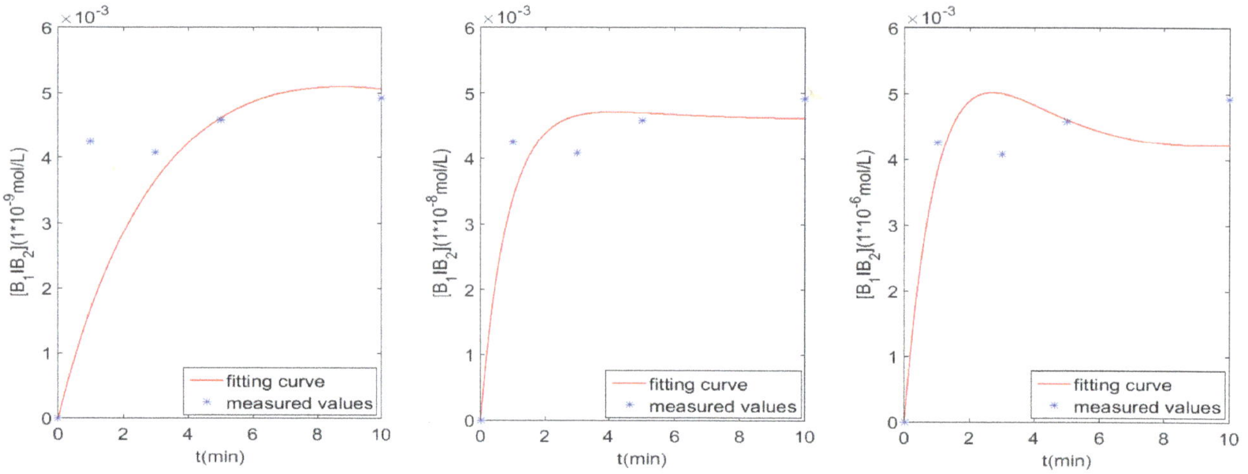

(a) (b) (c)

FIGURE 10: The fitting graphs of $[B_1IB_2]$ with the change of initial concentrations of β_1-AA (I) in interaction model. **(a)** $1 \times 10^{-9} mol/L$. **(b)** $1 \times 10^{-8} mol/L$. **(c)** $1 \times 10^{-6} mol/L$.

5. Conclusion

We analyzed the two types of mechanisms that cause HF; it can be concluded that conformation changes and interactions between β_1-AR and β_2-AR both contribute to the HF progression in rats and the interaction has the greater impact on it. In our study, for the first time, the model block diagrams described the causation of HF. By comparing the experimental group models with the control group model and then calculating the AIC_c, we concluded that the interaction model between β_1-AR and β_2-AR was the optimal model, which leads to the important role of β_2-AR in the progression of HF. β_2-AR and β_1-AR connect together and participate in a reaction, which then causes conformation changes in receptor β_1-AR. This results in endocytosis inhibition, which ultimately leads to β_1-AR non-desensitization and HF. Thus, β_2-AR is an important consideration in guiding the treatment of HF.

Previous studies have found that β_1-AR and β_2-AR could form heterodimers, although they also found that the autoantibody β_1-AA did not bind to β_2-AR [15]. We found that β_1-AA could inhibit heterodimerization of β_1/β_2-AR, observing laboratory experiments on animals at Capital Medical University. Therefore, we speculated that β_1-AA might indirectly affect the β_2-AR- C-terminal conformation and interfere with heterodimerization of β_1/β_2-AR. This would lead to β_1-AR endocytosis inhibition, to continuous signal activation, and ultimately to heart failure.

Because the interaction between β_1-AR and β_2-AR was found to be the trigger mechanism of heart failure progression, receptor β_2-AR should be further studied to determine if it could play a role in heart failure treatment. In the presence of β_1-AA-positive heart failure, β_2-AR can be used as a drug and therapeutic target to improve the interaction between β_1-AR and β_2-AR, thereby decreasing the risk of further heart failure.

Data Availability

The study conformed to AVMA Guidelines on Euthanasia and the Guide for the Care and Use of Laboratory Animals protocol published by the Ministry of Education of People's Republic of China. All studies were approved by Capital Medical University Committee on Animal Care. According to the data provided by Capital Medical University, we extracted the original data and established the relationship between experimental data and mathematical models to facilitate our research.

Conflicts of Interest

The authors declare that there are no conflicts of interest.

Acknowledgments

This research is supported by National Natural Science Foundation of China (91539205), Natural Science Foundation of Shanxi (201601D102002, 201601D021015), Special Foundation of Taiyuan University of Technology (2015MS033), Talent Introduction Research Fund of Taiyuan University of Technology (tyut-rc201317a), and China Scholarship Council.

References

[1] S. S. Mitter and C. W. Yancy, "Contemporary Approaches to Patients with Heart Failure," *Cardiology Clinics*, vol. 35, no. 2, pp. 261–271, 2017.

[2] P. Chowdhury, D. Kehl, R. Choudhary, and A. Maisel, "The use of biomarkers in the patient with heart failure," *Current Cardiology Reports*, vol. 15, no. 6, article no. 372, 2013.

[3] C. D. Kemp and J. V. Conte, "The pathophysiology of heart failure," *Cardiovascular Pathology*, vol. 21, no. 5, pp. 365–371, 2012.

[4] D. O. Verschure, B. L. F. van Eck-Smit, G. A. Somsen, R. J. J. Knol, and H. J. Verberne, "Cardiac sympathetic activity in chronic heart failure: Cardiac123i-mIBG scintigraphy to improve patient selection for ICD implantation," *Netherlands Heart Journal*, vol. 24, no. 12, pp. 701–708, 2016.

[5] S. Andersen, A. Andersen, F. S. De Man, and J. E. Nielsen-Kudsk, "Sympathetic nervous system activation and β-adrenoceptor blockade in right heart failure," *European Journal of Heart Failure*, vol. 17, no. 4, pp. 358–366, 2015.

[6] L. C. Harrison, J. Callaghan, J. C. Venter, C. M. Fraser, and M. L. Kaliner, "Atopy, Autonomic Function and β-Adrenergic Receptor Autoantibodies," in *Ciba Foundation Symposium 90 - Receptors, Antibodies and Disease*, Novartis Foundation Symposia, pp. 248–262, John Wiley & Sons, Ltd., Chichester, UK, 1982.

[7] G. Wallukat and A. Wollenberger, "Effects of the serum gamma globulin fraction of patients with allergic asthma and dilated cardiomyopathy on chronotropic beta adrenoceptor function in cultured neonatal rat heart myocytes.," *Biomedica Biochimica Acta*, vol. 46, no. 8-9, pp. S634–639, 1987.

[8] A. Castaldi, T. Zaglia, and V D. Mauro, *MicroRNA-133 Modulates the β1-Adrenergic Receptor Transduction CascadeNovelty and Significance*, vol. 115, Circulation Research, 2014.

[9] Y. Magnusson, G. Wallukat, F. Waagstein, A. Hjalmarson, and J. Hoebeke, "Autoimmunity in idiopathic dilated cardiomyopathy: Characterization of antibodies against the β1-adrenoceptor with positive chronotropic effect," *Circulation*, vol. 89, no. 6, pp. 2760–2767, 1994.

[10] V. K. Parmar, E. Grinde, J. E. Mazurkiewicz, and K. Herrick-Davis, "Beta2-adrenergic receptor homodimers: Role of transmembrane domain 1 and helix 8 in dimerization and cell surface expression," *Biochimica et Biophysica Acta*, vol. 1859, no. 9, pp. 1445–1455, 2017.

[11] D. Pétrin and T. E. Hébert, "The functional size of GPCRs - monomers, dimers or tetramers?" *Subcellular Biochemistry*, vol. 63, pp. 67–81, 2012.

[12] Y. K. Xiang, "Compartmentalization of β-adrenergic signals in cardiomyocytes," *Circulation Research*, vol. 109, no. 2, pp. 231–244, 2011.

[13] A. Y. Woo, Y. Song, R. Xiao, and W. Zhu, "Biased β2-adrenoceptor signalling in heart failure: Pathophysiology and drug discovery," *British Journal of Pharmacology*, vol. 172, no. 23, pp. 5444–5456, 2015.

[14] M. Suzuki, N. Ohte, Z.-M. Wang, D. L. Williams Jr., W. C. Little, and C.-P. Cheng, "Altered inotropic response of endothelin-1 in cardiomyocytes from rats with isoproterenol-induced cardiomyopathy," *Cardiovascular Research*, vol. 39, no. 3, pp. 589–599, 1998.

[15] N. Cao, H. Chen, Y. Bai et al., "β2-adrenergic receptor autoantibodies alleviated myocardial damage induced by β1-adrenergic receptor autoantibodies in heart failure," *Cardiovascular Research*, 2018.

[16] A. Martinsson, K. Lindvall, A. Melcher, and P. Hjemdahl, "Beta-adrenergic receptor responsiveness to isoprenaline in humans: concentration-effect, as compared with dose-effect evaluation and influence of autonomic reflexes.," *British Journal of Clinical Pharmacology*, vol. 28, no. 1, pp. 83–94, 1989.

[17] J. De Las Rivas, C. Fontanillo, and F. Lewitter, "Protein-protein interactions essentials: key concepts to building and analyzing interactome networks," *PLoS Computational Biology*, vol. 6, no. 6, Article ID e1000807, 2010.

[18] N. F. Britton, "Essential mathematical biology," *Physics Today*, vol. 57, no. 3, pp. 80–82, 2004.

[19] N. B. Janson, "Non-linear dynamics of biological systems," *Contemporary Physiscs*, vol. 53, no. 2, pp. 137–168, 2012.

[20] H. Akaike, "A new look at the statistical model identification," *IEEE Transactions on Automatic Control*, vol. 19, pp. 716–723, 1974.

[21] H. Akaike, "An information criterion (AIC)," *Mathematical Sciences*, vol. 14, no. 153, pp. 5–9, 1976.

[22] H. Akaike, "Likelihood and the Bayes procedure," *Trabajos de Estadistica y de Investigacion Operativa*, vol. 31, no. 1, pp. 143–166, 1980.

12

Wall Shear Stress Estimation of Thoracic Aortic Aneurysm using Computational Fluid Dynamics

J. Febina,[1] Mohamed Yacin Sikkandar,[2] and N. M. Sudharsan[3]

[1]*Department of Biomedical Engineering, GRT Institute of Engineering and Technology, Tiruttani, India*
[2]*Department of Medical Equipment Technology, College of Applied Medical Sciences, Majmaah University, Al Majmaah 11952, Saudi Arabia*
[3]*Department of Mechanical Engineering, Rajalakshmi Engineering College, Chennai, India*

Correspondence should be addressed to Mohamed Yacin Sikkandar; m.sikkandar@mu.edu.sa

Academic Editor: Dominique J. Monlezun

An attempt has been made to evaluate the effects of wall shear stress (WSS) on thoracic aortic aneurysm (TAA) using Computational Fluid Dynamics (CFD). Aneurysm is an excessive localized swelling of the arterial wall due to many physiological factors and it may rupture causing shock or sudden death. The existing imaging modalities such as MRI and CT assist in the visualization of anomalies in internal organs. However, the expected dynamic behaviour of arterial bulge under stressed condition can only be effectively evaluated through mathematical modelling. In this work, a 3D aneurysm model is reconstructed from the CT scan slices and eventually the model is imported to Star CCM+ (Siemens, USA) for intensive CFD analysis. The domain is discretized using polyhedral mesh with prism layers to capture the weakening boundary more accurately. When there is flow reversal in TAA as seen in the velocity vector plot, there is a chance of cell damage causing clots. This is because of the shear created in the system due to the flow pattern. It is observed from the proposed mathematical modelling that the deteriorating WSS is an indicator for possible rupture and its value oscillates over a cardiac cycle as well as over different stress conditions. In this model, the vortex formation pattern and flow reversals are also captured. The non-Newtonian model, including a pulsatile flow instead of a steady average flow, does not overpredict the WSS (15.29 Pa compared to 16 Pa for the Newtonian model). Although in a cycle the flow behaviour is laminar-turbulent-laminar (LTL), utilizing the non-Newtonian model along with LTL model also overpredicted the WSS with a value of 20.1 Pa. The numerical study presented here provides good insight of TAA using a systematic approach to numerical modelling and analysis.

1. Introduction

Aorta is the major artery that carries blood from heart to all parts of the body and part of the aorta that runs through the chest is called thoracic aorta [1]. When an area of thoracic aorta expands or bulges, it is called a thoracic aortic aneurysm (TAA). According to the study of incidence and mortality rate of TAA, the incidence of ruptured thoracic aneurysms in individuals aged 60–69 years is about 100 cases per 10,000; in those aged 70–79 years, it is about 300 cases per 10,000 and in those aged 80–89 years, it is about 550 cases per 10,000 people [1]. TAA causes plaque formation, which is a serious health risk as it can burst or rupture the inner wall intima continuing to the outer wall adventitia. However, plaque cap rupture per se does not lead to stoppage of blood flow. Rather, plaque cap rupture provides a surface that initiates thrombosis, which may then grow to occlude the vessel and stop blood flow [2]. TAA exists in both saccular shape and fusiform shape. The saccular shape aneurysm is eccentric, involving only one portion of the circumference of an aortic wall. The fusiform aneurysm is concentric and involves the full circumference of the vessel wall. The effect of high shear hemodynamics on thrombus growth has profound implications for the understanding of all acute thrombotic cardiovascular events as well as for vascular reconstructive techniques and vascular device design, testing, and clinical performance [3]. In the present work, saccular shape TAA is considered in detail due to the fact that it has caused

TABLE 1: Derived values of aortic diameter, average velocity, and Reynolds number.

Patient No. *	D = (Re∗μ)/(Vpeak) Aortic diameter (D) (m)	Vavg = Q/A Average velocity (m/sec) (V avg)	Reavg = (ρ∗D∗Vavg)/μ Average Reynolds number (Re avg)
2	0.0302	0.1229	730.03
3	0.0287	0.1333	797.38
4	0.0262	0.1629	856.39
5	0.0261	0.1674	844.23
6	0.0304	0.1281	811.12

*Table 1 of Stein et al. [4].

greater rupture risks than fusiform aneurysm [3]. This work aims to show that Computational Fluid Dynamics (CFD) is an effective tool that can provide better insights into TAA diagnosis with proper solver settings and a numerical protocol.

The viscosity values for a group of five normal people were estimated by Stein et al. [4] to be in the range of 0.0051 to 0.0055 Ps s (average value of 0.0053 Pa s) and the same has been used in the present study (Table 1). The aorta diameter was computed using the peak Reynolds number, peak velocity, and viscosity. This value was then used to obtain the average velocity and Reynolds number. The density value of blood is taken to be $\rho = 1060\ \mathrm{kg/m^3}$. It can be seen from table that the flow of blood inside aorta is predominantly laminar in nature. Owing to the pulsatile nature, the flow is sometimes (locally) turbulent. The derived values obtained from Stein et al. [4] are shown in Table 1.

From Table 1, it is clear that turbulent flow occurs only with peak blood flow velocity values. With average velocity values, the flow tends to be laminar with the average Reynolds number in the range of 730 to 856. A regular geometry profile that mimics an aneurysm was modelled and numerically solved by Berguer et al. [5]. Both laminar and turbulent pulsatile flows were studied. The actual diseased model was not studied. The effects of Newtonian and non-Newtonian behaviours of blood were compared. They concluded that non-Newtonian turbulent flow is to be considered in the study of aneurysms. It is to be noted that the pulsatile flow will be both laminar and turbulent based on the velocity attained at that instant of time. A transit model that could best handle both laminar and turbulent flow would be a better predictor of the flow phenomenon and provide more acceptable wall shear stress values.

A transitional flow model based on Menter et al. [6] was employed by Tan et al. [7] for predicting the blood flow patterns in a fusiform aneurysm region assuming the blood to be Newtonian in nature. In essence, although the flow was pulsatile with a major pulse component being laminar in nature, the transitional flow model solves the fluid flow in the near wall region as laminar and turbulent elsewhere. From the simulation results, they observed that the transitional model gave better inference compared with the laminar simulation. Highly disturbed, recirculating flow was observed within the bulged region of the aneurysm. High turbulence intensity values were particularly observed near the outlet of the aneurysm. It was also presented that the wall shear stress values obtained could be an overestimate. It would be of interest to investigate an appropriate transitional model considering blood to be non-Newtonian in nature on a saccular aneurysm of a diseased aorta. However, the effective implementation of this basic scheme requires a very fine grid resolution near the wall region. The suggested y^+ (nondimensional distance from wall) value is < 2. This is extremely fine and would be computationally intensive. The detailed significance and explanation of computation is presented under the numerical protocol section of this paper. An optimum solution to this would be to achieve a good prediction even with a comparative fine mesh having a selected wall y^+ value of 100, at the same time taking care to ensure that the laminar/turbulent transition is in a pulsatile flow instead of using the typical transitional flow model.

A. C. Benim et al. [8] observed that, for a normal human aorta, time averaged velocity field of pulsatile flow did not show remarkable differences in steady-state results. They indicated that the mobilization of atherosclerotic plaques needs to be considered as a very important issue for extracorporeal circulation. However, the effect of actual flow pattern on a diseased aorta was, however, not studied. A detailed lumen surface representation of aortic aneurysm is very important in the analysis of stress pattern [9]. However, the fluctuations of blood flow inside an aneurysm lumen region were not studied in detail. Qiao et al. described the formation and development of aortic plaque in an aneurysm region using CFD [10]. The simulation was performed for a fusiform aneurysm in the descending aorta with pulsatile flow but the cell refinement and grid independence test were not performed. Callaghan et al. presented a work that combined a 4D flow and CFD simulation of a thoracic aortic aneurysm case [11]. They reported that high wall shear stress values of 20 Pa were found in the ascending aorta during the turbulent flow and concluded that the CFD provides results supplementing the 4D flow data in the understanding of aneurysm development and risk; however, the laminar flow and significance of wall y+ in the aneurysm model were not studied. Numata et al. [12] and Markl et al. [13] reported that CFD simulation alone does not guarantee fidelity to reproduce in vivo hemodynamics due to inherent model limitations. They noted that the grid resolution errors were a possible source of uncertainty. In order to overcome this, mesh independence study was performed. Soudah et al. [14] provided a detailed methodology and the importance of wall y^+ for capturing the WSS. However, it was computed for the peak systolic instant time using flat inlet velocity profile for a normal aorta. Basri et al. [15] detailed the recent usage of CFD in biomedical applications. The authors reviewed several research papers that studied the use of CFD as a tool for determining the pathophysiology of a cardiovascular system. The abnormalities discussed by the authors included narrowing of aortic wall, leakage of blood from the valve opening, and stenosis conditions. However, the usage of CFD in aneurysm condition was not studied.

In summary, from the analysis of available literature, it is seen that it is necessary to consider a geometry model that is as close as possible to the real aorta. This can be ensured by using one of the several imaging modalities, like CT. This model has to be discretized (meshed) with proper refinement close to the wall and must be fine enough to avoid numerical errors. In this research work, an aorta having a saccular aneurysm is reconstructed from a CT image. The detailed discretization scheme is an extension of [14] with improvements in mesh topology which are explained in detail in the next section. As far as the physics is concerned, it is seen from literature that the flow should be considered as pulsatile and fluid (blood) as non-Newtonian. The discretization of the geometry is very important to obtain a solution with minimum numerical error. The protocol adopted is presented in detail in the next section. The numerical scheme is the key to accurate prediction. From the study of available literature, it is seen/noted that several schemes have been tried, namely, laminar, turbulent, and transitional models assuming a steady velocity profile and/or pulsatile profile with a Newtonian behaviour. A pulsatile flow with non-Newtonian fluid model has not been attempted thus far/yet and it is suggested that this improved method of approach with above-mentioned modelling parameters would provide a more accurate estimation of WSS values.

In this research work, an attempt is made to test the efficacy of the numerical scheme by comparing the results obtained using a pulsatile velocity profile for both Newtonian and non-Newtonian models considering the flow to be laminar. The reason for using the laminar flow model is that for a pulse of 0.8 seconds the flow is turbulent only from 0.02 to 0.2 seconds, where the Re values exceed 2200. The average Re is always less than 2200. To find an alternate to the transitional model that assumes the bulk of the fluid transport as fully turbulent (which it is not) and also requires a very fine mesh (a computationally intensive proposition), it is proposed to use a laminar-turbulent switch based on the Reynolds number. This is to see if the possibility of overprediction of WSS [8] can be mitigated. The velocity trace can be mapped to a laminar-turbulent-laminar flow from a cardiac cycle. In this model, the velocity trace is mapped to the Reynolds number. For all values of Re < 2200, the laminar flow solver is enabled, and for Re > 2200, the standard k-epsilon model is enabled.

2. Materials And Methods

2.1. Numerical Evaluation Protocol. The workflow followed in this study is pictorially represented in Figure 1 and is briefly explained below.

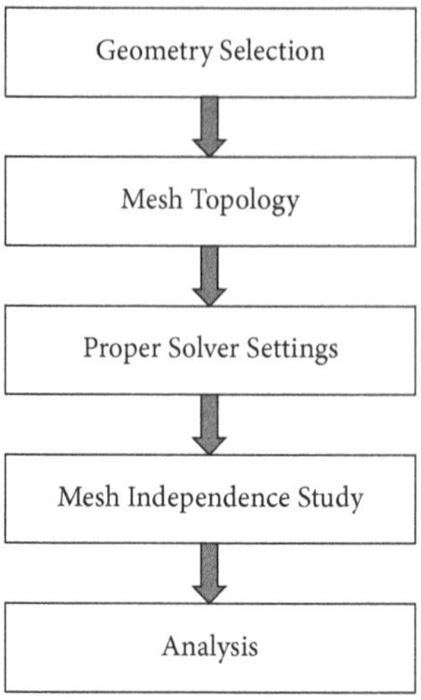

FIGURE 1: Workflow.

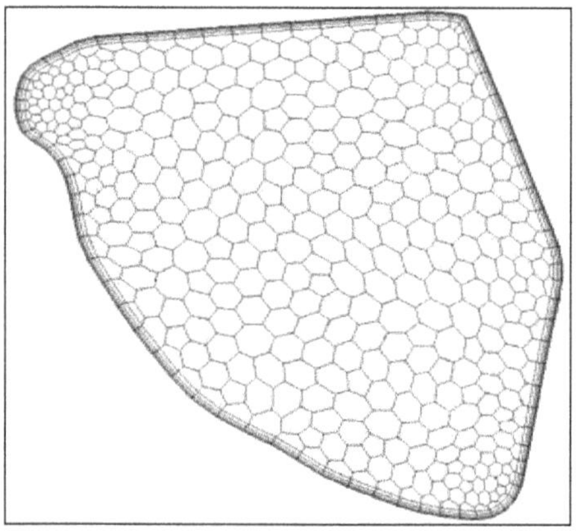
FIGURE 2: Prism layer at the outlet.

2.1.1. Geometry Selection. In this research, the 3D aneurysm model was reconstructed from the CT scan slices using MIMICS. The original CT image file format was DICOM. The total number of scanning slices is 600 and the range of scanning was from neck to legs. The distance between neighbouring layers was 1 mm. The CT data was imported into MIMICS software and data of the aortic vessel was extracted by means of 3D threshold segmentation. Then, the model is imported to Star CCM+ (Siemens, USA) for CFD analysis. The domain is discretized using polyhedral mesh with prism layers to capture the boundary more accurately based on the following reasons.

2.1.2. Polyhedral Mesh. Polyhedral meshes provide a balanced solution for complex mesh generation problems. They are relatively easy and efficient to build, requiring no more surface preparation than the equivalent tetrahedral mesh. They also contain approximately five times fewer cells than a tetrahedral mesh for a given starting surface. Multiregion meshes with a conformal mesh interface are allowed.

2.1.3. Prism Layer Mesh. The prism layer mesh model as shown in Figure 2 is used with a core volume mesh to generate orthogonal prismatic cells next to wall surfaces or boundaries. This layer of cells is necessary to improve the accuracy of the flow solution and provides a conformal mesh for the model. This helps in capturing the velocity across the boundary layer more accurately than depending on standard wall functions. This is decided from the wall y+ value that is discussed later in this section. It is to be noted that Figure 2 presents only the representation of the prismatic layer near wall with polyhedral cells in the center. The actual mesh is

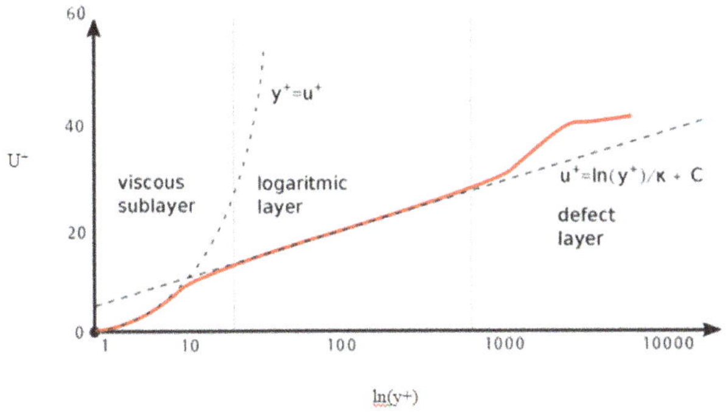

FIGURE 3: Nondimensional distance from wall y+ versus nondimensional velocity U+.

extremely fine (average distance from the wall to the adjacent grid is 0.0001 m.) and one would not be able to see the geometric progression of cell layer thickness from wall to the inner fluid region.

2.1.4. Significance of Wall y+ Value. To understand the actual physics of wall shear stress, the flow close to the boundary layer has to be accurately captured. Since the boundary layer thickness is extremely small, the first grid point must be very close to the wall. This distance from the wall is represented as nondimensionless wall y^+.

$$y^+ = \frac{y u_\tau}{\vartheta}, \quad u_\tau = \sqrt{\frac{\tau_w}{\rho}} \qquad (1)$$

where

y^+ is nondimensional distance from the wall,

y is the distance from the wall, m,

u_τ is frictional velocity,

ϑ is kinematic viscosity, m/s^2,

τ_w is wall shear stress, Pa,

ρ is density, kg/m^3.

The velocity profile close to the wall is generally assumed to be parabolic and the boundary layer variation is assumed to be parabolic. However, this is not the case. The nondimensional velocity u+ is plotted against the nondimensional distance from the wall and defined as y+ (Figure 3). As seen in Figure 3, the boundary layer can be divided into three regions and they are viscous sublayer, log layer, and defect layer. In the viscous sublayer y+ = u+ and this holds good for a value of y+ up to 5. It means that the viscous forces are as strong as the inertial forces. In the log layer, the u+ value increases exponentially in comparison to the distance from the wall and is linear when plotted in logarithmic scale.

Wall y+ value indicates the position of the grid inside the boundary layer. A value of less than five signifies that the first grid is in viscous sublayer and a value of 300 signifies that the first grid is in log layer. It is desirable that y+ be in this range to ensure that the physics of boundary layer are truly represented in this study's computation even though standard wall functions are enabled. In this case, y+ ranges from 3 to 100, respectively. This clearly satisfies the condition that, in the present simulation, the flow inside boundary layer is fully represented by the prism layer grid points.

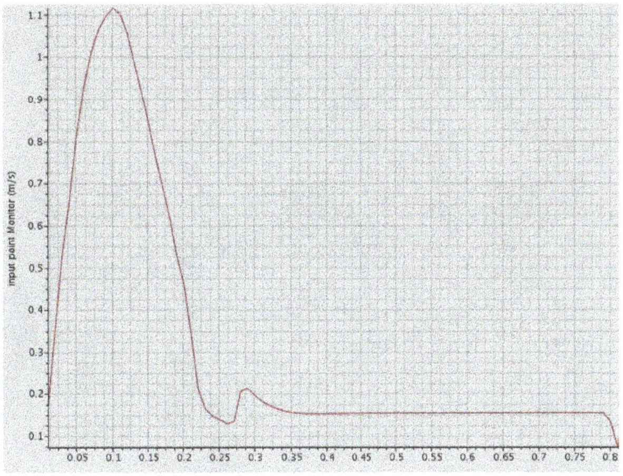

FIGURE 4: Velocity profile graph [15].

2.1.5. Mesh Independence Study. In order to avoid the grid resolution errors, three different mesh models are generated in the fluid domain. The number of cells generated is two, four, and eight hundred thousand, respectively. The number of prism layers is set to four for capturing the near-wall velocity profile. The simulations were performed for pulsatile velocity profile of a typical resting condition on the aneurysm region in thoracic aorta and the results presented are of a male person (age 61) in Figure 4. The velocity profile was obtained from the published literature [15].

The simulation is performed assuming Newtonian behaviour. The simulation is run for 6 cycles to allow the solver to stabilize and the results for the seventh cycle are plotted. Three points are monitored. Point 1 corresponds to inlet, point 2 corresponds to the location where the aneurysm is present, and point 3 refers to the outlet (Figure 5). Figures 6–8 present the velocity profile over time for various mesh counts. The negative value in the velocity is because the flow is considered to be positive in the upward direction in the inlet region. It can be seen from all the three figures that the mesh-independent solution is reached for a mesh count of 400,000. However, for ensuring fidelity, all further simulations are performed with a refined mesh having a mesh count of 800,000.

2.1.6. Solver Settings. Regarding physical conditions, they include unsteady, pulsatile, and laminar, segregated flows. The laminar flow is considered based on the value obtained from the Reynolds number. The average Reynolds number for pulsatile flow is 1405. From the velocity profile, it is found that 78% is laminar and 22% is turbulent. As the flow is predominantly laminar, the laminar flow model is chosen. However, the laminar-turbulent-laminar (LTL) model is also simulated for comparison.

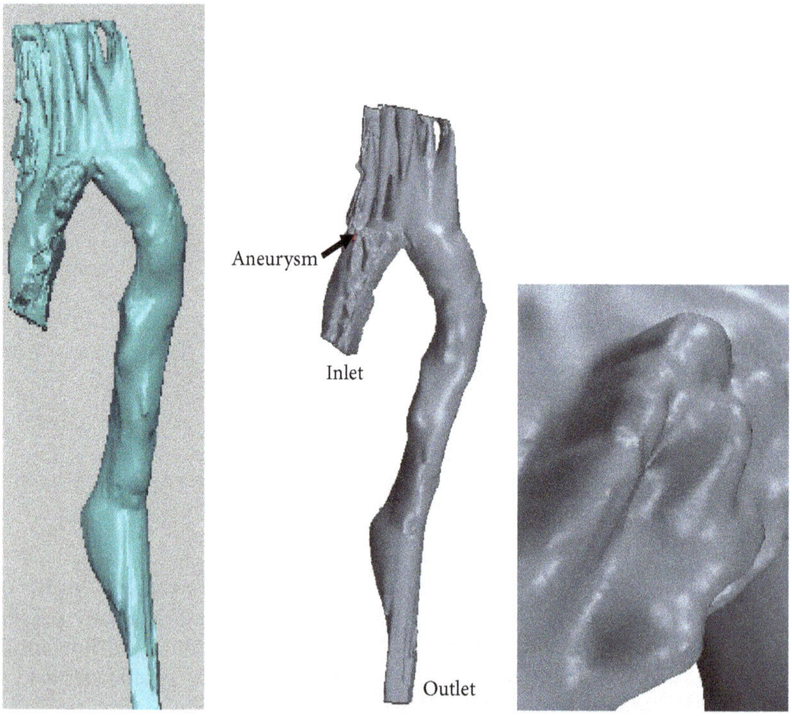

(a) CT DICOM image (b) Aorta model with three monitor points (c) Zoomed image of the aneurysm

FIGURE 5

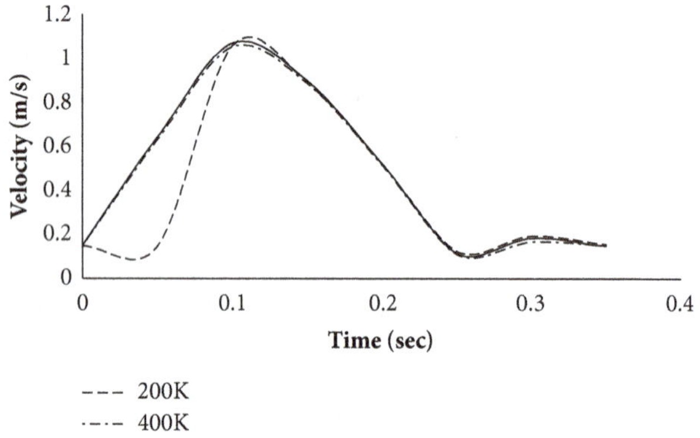

FIGURE 6: Velocity profile over time at monitoring point 1 (inlet) for various mesh counts.

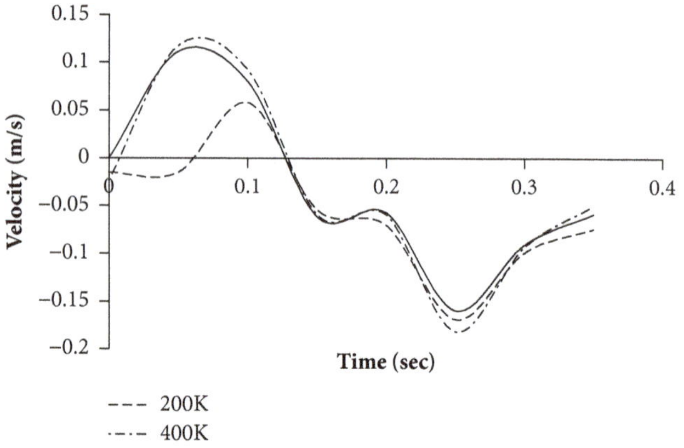

FIGURE 7: Velocity profile over time at monitoring point 2 (aneurysm) for various mesh counts.

Regarding boundary conditions, the inlet boundary condition is velocity inlet and the velocity profile given in the inlet is shown in Figure 5(a). For CFD analysis, the average velocity has to be set as an inlet boundary condition instead of using peak velocity value. The wall is assumed to be rigid and no slip condition is set in the wall. The outlet boundary condition is the pressure outlet.

For Newtonian or non-Newtonian fluid, generally, blood follows a Newtonian behaviour in large arteries and non-Newtonian behaviour in small arteries and capillaries. But in both medium and large sized blood vessels, non-Newtonian behaviour influences hemodynamic factors [16–18]. To understand this effect, non-Newtonian model of blood is also adopted and compared with the results obtained using Newtonian flow. The viscosity of the blood is set at 0.0052 Pa-s based on the experimental results reported in [4].

During the steady state, non-Newtonian behaviour affects the wall shear stress predicting larger values than the Newtonian model [16, 17, 19–21]. Solving this aorta model assuming a steady average velocity, WSS value is estimated as 13.2 Pa for non-Newtonian model, which is higher than the WSS value of Newtonian model (7.4 Pa). But when pulsatile flow is considered, Newtonian behaviour tends to provide larger WSS than the non-Newtonian behaviour as can be seen from the graph presented above (Figure 9) with average values

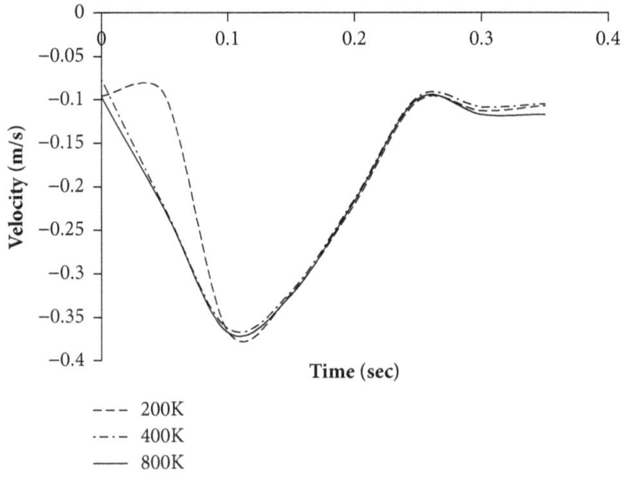

FIGURE 8: Velocity profile over time at monitoring point 3 (outlet) for various mesh counts.

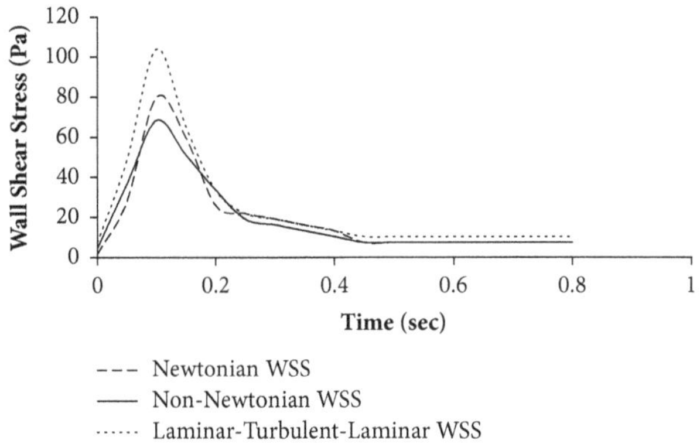

FIGURE 9: Pulsatile flow wall shear stress versus time for Newtonian and non-Newtonian WSS.

of 16 Pa and 15.29 Pa, respectively. The graph also shows the laminar-turbulent-laminar (LTL) model proposed in this paper. This model (LTL) overpredicts WSS with an average value of 20.10 Pa. In effect, it is amply evident from this work and others that considering blood flow as laminar is the right assumption/presumption.

The simulation was performed based on three conditions: during rest, light exercise, and moderate exercise. The velocity profile varies with the stress condition and the same is presented in Figure 10.

3. Result and Discussion

We consider the velocity profile and vorticity at the three peaks at 0.05, 0.25, and 0.75 time instants in the velocity profile of blood flow during rest, light exercise, and moderate exercise positions (Figure 10).

From Figure 10, it is observed that, for moderate exercise conditions, the velocity profile has peaks at 0.05, 0.25, 0.4, and 0.75 seconds and two peaks for the other two stress conditions. The corresponding velocity vector at these three time instants is plotted in Figure 10.

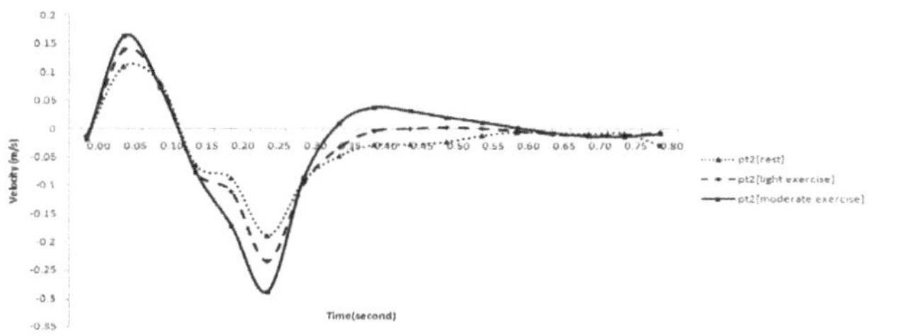

FIGURE 10: Velocity in the aneurysm region at different exercise conditions. Note: pt2 indicates the point in the aneurysm region.

Figures 11(a) and 11(b) indicate the vector scene represented during the first peak in Figure 10 at the aneurysm point for both laminar and laminar-turbulent-laminar methods. This shows that the flow is towards the left side, which makes the base for the formation of vortex. Figure 11(c) presents the vorticity plot at the same time instant. The vorticity value at the aneurysm using laminar method is 110.7285(/s) and for LTL method it is 221.6708 (/s). Although the pulsatile flow behaves as a laminar-turbulent-laminar based on the velocity profile, it overpredicts the values when compared to a laminar method. This again fortifies that the simulation needs to be performed using a non-Newtonian and laminar scheme.

Figure 12 indicates the flow reversal in the aneurysm region (i.e., flow towards the right). Figure 12(c) presents the vorticity plot at the same time instant. The vorticity value at the aneurysm using laminar method is 111.07(/s) and for LTL method it is 182.44 (/s).

In Figure 13, the flow is towards the left side and this vector scene is obtained during the second positive peak in Figure 10. Figure 13(c) presents the vorticity plot at the same time instant. The vorticity value at the aneurysm using laminar method is 19.39(/s) and for laminar-turbulent-laminar method it is 46.98 (/s).

In Figures 14(a) and 14(b), the flow vector direction is towards the right, indicating the flow reversal in the aneurysm region again. This flow reversal may have an effect on wall abrasion and the possibility of rupture. There is an increase in peak velocity of flow in the ascending aorta with exercise [22]. Figure 14(c) presents the vorticity plot at the same time instant. The vorticity value at the aneurysm using laminar method is 13.5542 (/s) and for laminar-turbulent-laminar method it is 31.3758(/s).

According to Taylor [23], for a normal person, reverse flow occurs in aorta during rest and reverse flow gets eliminated during exercise. The present model was carried out on subject with aneurysm and from the analysis it was found that there is reverse flow and flow fluctuations during exercise condition in the aneurysm region, which could lead to rupture.

Although the LTL scheme provides the same vector scene as non-Newtonian model, the WSS is comparatively high for the laminar-turbulent-laminar scheme. Also the vorticity value is high for the laminar-turbulent-laminar scheme when compared to the laminar scheme.

The WSS is associated with blood flow through an artery and also depends on the size and geometry of an aorta. The

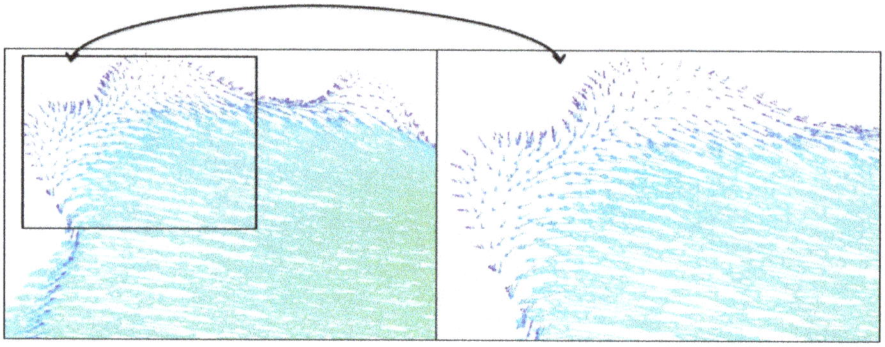

(a)

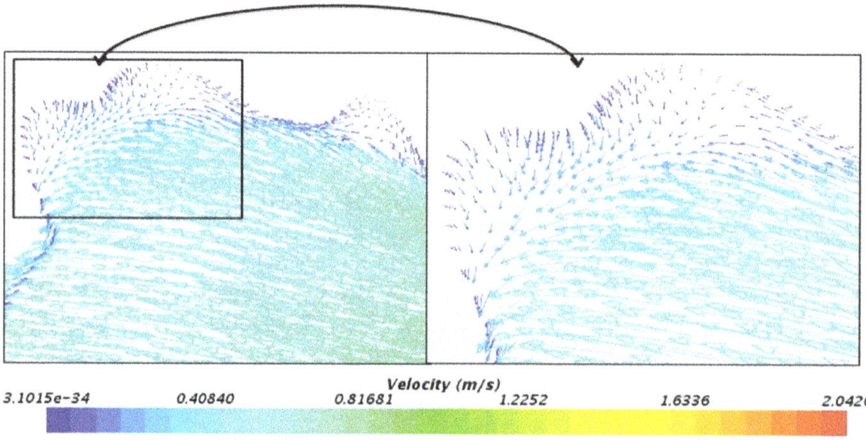

(b)

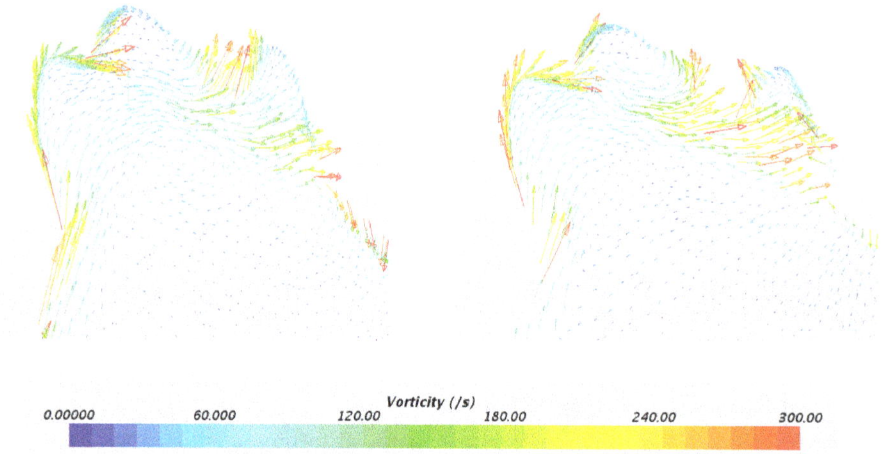

(c)

FIGURE 11: (a) Velocity profile at 0.05 sec using laminar method. (b) Velocity profile at 0.05 sec using laminar-turbulent-laminar scheme. (c) Vorticity profile using laminar and laminar-turbulent-laminar methods at 0.05 sec.

corresponding WSS during rest, light exercise, and moderate exercise are shown in Figures 15 and 16.

From this, it is clear that laminar-turbulent-laminar scheme overpredicts high WSS values. So, the alternate choice of the non-Newtonian model with laminar flow can provide better results among the different models discussed above.

WSS is an important factor for rupture and plaque formation. Results so far published in open literature have emphasised that the WSS is overpredicted in a numerical experiment. Numerical results heavily depend on the settings and these have not been well documented so far. In order to obtain solutions that match the physical experiments, there is

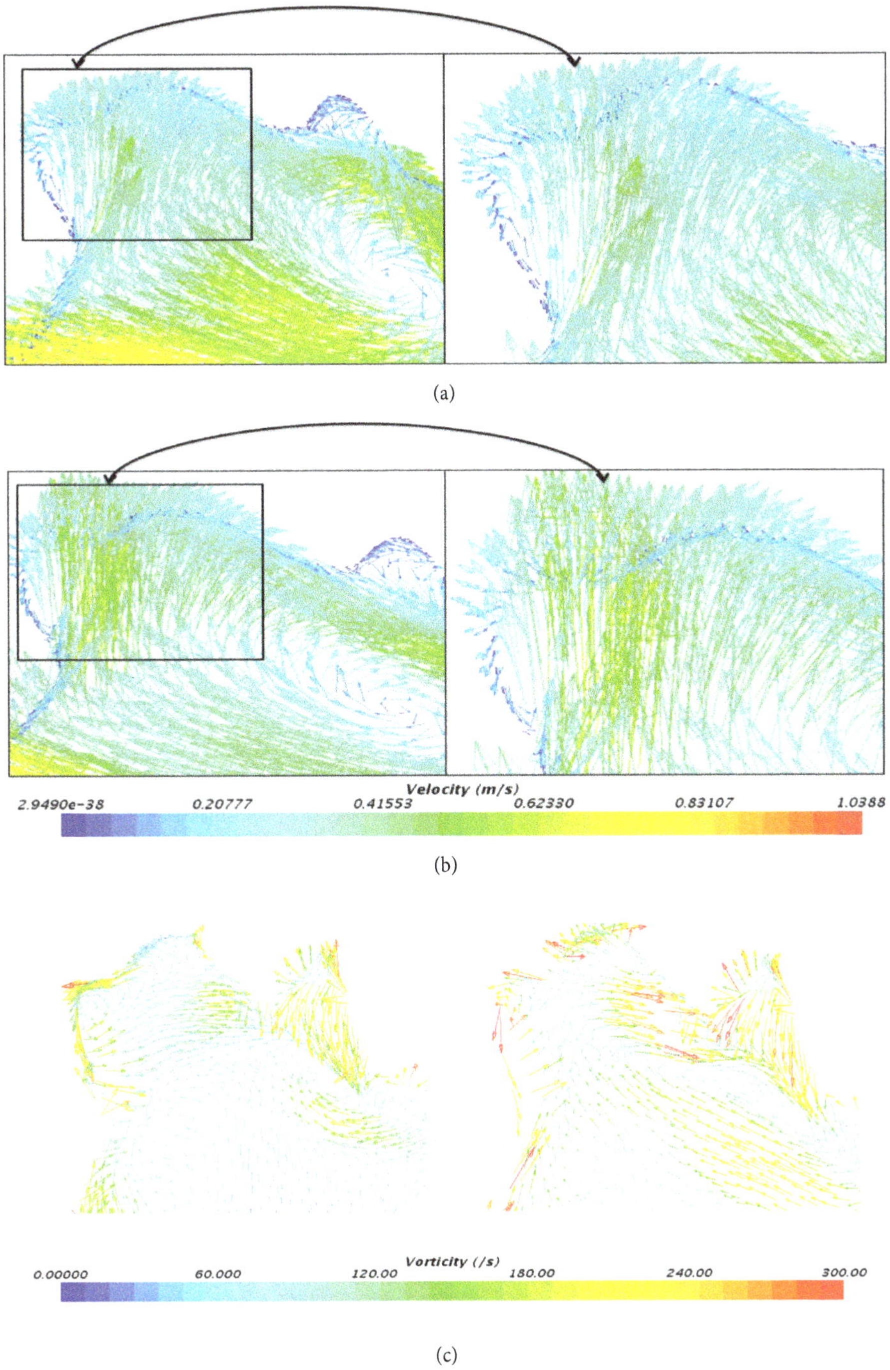

FIGURE 12: (a) Velocity profile at 0.25 sec using laminar method. (b) Velocity profile at 0.25 sec using laminar-turbulent-laminar scheme. (c) Vorticity profile using laminar and laminar-turbulent-laminar methods at 0.25 sec.

a need for (a) proper extraction of the geometry without loss of detail and a good discretization scheme; (b) choice of flow; and (c) choice of physics. These are explained in detail below.

The discretization of the geometry must follow a protocol in such a way that the near-wall region is adequately captured along with a mesh-independent study to check the fidelity of the solution. Although the flow behaviour is laminar-turbulent-laminar over a cardiac cycle, it has been seen that this model overpredicts WSS as well as the vorticity. Surprisingly, it is assumed that the flow to be laminar provides a better estimate for WSS. Also the physics of the fluid are taken as non-Newtonian and this provides a better result than Newtonian. It is to be noted that a pulsatile flow with non-Newtonian fluid model has not been attempted so far and seen as an improved method of approach with above-mentioned modelling parameters to estimate the WSS more accurately.

Also, the development of vortex and flow reversal is presented in this work, which is a possible reason for formation of plaque deposition. This is a cause for reduction

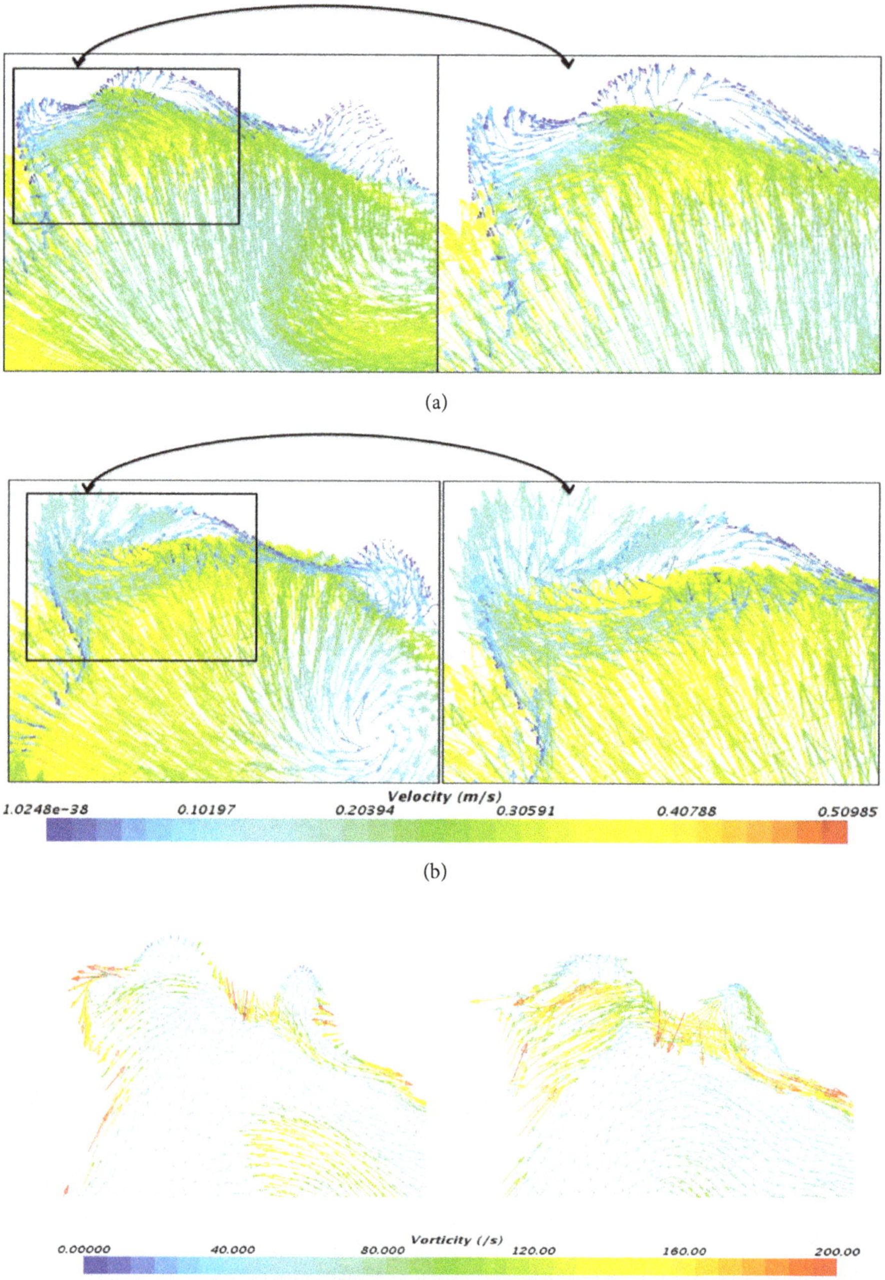

(c)

FIGURE 13: (a) Velocity profile at 0.4 sec using laminar method. (b) Velocity profile at 0.4 sec using laminar-turbulent-laminar scheme. (c) Vorticity profile using laminar and laminar-turbulent-laminar method at 0.4 sec.

in flow area and increase in internal pressure. This insight on the flow reversal and vortex development has not yet been explored based on the available literature to the best of the authors' knowledge. Chatzizisis et al. and Chen et al. have presented that, at locations where there is a presence of atherosclerotic lesions, oscillatory or low shear stress is predominantly observed [24, 25]. However, Chen et al. also observe that effect of stress on plaque is unknown [25].

4. Conclusion

The conformal mesh for the model is obtained using the polyhedral and prism layer mesh. The flow along the sides of

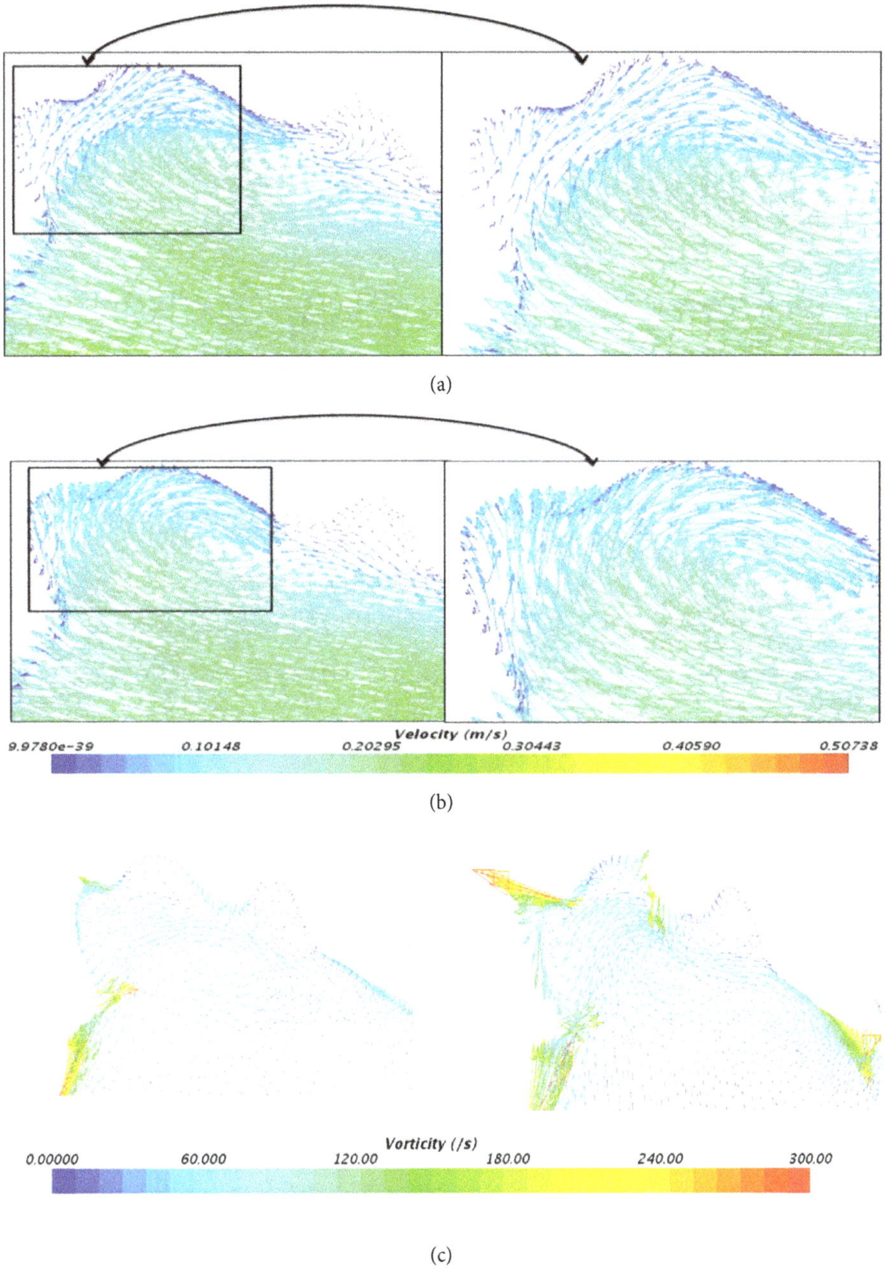

FIGURE 14: (a) Velocity profile at 0.75 sec using laminar method. (b) Velocity profile at 0.75 sec using laminar-turbulent-laminar scheme. (c) Vorticity profile using laminar and laminar-turbulent-laminar method at 0.75 sec.

the wall is captured well by using wall y+. It has been observed that considering pulsatile blood flow to be laminar is correct and it does not overpredict the WSS values. Moreover, it is also found necessary to consider the blood to be non-Newtonian even when the flow is in the larger blood vessel. The true representation of the geometry, discretization with fine meshes in the near wall region ($y^+ < 100$), and the proper choice of numerical scheme are the keys to correct prediction of flow and WSS. CFD as a mathematical tool can help in understanding the flow physics phenomena inside an artery. The advantage is that the model can be tested for varying stresses that an artery may be subjected (to) in day to day life. This tool will help in evaluating treatment methodology and suggest lifestyle modifications for the diseased patient. Thus, the relationship between CFD and cardiovascular hemodynamics was studied with different assumptions. It was found that CFD can provide better results with proper modelling, mesh, and solver settings. Limitation of this study is that the present findings are based on limited population (i.e., one particular case). In future, more CT data

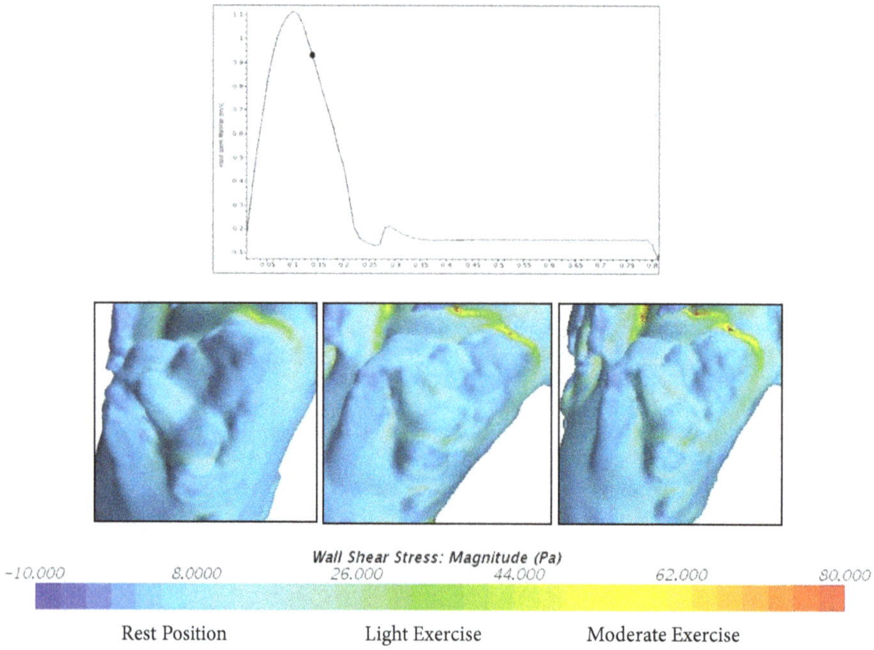

FIGURE 15: WSS during rest, light exercise, and moderate exercise at 0.15 sec.

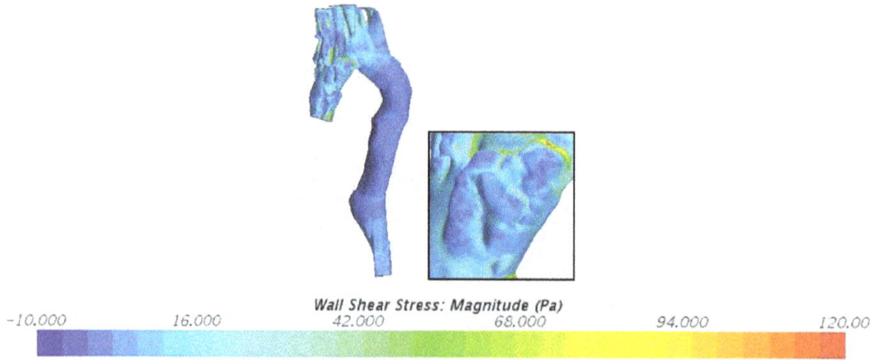

FIGURE 16: Wall shear stress during moderate exercise using the laminar-turbulent-laminar scheme.

of saccular shape thoracic aortic aneurysm patients can be obtained and then simulation can be done to provide more appropriate numerical results.

Conflicts of Interest

The authors declare that they have no conflicts of interest.

References

[1] R. Erbel and H. Eggebrecht, "Aortic dimensions and the risk of dissection," *Heart*, vol. 92, no. 1, pp. 137–142, 2006.

[2] L. D. C. Casa, D. H. Deaton, and D. N. Ku, "Role of high shear rate in thrombosis," *Journal of Vascular Surgery*, vol. 61, no. 4, pp. 1068–1080, 2015.

[3] E. K. Shang, D. P. Nathan, W. W. Boonn et al., "A modern experience with saccular aortic aneurysms," *Journal of Vascular Surgery*, vol. 57, no. 1, pp. 84–88, 2013.

[4] P. D. Stein and H. N. Sabbah, "Turbulent blood flow in the ascending aorta of humans with normal and diseased aortic valves," *Circulation Research*, vol. 39, no. 1, pp. 58–65, 1976.

[5] R. Berguer, J. L. Bull, and K. Khanafer, "Refinements in mathematical models to predict aneurysm growth and rupture," *Annals of the New York Academy of Sciences*, vol. 1085, pp. 110–116, 2006.

[6] F. R. Menter, R. B. Langtry, S. R. Likki, Y. B. Suzen, P. G. Huang, and S. Volker, "A correlation-based transition model using local variables, part i - model formulation," in *Proceedings of the ASME Turbo Expo 2004: Power for Land, Sea, and Air*, pp. 57–67, Vienna, Austria, 2004.

[7] F. P. P. Tan, A. Borghi, R. H. Mohiaddin, N. B. Wood, S. Thom, and X. Y. Xu, "Analysis of flow patterns in a patient-specific thoracic aortic aneurysm model," *Computers and Structures*, vol. 87, no. 11-12, pp. 680–690, 2009.

[8] A. C. Benim, A. Nahavandi, A. Assmann, D. Schubert, P. Feindt, and S. H. Suh, "Simulation of blood flow in human aorta with emphasis on outlet boundary conditions," *Applied Mathemati-*

cal Modelling: Simulation and Computation for Engineering and Environmental Systems, vol. 35, no. 7, pp. 3175–3188, 2011.

[9] A. Borghi, N. B. Wood, R. H. Mohiaddin, and X. Y. Xu, "3D geometric reconstruction of thoracic aortic aneurysms," *Biomedical Engineering Online*, vol. 5, article no. 59, 2006.

[10] A.-K. Qiao, W.-Y. Fu, and Y.-J. Liu, "Study on hemodynamics in patient-specific thoracic aortic aneurysm," *Theoretical and Applied Mechanics Letters*, vol. 1, Article ID 014001, 2011.

[11] F. M. Callaghan, J. Karkouri, K. Broadhouse, M. Evin, D. F. Fletcher, and S. M. Grieve, "Thoracic aortic aneurysm: 4D flow MRI and computational fluid dynamics model," *Computer Methods in Biomechanics and Biomedical Engineering*, vol. 18, pp. 1894-1895, 2015.

[12] S. Numata, K. Itatani, K. Kanda et al., "Blood flow analysis of the aortic arch using computational fluid dynamics," *European Journal of Cardio-Thoracic Surgery*, vol. 49, no. 6, pp. 1578–1585, 2016.

[13] M. Markl, G. J. Wagner, and A. J. Barker, "Re: Blood flow analysis of the aortic arch using computational fluid dynamics," *European Journal of Cardio-Thoracic Surgery*, vol. 49, no. 6, pp. 1586-1587, 2016.

[14] E. Soudah, J. Casacuberta, P. J. Gamez-Montero et al., "Estimation of wall shear stress using 4D flow cardiovascular MRI and computational fluid dynamics," *Journal of Mechanics in Medicine and Biology*, vol. 17, no. 3, Article ID 1750046, 2017.

[15] E. I. Basri, A. A. Basri, V. N. Riazuddin, S. F. Shahwir, Z. Mohammad, and K. A. Ahmad, "Computational Fluid Dynamics Study in Biomedical Applications: A Review," *International Journal of Fluids and Heat Transfer*, vol. 1, no. 2, 2016.

[16] S. S. Shibeshi and W. E. Collins, "The rheology of blood flow in a branced arterial system," *Applied Rheology*, vol. 15, no. 6, pp. 398–405, 2005.

[17] Y. I. Cho and K. R. Kensey, "Effects of the non-Newtonian viscosity of blood on flows in a diseased arterial vessel. Part 1: Steady flows," *Biorheology*, vol. 28, no. 3-4, pp. 241–262, 1991.

[18] F. J. H. Gijsen, E. Allanic, F. N. van de Vosse, and J. D. Janssen, "The influence of the non-Newtonian properties of blood on the flow in large arteries: unsteady flow in a 90∘ curved tube," *Journal of Biomechanics*, vol. 32, no. 7, pp. 705–713, 1999.

[19] J. P. W. Baaijens, A. A. Van Steenhoven, and J. D. Janssen, "Numerical analysis of steady generalized Newtonian blood flow in a 2D model of the carotid artery bifurcation," *Biorheology*, vol. 30, no. 1, pp. 63–74, 1993.

[20] P. Ballyk, D. Steinman, and C. Ethier, "Simulation of non-Newtonian blood flow in an end-to-side anastomosis," *Biorheology*, vol. 31, no. 5, pp. 565–586, 1994.

[21] D. N. Ku and D. Liepsch, "The effects of non-Newtonian viscoelasticity and wall elasticity on flow at a 90∘ bifurcation," *Biorheology*, vol. 23, no. 4, pp. 359–370, 1986.

[22] P. J. Daley, K. B. Sagar, and L. S. Wann, "Doppler echocardiographic measurement of flow velocity in the ascending aorta during supine and upright exercise," *British Heart Journal*, vol. 54, no. 6, pp. 562–567, 1985.

[23] C. A. Taylor and M. T. Draney, "Experimental and computational methods in cardiovascular fluid mechanics," in *Annual review of fluid mechanics. Vol. 36*, vol. 36 of *Annu. Rev. Fluid Mech.*, pp. 197–231, Annual Reviews, Palo Alto, CA, 2004.

[24] Y. S. Chatzizisis, A. U. Coskun, M. Jonas, E. R. Edelman, C. L. Feldman, and P. H. Stone, "Role of endothelial shear stress in the natural history of coronary atherosclerosis and vascular remodeling: molecular, cellular, and vascular behavior," *Journal of the American College of Cardiology*, vol. 49, no. 25, pp. 2379–2393, 2007.

[25] C. Cheng, D. Tempel, R. van Haperen et al., "Atherosclerotic lesion size and vulnerability are determined by patterns of fluid shear stress," *Circulation*, vol. 113, no. 23, pp. 2744–2753, 2006.

13

Automatic Extraction of the Centerline of Corpus Callosum from Segmented Mid-Sagittal MR Images

Wenpeng Gao,[1,2] Xiaoguang Chen,[3] Yili Fu,[1,2] and Minwei Zhu[4]

[1]*School of Life Science and Technology, Harbin Institute of Technology, Harbin, China*
[2]*State Key Laboratory of Robotics and System, Harbin Institute of Technology, Harbin, China*
[3]*Department of Neurosurgery, The Third People Hospital of Hainan Province, Sanya 572000, China*
[4]*Department of Neurosurgery, The First Affiliated Hospital of Harbin Medical University, Harbin 150001, China*

Correspondence should be addressed to Yili Fu; meylfu@hit.edu.cn and Minwei Zhu; zhumw2013@gmail.com

Academic Editor: Giancarlo Ferrigno

The centerline, as a simple and compact representation of object shape, has been used to analyze variations of the human callosal shape. However, automatic extraction of the callosal centerline remains a sophisticated problem. In this paper, we propose a method of automatic extraction of the callosal centerline from segmented mid-sagittal magnetic resonance (MR) images. A model-based point matching method is introduced to localize the anterior and posterior endpoints of the centerline. The model of the endpoint is constructed with a statistical descriptor of the shape context. Active contour modeling is adopted to drive the curve with the fixed endpoints to approximate the centerline using the gradient of the distance map of the segmented corpus callosum. Experiments with 80 segmented mid-sagittal MR images were performed. The proposed method is compared with a skeletonization method and an interactive method in terms of recovery error and reproducibility. Results indicate that the proposed method outperforms skeletonization and is comparable with and sometimes better than the interactive method.

1. Introduction

The corpus callosum (CC) is the main commissural bundle of fibers interconnecting the left and right cerebral hemispheres [1]. It facilitates interhemispheric communication in the human brain. Its special role has motivated imaging-based study of its size and shape to investigate the morphological correlation with various disorders, such as spastic cerebral palsy [2], fetal alcohol syndrome and fetal alcohol spectrum disorders [3], autism [4, 5], Turner syndrome [6, 7], HIV/AIDS [8], frontonasal dysplasia [9], dyslexia [10], attention-deficit hyperactivity disorder (ADHD) [11], and Alzheimer's disease [12, 13]. Most of these studies are based on the measurement of the CC's simplex geometric properties, such as the area [2, 6, 7, 12, 13] and circumference [11] of CC region, the angle between the CC and anterior-posterior commissure line [9]. However, these studies can only reveal the growth or atrophy of the entire CC but not exactly where the change occurs.

Recently, some researchers have focused on centerline-based analysis [3–5, 10], which is more powerful and comprehensive: centerline-based analysis can detect the exact position where the variation of thickness and angular change of the CC along the centerline occurs, which is more sensitive and discriminative in comparison with size- or area-based analysis. Nevertheless, the centerline is an implicit representation of the shape, and it is impossible to delineate the callosal centerline from magnetic resonance (MR) images manually. Many researchers have utilized skeletonization techniques to extract the skeleton as the main body of the centerline. The skeleton is a thin version of a shape, which is an important feature for shape description in image processing and computer vision. It is defined as the locus of centers of maximal inscribed disks in two dimensions (2D) [14]. In the technical literature, the concepts of skeleton and centerline are used interchangeably by some researchers, while others regard them as related, but not the same. In the view of anatomists, the centerline of the anatomy is not consistent with the skeleton, because the topology of the skeleton is uncertain, whereas the topology of the anatomical centerline is known. In general, the centerline starts and ends at boundary points. Taking the CC as an example, its centerline should be a curve that starts at the anterior pole of the rostrum and ends at the posterior pole of the splenium. Therefore, centerline extraction cannot completely depend on the techniques of skeletonization. However, the idea can be applied to extraction of the callosal centerline. Most previous centerline-based studies have adopted skeletonization techniques to extract the main part of the centerline and apply curve fitting after labeling the endpoints to obtain the centerline.

To date, diversified approaches have been proposed to extract the skeleton from an image. These approaches can be mainly classified into three categories: distance transformation based [15–19], Voronoi diagram based [20], and thinning based [21]. The distance transform computes the minimum distance of each pixel to the shape boundary. However, the distance transform is very sensitive to small perturbations of the boundary, as each value of the shape is assigned according to a single boundary point (the nearest point). The skeletons obtained by the distance transform require a pruning stage if the boundary is noisy [22]. To overcome the limitations of the distance transform, several smooth medial functions have been introduced based on Newton's law [23], electrostatic field [24], and Poisson's equation [25]. These methods consider several boundary points and therefore better reflect the global properties of the shape than does the distance transform. Thinning based methods involve a morphological operation that is used to remove object boundary pixels from binary images iteratively with a set of conditions, somewhat like erosion or gradual opening. Complex conditions are required to terminate this process and to preserve the topology and connectivity of the skeleton. In the Voronoi diagram-based approaches, the skeleton is extracted from a Voronoi diagram derived from the object boundaries. Existing skeletonization techniques suffer from at least one of the following shortcomings: dependence on the accuracy of determining the medial axis, computational complexity, lack of robustness, connectivity, spurious branches, or sensitivity to boundary noise. Therefore, the centerline cannot be precisely obtained through skeletonization alone.

Localization of the anterior and posterior endpoints is another issue. The anterior and posterior endpoints are at the anterior and posterior poles of the CC, respectively, as shown in Figure 1. In general, the skeleton extraction methods cannot localize these two points, because they are not part of the skeleton according to the definition of a skeleton. The endpoint at the anterior pole of the rostrum (see Figure 1) is usually associated with a local maximum curvature of the callosal boundary [4, 5, 7]. Owing to the existence of noise on the boundary, it is not easy to locate it uniquely using state-of-the-art corner detection methods. As for the posterior endpoint, the problem is even more complicated, because the geometric features around it are not obvious, and there is no sharp tip in the splenium as exists in the rostrum. In addition, anatomical variability makes it more complicated to locate the posterior endpoint. Thompson et al. [8] selected the lowest points of the genu and splenium as the endpoints. In [11], the endpoints of the CC were determined by extending the centerline to the boundary. Owing to the inconsistent criteria for locating the endpoints, the results of these studies may also be inconsistent. To the best of our knowledge, there is no effective method that localizes these two endpoints.

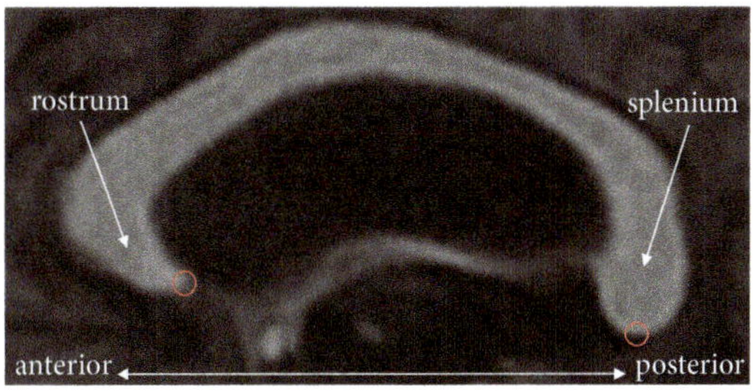

FIGURE 1: Endpoints (centers of the red circles) of the CC in a mid-sagittal MR image.

Centerline-based shape analysis has been widely used in CC. Most research has adopted the method of skeletonization to extract the centerline. However, there are few works on the evaluation and validation of these centerline extraction techniques, which poses a rather serious challenge when interpreting their results. In this paper, we propose a method for the callosal centerline extraction from segmented mid-sagittal MR images. The main contributions of this paper are as follows. First, a method of model-based point detection is proposed to localize the callosal endpoints. A model for each endpoint is generated using statistical shape context as the descriptor under a local coordinate system, in which point detection is robust to boundary noise and is rotation invariant (to a certain extent). Then, active contour model (ACM) based curve evolution with two fixed endpoints is applied to approximate the centerline, which guarantees the topology of the obtained centerline and tolerates the influence of boundary noise. Experiments with 80 segmented mid-sagittal MR images were performed to evaluate the effectiveness of the proposed method.

2. Methods

2.1. Automatic Localization of the Endpoints. To automatically localize the two endpoints, a statistical model-based point detection method is proposed, which consists of two steps: model construction and point localization.

2.1.1. Model Construction. The statistical models of the endpoints are generated using shape context [26], which is a robust, compact, and highly discriminative descriptor widely used in shape matching. The shape context of a point of interest is a measure of the distribution of other points in the shape relative to it under the log-polar coordinate system. Given a point p, the shape context of p is defined as a coarse histogram of the relative polar coordinates of the other points, written as

$$h(m,n) = \#\{q \neq p : (q-p) \in \text{bin}(m,n)\} \tag{1}$$

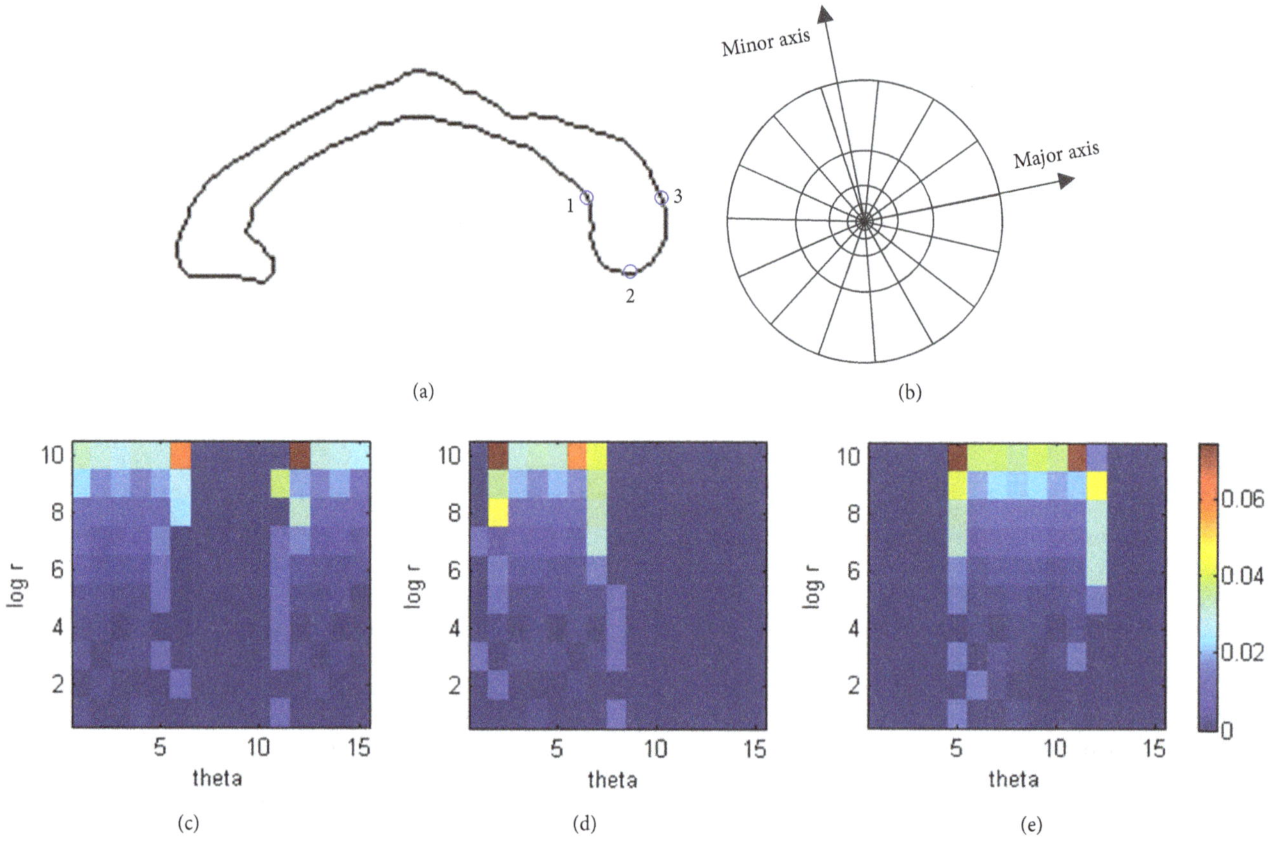

FIGURE 2: Shape context computation. (a) Contour of CC (black) and three boundary points marked by the centers of circles (blue). (b) Diagram of log-polar bins used in computing the shape contexts under the local log-polar coordinate system (10 bins for $\log r$ coordinate and 15 bins for angular coordinate in this work). (c–e) Histogram maps of three points marked in (a).

where q denotes the other points of the shape and $h(m, n)$ is a normalized $M \times N$ bins histogram in log-polar space at p. Each bin indicates the proportion of the points in this region with respect to the total adjacent points of p. Figure 2 illustrates the process of computing the shape context.

It is easy to make the shape context scale invariant, but we cannot guarantee rotation invariance by referring to the image coordinate system owing to different scanning directions and the existence of individual variability. Some methods obtain the shape context with respect to the tangent direction at the point, which may lose orientation information of the point and cause the shape context to be less sensitive when distinguishing similar boundary points. Alternatively, two local Cartesian coordinate systems with respect to the rostrum and splenium are defined for the computation of the two endpoints' shape contexts. Given a segmented CC, its bounding rectangle and major and minor axes are extracted using the method proposed by Chaudhuri and Samal [27]. Then, the CC is automatically divided into five subregions according to a modification of the Witelson partitioning scheme [28, 29]. Four radial dividers emanate from the midpoint of the inferior side of the bounding rectangle with equal angular interval and divide the CC into five subregions, i.e., the rostrum and genu (denoted as CC1), the rostral body (denoted as CC2), the mid-body (denoted as CC3), the isthmus (denoted as CC4), and the splenium (denoted as CC5) (see Figure 3). The log-polar coordinate system is defined on CC1 (and CC5) with its origin at the mass center of CC1 (and CC5) and radial axis parallel to the major axis of CC1 (and CC5) from anterior to posterior (see Figure 2(b)). The radial coordinate is divided by the height of the bounding rectangle of the CC for normalization, which guarantees scale invariance of the shape context.

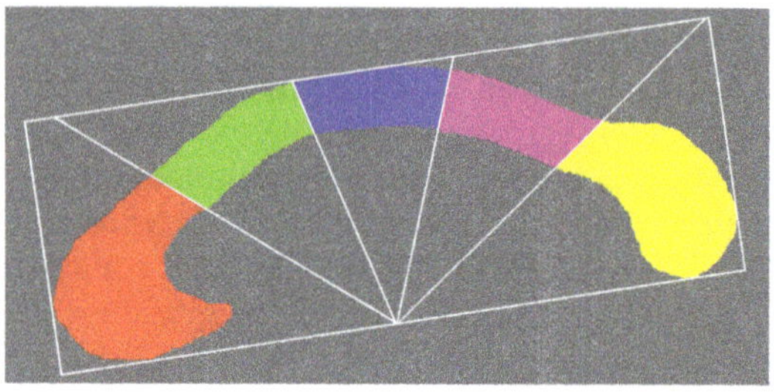

FIGURE 3: Subregions of CC. Red: rostrum and genu (CC1), green: rostral body (CC2), blue: mid-body (CC3), pink: isthmus (CC4), and yellow: splenium (CC5).

Results may be biased if the endpoint with its shape context is derived from only one individual's CC. Therefore, we create a statistical model using the mean shape context as the descriptor. Suppose there are K samples (i.e., segmented CC images) in the training sets. Two raters are asked to label the endpoints by mutual agreement. Then, the shape context of each sample (denoted as h_k) is calculated according to (1) and all shapes are aligned with respect to a local log-polar coordinate system. The mean shape context (denoted as $\bar{h}$) is then written as

$$\bar{h}(m,n) = \frac{1}{K}\sum_{k=1}^{K} h_i(m,n) \tag{2}$$

Here, a statistical model is created and used to detect the endpoint by matching the model with the shape contexts of the candidate points.

2.1.2. Point Localization. Given a segmented CC, p_j denotes a candidate point on the boundary. The process of locating the endpoints is to find a boundary point whose shape context is most similar to the model. As the shape context is represented as a histogram, the similarity is measured as the sum of the difference of two histograms according to

$$p^* = \arg\min_{p_j} \sum_m \sum_n \left| \bar{h}(m,n) - h_j(m,n) \right| \tag{3}$$

Here, $h_j(m,n)$ is the shape context of p_j and $\bar{h}(m,n)$ is the statistical model obtained from (2).

2.2. Active Contour Based Centerline Extraction. The invisible CC centerline is approximated using the ACM proposed by Kass et al. [30]. The advantage of ACM is that the topology of the curve can be preserved during its evolution, which means that spurious branches can be avoided. To allow the curve to approximate the invisible centerline of the CC, the representation of the centerline should be introduced in advance.

2.2.1. Representation of the Centerline. The centerline is depicted implicitly using a distance map [31], which labels each pixel with the distance to the nearest boundary pixel. If a pixel in the CC is labeled with a maximum distance, it means that this pixel is far from the boundary and in the center of the CC. Therefore, this pixel may be on the centerline. Let O denote the segmented CC region, and ∂O denote the boundary of O. We refer to $d(p,q)$ as the Euclidean distance between two pixels p and q. The distance map in the CC is defined as

$$D_O(p) = \begin{cases} \min\limits_{\forall q \in \partial O} d(p,q) & p \in O \\ 0 & p \notin O \end{cases} \tag{4}$$

2.2.2. Evolution of the Curve. To fit the centerline using ACM, a curve $\mathbf{x}(s) = [x(s), y(s)]$, $s \in [0,1]$ moves within the spatial domain of the distance map by minimizing the following energy function:

$$E = \int_0^1 \frac{1}{2}\left(\alpha \left|\mathbf{x}'(s)\right|^2 + \beta \left|\mathbf{x}''(s)\right|^2 + E_{ext}(\mathbf{x}(s))\right) ds \tag{5}$$

where α and β are weighting parameters that control the curve's tension and rigidity, respectively, and $\mathbf{x}'(s)$ and $\mathbf{x}''(s)$ denote the first and second derivatives of $\mathbf{x}(s)$ with respect to s. The external energy E_{ext} is a function derived from the distance map of the CC and is responsible for driving the curve to the maximum distance region where the centerline is located. The formulation of E_{ext} is

$$E_{ext} = \frac{2}{\left(1 - e^{|D(\mathbf{x}(s))|}\right)} \left|\nabla D(\mathbf{x}(s))\right| \tag{6}$$

where D is the normalized distance map. The gradient flow $\nabla D(\mathbf{x}(s))$ moves the curve toward to the centerline. The coefficient $2/(1 - e^{|D(\mathbf{x}(s))|})$ is used to modulate the force of the gradient flow of the distance map. When $\mathbf{x}(s)$ is near the boundary (or center) of the CC, the coefficient is close to 1.0 (or 0.0), and the external energy is increased (or decreased). This guarantees that the curve approximates the centerline more stably.

The model is initialized with a spline curve starting at the anterior endpoint, ending at the posterior endpoint, and passing through four control points in the CC. These four control points are on the four radial lines shown in Figure 3 (the maximum distance points). Then, a spline curve is interpolated with nearly equal distance intervals for initialization of the model. During the evolution of the curve, the endpoints of the curve are fixed at the detected endpoints.

3. Experiments and Results

The proposed method was implemented using the C++ language. The experiments were performed on an HP workstation with Intel Xeon CPU (E5540@ dual-core, 2.53 GHz) and 8 GB RAM. In the experiments, the weighted coefficients α and β in (5) were empirically set to 0.1 and 0.5, respectively.

To compare our method with existing methods, a skeletonization method and an interactive method were implemented. The skeletonization method (pfSkel-1.2.1.1) proposed by Chuang et al. [32] is publicly available (http://cocwww.rutgers.edu/www2/vizlab/NicuCornea/Skeletanization/skeletanization.html).pfSkel mainly consists of four steps. First, a 2D vector field in the segmented CC is calculated with respect to the boundary pixels. Second, the critical points of the vector field are detected as the core skeleton. Third, the first level skeleton is generated from the divergence of the vector field. Last and fourth, the second level skeleton is derived by connecting the boundary pixel with a certain percentage of curvature value to the core and first level skeleton. The interactive method is based on the pfSkel method and consists of three steps. First, the skeleton is extracted from the segmented CC. Then, the anterior and posterior endpoints are labeled manually. Finally, the centerline is obtained with a cubic spline connecting the endpoints and fitting the skeleton. For clarity, pfSkel is denoted as SKEL1 (which only generates the first level skeleton) and SKEL2 (which generates the first level plus second level skeletons). The interactive method and our method are denoted as CLM and CLA, respectively.

3.1. Data and Preprocessing. The data sets for evaluating the presented method contain high-resolution T1-weighted MR brain volumes of 80 subjects, including 50 healthy controls and 30 patients with various pathologies (infarctions); subject ages range from 12 to 60 years. The volume size varies from 192×256×256 to 256×181×256 voxels. The voxel size ranges from 0.897 mm to 1 mm in the sagittal plane, from 0.879 mm to 1.25 mm in the coronal plane, and from 0.67 mm to 1.5 mm in the axial directions.

The CC in the mid-sagittal plane was segmented with our self-developed software applying the following steps: (1) resampling each volume to make it isotropic; (2) extracting the mid-sagittal MR image using the method proposed by Hu and Nowinski [33]; (3) Binarizing the mid-sagittal MR image with upper and lower thresholds determined using Gaussian mixture modeling [34]; (4) extracting the bounding rectangle of each region and calculating geometric parameters (such as length and width) using the method proposed by Chaudhrui and Samal [27]; (5) selecting the CC region according to its anatomic characteristics: (a) length (from the anterior point to posterior point) of 7 to 9 cm, (b) width (from the superior point to the inferior point) of 2 to 4 cm, (c) orientation (angle of the major axis with respect to the horizontal axis) from 5° to 40°, and (d) area > 2 cm^2; and (6) manually rectifying any mis-segmentation or oversegmentation by two raters in mutual agreement. After the segmentation, the centerline endpoints were manually identified on the boundary of the CC by two experts according to their anatomical knowledge after mutual agreement.

3.2. Accuracy of Endpoint Localization. To validate the accuracy of the presented endpoint localization method, statistical models were generated with 15 samples in the datasets using the method described in Section 2.1.1. Then, the statistical models were used to localize the endpoints in the other 65 samples in the datasets. The endpoint localization error is measured as the distance between the detected point and the manually labeled point. The endpoint localization error was 0.85±0.12 mm in this case.

3.3. Qualitative (Visual) Evaluation. We present the results of SKEL1, SKEL2, CLM, and CLA to illustrate the difference in the centerline extraction in Figure 4. The top row illustrates the mid-sagittal MR images. Owing to the existence of intersubject variability, the shape of the CC varies significantly among the eight subjects. The results of SKEL1 are shown in the second row. The skeletons are not continuous and do not start and end at the anterior and posterior poles of the CC (see Figures 4(c) and 4(g)). The third row illustrates the results of SKEL2, in which the percentage was set to 0.001 experimentally. It generates fewer branches and more skeletons near the centerline. Even though the parameter has been adjusted to reduce the number of branches, there are still some spurious branches present (see Figures 4(b), 4(d), 4(e), 4(g), and 4(h)). The fourth row demonstrates the centerline extracted by an experienced and well-trained rater with the interactive method. The bottom row exhibits the results of the proposed method. The extracted centerlines are continuous curves connecting the anterior pole to the posterior pole and are centered in the region of the CC.

3.4. Quantitative Evaluation. The centerline is a geometric feature of a shape and is essentially invisible to the naked eye. Given a segmented CC, no radiologist or anatomist can manually delineate a centerline as the ground truth. Hence, it is difficult to validate the accuracy of the proposed method straightforwardly. In this paper, we adopted a technique used in assessing skeletonization results as proposed by Direkoglu et al. [35].

Suppose a point set P represents the extracted centerline. According to the definition of the centerline, a point p on the centerline must be the center of a maximum disk inscribed in the CC's shape. Let $r_{\max}(p)$ denote the radius of the maximal disk $B(s, r(p))$ centered at the point p. The reconstruction of the CC region is given by

$$R(P) = \bigcup_{p \in P} B(s, r(p)) \tag{7}$$

where $R(P)$ is the reconstructed CC region. The quality of the extracted centerline is evaluated using a reconstruction error rate (RER) between the reconstructed and the segmented regions of the CC, which is calculated as follows:

$$RER = \frac{A(O) - A(R(P))}{A(O)} \tag{8}$$

where $A(*)$ is a function used to calculate the area measured in pixels. O and R represent the images that contain the segmented and reconstructed regions of the CC, respectively.

We reconstructed the regions of the CC using the centerlines obtained by SKEL1, SKEL2, CLM, and CLA, respectively. RER is calculated using (8). Figure 5 shows the RERs of SKEL1, SKEL2, CLM, and CLA. The mean and standard deviation of the RERs of CLA, SKEL1, SKEL2, and CLM are 0.12±0.01, 0.24±0.08, 0.15±0.04, and 0.14±0.02, respectively. The presented method outperforms the skeletonization methods (SKEL1 and SKEL2) and is comparable with or even better than CLM in terms of the RER.

3.5. Reproducibility Evaluation. To compare the presented method with CLM in terms of reproducibility, we randomly selected 10 samples in the dataset. For each sample, we extracted the centerline 10 times with the presented method and CLM, respectively. Five knowledgeable raters were asked to extract the centerline of each case with CLM once per day to guarantee that the raters were not influenced by previous results. Then, we obtained two groups of centerlines, i.e., one group with our method and another one with CLM. In each group, the distance between any two centerlines was calculated, and the mean distance was denoted as the reproducibility error.

Owing to the discretization of the centerline, the distance between two centerlines is measured as the distance between two point sets representing the centerlines. Given two centerline point sets $P = \{p_1, p_2, \ldots, p_M\}$ and $Q = \{q_1, q_2, \ldots, q_N\}$,

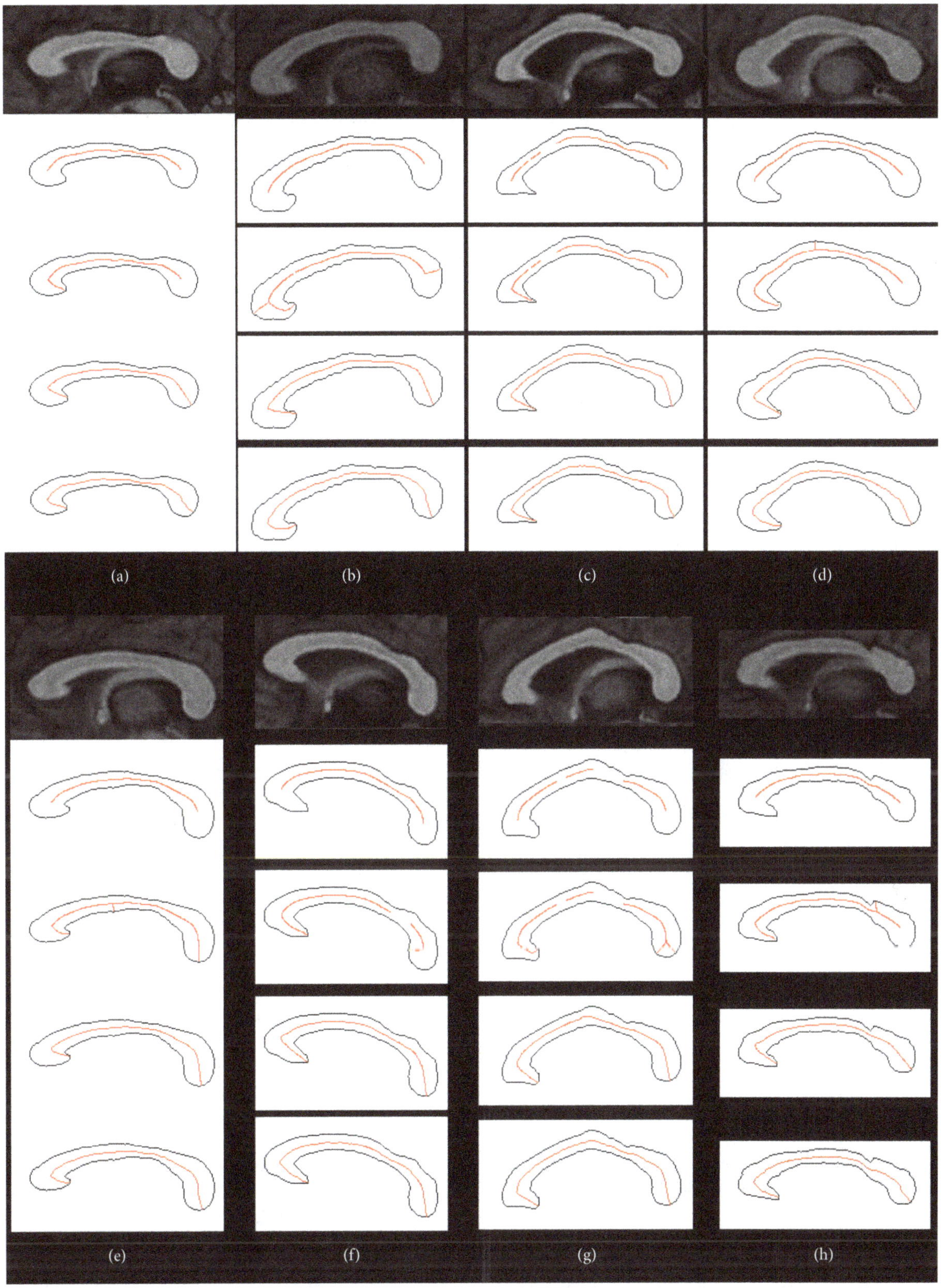

FIGURE 4: Results (red curves) for eight mid-sagittal MR images. Top row: mid-sagittal MR images, second row: results of SKEL1, third row: results of SKEL2, fourth row: results of CLM, and bottom row: results of CLA.

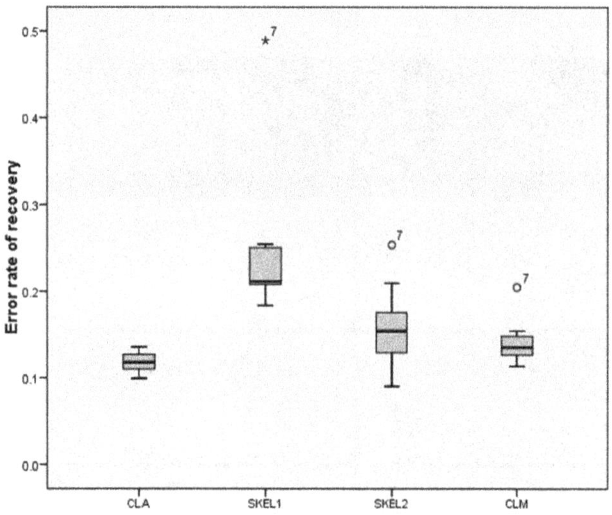

FIGURE 5: Boxplot chart of the RERs of SKEL1, SKEL2, CLA, and CLM.

TABLE 1: Reproducibility errors of CLM (unit: mm).

	Mean	SD.	Max	Min
Sample 1	0.012	0.003	0.034	0.002
Sample 2	0.023	0.009	0.067	0.001
Sample 3	0.071	0.010	0.106	0.015
Sample 4	0.044	0.009	0.082	0.009
Sample 5	0.042	0.007	0.067	0.014
Sample 6	0.072	0.014	0.139	0.021
Sample 7	0.119	0.015	0.214	0.039
Sample 8	0.072	0.089	0.113	0.025
Sample 9	0.063	0.009	0.106	0.021
Sample 10	0.066	0.008	0.103	0.030

the mean distance between them using Euclidean distance is

$$d(P,Q) = \frac{1}{2}\left[\frac{1}{M}\sum_{i=1}^{M}\min_{j=1,2,\ldots,N}\left\|p_i - q_j\right\| + \frac{1}{N}\sum_{j=1}^{N}\min_{i=1,2,\ldots,N}\left\|p_i - q_j\right\|\right] \quad (9)$$

There was no reproducibility error with our method and an average reproducibility error of 0.047±0.003 mm with CLM. Table 1 shows the results of CLM in detail.

4. Discussion

The corpus callosum plays an important role in the communication between the left and right cerebrums. Due to its essential role, its dysfunction may cause various neuropsychological or neuropathological diseases, while the progression of these diseases may also cause it to physically change shape and/or thickness. MRI-based morphology analysis of the CC has become an effective technique to investigate the variation of the CC in relation to these diseases in vivo. Most studies are based on area measurement [2, 13]. These methods can only detect the whole body change of the CC, which cannot describe the shape change in detail, and their findings are not sensitive or discriminative to specific diseases. To reduce this limitation, some researchers proposed measuring the area of the CC's subregions, which are obtained according to its geometric features [1, 12]. There are several rules to divide the CC [29, 36–38]. More recent studies based on these schemes have generated controversial results concerning the assumed topography of the callosal fiber tracts. Recently, several groups have focused on centerline-based analysis of the CC [3–5, 10], which is a promising way to investigate the variation of the CC in relation to specific diseases. The centerline, as a compact representation of the CC's shape, can be used to measure the thickness of the CC and the curvature at any centerline point; these descriptors provide comprehensive information regarding the CC's shape. In addition, the correspondence information among samples can be achieved easily, which facilitates population-based analysis, also known as centerline-based morphological analysis.

The presented method consists of two steps: automatic localization of the endpoints and ACM-based centerline extraction. There are three advantages to the presented method. First, the endpoint localization method is robust to boundary noise in comparison with methods based on curvature because the statistical shape context as a descriptor of local shape features can avoid the disturbances caused by noise. Second, the endpoints localization method is scale invariant due to normalization of the shape context. In addition, the endpoints localization method is rotation invariant to some extent. This is owing to the adoption of the local coordinate system, which makes our method robust to the rotation derived from not only the scanning direction but also individual variability in the CCs of different people. Despite the CC inclining forward and backward with respect to the horizontal line in Figures 4(b) and 4(f), our method can localize the endpoints accurately. The shape context is calculated with 15 bins in (1) (see Figure 2). In theory, the presented method can accommodate an angle between the model and the sample if less than 24° (= 360°/15). Figures 4(d) and 4(e) show the case for different angles between the rostrum and the body owing to the existence of intersubject variability. Finally, our method preserves topology by utilizing ACM to fit the centerline: a smooth centerline with no branches is obtained. In contrast, it is difficult to control the topology of the centerline using skeletonization. There is also no gap in the extracted centerline using our method, while gaps may exist in the skeletonization centerline (see Figures 4(c) and 4(g)).

The presented method has a lower RER in comparison with SKEL1, SKEL2, and CLM. This contributes to an automatic, accurate, and robust method for locating the endpoints and reproducing the centerline using ACM-based curve evolution. However, the recovery error cannot reach zero due to the irregular shape of any CC. In terms of reproducibility, the presented method has a higher accuracy in comparison with CLM because the endpoints localization method is more consistent in contrast to manual labeling by raters' subjective analysis.

The accuracy of the endpoint localization will affect that of the centerline extraction. However, the influence is limited owing to the movement of the curve in ACM mainly driven by the gradient flow of the distance map. The endpoint localization error merely interferes in the curve's behavior near the endpoints. The movement of the curve's main body is still under the supervision of the gradient flow. Moreover, the proposed method presents high accuracy (0.85±0.12mm) and robustness (see Figure 4) in the endpoint localization.

The prerequisite of the presented method is that the CC should be segmented from a mid-sagittal MR image in advance. To date, there are several techniques available to extract the mid-sagittal MR image automatically [33, 39–41] and various methods to delineate the corpus callosum, such as mathematical morphology-based methods [42], cluster-based methods [43, 44], deformable mode-based methods [45], tractography-based methods [46, 47], and template-based methods [48]. Any of these methods can be integrated into the presented method for convenience.

5. Conclusions

The centerline of the CC can depict the CC's shape variation in more detail when compared to size or area measurements. In this paper, we proposed a method of automatic extraction of the callosal centerline. The anterior and posterior endpoints are localized using statistical model-based point matching, which is robust to boundary noise and is rotation invariant to a certain extent. The centerline is fitted using the active contour model driven by a gradient of the distance map to produce an implicit representation of the centerline. Experiments with segmented MR images were performed to validate this method and the results indicate that our method outperforms skeletonization and is comparable with and sometimes better than the interactive method.

In the future, neurological or neuropathological diseases related to changes in the corpus callosum can be analyzed with centerline-based measurements, such as variation of thickness and curvature.

Conflicts of Interest

The authors declare that they have no conflicts of interest.

Acknowledgments

This work was supported by the National Natural Science Foundation of China (Grants nos. 81500924, 81171304, and 81201150). It was also supported by Sanya Key Laboratory Construction (Grant no. L1232), Natural Science Foundation of Hainan Province of China (Grant no. 20158306), and Postdoctoral Scientific Research Developmental Fund of Heilongjiang Province of China (Grant no. LBH-Q17012).

References

[1] J. N. Giedd, J. M. Rumsey, F. X. Castellanos et al., "A quantitative MRI study of the corpus callosum in children and adolescents," *Developmental Brain Research*, vol. 91, no. 2, pp. 274–280, 1996.

[2] W. Kułak, W. Sobaniec, B. Kubas, and J. Walecki, "Corpus callosum size in children with spastic cerebral palsy: Relationship to clinical outcome," *Journal of Child Neurology*, vol. 22, no. 4, pp. 371–374, 2007.

[3] L. Li, C. D. Coles, M. E. Lynch, and X. Hu, "Voxelwise and skeleton-based region of interest analysis of fetal alcohol syndrome and fetal alcohol spectrum disorders in young adults," *Human Brain Mapping*, vol. 30, no. 10, pp. 3265–3274, 2009.

[4] M. F. Casanova, A. El-Baz, A. Elnakib et al., "Quantitative analysis of the shape of the corpus callosum in patients with autism and comparison individuals," *Autism*, vol. 15, no. 2, pp. 223–238, 2011.

[5] A. El-Baz, A. Elnakib, M. F. Casanova et al., "Accurate automated detection of autism related corpus callosum abnormalities," *Journal of Medical Systems*, vol. 35, no. 5, pp. 929–939, 2011.

[6] S. L. Fryer, H. Kwon, S. Eliez, and A. L. Reiss, "Corpus callosum and posterior fossa development in monozygotic females: A morphometric MRI study of Turner syndrome," *Developmental Medicine & Child Neurology*, vol. 45, no. 5, pp. 320–324, 2003.

[7] K. J. Plessen, T. Wentzel-Larsen, K. Hugdahl et al., "Altered interhemispheric connectivity in individuals with Tourette's disorder," *The American Journal of Psychiatry*, vol. 161, no. 11, pp. 2028–2037, 2004.

[8] P. M. Thompson, R. A. Dutton, K. M. Hayashi et al., "3D mapping of ventricular and corpus callosum abnormalities in HIV/AIDS," *NeuroImage*, vol. 31, no. 1, pp. 12–23, 2006.

[9] S. D. A. Giffoni, V. M. Gimenes Gonçalves, V. A. Zanardi, and V. L. Gil Da Silva Lopes, "Angular analysis of corpus callosum in 18 patients with frontonasal dysplasia," *Arquivos de Neuro-Psiquiatria*, vol. 62, no. 2 A, pp. 195–198, 2004.

[10] A. Elnakib, M. F. Casanova, G. Gimelrfarb, A. E. Switala, and A. El-Baz, "Dyslexia diagnostics by 3-D shape analysis of the corpus callosum," *IEEE Transactions on Information Technology in Biomedicine*, vol. 16, no. 4, pp. 700–708, 2012.

[11] M. A. McNally, D. Crocetti, E. M. Mahone, M. B. Denckla, S. J. Suskauer, and S. H. Mostofsky, "Corpus callosum segment circumference is associated with response control in children with attention-deficit hyperactivity disorder (ADHD)," *Journal of Child Neurology*, vol. 25, no. 4, pp. 453–462, 2010.

[12] M. Zhu, W. Gao, X. Wang, C. Shi, and Z. Lin, "Progression of Corpus Callosum Atrophy in Early Stage of Alzheimer's Disease. MRI Based Study," *Academic Radiology*, vol. 19, no. 5, pp. 512–517, 2012.

[13] M. Zhu, X. Wang, W. Gao et al., "Corpus callosum atrophy and cognitive decline in early Alzheimer's disease: Longitudinal MRI study," *Dementia and Geriatric Cognitive Disorders*, vol. 37, no. 3-4, pp. 214–222, 2014.

[14] A. Lieutier, "Any open bounded subset of ℝn has the same homotopy type than its Medial Axis," in *Proceedings of the Eighth ACM Symposium on Solid Modeling and Applications*, pp. 65–75, usa, June 2003.

[15] C. Arcelli and G. Sanniti di Baja, "Ridge points in Euclidean distance maps," *Pattern Recognition Letters*, vol. 13, no. 4, pp. 237–243, 1992.

[16] R. Kimmel, D. Shaked, N. Kiryati, and A. M. Bruckstein, "Skeletonization via Distance Maps and Level Sets," *Computer Vision and Image Understanding*, vol. 62, no. 3, pp. 382–391, 1995.

[17] G. Malandain and S. Fernández-Vidal, "Euclidean skeletons," *Image and Vision Computing*, vol. 16, no. 5, pp. 317–327, 1998.

[18] W. H. Hesselink and J. B. T. M. Roerdink, "Euclidean skeletons of digital image and volume data in linear time by the integer medial axis transform," *IEEE Transactions on Pattern Analysis and Machine Intelligence*, vol. 30, no. 12, pp. 2204–2217, 2008.

[19] A. D. Ward and G. Hamarneh, "The groupwise medial axis transform for fuzzy skeletonization and pruning," *IEEE Transactions on Pattern Analysis and Machine Intelligence*, vol. 32, no. 6, pp. 1084–1096, 2010.

[20] R. L. Ogniewicz and O. Kübler, "Hierarchic Voronoi skeletons," *Pattern Recognition*, vol. 28, no. 3, pp. 343–359, 1995.

[21] L. Lam and C. Y. Suen, "Thinning methodologies—a comprehensive survey," *IEEE Transactions on Pattern Analysis and Machine Intelligence*, vol. 14, no. 9, pp. 869–885, 1992.

[22] X. Bai, L. J. Latecki, and W.-Y. Liu, "Skeleton pruning by contour partitioning with discrete curve evolution," *IEEE Transactions on Pattern Analysis and Machine Intelligence*, vol. 29, no. 3, pp. 449–462, 2007.

[23] K. Siddiqi, S. Bouix, A. Tannenbaum, and S. W. Zucker, "Hamilton-Jacobi skeleton," in *Proceedings of the 1999 7th IEEE International Conference on Computer Vision (ICCV'99)*, pp. 828–834, September 1999.

[24] T. Grogorishin, G. Abdel-Hamid, and Y. Yang, "Skeletonization, an electrostatic field-based approach," in *Pattern Analysis and Applications*, vol. 1, pp. 163–177, 163-177, 1, 1996.

[25] L. Gorelick, M. Galun, E. Sharon, R. Basri, and A. Brandt, "Shape representation and classification using the poisson equation," *IEEE Transactions on Pattern Analysis and Machine Intelligence*, vol. 28, no. 12, pp. 1991–2004, 2006.

[26] S. Belongie, J. Malik, and J. Puzicha, "Shape matching and object recognition using shape contexts," *IEEE Transactions on Pattern Analysis and Machine Intelligence*, vol. 24, no. 4, pp. 509–522, 2002.

[27] D. Chaudhuri and A. Samal, "A simple method for fitting of bounding rectangle to closed regions," *Pattern Recognition*, vol. 40, no. 7, pp. 1981–1989, 2007.

[28] C. Ryberg, E. Rostrup, M. B. Stegmann et al., "Clinical significance of corpus callosum atrophy in a mixed elderly population," *Neurobiology of Aging*, vol. 28, no. 6, pp. 955–963, 2007.

[29] S. F. Witelson, "Hand and sex differences in the isthmus and genu of the human corpus callosum. A postmortem morphological study," *Brain*, vol. 112, no. 3, pp. 799–835, 1989.

[30] M. Kass, A. Witkin, and D. Terzopoulos, "Snakes: active contour models," *International Journal of Computer Vision*, vol. 1, no. 4, pp. 321–331, 1988.

[31] H. Blum, *A transformation for extracting new descriptors of shape*, The MIT Press, Cambridge, MA, 1967.

[32] J.-H. Chuang, C.-H. Tsai, and M.-C. Ko, "Skeletonization of three-dimensional object using generalized potential field," *IEEE Transactions on Pattern Analysis and Machine Intelligence*, vol. 22, no. 11, pp. 1241–1251, 2000.

[33] Q. Hu and W. L. Nowinski, "A rapid algorithm for robust and automatic extraction of the midsagittal plane of the human cerebrum from neuroimages based on local symmetry and outlier removal," *NeuroImage*, vol. 20, no. 4, pp. 2153–2165, 2003.

[34] A. P. Dempster, N. M. Laird, and D. B. Rubin, "Maximum likelihood from incomplete data via the EM algorithm," *Journal of the Royal Statistical Society: Series B (Statistical Methodology)*, vol. 39, no. 1, pp. 1–38, 1977.

[35] C. Direkoglu, R. Dahyot, and M. Manzke, "On using anisotropic diffusion for skeleton extraction," *International Journal of Computer Vision*, vol. 100, no. 2, pp. 170–189, 2012.

[36] S. Weis, K. Jellinger, and E. Wenger, "Morphometry of the corpus callosum in normal aging and Alzheimer's disease," *Journal of Neural Transmission. Supplementa*, no. 33, pp. 35–38, 1991.

[37] H. Hampel, S. J. Teipel, G. E. Alexander et al., "Corpus callosum atrophy is a possible indicator of region- and cell type-specific neuronal degeneration in Alzheimer disease: A magnetic resonance imaging analysis," *JAMA Neurology*, vol. 55, no. 2, pp. 193–198, 1998.

[38] A. Hensel, H. Wolf, F. Kruggel et al., "Morphometry of the corpus callosum in patients with questionable and mild dementia," *Journal of Neurology, Neurosurgery & Psychiatry*, vol. 73, no. 1, pp. 59–61, 2002.

[39] H. Wu, D. Wang, L. Shi, Z. Wen, and Z. Ming, "Midsagittal plane extraction from brain images based on 3D SIFT," *Physics in Medicine and Biology*, vol. 59, no. 6, pp. 1367–1387, 2014.

[40] I. Volkau, K. N. Bhanu Prakash, A. Ananthasubramaniam, A. Aziz, and W. L. Nowinski, "Extraction of the midsagittal plane from morphological neuroimages using the Kullback-Leibler's measure," *Medical Image Analysis*, vol. 10, no. 6, pp. 863–874, 2006.

[41] Y. Liu, R. T. Collins, and W. E. Rothfus, "Robust midsagittal plane extraction from normal and pathological 3-D neuroradiology images," *IEEE Transactions on Medical Imaging*, vol. 20, no. 3, pp. 175–192, 2001.

[42] C. Adamson, R. Beare, M. Walterfang, and M. Seal, "Software Pipeline for Midsagittal Corpus Callosum Thickness Profile Processing: Automated Segmentation, Manual Editor, Thickness Profile Generator, Group-Wise Statistical Comparison and Results Display," *Neuroinformatics*, vol. 12, no. 4, pp. 595–614, 2014.

[43] S. Içer, "Automatic segmentation of corpus collasum using Gaussian mixture modeling and Fuzzy C means methods," *Computer Methods and Programs in Biomedicine*, vol. 112, no. 1, pp. 38–46, 2013.

[44] Y. Li, M. Mandal, and S. N. Ahmed, "Fully automated segmentation of corpus callosum in midsagittal brain MRIs," in *Proceedings of the 2013 35th Annual International Conference of the IEEE Engineering in Medicine and Biology Society (EMBC)*, pp. 5111–5114, Osaka, July 2013.

[45] M. Kubicki, M. Styner, S. Bouix et al., "Reduced interhemispheric connectivity in schizophrenia-tractography based segmentation of the corpus callosum," *Schizophrenia Research*, vol. 106, no. 2-3, pp. 125–131, 2008.

[46] C. Cascio, M. Styner, R. G. Smith et al., "Reduced relationship to cortical white matter volume revealed by tractography-based segmentation of the corpus callosum in young children with developmental delay," *The American Journal of Psychiatry*, vol. 163, no. 12, pp. 2157–2163, 2006.

[47] I. Liu, C. Chiu, C. Chen, L. Kuo, Y. Lo, and W. I. Tseng, "The microstructural integrity of the corpus callosum and associated impulsivity in alcohol dependence: A tractography-based segmentation study using diffusion spectrum imaging," *Psychiatry Research: Neuroimaging*, vol. 184, no. 2, pp. 128–134, 2010.

[48] N. Changizi, G. Hamarneh, O. Ishaq, A. Ward, and R. Tam, "Extraction of the plane of minimal cross-sectional area of the corpus callosum using template-driven segmentation.," *Medical image computing and computer-assisted intervention : MICCAI ... International Conference on Medical Image Computing and Computer-Assisted Intervention*, vol. 13, no. 3, pp. 17–24, 2010.

14

Biomedical Text Categorization based on Ensemble Pruning and Optimized Topic Modelling

Aytuğ Onan

Celal Bayar University, Department of Software Engineering, 45400 Turgutlu, Manisa, Turkey

Correspondence should be addressed to Aytuğ Onan; aytugonan@gmail.com

Academic Editor: Federico Divina

Text mining is an important research direction, which involves several fields, such as information retrieval, information extraction, and text categorization. In this paper, we propose an efficient multiple classifier approach to text categorization based on swarm-optimized topic modelling. The Latent Dirichlet allocation (LDA) can overcome the high dimensionality problem of vector space model, but identifying appropriate parameter values is critical to performance of LDA. Swarm-optimized approach estimates the parameters of LDA, including the number of topics and all the other parameters involved in LDA. The hybrid ensemble pruning approach based on combined diversity measures and clustering aims to obtain a multiple classifier system with high predictive performance and better diversity. In this scheme, four different diversity measures (namely, disagreement measure, *Q*-statistics, the correlation coefficient, and the double fault measure) among classifiers of the ensemble are combined. Based on the combined diversity matrix, a swarm intelligence based clustering algorithm is employed to partition the classifiers into a number of disjoint groups and one classifier (with the highest predictive performance) from each cluster is selected to build the final multiple classifier system. The experimental results based on five biomedical text benchmarks have been conducted. In the swarm-optimized LDA, different metaheuristic algorithms (such as genetic algorithms, particle swarm optimization, firefly algorithm, cuckoo search algorithm, and bat algorithm) are considered. In the ensemble pruning, five metaheuristic clustering algorithms are evaluated. The experimental results on biomedical text benchmarks indicate that swarm-optimized LDA yields better predictive performance compared to the conventional LDA. In addition, the proposed multiple classifier system outperforms the conventional classification algorithms, ensemble learning, and ensemble pruning methods.

1. Introduction

The immense quantity of biomedical text documents can serve as an essential source of information for biomedical research. Biomedical text documents are characterized by an immense quantity of unstructured and sparse information in a wide range of forms, such as scientific articles, biomedical datasets, and case reports. Text mining aims to identify valuable information from unstructured text documents with the use of tools and techniques from several disciplines, such as machine learning, information retrieval, and computational linguistics. The use of text mining is one of the most promising tools in the biomedical domain that has attracted a lot of research interest. Text mining in biomedical domain can be successfully applied in a wide range of applications, including identification of disease-specific knowledge [1], diagnosis, treatment, and prevention of cancer [2], identification of obesity status of patients [3], identification of risk factors for heart disease [4], annotation of gene expression [5], and identification of drug targets and candidates [6].

Biomedical text mining follows the same stages (namely, format conversation, tokenization, stop word removal, normalization, stemming, dictionary construction, and vector space construction) utilized in the text processing from other domains [7]. To build accurate classification schemes on text documents, one pivotal issue is to identify an appropriate representation model for the documents [8]. The vector space model (also known as term vector model) is one of the most commonly employed representation schemes to process text documents, owing to its simple structure [9]. In this model, each text document is represented as vectors of identifiers (index terms). The vector space model suffers from high dimensional feature space, irrelevancy, and sparsity of features. Since each document is represented as a bag of words with the corresponding frequencies, words are regarded as statistically independent. Hence, word order is not taken into consideration [10].

Considering the limitations of the vector space model and the high dimensional unstructured nature of biomedical text documents, there are a number of representation schemes (such as the latent semantic analysis, the probabilistic latent semantic analysis, and the latent Dirichlet allocation) employed to process biomedical text documents [7]. The latent semantic analysis (LSA) is a scheme to extract and represent the contextual meaning of words with the use of statistical computations utilized on a large amount of text [11]. LSA can represent the semantic relations within the text. It can find the latent classes, while reducing the dimensionality of vector space model [12]. However, LSA has no strong statistical foundation and can suffer from high mathematical complexity [13]. The probabilistic latent semantic analysis (PLSA) is a statistical method for analysis of data which is based on a latent class model. PLSA has a strong statistical foundation. It can find latent topics and it can yield better performance compared to LSA [13].

The latent Dirichlet allocation (LDA) is an efficient generative probabilistic topic model, where each document is represented as a random mixture of latent topics. LDA can find latent topics, reduce the high dimensionality of vector space model, and can outperform other linguistic representation schemes, such as latent semantic analysis and probabilistic latent semantic analysis [14]. LDA involves several parameter values, such as the number of topics, the number of iterations for Gibbs sampling, α parameter to control the topic distribution per document, and β parameter to model distributions of terms per topic (Panichella et al., 2003). For unstructured text documents, information about the document-wise content and number of relevant topics is not known in advance (Zhao et al., 2005). Hence, the identification of an appropriate value for the number of topics is a challenging problem for unstructured text documents. An insufficient or excessive number of topics can degrade the predictive performance of machine learning algorithms built on LDA-based topic modelling. In addition to the number of topics, LDA requires several other parameters. Therefore, finding an optimal configuration for LDA-based topic modelling involves extensive empirical analysis with different configurations.

In order to build robust classification schemes, multiple classifier systems (also known as ensemble classifiers) have been widely employed in the field of pattern recognition, owing to its remarkable improvement in generalization ability and predictive performance [15]. There are three main stages of the ensemble learning process, namely, ensemble generation, ensemble pruning, and ensemble combination [16, 17]. The ensemble generation stage is the phase, in which base learning algorithms to be utilized in the multiple classifier system are generated. The base learning algorithms can be generated either homogeneously or heterogeneously. The ensemble combination stage seeks to integrate the individual predictions of base learning algorithms. The ensemble pruning stage aims to identify an optimal subset of base learning algorithms from the ensemble to enhance the predictive performance and computational efficiency. It has been empirically validated that ensemble pruning can yield more robust classification schemes [18].

Considering these issues, we propose a multiple classifier approach to biomedical text categorization based on swarm-optimized topic modelling and ensemble pruning. In the presented scheme, swarm-optimized approach is employed to estimate the parameters of LDA, including the number of topics and all the other parameters involved in LDA. Motivated by the success of hybrid ensemble pruning schemes [19–21], the proposed approach combines diversity measures and clustering. In this scheme, four different diversity measures (namely, disagreement measure, Q-statistics, the correlation coefficient, and the double fault measure) are computed to capture the diversities within the ensemble. Based on these diversity measures, a combined diversity matrix is obtained. Based on this matrix, a swarm intelligence based clustering algorithm partitions the classification algorithms into a number of disjoint groups and one algorithm (with the highest predictive performance) from each cluster is selected to build the multiple classifier system. In the empirical analysis, five biomedical text benchmarks have been utilized. In the swarm-optimized LDA, different metaheuristic algorithms (such as genetic algorithms, particle swarm optimization, firefly algorithm, cuckoo search algorithm, and bat algorithm) are considered. In addition, five different metaheuristic clustering algorithms are considered in the ensemble pruning stage. The empirical analysis on biomedical text benchmarks indicates that swarm-optimized LDA yields better predictive performance compared to the conventional LDA. In addition, the proposed hybrid ensemble pruning scheme outperforms the conventional classification algorithms and ensemble learning methods.

The main contributions of our proposed categorization scheme can be summarized as follows:

(i) We introduced a metaheuristic approach to optimize the set of parameters utilized in LDA-based topic modelling. In this regard, the number of topics (k), the number of Gibbs iterations (n), α parameter to control the topic distribution per document, and β parameter to model distributions of terms per topic are considered. We conducted several experiments on swarm-optimized LDA with different metaheuristic algorithms (namely, genetic algorithms, particle swarm optimization, firefly algorithm, cuckoo search algorithm, and bat algorithm). To the best of our knowledge, this is the first comprehensive empirical analysis devoted to metaheuristic algorithms on LDA-based topic modelling.

(ii) We introduced an ensemble pruning approach based on combined diversity measures and metaheuristic clustering. To the best of our knowledge, this is the first study in ensemble pruning, which utilizes metaheuristic clustering algorithms to obtain diversified base learning algorithms.

(iii) The presented classification scheme, which integrates swarm-optimized LDA-based modelling with the hybrid ensemble pruning scheme, is employed on biomedical text categorization. To the best of our knowledge, this is the first comprehensive study on LDA-based topic modelling and ensemble pruning on biomedical text categorization.

The rest of this paper is structured as follows. In Section 2, related work on topic modelling and multiple classifier systems have been presented. Section 3 presents the theoretical foundations, Section 4 presents the proposed text categorization framework, Section 5 presents the experimental results, and Section 6 presents the concluding remarks.

2. Related Work

This section presents the related work on topic modelling and multiple classifier systems in biomedical text categorization.

2.1. Related Work on Topic Modelling. Topic modelling models have been successfully employed to summarize large-scale collections of text documents. Probabilistic topic modelling methods can be utilized to identify the core topics of text collections. In addition, topic modelling schemes can be utilized in a variety of tasks in computational linguistics, such as analysis of source code documents [23], summarizing opinions of product reviews [24], identification of topic evolution [25], aspect detection in review documents [26], analysis of Twitter messages [27], and sentiment analysis [28, 29].

Probabilistic topic modelling has attracted the attention of researchers on biomedical domain. Biomedical text collections suffer from high dimensionality and topic modelling methods are effective tools to handle with large-scale collections of documents. Hence, topic modelling can yield promising results on biological and biomedical text mining [30]. For instance, Wang et al. [31] presented a probabilistic topic modelling scheme to identify protein-protein interactions from the biological literature. In this scheme, the correlation between different methods and related words is modelled in a probabilistic way to extract the detection methods. In another study, Arnold et al. [32] utilized the latent Dirichlet allocation method to identify relevant clinical topics and to structure clinical text reports. Song and Kim [33] employed the latent Dirichlet allocation method to conduct bibliometric analysis on bioinformatics from full-text text collections of PubMed Central articles. In another study, Sarioglu et al. [34] utilized topic modelling to represent clinical reports in a compact way, so that these collections can be efficiently processed. In another study, Bisgin et al. [35] applied topic modelling to drug labelling, which is a human-intensive task with many ambiguous semantic descriptions. In this way, manual annotation challenges can be eliminated. Likewise, Wang et al. [36] introduced a topic modelling based scheme to identify literature-driven annotations for gene sets. In this scheme, the number of topics to be utilized in topic modelling is empirically inferred through the analysis with various parameter values (5, 10, 15, 20, etc.) for the number of topics. In another study, Bisgin et al. [37] employed the latent Dirichlet allocation based topic modelling to identify interdependencies between cellular endpoints. The experimental analysis indicated that LDA can substantially enhance the understanding of systems biology. Probabilistic topic modelling has also been employed to identify drug repositioning strategies [38]. Wang et al. [39] utilized topic modelling to analyze 17,723 abstracts from PubMed publications related to adolescent substance use and depression. In this study, topic modelling was employed to identify the literature and to capture other relevant topics. In another study, Wang et al. [40] presented a topic modelling based scheme to mine biomedical text collections. In this scheme, topic modelling was employed as a fine-grained preprocessing model. Recently, Sullivan et al. [41] utilized topic modelling to identify unsafe nutritional supplements from review documents. In another study, Chen et al. [42] employed probabilistic topic modelling to represent hospital admission processes in a compact way.

2.2. Related Work on Multiple Classifier Systems. Multiple classifier systems have been successfully employed in a wide range of applications in pattern recognition, including biomedical domain. Empirical analysis on multiple classifier systems indicates that ensemble pruning can enhance the predictive performance of multiple classifier systems [18]. Ensemble pruning approaches can be mainly divided into five groups, as exponential search, randomized search, sequential search, ranking-based, and clustering based methods [16]. Exponential approaches to ensemble pruning seek to examine all possible subsets of base learning algorithms within the multiple classifier system. For instance, Aksela [43] examined the predictive performance of several evaluation metrics (namely, correlation between errors, Q-statistics, and mutual information) in ensemble pruning. Randomized approaches to ensemble pruning aim to explore the search space of candidate classifiers with the use of metaheuristic algorithms. A wide range of metaheuristics, such as genetic algorithms, tabu search, and population based incremental learning, have been successfully utilized for ensemble pruning [44, 45]. For instance, Sheen and Sirisha [46] introduced an ensemble pruning scheme for malware detection based on harmony search. Likewise, Mendialdua et al. [47] utilized the estimation of distribution algorithm for ensemble pruning. In sequential search based methods, the search space of candidate classifiers has been explored in forward, backward, or forward-backward direction. For instance, Margineantu and Dietterich [48] introduced a sequential approach for ensemble pruning based on reduced error pruning with backfitting. Similarly, Caruana et al. [49] presented a forward stepwise selection based approach for ensemble pruning. Recently, Dai et al. [50] introduced a reverse reduced error-based ensemble pruning algorithm based on subtraction operation. Ranking-based approaches to ensemble pruning aim to identify an optimal subset of classifiers based on a ranking obtained by a particular evaluation measure. For instance, Kotsiantis and Pintelas [51] presented a t-test based ranking scheme for ensemble pruning. More recently, Galar et al. [52] presented an ordering-based metric for ensemble pruning. Clustering based approaches to ensemble pruning partition the base learning algorithms of ensemble into clusters. For instance, Zhang and Cao [53] presented a spectral clustering based algorithm for ensemble pruning. In this scheme, the base learning algorithms were grouped into two clusters based on predictive performance and diversity. Then, one cluster of ensemble was pruned and one cluster of ensemble was retained as the pruned subset of classifiers.

2.3. Motivation and Contribution of the Study. As outlined in advance, probabilistic topic modelling methods are essential tools to identify hidden topics in large-scale collections of text documents. In order to enhance the performance of LDA, there are a number of extensions on the basic model. For instance, Griffiths and Tenenbaum [54] introduced a hierarchical latent Dirichlet allocation model. In this model, topic distributions are identified from hierarchies of topics, where each hierarchy is modelled by a nested Chinese restaurant process. Each node of tree corresponds to a particular topic, where each topic is associated with a distribution. In another study, Teh et al. [55] presented a hierarchical latent Dirichlet allocation scheme, in which parameter value for the number of topics is inferred through the use of posterior inference. Grant and Cordy [56] introduced a heuristic approach to estimate the number of topics in source code analysis. In another study, Panichella et al. [57] presented a genetic algorithm based scheme to identify optimal configurations for latent Dirichlet allocation. In this scheme, parameter set for topic modelling was estimated with the use of genetic algorithm. The presented scheme was employed on three different tasks of software engineering, namely, traceability link recovery, feature location, and software artifact labelling. Likewise, Zhao et al. [58] introduced a heuristic approach to estimate the appropriate number of topics for latent Dirichlet allocation. In this scheme, the appropriate number of topics is identified through the use of ratio for perplexity change. Recently, Karami et al. [59] presented a fuzzy approach to topic modelling. In this scheme, fuzzy clustering was employed to identify optimal number of topics.

In addition to the aforementioned five ensemble pruning approaches, hybrid methods have attracted research attention in the pattern recognition. Hybrid approaches to ensemble pruning seek to integrate several ensemble pruning paradigms. For instance, Lin et al. (2014) introduced a hybrid ensemble pruning algorithm which integrates k-means clustering and dynamic selection. Similarly, Mousavi and Eftekhari [60] presented a hybrid ensemble pruning scheme which integrates static and dynamic ensemble selection with NSGA-II multiobjective genetic algorithm. In another study, Cavalcanti et al. [21] presented a hybrid ensemble pruning algorithm based on genetic algorithm and graph coloring. In this scheme, several different diversity measures (such as Q-statistics, correlation coefficient, Kappa statistics, and double fault measure) are combined via a genetic algorithm. Similarly, Onan et al. [19, 20] introduced a hybrid ensemble pruning algorithm based on consensus clustering and multiobjective evolutionary algorithm. In this scheme, classifiers are assigned into clusters based on their predictive performance and the set of candidate classifiers are explored through the use of evolutionary algorithm.

Recent studies on topic modelling indicate that the identification of an appropriate parameter value for the number of topics is an essential task to build robust classification schemes. In addition, hybrid ensemble pruning schemes can outperform conventional classifiers, ensemble learning methods, and ensemble pruning methods. Through their potential use on text classification, the number of works that utilize metaheuristic algorithms to optimize parameters of LDA and the number of works that utilize ensemble pruning schemes are very limited. To fill this gap, this paper presents a classification scheme based on swarm-optimized topic modelling and hybrid ensemble pruning for text categorization.

3. Theoretical Foundations

This section summarizes the theoretical foundations of the study. Namely, the latent Dirichlet allocation method, swarm-based optimization algorithms, ensemble learning methods, ensemble pruning methods, cluster validity indices, and pairwise diversity measures are presented.

3.1. The Latent Dirichlet Allocation. The latent Dirichlet allocation model (LDA) is a widely employed generative probabilistic model to identify the latent topics in text documents [22]. In LDA, each document is represented as a random mixture of latent topics and each topic is represented as a mixture of words. The mixture distributions are Dirichlet-distributed random variables to be inferred. In this scheme, each document exhibits the topics in different proportions, each word in each document is drawn among the topics, and topics are chosen based on per-document distribution over topics [61]. LDA attempts to determine the underlying latent topic structure based on the observed data. In LDA, the words of each document correspond to the observed data. For each document in the corpus, words are obtained by following a two-staged procedure. Initially, a distribution over topics is randomly chosen for each word of the document [22]. In LDA, a word is a discrete data from a vocabulary indexed by $\{1,\ldots,V\}$, a sequence of N words $w=(w_1, w_2, \ldots, w_n)$, and a corpus is a collection of M documents denoted by $D=\{\mathrm{w}_1, \mathrm{w}_2, \ldots, \mathrm{w}_M\}$. The generative process of LDA is summarized in Box 1.

LDA process can be modelled by a three-level Bayesian graphical model, as given in Figure 1. In this graphical model, nodes are used to represent random variables and edges are used to denote the possible dependencies between the variables. In this notation, α refers to Dirichlet parameter, Θ refers to document-level topic variables, z refers to per-word topic assignment, w refers to the observed word, and β indicates the topics [61].

Based on this notation, the generative process of LDA corresponds to a joint distribution of the hidden and observed variables. The probability density function of a k-dimensional Dirichlet random variable is computed as given by (1), the joint distribution of a topic mixture is computed as given by

For each document w in a corpus D:
(1) Choose $N \sim$ Poisson (ξ).
(2) Choose $\Theta \sim$ Dir (α).
(3) For each of the N words w_n:
(a) Choose a topic $z_n \sim$ Multinomial (Θ).
Choose a word w_n from $p(w_n \mid z_n, \beta)$, a multinomial probability conditioned on the topic z_n.

Box 1: The generative process of LDA (Blei et al., 2013; [19, 20]).

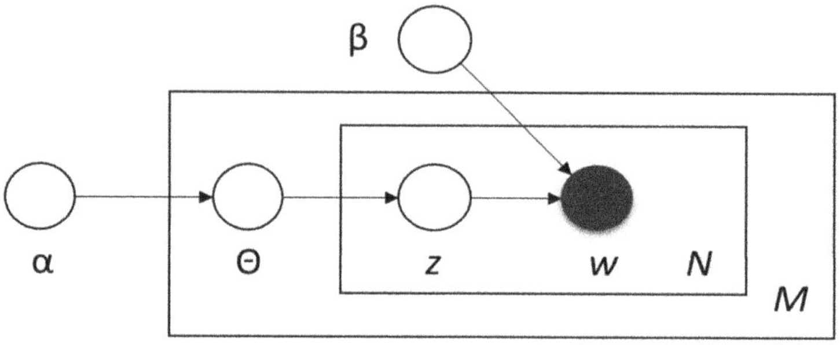

FIGURE 1: The graphical representation of LDA [22].

(2), and the probability of a corpus is computed as given by (3) [22]:

$$p(\Theta \mid \alpha) = \frac{\Gamma\left(\sum_{i=1}^{k} \alpha_i\right)}{\prod_{i=1}^{k} \Gamma(\alpha_i)} \Theta_1^{\alpha_1 - 1} \ldots \Theta_k^{\alpha_k - 1} \quad (1)$$

$$p(\Theta, z, w \mid \alpha, \beta) = p(\Theta \mid \alpha) \prod_{n=1}^{N} p(z_n \mid \Theta)\, p(w_n \mid z_n, \beta) \quad (2)$$

$$p(D \mid \alpha, \beta) = \prod_{d=1}^{M} \int p(\Theta_d \mid \alpha) \cdot \left(\prod_{n=1}^{N_d} \sum_{Z_{dn}} p(z_{dn} \mid \Theta_d)\, p(w_{dn} \mid z_{dn}, \beta) \right) d\Theta_d \quad (3)$$

In LDA, the computation of the posterior distribution of the hidden variables is an important inferential task. The exact inference of hidden variables is exponentially large. Hence, approximation algorithms (such as Laplace approximation, variational approximation, and Gibbs sampling) have been utilized in LDA process [61].

3.2. Ensemble Learning Methods. Ensemble learning methods aim to combine the predictions of multiple classification algorithms so that a classification model with higher predictive performance can be achieved [62]. In dependent methods, the outputs of former classifiers determine the outputs of following classifiers. In contrast, the outputs of classifiers are individually identified and combined to produce the final prediction in independent methods. Dependent ensemble methods include Boosting (e.g., AdaBoost algorithm) and independent methods include Bagging, Dagging, and Random Subspace. To examine the predictive performance of the proposed scheme, four well-known ensemble learning methods (namely, AdaBoost [63], Bagging [64], Random Subspace [65], and Stacking [66]) are considered.

3.3. Ensemble Pruning Methods. The ensemble pruning methods aim to identify optimal subset of classification algorithms to improve the predictive performance and computational efficiency of multiple classifier systems. To examine the predictive performance of proposed ensemble pruning algorithm, we have employed four ensemble pruning algorithms. These methods are the ensemble pruning methods from libraries of models [49], Bagging ensemble selection [67], LibD3C algorithm [68], and ensemble pruning based on combined diversity measures [21].

3.4. Swarm-Based Optimization Algorithms. Swarm-based optimization algorithms, including genetic algorithms, particle swarm optimization, firefly algorithm, cuckoo search algorithm, and bat algorithm, have been successfully employed on applications of data science, such as data clustering and data categorization [68]. In the proposed scheme, swarm-based optimization algorithms have been utilized to optimize the set of parameters of LDA-based topic modelling. In addition, the proposed ensemble pruning algorithm employs swarm-based optimization algorithms to group classifiers into clusters. In the empirical analysis, genetic algorithms [69], particle swarm optimization algorithm [70], firefly algorithm [71], cuckoo search algorithm [72], and bat algorithm [73] are utilized.

3.5. Cluster Validity Indices. This section briefly introduces four cluster validity indices (namely, the Bayesian information criterion, Calinski-Harabasz index, Davies-Bouldin index, and Silhouette index), which are utilized to evaluate the clustering quality of different configurations of LDA.

The Bayesian information criterion (BIC) is computed as given below:

$$\mathrm{BIC} = -\ln(\mathrm{L}) + \mathrm{v}\ln(\mathrm{n}) \quad (4)$$

where n denotes the number of topics, L denotes the likelihood of parameters to generate data in the model, and v denotes the number of free parameters in Gaussian model [74]. The smaller the Bayesian information criterion, the better the generated model.

The Calinski-Harabasz index (CH) is the ratio of the traces of between cluster scatter matrix and the internal scatter matrix, which is computed as given below [74]:

$$\mathrm{CH}(K) = \frac{[trace\ B/K - 1]}{[trace\ W/N - K]} \quad (5)$$

$$\text{trace B} = \sum_{k=1}^{K} |C_k| \left\|\overline{c_k} - \overline{x}\right\|^2 \quad (6)$$

$$\text{trace C} = \sum_{k=1}^{K}\sum_{i=1}^{N} w_{k,i} \left\|x_i - \overline{C_k}\right\|^2 \quad (7)$$

where K denotes the number of clusters, N denotes the number of data instances, $|C_k|$ denotes the number of elements in cluster C_k, x_i denotes a point within cluster C_k, B denotes the between-cluster scatter matrix, which represents the error sum of squares between different clusters, and W denotes the internal scatter matrix, which represents the squared differences of instances in a cluster. Here, trace of an n-by-n square matrix corresponds to the sum of the elements on the main diagonal [75].

The Davies-Bouldin index (DB) is a cluster validity index, which aims to maximize between-cluster distance and to minimize the distance between centroids of clusters and the other data points, that is defined as given by the following equation:

$$\mathrm{BD} = \frac{1}{c}\sum_{i=1}^{c} \max_{i \neq j} \left\{ \frac{d(X_i) + d(X_j)}{d(c_i, c_j)} \right\} \quad (8)$$

where c denotes the number of clusters, i and j correspond to cluster labels, $d(c_i, c_j)$ corresponds to distance between centroids of clusters, and X_i corresponds to a data point within cluster C_i. The smaller the DB criterion, the better the generated model.

The Silhouette index (SI) is defined as given by (9):

$$\mathrm{SI} = \frac{1}{N}\sum_i \left(\frac{1}{n_i} \sum_{x \in C_i} \frac{b(x) - a(x)}{\max[b(x), a(x)]} \right) \quad (9)$$

$$a(x) = \frac{1}{n_i - 1} \sum_{y \in C_{i, y \neq x}} d(x, y) \quad (10)$$

$$b(x) = \min_{j \neq i} \left[\frac{1}{n_i} \sum_{y \in C_j} d(x, y) \right] \quad (11)$$

where N denotes the number of clusters, n_i denotes the size of cluster C_i, $a(x)$ denotes the average distance between the ith instance and all instances in X_j, $b(x)$ denotes the minimum distance from i to the centroids of clusters not containing i.

3.6. Pairwise Diversity Measures. This section briefly introduces four diversity measures (namely, disagreement measure, Q-statistics, the correlation coefficient, and the double fault measure) which are utilized in the proposed ensemble classification scheme.

Q-statistics, the correlation coefficient ($p_{i,k}$), the disagreement measure (Dis), and the double fault measure (DF) among two classifiers D_i and D_k are computed using (12), (13), (14), and (15), respectively [76]:

$$Q_{i,k} = \frac{N^{11}N^{00} - N^{01}N^{10}}{N^{11}N^{00} + N^{01}N^{10}} \quad (12)$$

$$\rho_{i,k} = \frac{N^{11}N^{00} - N^{01}N^{10}}{\sqrt{(N^{11} + N^{10})(N^{01} + N^{00})(N^{11} + N^{01})(N^{10} + N^{00})}} \quad (13)$$

$$Dis_{i,k} = \frac{N^{01} + N^{10}}{N^{11} + N^{10} + N^{01} + N^{00}} \quad (14)$$

$$DF_{i,k} = \frac{N^{00}}{N^{11} + N^{10} + N^{01} + N^{00}} \quad (15)$$

where N^{11}, N^{00}, N^{10}, and N^{01} denote the number of correctly classified instances by the two classifiers, the number of incorrectly classified instances by the two classifiers, the number of instances correctly classified by D_i and incorrectly classified by D_k, and the number of instances correctly classified by D_k and incorrectly classified by D_i, respectively.

4. The Proposed Text Categorization Framework

The proposed text categorization framework combines the swarm-optimized Latent Dirichlet allocation and diversity-based hybrid ensemble pruning scheme. The rest of this section explains the methods utilized in the proposed biomedical text categorization framework.

4.1. Swarm-Optimized Latent Dirichlet Allocation. The latent Dirichlet allocation (LDA) is an efficient generative probabilistic model that can be employed to represent unstructured text documents in an efficient way. In general, LDA-based topic modelling involves the calibration of several parameters, summarized as follows:

(i) Number of topics in LDA-based topic modelling (k).

(ii) α parameter to control the topic distribution per document. A higher value for α parameter denotes better smoothing of topics for each document.

(iii) β parameter to model distributions of terms per topic.

In order to improve the computational complexity of LDA, LDA is usually employed in conjunction with an approximation method. In this work, we utilized Gibbs sampling method in conjunction with LDA. In this way, the number of iterations (N) for sampling is also involved as an additional parameter value. Identifying appropriate parameter values of LDA with the optimal configuration is a challenging task. Without setting appropriate parameter values, LDA-based representation may degrade the predictive performance of classification schemes. Too low or too much number of topics can result in a poor predictive performance. Hence, finding an optimal configuration for LDA-based topic modelling involves extensive empirical analysis. Exhaustively enumerating possible parameter values for LDA to identify an optimal configuration involves high computational analysis with a wide range of parameter values.

In this paper, five metaheuristic algorithms (namely, genetic algorithms, particle swarm optimization, firefly algorithm, cuckoo search algorithm, and bat algorithm) are utilized to calibrate the parameters of LDA. In this scheme, values of all parameters of LDA are taken into consideration. Hence, various values for each parameter are evaluated to find an optimal configuration. In the presented problem, the first issue is to examine the merit of a particular LDA-based configuration. In order to evaluate the merit of a particular configuration of LDA before employing on a particular task, we have employed four internal cluster validity indices, namely, the Bayesian information criterion, Calinski-Harabasz index, Davies-Bouldin index, and Silhouette index. Higher clustering quality of a particular LDA-based configuration tends to yield higher predictive performance on LDA-based categorization tasks [19, 20]. For this reason, we seek to identify an LDA configuration which maximizes the overall clustering quality of LDA configuration.

Since exhaustively enumerating possible configurations for LDA can be computationally infeasible task, the identification of a parameter set which maximizes the overall clustering quality can be modelled as an optimization problem. In the presented scheme, five swarm-based optimization algorithms (namely, genetic algorithms, particle swarm optimization, firefly algorithm, cuckoo search algorithm, and bat algorithm) have been considered. The presented approach seeks to find an LDA configuration $[k, \alpha, \beta, N]$ which maximizes the clustering quality in terms of internal cluster validity indices (Bayesian information criterion, Calinski-Harabasz index, Davies-Bouldin index, and Silhouette index). The presented scheme starts with a randomly generated population of initial configuration. Then, randomly generated LDA configurations are utilized to cluster text documents. The merit of clusters is evaluated using four internal clustering validity indices and the swarm-based optimization algorithms have been utilized to optimize the parameter values. In Figure 2, the general structure of swarm-optimized LDA is summarized.

4.2. Diversity-Based Ensemble Pruning. Diversity-based ensemble pruning approach is a hybrid ensemble pruning scheme, which integrates combined pairwise diversity measures and swarm-based clustering algorithms. The presented ensemble pruning method consists of two main stages, namely, computation of pairwise diversity matrices among the base learning algorithms of the ensemble and swarm-based clustering on combined pairwise diversity matrix to obtain final base learning algorithms of the pruned ensemble.

The general structure of diversity-based ensemble pruning algorithm is presented in Figure 3. Initially, many different base learning algorithms (classification algorithms) from the model library with varying parameter values have been taken as the initial set of classifiers. The model library contains classification algorithms from five groups, namely, five Bayesian classifiers, fourteen function based classifiers, ten instance based classifiers, three rule based classifiers, and eight decision tree classifier which have been considered. The detailed description regarding the classification algorithms of the model library is presented in Table 2. Classification algorithms of the model library have been trained on the training set. In this way, the predictive characteristics of different learning algorithms have been obtained.

After training classification algorithms, pairwise diversity matrices are computed. The diversity and accuracy are two essential factors to build multiple classifier systems with high predictive performance. There are many pairwise and nonpairwise diversity measures presented in the literature. Different diversity measures concentrate on different aspects of the diversity and there is not a widely accepted definition for the term. Motivated by the success of the combined diversity measures in the ensemble pruning [21], we seek to find an appropriate subset of diversity measures. In this regard, we have conducted an experimental analysis with five widely utilized diversity measures (namely, Q-statistics, correlation coefficient, disagreement measure, double fault measure, and kappa statistics). Since there are five diversity measures, we have evaluated 2^5-1=31 different subset cases. The values obtained for each measure are normalized. Since the highest predictive performance is obtained by averaging the four diversity measures (Q-statistics, correlation coefficient, disagreement measure, and double fault measure), this configuration is utilized in the proposed ensemble pruning. For four pairwise diversity measures mentioned above, the diversity values of each pair of classifiers are computed using the validation set. Then, the combined pairwise diversity matrix is obtained from the four pairwise diversity matrices by averaging the diversity values of the individual diversity matrices.

After computation of the combined pairwise diversity matrix, clustering has been employed on the combined diversity matrix. Clustering has been widely employed technique for ensemble pruning, which aims to group classification algorithms into clusters such that the classifiers with the similar characteristics are assigned into the same cluster. By obtaining classifiers from the different clusters, a multiple classifier system with high diversity can be achieved. In this study, five metaheuristic clustering algorithms (namely, genetic algorithm based clustering, particle swarm clustering, firefly clustering, cuckoo clustering, and bat clustering) have been employed on the combined diversity matrix. Based on the clustering results, the classification algorithms have been assigned into a number of clusters.

On the empirical analysis with five metaheuristic clustering algorithms, the highest predictive performance is

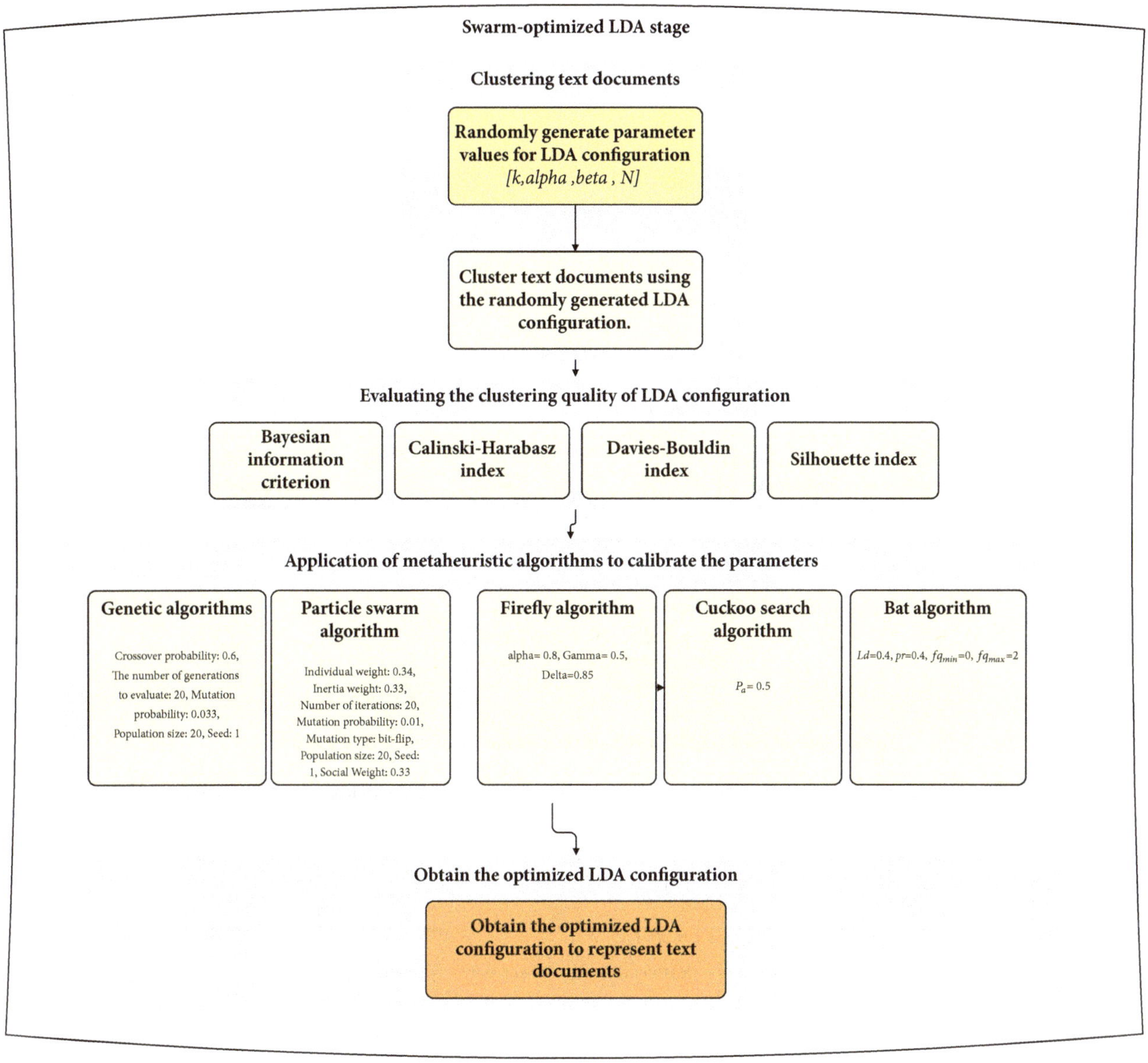

FIGURE 2: Swarm-optimized latent Dirichlet allocation.

achieved by firefly clustering algorithm. Hence, we utilized firefly clustering scheme to cluster classification algorithms on the combined diversity matrix based on their predictive characteristics. Let A denote an agent that consists of m n-dimensional points, a_i denote n-dimensional points in A, P denote a set containing of l n-dimensional points, p_i denote n-dimensional point contained in P, and $Dist(A,P)$ denote the distance between A and p; the general structure of firefly clustering algorithm utilized in the proposed scheme is outlined in Box 2.

After applying clustering algorithm on the combined pairwise diversity matrix, clustering results are utilized to select the classifiers of the pruned ensemble. In order to do so, classifiers of each cluster are ranked based on their predictive performance (in terms of classification accuracy). Then, one classifier with the highest predictive performance is selected from each cluster. Let N denote the number of clusters obtained at the end of firefly clustering algorithms, and one classifier has been selected from each classifier. In this way, N classifiers constitute the pruned ensemble. In order to combine the predictions of the selected classifiers, majority voting scheme is employed.

5. Experimental Analysis

In order to examine the predictive performance of the proposed biomedical text categorization scheme, an extensive empirical analysis has been performed. This section presents the datasets utilized in the analysis, the experimental procedure, and the experimental results.

5.1. Dataset. The experimental analysis has been conducted on five public biomedical text categorization datasets. These datasets are Oh5 collection, Oh10 collection, Oh15 collection,

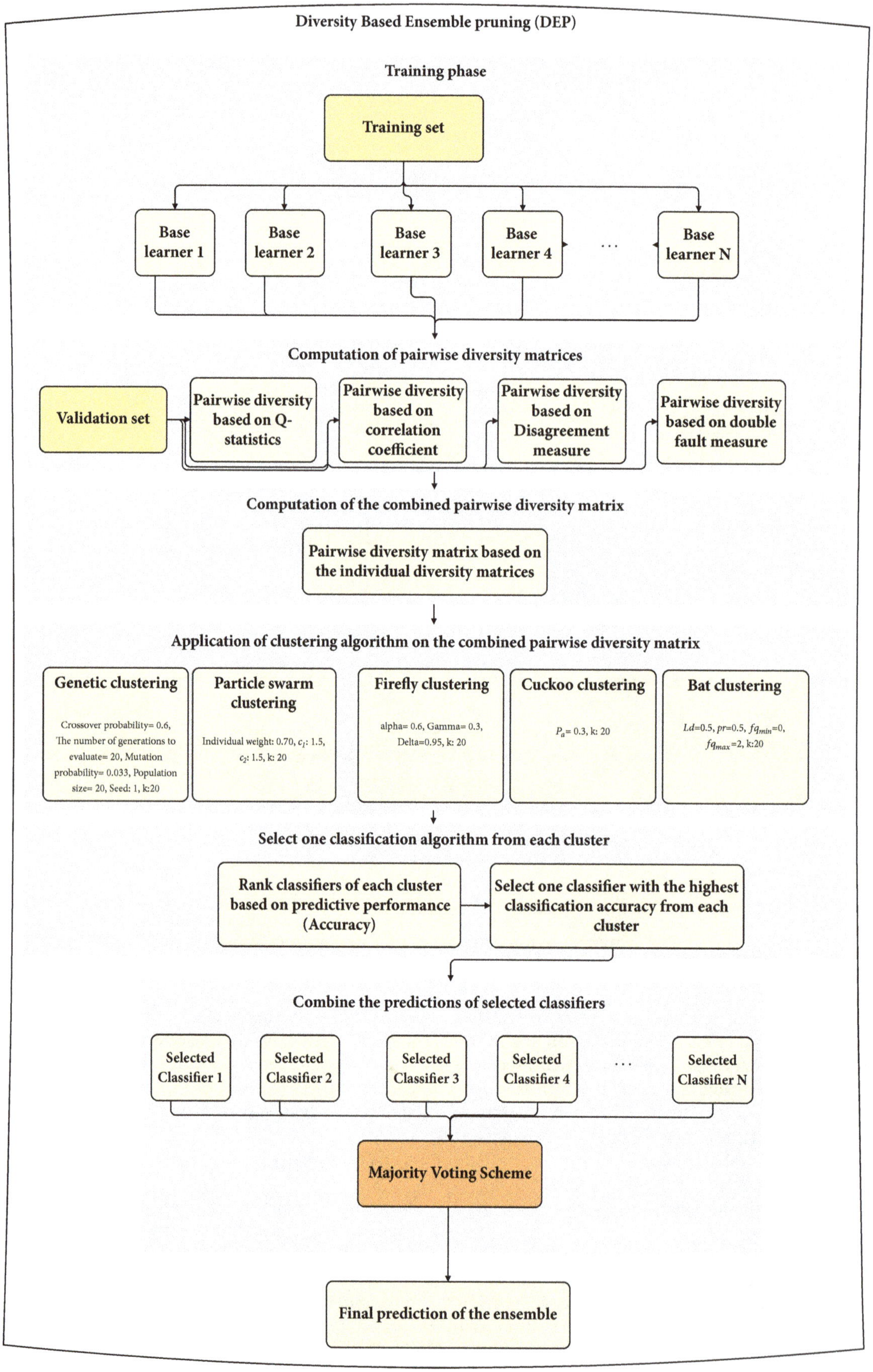

FIGURE 3: Diversity-based ensemble pruning approach.

Input: Data points: $P=\{p_1, p_2, \ldots, p_l\}$, α, δ and γ parameters.
Output: An agent A with the highest fitness value.
Initialize $A=\{A_1, A_2, \ldots, A_k\}$ agents,
for before stopping criterion has been met do
(i) For each A_i agent, calculate fitness function value F_i based on the following equation:

$$F(A) = \sum_{i=1}^{l} Distance(A, p_i)$$

$$Distance(A, p) = \min(\|a_1 - p\|, \|a_2 - p\|, \ldots, \|a_m - p\|).$$

(ii) For each A_i agent, compare fitness value of A_i with fitness value of A_j agent. If $F_i > F_j$ then, Update A_i agent based on the following equations:

$$a_j^i = a_j^i + d * e^{-\gamma * d^2} + \alpha * r$$

$$d = (a_j^x - a_j^i)$$

(iii) Update $\alpha=\alpha * \delta$.

Box 2: The general structure of firefly clustering algorithm.

Table 1: Descriptive information for the datasets.

Dataset	Number of documents	Number of terms	Average occurrence of terms	Number of classes
Oh5	918	3013	54.43	10
Oh10	1050	3239	55.63	10
Oh15	3101	54142	17.46	10
Ohscal	11162	11466	60.38	10
Ohsumed-400	9200	13512	55.14	12

Ohscal collection, and Ohsumed-400 collection [77]. Oh5, Oh10, Oh15, Ohscal, and Ohsumed-400 collections are part of OHSUMED collection. Each collection contains biomedical text collections. The basic descriptive information about biomedical text collections utilized in the empirical analysis has been summarized in Table 1, and the number of terms extracted after preprocessing is given.

5.2. Evaluation Metrics. In order to evaluate the predictive performance of the presented biomedical text categorization scheme, classification accuracy (ACC) and F-measure have been employed as the evaluation measure.

Classification accuracy is one of the most widely utilized measures in performance evaluation of classification algorithms. It is the proportion of the number of true positives and true negatives obtained by the classifiers in the total number of instances as given by the following equation:

$$ACC = \frac{TN + TP}{TP + FP + FN + TN} \quad (16)$$

where TN, TP, FP, and FN represent the number of true negatives, true positives, false positives, and false negatives, respectively.

F-measure is another common measure in performance evaluation of classification algorithms. F-measure is the harmonic mean of the precision and recall of a classification algorithm. It can take values between 0 and 1 and the higher values of F-measure indicate a better predictive performance. Based on the characteristics of datasets utilized in the empirical analysis, there are two variants of F-measure, namely, micro-averaged F-measure and macro-averaged F-measure. The micro-averaged F-measure extends F-measure to multiclass problems by averaging precision and recall values across all classes. However, F-measure and micro-averaged F-measure cannot focus entirely on rare classes [78]. Since some of the datasets utilized in the empirical analysis are imbalanced dataset, the macro-averaged F-measure is also utilized as another evaluation measure. The macro-averaged F-measure, which determines the average F-measure across all one-versus-all classes, is computed as given by (17):

$$\text{Macro} - \text{averaged F} - \text{measure} = \frac{1}{n}\sum_{i=1}^{n} \frac{2 \times Precision_i \times Recall_i}{Precision_i + Recall_i} \quad (17)$$

$$\text{Precision} = \frac{TP}{TP + FP} \quad (18)$$

$$\text{Recall} = \frac{TP}{TP + FN} \quad (19)$$

where TP, FP, and FN represent the number of true positives, false positives, and false negatives, respectively.

5.3. Experimental Procedure. In the experimental analysis, dataset is divided into tenfold (parts). In this scheme, sixfold is utilized for training, twofold is utilized for validation, and twofold is utilized for test. The experimental analysis is performed with the machine learning toolkit WEKA

Table 2: Classification algorithms used to build the model library.

Classifier Group	Classification Algorithms
Bayesian Classifiers (5)	Bayesian logistic regression (with Norm-based hyper-parameter selection), Bayesian logistic regression (with Cross-validated hyper-parameter selection), Bayesian logistic regression (with Specific value based hyper-parameter selection), Naive Bayes, Naive Bayes Multinomial
Function based classifiers (14)	FLDA, Kernel Logistic Regression (with Poly Kernel), Kernel Logistic Regression (with Normalized Poly Kernel), LibLINEAR (with L2-regularized logistic regression), LibLINEAR (with L2-regularized L2-loss support vector classification), LibLINEAR (with L1-regularized logistic regression), LibSVM (with radial basis function), LibSVM (with linear kernel), LibSVM (with polynomial kernel), LibSVM (with sigmoid kernel), Multi-layer perceptron, radial basis function networks, Logistic regression, Gaussian radial basis function networks
Instance based classifiers (10)	KNN (with K: 1), KNN (with K:2), KNN (with K:3), KNN (with K: 4), KNN (with K:5), KNN (with K:6), KNN (with K:7), KNN (with K:8), KNN (with K:9), KNN (with K:10)
Rule based classifiers (3)	FURIA (with Product T-norm), FURIA (with Minimum T-norm), RIPPER
Decision tree classifiers (8)	BFTree (Unpruned), BFTree (Post-pruning), BFTree (Pre-pruning), Functional Tree, C4.5 (J48), NBTree, Random Forest, Random Tree

Table 2 is reproduced from ONAN et al. [19, 20] (under the Creative Commons Attribution License/public domain).

(Waikato Environment for Knowledge Analysis) version 3.9, which is an open-source platform with many machine learning algorithms implemented in Java [79]. The presented classification scheme is also implemented in Java. In the empirical analysis on swarm-based latent Dirichlet allocation, Naïve Bayes algorithm and support vector machines are utilized as the base learning algorithms. In order to compare the presented multiple classifier system, four well-known ensemble methods (namely, AdaBoost, Bagging, Random Subspace, and Stacking) have been considered. For AdaBoost, Bagging, and Random Subspace algorithms, Naïve Bayes and support vector machines are utilized as the base learners. In the Stacking (stacked generalization), the classifier ensemble consisted of five base learners (namely, Naïve Bayes, support vector machines, logistic regression, Bayesian logistic regression, and linear discriminant analysis). For ensemble selection from libraries of models (ESM) and Bagging ensemble selection (BES), the same model library presented in Table 2 has been utilized [19, 20].

For evaluating ensemble pruning schemes, we have adopted the scheme outlined in [19, 20]. In the experimental analysis, ESM, BES, and LibD3C algorithms are considered with different parameter values. For ESM algorithm, four different schemes (namely, forward selection, backward elimination, forward-backward selection, and the best model scheme) have been considered. In ESM algorithm, root mean squared error (RMSE), classification accuracy (ACC), ROC area, precision, recall, and F-measure are considered as the evaluation measures. For BES algorithm, different bag sizes ranging from 10 to 100 are considered. In this algorithm, root mean squared error (RMSE), accuracy (ACC), ROC area, precision, recall, F-measure, and the combination of all metrics are employed as the evaluation measures. For LibD3C algorithm, five different ensemble combination rules (namely, average of probabilities, product of probabilities, majority voting, minimum probability, and maximum probability) are considered. In the experimental analysis, the highest predictive performances obtained from these algorithms are reported. In Table 3, the parameter values of metaheuristic algorithms utilized in swarm-based LDA are presented. In Table 4, parameters of metaheuristic clustering algorithms utilized in the ensemble pruning stage are given. The parameters of the metaheuristic algorithms utilized in the swarm-based LDA stage and the parameters of the metaheuristic algorithms utilized in the ensemble pruning stage are determined based on the benchmark empirical results for the algorithms [80, 81].

5.4. Experimental Results and Discussion. The presented biomedical text categorization framework consists of two main stages, namely, swarm-optimized latent Dirichlet allocation stage and diversity-based ensemble pruning stage.

Swarm-optimized latent Dirichlet allocation stage aims to estimate the parameters of LDA. In the empirical analysis on LDA, five different metaheuristic algorithms (namely, genetic algorithms, particle swarm optimization, firefly algorithm, cuckoo search algorithm, and bat algorithm) are considered. To evaluate the clustering quality of different configurations of LDA, four internal cluster validity indices (namely, the Bayesian information criterion, Calinski-Harabasz index, Davies-Bouldin index, and Silhouette index) are considered. In addition, the proposed scheme presents an ensemble pruning based on combined diversity measures and metaheuristic clustering. In the tables, the highest (the best) results achieved by a particular configuration are indicated as both boldface and underline and the second best results are indicated as both boldface and italics.

In order to evaluate the merit of swarm-optimized topic modelling in LDA, Table 5 presents the classification accuracies obtained by different LDA-based configurations with Naïve Bayes and support vector machine classifiers. To verify the impact of ensemble pruning method in the presented scheme, Table 6 presents the classification results obtained by conventional algorithms, ensemble learning methods, conventional ensemble pruning methods, and the proposed diversity-based ensemble pruning method. For the

Table 3: Parameters of the metaheuristics algorithms utilized in swarm-based LDA.

Metaheuristic algorithm	Parameter Values
Genetic algorithms	Crossover probability: 0.6, The number of generations to evaluate: 20, Mutation probability: 0.033, Population size: 20, Seed: 1
Particle swarm optimization	Individual weight: 0.34, Inertia weight: 0.33, Number of iterations: 20, Mutation probability: 0.01, Mutation type: bit-flip, Population size: 20, Seed: 1, Social Weight: 0.33
Firefly algorithm	α= 0.8, γ= 0.5, δ=0.85
Cuckoo search algorithm	P_a= 0.5
Bat algorithm	Ld=0.4, pr=0.4, fq_{min}=0, fq_{max}=2

Table 4: Parameters of the metaheuristics algorithms utilized in ensemble pruning.

Metaheuristic algorithm	Parameter Values
Genetic clustering	Crossover probability= 0.6, The number of generations to evaluate= 20, Mutation probability= 0.033, Population size= 20, Seed: 1, k:20
Particle swarm clustering	Individual weight: 0.70, c_1: 1.5, c_2: 1.5, k: 20
Firefly clustering	α= 0.6, γ= 0.3, δ=0.95, k: 20
Cuckoo clustering	P_a= 0.3, k: 20
Bat clustering	Ld=0.5, pr=0.5, fq_{min}=0, fq_{max}=2, k:20

Table 5: Classification accuracies obtained with different LDA-based configurations.

	Naive Bayes (NB)					Support Vector Machines (SVM)				
Configuration	oh5	oh10	oh15	ohscal	Ohsu-med	oh5	oh10	oh15	ohscal	Ohsu-med
LDA (k=50)	74.38	66.66	69.40	59.27	28.35	76.24	78.73	83.17	70.62	34.64
LDA (k=100)	70.85	63.64	67.44	60.05	29.56	78.28	78.25	83.23	73.23	38.82
LDA (k=150)	69.02	65.24	65.51	59.01	29.43	76.72	79.09	84.74	73.8	41.27
LDA (k=200)	66.17	64.01	63.61	58.93	27.99	77.33	77.93	84	74.19	41.82
GA-LDA (BIC)	75.16	67.24	74.70	71.66	35.45	77.98	69.03	75.12	73.62	35.83
PSO-LDA (BIC)	75.40	68.60	76.90	72.43	35.46	78.22	72.56	75.17	75.89	36.23
FA-LDA (BIC)	75.48	71.26	77.48	72.80	35.60	79.50	74.73	76.63	76.90	37.69
CSA-LDA (BIC)	76.66	71.96	78.77	72.94	35.65	79.56	75.97	77.96	77.02	37.94
BA-LDA (BIC)	78.82	72.21	79.77	73.02	36.58	79.85	76.53	78.89	77.34	38.89
GA-LDA (CH)	79.02	72.88	80.11	74.53	36.85	80.62	77.72	80.31	78.17	38.96
PSO-LDA (CH)	80.20	72.93	80.66	74.76	37.03	81.50	77.91	80.50	78.99	39.03
FA-LDA (CH)	81.20	72.99	80.72	75.13	37.75	81.80	77.99	80.55	79.09	39.03
CSA-LDA (CH)	81.40	73.12	81.71	76.02	38.34	82.61	78.01	80.78	79.82	39.03
BA-LDA (CH)	81.46	73.49	81.82	76.21	39.24	82.87	78.93	81.01	79.89	39.52
GA-LDA (DB)	84.46	76.22	84.13	78.71	40.50	84.73	80.95	85.88	82.46	43.02
PSO-LDA (DB)	84.60	80.07	85.14	79.21	42.57	85.13	81.11	86.17	84.22	43.51
FA-LDA (DB)	85.89	80.82	85.17	80.83	44.60	86.22	81.88	86.73	84.62	44.61
CSA-LDA (DB)	***86.42***	***80.97***	***86.10***	***81.69***	***45.21***	***86.79***	***82.00***	***86.96***	***85.07***	***46.67***
BA-LDA (DB)	**87.60**	**81.36**	**87.32**	**83.56**	**47.00**	**88.86**	**82.09**	**88.05**	**85.24**	**50.08**
GA-LDA (SI)	81.57	73.57	82.03	76.48	39.36	83.21	79.00	82.24	79.93	40.58
PSO-LDA (SI)	82.61	73.76	82.50	76.61	39.66	83.58	79.33	83.03	80.36	40.87
FA-LDA (SI)	83.19	74.18	82.88	77.47	39.68	83.69	79.41	83.11	80.95	40.95
CSA-LDA (SI)	83.78	75.11	83.01	78.06	39.69	83.84	80.83	84.47	81.82	41.12
BA-LDA (SI)	84.11	76.08	83.03	78.13	40.08	84.49	80.90	85.52	81.99	42.65

LDA: latent Dirichlet allocation, GA-LDA: genetic algorithm based LDA, PSO-LDA: particle swarm optimization based LDA, FA-LDA: firefly algorithm based LDA, CSA-LDA: cuckoo search algorithm based LDA, BA-LDA: bat algorithm based LDA, BIC: Bayesian information criterion, CH: Calinski-Harabasz index, DB: Davies-Bouldin index, and SI: Silhouette index.

Table 6: Classification results obtained by conventional algorithms and the proposed diversity-based ensemble pruning (with LDA (k=50) based representation).

Classification algorithm	oh5	oh10	oh15	ohscal	ohsumed
NB	75.19	67.43	70.77	60.24	29.41
SVM	77.59	80.29	84.47	71.58	34.72
Bagging+NB	76.08	69.77	70.94	60.21	29.21
Bagging+SVM	84.36	77.20	79.07	71.92	35.98
AdaBoost+NB	73.53	68.07	70.26	60.09	29.60
AdaBoost+SVM	84.06	77.19	78.88	72.08	35.03
RandomSubspace+NB	74.75	67.29	68.51	57.58	28.60
RandomSubspace+SVM	78.02	69.89	71.22	67.65	31.80
Stacking	83.78	81.32	81.69	60.02	40.76
ESM	79.25	79.07	78.91	72.52	37.84
BES	80.11	80.61	81.08	73.02	40.04
LibD3C	82.86	82.93	84.51	74.86	41.17
CDM	84.77	84.13	85.32	76.45	43.55
DEP (Genetic clustering)	81.61	81.96	84.64	74.21	43.27
DEP (PSO clustering)	80.91	81.41	83.31	73.98	***45.73***
DEP (Firefly clustering)	**86.52**	**86.08**	**86.29**	**77.47**	**47.48**
DEP (Cuckoo clustering)	***85.06***	83.00	***85.84***	***76.81***	45.43
DEP (Bat clustering)	84.47	***84.18***	82.11	72.70	44.13

NB: Naïve Bayes algorithm, SVM: support vector machines, ESM: ensemble selection from libraries of models, BES: Bagging ensemble selection, LibD3C: hybrid ensemble pruning based on k-means and dynamic selection, CDM: ensemble pruning based on combined diversity measures, and DEP: the proposed diversity-based ensemble pruning.

Table 7: Comparison of the proposed text categorization scheme with conventional classifiers, ensemble learners, and ensemble pruning method (with BA-LDA (DB) based representation).

Classification algorithm	oh5	oh10	oh15	ohscal	ohsumed
NB	87.67	81.42	87.44	83.64	47.09
SVM	88.97	82.22	88.16	85.32	50.08
Bagging+NB	89.32	83.35	88.87	83.47	48.52
Bagging+SVM	88.03	84.84	87.86	83.92	50.73
AdaBoost+NB	89.77	83.60	87.48	86.18	51.18
AdaBoost+SVM	88.18	84.95	87.35	86.29	51.85
RandomSubspace+NB	88.32	83.96	86.66	88.09	50.70
RandomSubspace+SVM	88.56	84.11	89.58	88.29	50.29
Stacking	88.28	86.87	88.93	84.90	53.84
ESM	88.58	86.66	90.25	88.48	51.94
BES	89.29	86.00	90.98	89.12	52.47
LibD3C	90.35	87.95	91.27	90.48	53.41
CDM	***91.51***	***89.61***	***93.17***	***91.33***	***54.47***
Proposed scheme	**93.14**	**91.29**	**93.76**	**92.14**	**58.17**

NB: Naïve Bayes algorithm, SVM: support vector machines, ESM: ensemble selection from libraries of models, BES: Bagging ensemble selection, LibD3C: hybrid ensemble pruning based on k-means and dynamic selection, and CDM: ensemble pruning based on combined diversity measures.

results reported in Table 6, the biomedical text categorization datasets are represented with LDA (k=50); i.e., swarm-optimized latent Dirichlet allocation stage has not been applied for the results presented in Table 6 to examine the predictive performance of the proposed ensemble pruning scheme. Finally, Table 7 compares the predictive performance of conventional algorithms, ensemble learning methods, conventional ensemble pruning methods, and the proposed diversity-based ensemble pruning method when swarm-optimized latent Dirichlet allocation stage has been applied to represent the dataset.

As can be observed from the classification accuracies presented in Table 5, the performance of LDA-based representation schemes generally enhances with the use of metaheuristic algorithms in conjunction with LDA to estimate the parameters of it. Among the different metaheuristic algorithms, the highest predictive performance is obtained by bat algorithm based LDA with Davies-Bouldin index based evaluation. The second highest predictive performance is obtained by cuckoo search algorithm based LDA with Davies-Bouldin index based evaluation. Regarding the performance of different evaluation measures, the highest performance is achieved by Davies-Bouldin index based configurations. The second predictive performance is achieved by Silhouette index based configurations, which is followed by Calinski-Harabasz index based configurations. Regarding the performance of conventional LDA-based representation schemes, the highest predictive performance is generally achieved when k=50. The predictive performance patterns obtained by different LDA-based configurations with Naïve Bayes algorithm are valid for LDA-based configurations with support vector machines algorithm.

In the empirical analysis on the ensemble pruning, five swarm-based clustering algorithms (namely, genetic clustering, particle swarm-based clustering, firefly clustering, cuckoo clustering, and bat clustering) have been considered. Regarding the predictive performance obtained by conventional classification algorithms, support vector machines algorithm outperforms Naïve Bayes algorithm for the compared datasets. In addition, Bagging ensemble of Naïve Bayes algorithm yields better predictive performance compared to Naïve Bayes algorithm. In general, the predictive performance is enhanced with the use of conventional ensemble learning methods (namely, Bagging, AdaBoost, and Random Subspace algorithm). As can be seen from the results reported in Table 6, conventional ensemble pruning methods outperform the conventional classification algorithms and ensemble learning schemes. In addition, hybrid ensemble pruning schemes (the proposed diversity-based ensemble pruning method, LibD3C algorithm, and ensemble pruning based on combined diversity measures) outperform the other ensemble pruning schemes (ensemble selection from libraries of models and Bagging ensemble selection). The highest predictive performance is obtained by the proposed diversity-based ensemble pruning scheme with firefly clustering. The second highest predictive performance is generally obtained by the proposed diversity-based ensemble pruning scheme with cuckoo clustering.

Based on the extensive empirical analysis with different metaheuristic algorithms in swarm-based LDA and with different clustering algorithms in diversity-based ensemble pruning algorithm, the highest predictive performance is obtained by bat algorithm based LDA with Davies-Bouldin index and diversity-based ensemble pruning with firefly clustering. In Table 7, the predictive performance of the proposed biomedical text categorization scheme is compared with two classification algorithms (namely, Naïve Bayes algorithm and support vector machines), four ensemble methods (namely, Bagging, AdaBoost, Random Subspace, and Stacking), and four ensemble pruning methods (namely, ensemble selection from libraries of models, Bagging ensemble selection, LibD3C algorithm, and ensemble pruning based on combined diversity measures). For the results reported in Table 7, the biomedical text categorization datasets are represented with bat algorithm based LDA with Davies-Bouldin index (BA-LDA (DB)). As can be observed from the results outlined in Table 7, the proposed scheme outperforms the conventional classifiers, ensemble learning methods, and ensemble pruning methods.

In addition to classification accuracy, the predictive performances of classification algorithms, ensemble learning methods, and ensemble pruning methods have been also examined in terms of the macro-averaged F-measure. In Table 8, the macro-averaged F-measure results obtained by different LDA-based configurations with Naïve Bayes and support vector machine classifiers are presented. Regarding the macro-averaged F-measure results presented in Table 8, the highest predictive performance is obtained by bat algorithm based LDA with Davies-Bouldin index based representation. The same patterns obtained in terms of classification accuracies presented in Table 5 are also valid for F-measure based results. Hence, the utilization of metaheuristic optimization algorithms in conjunction with LDA to calibrate its hyper-parameters enhances the predictive model.

To examine the performance improvement achieved by the proposed ensemble pruning scheme, Table 9 presents the macro-averaged F-measure values obtained by conventional algorithms, ensemble learning methods, conventional ensemble pruning methods, and the proposed diversity-based ensemble pruning method. For the results reported in Table 9, the biomedical text categorization datasets are represented with LDA (k=50); i.e., swarm-optimized latent Dirichlet allocation stage has not been applied for the results presented in Table 9. Regarding the macro-averaged F-measure results presented in Table 9, the highest predictive performance is obtained by the proposed diversity-based ensemble pruning scheme with firefly clustering. The second highest predictive performance is generally obtained by the proposed diversity-based ensemble pruning scheme with cuckoo clustering and ensemble pruning based on combined diversity.

In Table 10, the macro-averaged F-measure results obtained by classification algorithms, ensemble learning methods, and ensemble pruning methods are presented. For the results reported in Table 10, the biomedical text categorization datasets are represented with bat algorithm based LDA with Davies-Bouldin index (BA-LDA (DB)). Regarding the macro-averaged F-measure results, the proposed scheme outperforms the conventional classifiers, ensemble learning methods, and ensemble pruning methods.

To statistically validate the results obtained in the empirical analysis, we have performed the two-way ANOVA (analysis of variance) test in the Minitab statistical program. The two-way ANOVA test is an extension of the one-way ANOVA test, which aims to evaluate the effect of two different categorical independent variables on one dependent variable. In two-way ANOVA test, both the main effect of each independent variable and their interactions are taken into assessment. The results for the two-way ANOVA test of overall results (in terms of classification accuracy) are presented in Table 11, where DF, SS, MS, F, and P denote degrees of freedom,

Table 8: The macro-averaged F-measure results obtained with different LDA-based configurations.

	Naive Bayes (NB)					Support Vector Machines (SVM)				
Configuration	oh5	oh10	oh15	ohscal	Ohsu-med	oh5	oh10	oh15	ohscal	Ohsu-med
LDA (k=50)	0.75	0.68	0.71	0.61	0.30	0.77	0.80	0.85	0.73	0.36
LDA (k=100)	0.72	0.65	0.69	0.62	0.31	0.79	0.80	0.85	0.75	0.40
LDA (k=150)	0.70	0.67	0.67	0.61	0.31	0.77	0.81	0.86	0.76	0.43
LDA (k=200)	0.67	0.65	0.65	0.61	0.29	0.78	0.80	0.86	0.76	0.44
GA-LDA (BIC)	0.76	0.69	0.76	0.74	0.37	0.79	0.70	0.77	0.76	0.37
PSO-LDA (BIC)	0.76	0.70	0.78	0.75	0.37	0.79	0.74	0.77	0.78	0.38
FA-LDA (BIC)	0.76	0.73	0.79	0.75	0.37	0.80	0.76	0.78	0.79	0.39
CSA-LDA (BIC)	0.77	0.73	0.80	0.75	0.37	0.80	0.78	0.80	0.79	0.40
BA-LDA (BIC)	0.80	0.74	0.81	0.75	0.38	0.81	0.78	0.81	0.80	0.41
GA-LDA (CH)	0.80	0.74	0.82	0.77	0.38	0.81	0.79	0.82	0.81	0.41
PSO-LDA (CH)	0.81	0.74	0.82	0.77	0.39	0.82	0.79	0.82	0.81	0.41
FA-LDA (CH)	0.82	0.74	0.82	0.77	0.39	0.83	0.80	0.82	0.82	0.41
CSA-LDA (CH)	0.82	0.75	0.83	0.78	0.40	0.83	0.80	0.82	0.82	0.41
BA-LDA (CH)	0.82	0.75	0.83	0.79	0.41	0.84	0.81	0.83	0.82	0.41
GA-LDA (DB)	0.85	0.78	0.86	0.81	0.42	0.86	0.83	0.88	0.85	0.45
PSO-LDA (DB)	0.85	***0.82***	0.87	0.82	0.44	0.86	0.83	0.88	0.87	0.45
FA-LDA (DB)	***0.87***	***0.82***	0.87	0.83	0.46	0.87	***0.84***	***0.89***	0.87	0.46
CSA-LDA (DB)	***0.87***	**0.83**	***0.88***	***0.84***	***0.47***	***0.88***	***0.84***	***0.89***	***0.88***	***0.49***
BA-LDA (DB)	**0.88**	**0.83**	**0.89**	**0.86**	**0.49**	**0.90**	**0.84**	**0.90**	**0.88**	**0.52**
GA-LDA (SI)	0.82	0.75	0.84	0.79	0.41	0.84	0.81	0.84	0.82	0.42
PSO-LDA (SI)	0.83	0.75	0.84	0.79	0.41	0.84	0.81	0.85	0.83	0.43
FA-LDA (SI)	0.84	0.76	0.85	0.80	0.41	0.85	0.81	0.85	0.83	0.43
CSA-LDA (SI)	0.85	0.77	0.85	0.80	0.41	0.85	0.82	0.86	0.84	0.43
BA-LDA (SI)	0.85	0.78	0.85	0.81	0.42	0.85	0.83	0.87	0.85	0.44

LDA: latent Dirichlet allocation, GA-LDA: genetic algorithm based LDA, PSO-LDA: particle swarm optimization based LDA, FA-LDA: firefly algorithm based LDA, CSA-LDA: cuckoo search algorithm based LDA, BA-LDA: bat algorithm based LDA, BIC: Bayesian information criterion, CH: Calinski-Harabasz index, DB: Davies-Bouldin index, and SI: Silhouette index.

adjusted sum of squares, adjusted mean square, F-Value, and probability value, respectively. Degrees of freedom are the amount of information in the data. The adjusted sum of squares term (SS) denotes the amount of variation in the response data that is explained by each term of the model. F-statistics (F) is the test statistic to identify whether a term is associated with the response and the probability value (P) is used to determine the statistical significance of the terms and model. The results presented in Table 11 are divided into three parts. The upper part of the table denotes the statistical analysis of results on the different LDA-based configurations, the middle part of the table denotes the statistical analysis of results on ensemble pruning, and the lower part of the table denotes the statistical analysis of results on conventional classifiers, ensemble learning methods, and ensemble pruning methods. For two-way ANOVA test, two different factors (different datasets and different algorithmic configurations) are taken as categorical independent variables. In addition, the interaction among these factors is also taken into consideration. According to the results presented in Table 11, probability value is $P<0.001$ for different factors and their interactions. Hence, there are statistically meaningful differences between the predictive performances of compared methods. The performance gain obtained by swarm-optimized LDA is statistically meaningful. Similarly, the performance gain obtained by the proposed ensemble pruning method is also statistically meaningful ($P<0.001$).

The results for the two-way ANOVA test of overall results (in terms of the macro-averaged F-measure values) are presented in Table 12. According to the results presented in Table 12, there are statistically meaningful differences between the predictive performances of compared methods ($P<0.001$).

In Figure 4, the confidence intervals for the mean values of classification accuracies obtained by the different LDA-based configuration schemes are presented. Similarly, in Figure 5, the confidence intervals for the mean values of classification accuracies obtained by the conventional classifiers, ensemble learners, and ensemble pruning methods are presented. For results depicted in Figure 5, the biomedical text categorization datasets are represented with LDA (k=50); i.e., swarm-optimized latent Dirichlet allocation stage has not been applied. In contrast, in Figure 6, the confidence intervals for the mean values of classification accuracies obtained by the conventional classifiers, ensemble learners, and ensemble pruning methods are given. In Figure 6, swarm-optimized latent Dirichlet allocation stage has been applied to represent the dataset. For the statistical significance of results,

TABLE 9: The macro-averaged F-measure results obtained by conventional algorithms and the proposed diversity-based ensemble pruning (with LDA (k=50) based representation).

Classification algorithm	oh5	oh10	oh15	ohscal	ohsumed
NB	0.76	0.68	0.72	0.61	0.30
SVM	0.78	0.81	0.86	0.73	0.35
Bagging+NB	0.77	0.70	0.72	0.61	0.30
Bagging+SVM	0.85	0.78	0.81	0.73	0.37
AdaBoost+NB	0.74	0.69	0.72	0.61	0.31
AdaBoost+SVM	0.85	0.78	0.80	0.74	0.36
RandomSubspace+NB	0.76	0.68	0.70	0.59	0.29
RandomSubspace+SVM	0.79	0.71	0.73	0.69	0.33
Stacking	0.84	0.80	0.81	0.72	0.38
ESM	0.80	0.81	0.81	0.74	0.39
BES	0.81	0.82	0.83	0.75	0.41
LibD3C	0.84	0.85	0.86	0.76	0.42
CDM	***0.86***	***0.86***	***0.87***	***0.78***	0.45
DEP (Genetic clustering)	0.82	0.84	0.86	0.76	0.45
DEP (PSO clustering)	0.82	0.83	0.85	0.75	***0.47***
DEP (Firefly clustering)	**0.87**	**0.88**	**0.88**	**0.79**	**0.49**
DEP (Cuckoo clustering)	***0.86***	0.85	**0.88**	***0.78***	***0.47***
DEP (Bat clustering)	0.85	***0.86***	0.84	0.74	0.45

NB: Naïve Bayes algorithm, SVM: support vector machines, ESM: ensemble selection from libraries of models, BES: Bagging ensemble selection, LibD3C: hybrid ensemble pruning based on k-means and dynamic selection, CDM: ensemble pruning based on combined diversity measures, and DEP: the proposed diversity-based ensemble pruning.

TABLE 10: The macro-averaged F-measure results of methods (with BA-LDA (DB) based representation).

Classification algorithm	oh5	oh10	oh15	ohscal	ohsumed
NB	0.89	0.82	0.88	0.84	0.48
SVM	0.90	0.83	0.89	0.86	0.51
Bagging+NB	0.90	0.84	0.90	0.84	0.49
Bagging+SVM	0.89	0.86	0.89	0.85	0.51
AdaBoost+NB	0.91	0.84	0.88	0.87	0.52
AdaBoost+SVM	0.89	0.86	0.88	0.87	0.52
RandomSubspace+NB	0.90	0.86	0.88	0.90	0.52
RandomSubspace+SVM	0.90	0.86	0.91	0.90	0.51
Stacking	0.90	0.87	0.91	0.88	0.54
ESM	0.90	0.88	0.92	0.90	0.53
BES	0.93	0.90	0.95	0.93	0.55
LibD3C	0.94	0.92	0.95	0.94	0.56
CDM	***0.95***	***0.93***	***0.97***	***0.95***	***0.57***
Proposed scheme	**0.97**	**0.95**	**0.98**	**0.96**	**0.61**

NB: Naïve Bayes algorithm, SVM: support vector machines, ESM: ensemble selection from libraries of models, BES: Bagging ensemble selection, LibD3C: hybrid ensemble pruning based on k-means and dynamic selection, and CDM: ensemble pruning based on combined diversity measures.

confidence intervals are divided into regions denoted by red dashed lines. As the interval plots indicate, the predictive performances obtained by the swarm-optimized LDA (BA-LDA (DB)) and DEP (firefly clustering) are statistically significant.

In Figure 7, average execution times of compared algorithms have been presented in seconds. As can be observed from Figure 7, average execution times on base learning algorithms (Naïve Bayes and support vector machines) are the lowest. Conventional ensemble learning methods generally enhance the predictive performance of the conventional base learning algorithms. However, ensemble learning methods involve more execution times. Compared to the ensemble learning methods, ensemble pruning schemes have more execution time. The highest execution time is involved in ensemble pruning based on combined diversity measures (CDM) and the second highest execution time is required in the proposed classification scheme (DEP-firefly clustering).

Table 11: Two-way ANOVA test results of classification accuracy values.

Statistical analysis of results on different LDA-based configurations

Source	DF	SS	MS	F	P
Configuration	23	4073.9	177.1	90.50	P<0.001
Dataset	4	60336.7	15084.2	7707.50	P<0.001
Classifier	1	881.0	881.0	450.15	P<0.001
Configuration∗Dataset	92	334.0	3.6	1.85	P<0.001
Configuration∗Classifier	23	932.9	40.6	20.73	P<0.001
Dataset∗Classifier	4	106.3	26.6	13.57	P<0.001
Error	92	180.1	2.0		
Total	239	66844.8			

Statistical analysis of results on classifiers and ensemble pruning methods (with LDA (k=50) based representation).

Source	DF	SS	MS	F	P
Configuration	17	2691.7	158.34	25.86	P<0.001
Dataset	4	23128.7	5782.17	944.48	P<0.001
Error	68	416.3	6.12		
Total	89				

Statistical analysis of results on conventional classifiers, ensemble learners, and ensemble pruning methods (with BA-LDA (DB) based representation).

Source	DF	SS	MS	F	P
Configuration	13	324.5	24.96	17.81	P<0.001
Dataset	4	14736.0	3684.00	2628.98	P<0.001
Error	52	72.9	1.40		
Total	69	15133.4			

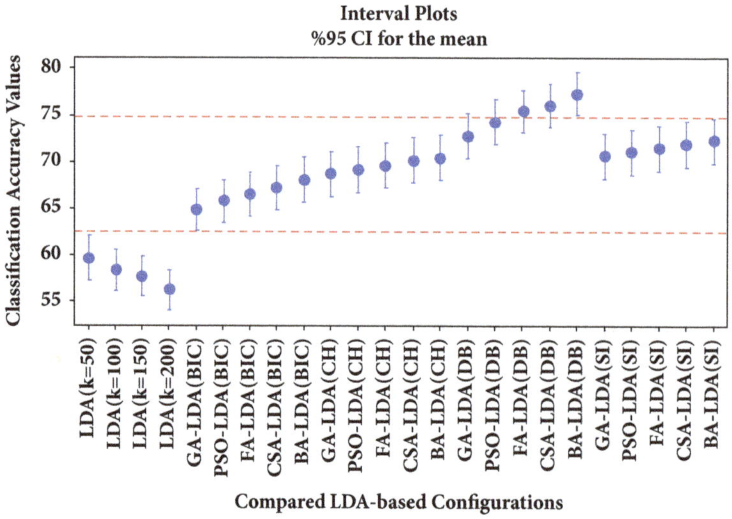

Figure 4: Interval plots for compared LDA-based configurations.

TABLE 12: Two-way ANOVA test results of the macro-averaged F-measure.

Statistical analysis of results on different LDA-based configurations					
Source	**DF**	**SS**	**MS**	**F**	**P**
Configuration	23	0.42777	0.01860	91.27	P<0.001
Dataset	4	5.99867	1.49967	7359.42	P<0.001
Classifier	1	0.09263	0.09263	454.58	P<0.001
Configuration*Dataset	92	0.03536	0.00038	1.89	P<0.001
Configuration*Classifier	23	0.09800	0.00426	20.91	P<0.001
Dataset*Classifier	4	0.01123	0.00281	13.78	P<0.001
Error	92	0.01875	0.00020		
Total	239	6.68241			
Statistical analysis of results on classifiers and ensemble pruning methods (with LDA (k=50) based representation).					
Source	**DF**	**SS**	**MS**	**F**	**P**
Configuration	17	0.27733	0.016314	23.26	P<0.001
Dataset	4	2.41143	0.692858	859.46	P<0.001
Error	68	0.04770	0.000701		
Total	89	2.73646			
Statistical analysis of results on conventional classifiers, ensemble learners, and ensemble pruning methods (with BA-LDA (DB) based representation).					
Source	**DF**	**SS**	**MS**	**F**	**P**
Configuration	13	0.03613	0.002780	14.68	P<0.001
Dataset	4	1.53718	0.384296	2029.89	P<0.001
Error	52	0.00984	0.000189		
Total	69	1.58316			

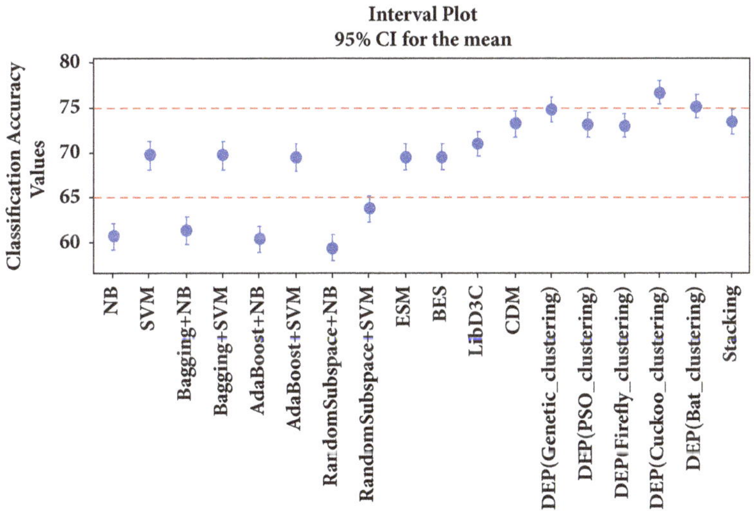

FIGURE 5: Interval plots for classifiers and ensemble pruning methods.

Metaheuristic optimization methods are well-established techniques on tuning the parameters. Hence, there is a trade-off between predictive performance and execution times.

6. Conclusion

In this work, we propose a novel biomedical text classification scheme based on swarm-optimized latent Dirichlet allocation and diversity-based ensemble pruning. Biomedical text categorization is an important research direction due to the immense quantity of unstructured information available. The latent Dirichlet allocation (LDA) is a popular representation scheme for text documents, which can yield better performance than other linguistic representation schemes, such as latent semantic analysis and probabilistic latent semantic analysis. We found out that the identification of appropriate parameter values is very important to the performance of LDA. In addition, it has been experimentally validated

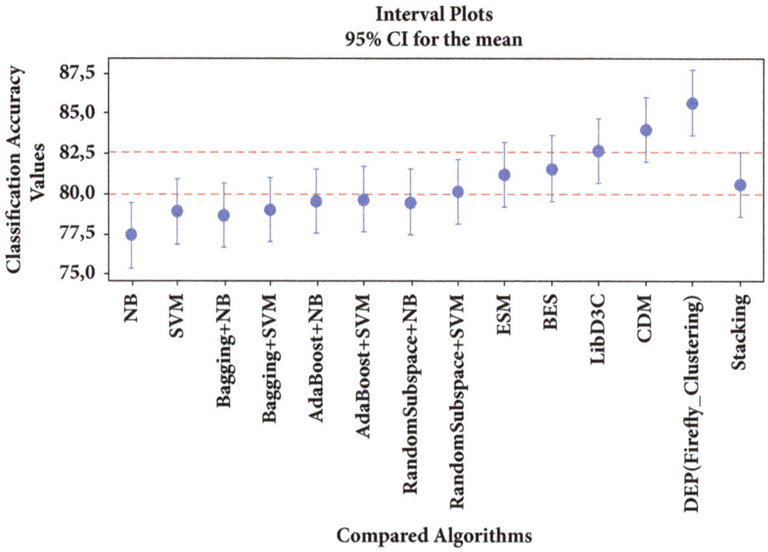

FIGURE 6: Interval plots for compared algorithms.

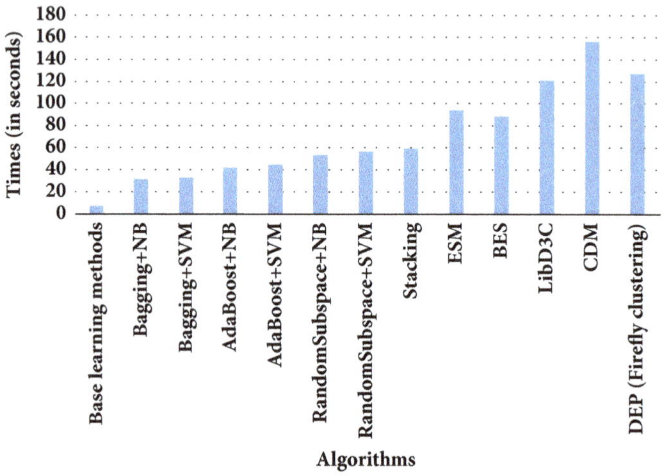

FIGURE 7: Average execution times (in seconds) for compared algorithms.

that the use of metaheuristic optimization algorithms to calibrate the parameters of LDA yields promising results on biomedical text categorization. The presented text classification scheme also employs an ensemble pruning approach based on combined diversity measures to identify a robust multiple classifier system with high predictive performance. The presented ensemble pruning approach combines four different diversity measures (namely, disagreement measure, Q-statistics, the correlation coefficient, and the double fault measure). In addition, the scheme employs the swarm-based clustering algorithm. The experimental results indicate that the proposed multiple classifier system outperforms the conventional classification algorithms, ensemble learning, and ensemble pruning methods.

Conflicts of Interest

The authors declare that they have no conflicts of interest.

References

[1] E. S. Chen, G. Hripcsak, H. Xu, M. Markatou, and C. Friedman, "Automated acquisition of disease–drug knowledge from biomedical and clinical documents: an initial study," *Journal of the American Medical Informatics Association*, vol. 15, no. 1, pp. 87–98, 2008.

[2] R. Rodriguez-Esteban, "Biomedical text mining and its applications," *PLoS Computational Biology*, vol. 5, no. 12, Article ID e1000597, 2009.

[3] R. L. Figueroa and C. A. Flores, "Extracting Information from Electronic Medical Records to Identify the Obesity Status of

a Patient Based on Comorbidities and Bodyweight Measures," *Journal of Medical Systems*, vol. 40, no. 8, pp. 1–9, 2016.

[4] J. Urbain, "Mining heart disease risk factors in clinical text with named entity recognition and distributional semantic models," *Journal of Biomedical Informatics*, vol. 58, pp. S143–S149, 2015.

[5] T. G. Soldatos, S. I. O'Donoghue, V. P. Satagopam et al., "Martini: using literature keywords to compare gene sets," *Nucleic Acids Research*, vol. 38, no. 1, pp. 26–38, 2010.

[6] C. A. Trugenberger, C. Wälti, D. Peregrim, M. E. Sharp, and S. Bureeva, "Discovery of novel biomarkers and phenotypes by semantic technologies," *BMC Bioinformatics*, vol. 14, no. 1, article 51, 2013.

[7] A. Holzinger, J. Schantl, M. Schroettner, C. Seifert, and K. Verspoor, "Biomedical text mining: state-of-the-art, open problems and future challenges," in *Interactive Knowledge Discovery and Data Mining in Biomedical Informatics*, pp. 271–300, Springer, Berlin, Germany, 2014.

[8] A. Onan and S. Korukoğlu, "A feature selection model based on genetic rank aggregation for text sentiment classification," *Journal of Information Science*, 2017.

[9] C. D. Manning, P. Raghavan, and H. Schütze, *Introduction to information retrieval*, vol. 1, No. 1, p. 496, Cambridge University Press, Cambridge, UK, 2008.

[10] T. Joachims, "Text categorization with support vector machines: Learning with many relevant features," *Machine Learning: ECML-98*, pp. 137–142, 1998.

[11] T. K. Landauer, D. Laham, B. Rehder, and M. E. Schreiner, "How well can passage meaning be derived without using word order? A comparison of Latent Semantic Analysis and humans," in *Proceedings of the 19th annual meeting of the Cognitive Science Society*, pp. 412–417, 1997.

[12] S. Deerwester, S. T. Dumais, G. W. Furnas, T. K. Landauer, and R. Harshman, "Indexing by latent semantic analysis," *Journal of the American Society for Information Science*, vol. 41, no. 6, article 391, 1990.

[13] T. Hofmann, "Probabilistic latent semantic indexing," in *Proceedings of the 22nd Annual International ACM SIGIR Conference on Research and Development in Information Retrieval, SIGIR 1999*, pp. 50–57, ACM, August 1999.

[14] M. Girolami and A. Kabán, "Sequential activity profiling: Latent dirichlet allocation of Markov chains," *Data Mining and Knowledge Discovery*, vol. 10, no. 3, pp. 175–196, 2005.

[15] T. G. Dietterich, "Ensemble methods in machine learning," in *International workshop on multiple classifier systems*, pp. 1–15, Springer, Berlin, Germany, 2000.

[16] J. Mendes-Moreira, C. Soares, A. M. Jorge, and J. F. D. Sousa, "Ensemble approaches for regression: A survey," *ACM Computing Surveys (CSUR)*, vol. 45, no. 1, article 10, 2012.

[17] F. Roli, G. Giacinto, and G. Vernazza, "Methods for designing multiple classifier systems," *Lecture Notes in Computer Science*, vol. 2096, pp. 78–87, 2001.

[18] Z. Zhou, J. Wu, and W. Tang, "Ensembling neural networks: many could be better than all," *Artificial Intelligence*, vol. 137, no. 1-2, pp. 239–263, 2002.

[19] A. Onan, H. Bulut, and S. Korukoglu, "An improved ant algorithm with LDA-based representation for text document clustering," *Journal of Information Science*, vol. 43, no. 2, pp. 275–292, 2017.

[20] A. Onan, S. Korukoğlu, and H. Bulut, "A hybrid ensemble pruning approach based on consensus clustering and multi-objective evolutionary algorithm for sentiment classification," *Information Processing & Management*, vol. 53, no. 4, pp. 814–833, 2017.

[21] G. D. C. Cavalcanti, L. S. Oliveira, T. J. M. Moura, and G. V. Carvalho, "Combining diversity measures for ensemble pruning," *Pattern Recognition Letters*, vol. 74, pp. 38–45, 2016.

[22] D. M. Blei, A. Y. Ng, and M. I. Jordan, "Latent Dirichlet allocation," *Journal of Machine Learning Research*, vol. 3, no. 4-5, pp. 993–1022, 2003.

[23] K. Tian, M. Revelle, and D. Poshyvanyk, "Using latent dirichlet allocation for automatic categorization of software," in *Proceedings of the 6th IEEE International Working Conference on Mining Software Repositories, 2009. MSR'09*, pp. 163–166, IEEE, 2009.

[24] Z. Zhai, B. Liu, H. Xu, and P. Jia, "Constrained LDA for grouping product features in opinion mining," *Advances in Knowledge Discovery and Data Mining*, pp. 448–459, 2011.

[25] Q. Wu, C. Zhang, Q. Hong, and L. Chen, "Topic evolution based on LDA and HMM and its application in stem cell research," *Journal of Information Science*, vol. 40, no. 5, pp. 611–620, 2014.

[26] A. Bagheri, M. Saraee, and F. De Jong, "ADM-LDA: An aspect detection model based on topic modelling using the structure of review sentences," *Journal of Information Science*, vol. 40, no. 5, pp. 621–636, 2014.

[27] L. Hong and B. D. Davison, "Empirical study of topic modeling in twitter," in *Proceedings of the first workshop on social media analytics*, pp. 80–88, ACM, 2010.

[28] Z. Chen, Y. Huang, J. Tian, X. Liu, K. Fu, and T. Huang, "Joint model for subsentence-level sentiment analysis with Markov logic," *Journal of the Association for Information Science and Technology*, vol. 66, no. 9, pp. 1913–1922, 2015.

[29] A. Onan, S. Korukoglu, and H. Bulut, "LDA-based Topic Modelling in Text Sentiment Classification: An Empirical Analysis," *International Journal of Computational Linguistics and Applications*, vol. 7, no. 1, pp. 101–119, 2016.

[30] L. Liu, L. Tang, W. Dong, S. Yao, and W. Zhou, "An overview of topic modeling and its current applications in bioinformatics," *SpringerPlus*, vol. 5, no. 1, article 1608, 2016.

[31] H. Wang, M. Huang, and X. Zhu, "Extract interaction detection methods from the biological literature," *BMC Bioinformatics*, vol. 10, no. 1, article S55, 2009.

[32] C. W. Arnold, S. M. El-Saden, A. A. Bui, and R. Taira, "Clinical case-based retrieval using latent topic analysis," in *AMIA annual symposium proceedings*, vol. 2010, p. 26, American Medical Informatics Association, 2010.

[33] M. Song and S. Y. Kim, "Detecting the knowledge structure of bioinformatics by mining full-text collections," *Scientometrics*, vol. 96, no. 1, pp. 183–201, 2013.

[34] E. Sarioglu, K. Yadav, and H. A. Choi, "Topic Modeling Based Classification of Clinical Reports," in *ACL (Student Research Workshop)*, pp. 67–73, 2013.

[35] H. Bisgin, Z. Liu, H. Fang, X. Xu, and W. Tong, "Mining FDA drug labels using an unsupervised learning technique-topic modeling," *BMC Bioinformatics*, vol. 12, no. 10, article no. S11, 2011.

[36] V. Wang, L. Xi, A. Enayetallah, E. Fauman, and D. Ziemek, "GeneTopics - interpretation of gene sets via literature-driven topic models," *BMC Systems Biology*, vol. 7, no. 5, article no. S10, 2013.

[37] H. Bisgin, M. Chen, Y. Wang et al., "A systems approach for analysis of high content screening assay data with topic modeling," *BMC Bioinformatics*, vol. 14, no. 14, article no. S11, 2013.

[38] H. Bisgin, Z. Liu, R. Kelly, H. Fang, X. Xu, and W. Tong, "Investigating drug repositioning opportunities in FDA drug labels through topic modeling," *BMC Bioinformatics*, vol. 13, no. 15, article S6, 2012.

[39] S.-H. Wang, Y. Ding, W. Zhao et al., "Text mining for identifying topics in the literatures about adolescent substance use and depression," *BMC Public Health*, vol. 16, no. 1, article no. 279, 2016.

[40] X. Wang, P. Zhu, T. Liu, and K. Xu, "BioTopic: A topic-driven biological literature mining system," *International Journal of Data Mining and Bioinformatics*, vol. 14, no. 4, pp. 373–386, 2016.

[41] R. Sullivan, A. B. E. E. D. Sarker, OK. A. R. E. N. Connor, A. M. A. N. D. A. Goodin, M. A. R. K. Karlsrud, and G. R. A. C. I. E. L. A. Gonzalez, "Finding potentially unsafe nutritional supplements from user reviews with topic modeling," in *Pacific Symposium on Biocomputing*, vol. 21, pp. 528–539, World Scientific, Kohala Coast, Hawaii, 2016.

[42] J. H. Chen, M. K. Goldstein, S. M. Asch, L. Mackey, and R. B. Altman, "redicting inpatient clinical order patterns with probabilistic topic models vs conventional order sets," *Journal of the American Medical Informatics Association*, ocw136, 2016.

[43] M. Aksela, "Comparison of classifier selection methods for improving committee performance," in *International Workshop on Multiple Classifier Systems*, pp. 84–93, Springer, Berlin, Germany, 2003.

[44] D. Ruta and B. Gabrys, "Application of the evolutionary algorithms for classifier selection in multiple classifier systems with majority voting," in *International Workshop on Multiple Classifier Systems*, pp. 399–408, Springer, Berlin, Germany.

[45] Z. H. Zhou and W. Tang, "Selective ensemble of decision trees," *Rough Sets, Fuzzy Sets, Data Mining, and Granular Computing*, pp. 589-589, 2003.

[46] S. Sheen and A. P. Sirisha, "Malware detection by pruning of parallel ensembles using harmony search," *Pattern Recognition Letters*, vol. 34, pp. 1679–1686, 2013.

[47] I. Mendialdua, A. Arruti, E. Jauregi, E. Lazkano, and B. Sierra, "Classifier Subset Selection to construct multi-classifiers by means of estimation of distribution algorithms," *Neurocomputing*, vol. 157, pp. 46–60, 2015.

[48] D. D. Margineantu and T. G. Dietterich, "Pruning adaptive boosting," in *Proceedings of the Fourteenth International Conference on Machine Learning*, pp. 211–218, San Francisco, Calf, USA, 1997.

[49] R. Caruana, A. Niculescu-Mizil, G. Crew, and A. Ksikes, "Ensemble selection from libraries of models," in *Proceedings of the 21st International Conference on Machine Learning (ICML '04)*, pp. 18–39, Banff, Canada, July 2004.

[50] Q. Dai, T. Zhang, and N. Liu, "A new reverse reduce-error ensemble pruning algorithm," *Applied Soft Computing*, vol. 28, pp. 237–249, 2015.

[51] S. B. Kotsiantis and P. E. Pintelas, "Selective averaging of regression models," *Annals of Mathematics, Computing & Teleinformatics*, vol. 1, no. 3, pp. 65–74, 2005.

[52] M. Galar, A. Fernández, E. Barrenechea, H. Bustince, and F. Herrera, "Ordering-based pruning for improving the performance of ensembles of classifiers in the framework of imbalanced datasets," *Information Sciences*, vol. 354, pp. 178–196, 2016.

[53] H. Zhang and L. Cao, "A spectral clustering based ensemble pruning approach," *Neurocomputing*, vol. 139, pp. 289–297, 2014.

[54] T. L. Griffiths, M. I. Jordan, J. B. Tenenbaum, and D. M. Blei, "Hierarchical topic models and the nested chinese restaurant process," in *Advances in neural information processing systems*, pp. 17–24, 2004.

[55] Y. W. Teh, M. I. Jordan, M. J. Beal, and D. M. Blei, "Sharing clusters among related groups: Hierarchical Dirichlet processes," in *Advances in Neural Information Processing Systems*, pp. 1385–1392, 2005.

[56] S. Grant and J. R. Cordy, "Estimating the optimal number of latent concepts in source code analysis," in *Proceedings of the 10th IEEE International Working Conference on Source Code Analysis and Manipulation (SCAM '10)*, pp. 65–74, IEEE, September 2010.

[57] A. Panichella, B. Dit, R. Oliveto, M. Di Penta, D. Poshynanyk, and A. De Lucia, "How to effectively use topic models for software engineering tasks? An approach based on genetic algorithms," in *Proceedings of the 35th International Conference on Software Engineering (ICSE '13)*, pp. 522–531, IEEE Press, May 2013.

[58] W. Zhao, J. J. Chen, R. Perkins et al., "A heuristic approach to determine an appropriate number of topics in topic modeling," *BMC Bioinformatics*, vol. 16, no. 13, article no. S8, 2015.

[59] A. Karami, A. Gangopadhyay, B. Zhou, and H. Kharrazi, "Fuzzy Approach Topic Discovery in Health and Medical Corpora," *International Journal of Fuzzy Systems*, pp. 1–12, 2017.

[60] R. Mousavi and M. Eftekhari, "A new ensemble learning methodology based on hybridization of classifier ensemble selection approaches," *Applied Soft Computing*, vol. 37, pp. 652–666, 2015.

[61] M. Jordan, *Learning in graphical models*, MIT Press, Cambridge, Mass, USA, 1999.

[62] L. Rokach, "Ensemble-based classifiers," *Artificial Intelligence Review*, vol. 33, no. 1-2, pp. 1–39, 2010.

[63] Z.-H. Zhou, *Ensemble Methods: Foundations and Algorithms*, Chapman and Hall, New York, NY, USA, 2012.

[64] L. Breiman, "Bagging predictors," *Machine Learning*, vol. 4, no. 2, pp. 123–140, 1996.

[65] T. K. Ho, "The random subspace method for constructing decision forests," *IEEE Transactions on Pattern Analysis and Machine Intelligence*, vol. 20, no. 8, pp. 832–844, 1998.

[66] D. H. Wolpert, "Stacked generalization," *Neural Networks*, vol. 5, no. 2, pp. 241–259, 1992.

[67] Q. Sun and B. Pfahringer, "Bagging ensemble selection," in *Proceedings of the 24th Australasian Joint Conference on Artificial Intelligence*, pp. 251–260, Australia, 2011.

[68] S. Cheng, B. Liu, T. O. Ting, Q. Qin, Y. Shi, and K. Huang, "Survey on data science with population-based algorithms," *Big Data Analytics*, vol. 1, no. 1, article 3, 2016.

[69] J. H. Holland, *Adaptation in natural and artificial systems: an introductory analysis with applications to biology, control, and artificial intelligence*, MIT press, 1992.

[70] J. Kennedy and R. Eberhart, "Particle swarm optimization," in *Proceedings of the IEEE International Conference on Neural Networks*, pp. 1942–1948, Perth, Australia, December 1995.

[71] X.-S. Yang, "A new metaheuristic bat-inspired algorithm," in *Nature Inspired Cooperative Strategies for Optimization (NICSO 2010)*, pp. 65–74, 2010.

[72] X.-S. Yang and S. Deb, "Engineering optimisation by Cuckoo search," *International Journal of Mathematical Modelling and Numerical Optimisation*, vol. 1, no. 4, pp. 330–343, 2010.

[73] X. S. Yang, *Nature-inspired metaheuristic algorithms*, Luniver press, 2010.

[74] E. Rendón, I. M. Abundez, C. Gutierrez et al., "A comparison of internal and external cluster validation indexes," in *Proceedings of the 2011 American Conference*, vol. 29, San Francisco, Calf, USA, 2011.

[75] D. J. Poirier, *Intermediate statistics and econometrics: a comparative approach*, MIT Press, 1995.

[76] L. I. Kuncheva and C. J. Whitaker, "Measures of diversity in classifier ensembles and their relationship with the ensemble accuracy," *Machine Learning*, vol. 51, no. 2, pp. 181–207, 2003.

[77] R. G. Rossi, R. M. Marcacini, and S. O. Rezende, *Benchmarking text collections for classification and clustering tasks*, Institute of Mathematics and Computer Sciences, University of Sao Paulo, 2013.

[78] H. Narasimhan, W. Pan, P. Kar, P. Protopapas, and H. G. Ramaswamy, "Optimizing the Multiclass F-Measure via Biconcave Programming," in *Proceedings of the IEEE 16th International Conference on Data Mining (ICDM)*, pp. 1101–1106, IEEE, 2016.

[79] M. Hall, E. Frank, G. Holmes, B. Pfahringer, P. Reutemann, and I. H. Witten, "The WEKA data mining software: an update," *ACM SIGKDD explorations newsletter*, vol. 11, no. 1, pp. 10–18, 2009.

[80] X. Min, L. Liu, Y. He et al., *Benchmarking swarm intelligence clustering algorithms with case study of medical data*, 2016.

[81] P. Das, D. K. Das, and S. Dey, "A New Class Topper Optimization Algorithm with an Application to Data Clustering," *IEEE Transactions on Emerging Topics in Computing*, 2018.

15

Understanding Dynamic Status Change of Hospital Stay and Cost Accumulation via Combining Continuous and Finitely Jumped Processes

Yanqiao Zheng,[1] Xiaobing Zhao,[2] and Xiaoqi Zhang[1]

[1] *School of Finance, Zhejiang University of Finance and Economics, China*
[2] *School of Data Sciences, Zhejiang University of Finance and Economics, China*

Correspondence should be addressed to Xiaoqi Zhang; xiaoqizh@buffalo.edu

Academic Editor: Kazuhisa Nishizawa

The Coxian phase-type models and the joint models of longitudinal and event time have been extensively used in the studies of medical outcome data. Coxian phase-type models have the finite-jump property while the joint models usually assume a continuous variation. The gap between continuity and discreteness makes the two models rarely used together. In this paper, a partition-based approach is proposed to jointly model the charge accumulation process and the time to discharge. The key construction of our new approach is a set of partition cells with their boundaries determined by a family of differential equations. Using the cells, our new approach makes it possible to incorporate finite jumps induced by a Coxian phase-type model into the charge accumulation process, therefore taking advantage of both the Coxian phase-type models and joint models. As a benefit, a couple of measures of the "cost" of staying in each medical stage (identified with phases of a Coxian phase-type model) are derived, which cannot be approached without considering the joint models and the Coxian phase-type models together. A two-step procedure is provided to generate consistent estimation of model parameters, which is applied to a subsample drawn from a well-known medical cost database.

1. Introduction

Rising expenditures and constraints on health care budgets have prompted the development of a variety of methods for the analyses of hospital charge and length of stay (LOS) as discussed in Gold [1], Lipscomb et al. [2], and Lin et al. [3]. Correctly fitting the charge and LOS data is a critical step in optimizing the allocation of healthcare resources. But due to the protection of private information, the detailed information regarding the treatment process that patient experience in hospital is not available from many well-known medical outcome databases, like the New York State's Statewide Planning and Research Cooperative System. The missing longitudinal information of the treatment process makes it more challenging to generate good fitting; meanwhile it becomes demanding to have a dynamic model, through which effective inference can be made against the hidden treatment process. To that goal, a bunch of stochastic-process-based models have been well developed and applied to analyze the medical datasets.

The continuous-time Phase-Type (PH) model has been widely used in the study of hospital charge and LOS data. Many authors focus in particular on a special subclass of PH model/distribution, namely, the Coxian phase-type (CPH) model/distribution Tang [4]; Faddy et al. [5]; Marshall et al. [6–8]; Fackrell [9]. Unlike other popular theoretical distributions widely used in inpatient data, such as log-normal and gamma distribution, the CPH model/distribution not only provides a theoretical distribution that can be used to fit the empirical data, but also gives us a sketch of the treatment dynamics that patient experience in hospital. In fact, from CPH models, we can track the pathways that patient went through in different medical stages (characterized by the discrete set of phases in the PH model) during a hospital stay.

The pathway information makes it possible to cluster patients and facilitate the use of healthcare process improvement technologies, such as Lean Thinking or Six Sigma McClean et al. [10, 11].

The other popular approach to study hospital charge and LOS is through dynamically modelling the charge accumulation process and the determination of the time to discharge, which belongs to a more general class of joint models of the longitudinal measurements and time to event, Ibrahim et al. [12]; Tsiatis and Davidian [13]; Henderson et al. [14]; Kim et al. [15]; Sousa [16]; Lawrence Gould et al. [17]. In medical cost studies, the charge accumulation is a monotonic nondecreasing process; the joint model used in this case is reduced to a class of random growth with random stopping time (RGRST) models.

Like CPH models, the RGRST models do also capture the treatment dynamics that patient experience in hospital. But in contrast to tracking the pathways of patient moving through different medical stages, the RGRST models focus more on describing how patient and/or doctor makes the discharge decision in reaction to the change of actual charge level and the length of time that patient has stayed in hospital. Therefore, the story of RGRST models is more about the behavioural patterns of patient/doctor behind the treatment dynamics, while the story of CPH models is more on the medical side.

It is natural in this paper to think of the possibility of combining CPH models and RGRST models together in order to extract more information regarding the discharge decision-making on different medical stages. However, there is a natural gap between the two models. The CPH model is a finitely jumped stochastic process in essence, while the charge accumulation in the RGRST model is continuous. It is not trivial to combine a jump process with a continuous process. To deal with that difficulty, we propose a partition-based approach with each partition cell determined by solving a boundary differential equation. These boundary differential equations are subtly designed to merge the continuous charge into discrete "phases" involved in a Coxian phase-type model. In sum, the main contributions of this paper are as follows:

(i) We show that there is a natural way to convert a special subclass of RGRST models to CPH models.

(ii) We propose an algorithm to estimate the transition matrix of the CPH model converted from a given RGRST model and the parameters involved in that RGRST model.

(iii) Based on the correspondence between RGRST models and CPH models, we derive a variety of different measures of the "cost" of staying in a medical stage at each time. That "cost" information is important for the purpose of insurance payment and healthcare process improvement.

McClean et al. [11] tried a different way to incorporate the charge accumulation process into a CPH model. But in their work only the case that the charge accumulation process adopts a piece-wise linear form was discussed. It turns out that the piece-wise linear assumption is quite restrictive while crucial to their main result. Without it, the matrix technique in McClean et al. [11] is no longer applicable to achieve the nth order moments of total charge for $n > 1$, while our differential-equation-based approach does still work. In fact, we believe our method extends the work of McClean et al. [11] in the following two aspects.

(1) Instead of being piece-wise linear, we consider a much more general situation in which the charge accumulation process can take arbitrary forms as long as a conditional expectation function of that process satisfies a general regularity condition. In particular, within our framework, it is possible to consider the potential influence of the current charge level on the future charge accumulation which is neglected by the piece-wise linear assumption.

(2) In addition to the moments of total charge, it is derivable from our model of the joint distribution of the total charge and LOS, and the joint distribution of the costs and time being spent on every stage by every fixed time t. Therefore, our model provides more detailed information of the treatment that the patient experiences in hospital.

Although the motivation of our work is the analysis of the charge accumulation and the determination of hospital length of stay, it turns out that the proposed method is useful for many other problems where the relation among the time to event and a hidden continuous process as well as a jump process is in interest. For example, in the field of investment risk management, it is always important to detect how the default probability of the corporate bond issued by a firm is affected by the growth stage and profitability (say measured by the flow of revenue) of that firm. In this case, our model can definitely provide some insights if we identify the default as the event in interest and consider the revenue flow as determined by a continuous process similar to the charge accumulation and the transition among different growth stages of the firm as described by a CPH process. In addition to problems of the survival-type, it is also natural to extend our work to the case of competing risks, of which every stage in our model can be identified with a type of risk. Although in competing risk models, the CPH transition matrix is no longer sufficient, it turns out that the partition-based technique introduced below is extendible to derive the joint distributions of a wide class of the competing risk models, the details of which will be discussed in a related paper by the authors.

This paper is organized as follows. In Section 2, after a short review of the CPH models and RGRST models, we present the correspondence between them and briefly introduce the estimation algorithm. In Section 3, we conduct numerical studies to show the validity and usefulness of our model. A couple of interesting findings toward the medical outcome database, the New York State's Statewide Planning and Research Cooperative System 2013, are discussed. Section 4 concludes the paper.

2. Model

In this section, a new model (denoted as CPH-RGRST model) is constructed that connects the CPH models to RGRST models in the sense that

(1) a CPH-RGRST model is a RGRST model;

(2) charges in a CPH-RGRST model can be classified into a number of stages such that every stage is identified with a

phase in a given CPH model in the sense that, at every time t, the probability of staying in a stage i is exactly given by the probability in the ith phase of the CPH model.

In particular, the marginal distribution of LOS induced by a CPH-RGRST model is a CPH distribution. We shall state the detailed construction of the CPH-RGRST models after a brief review of the definition and some basic properties of RGRST models and CPH models.

2.1. the Joint Model (RGRST) versus the CPH Model. A RGRST model can be formally defined as follows as discussed in Gardiner et al. [18, 19] and Polverejan et al. [20]:

$$Y(t) = Y_0 + \int_0^t I(T > s)\epsilon(s)\,ds, \tag{1}$$

where the process $\{Y(t) : t \in [0,\infty)\}$ represents the actual charge level at each time. The random variable T indicates the LOS, and I is the indicator function. $\{I(T > t) : t \in [0,\infty)\}$ ($I(t)$ for short) is the event process representing whether or not to stay in hospital for longer time at each time point t. $\{\epsilon(t)\}$ is a nonnegative process characterizing the potential increment rate of charge per unit time provided that patient decides to stay, and Y_0 is a nonnegative random variable representing the charge at the initial time. We shall denote by $G(t) = Y_0 + \int_0^t \epsilon(s)\,ds$ the potential charge accumulation process in distinguishing the actual charge process $\{Y(t)\}$.

As shown in the supplementary materials (available here) note that a RGRST model can be completely specified by the initial probability density function (pdf), $p(y,0)$, induced by the initial charge Y_0 and the following two conditional expectation functions:

$$\begin{aligned} q(y,t) &= E(\epsilon(t) \mid G(t) = y) \\ \rho(y,t) &= E(I(T > t) \mid G(t) = y). \end{aligned} \tag{2}$$

And using (2), the joint probability density function (pdf) of the LOS (T) and the total charge (Y_T) at the discharge time T can be expressed as follows:

$$f(y,t) = p(y,t)\cdot\left(-\frac{\partial q}{\partial y}\cdot q - \frac{\partial q}{\partial t}\right)(y,t), \tag{3}$$

where the function $p(y,t)$ in variable y is the time-dependent pdf induced by $G(t)$. The detailed derivation of (3) can be found in the supplementary materials. Expression (3) is useful in the estimation algorithm stated in the next section as it is the key component of the likelihood function.

To associate RGRST models with the CPH models, the hospital length of stay, represented as the random variable T in (1), should induce a CPH distribution generated from a CPH model, which is a finite-state continuous-time stationary Markovian process with only one absorbing state/phase (we shall use the term "phase", by convention, in place of "state"). A CPH model is determined by an initial probability mass vector α with $\alpha_i \geq 0$ and $\sum_{i=1}^{n} \alpha_i = 1$, and the transition intensity matrix

$$A = \begin{bmatrix} -c_1-\lambda_1 & \lambda_1 & 0 & \cdots & 0 & c_1 \\ 0 & -c_2-\lambda_2 & \lambda_2 & \cdots & 0 & c_2 \\ 0 & 0 & \ddots & \ddots & \vdots & \vdots \\ \vdots & \ddots & \ddots & \ddots & \lambda_{n-1} & c_{n-1} \\ 0 & 0 & \cdots & 0 & -c_n & c_n \\ 0 & 0 & \cdots & 0 & 0 & 0 \end{bmatrix}, \tag{4}$$

where $\lambda_k, c_k > 0$ and the entry $a_{i,j}$ of A represents the transition intensity of a patient ω from phase S_i to phase S_j at every time $t > 0$; formally:

$$a_{i,j} = \lim_{\delta\downarrow 0}\frac{\text{Prob}\left(\omega \in S_j \text{ at } t+\delta \mid \omega \in S_i \text{ at } t\right)}{\delta}. \tag{5}$$

As suggested in McClean et al. [10], a phase in a CPH model can be identified with a treatment stage during hospital stay, such as diagnosis, acute care, assessment, rehabilitation, and long-stay care. The transition of patients among these stages characterizes the treatment progress.

2.2. Correspondence between CPH and RGRST Models. The main result of this section is that there does exist a correspondence between CPH and RGRST models. The correspondence is built through converting the continuous variable, charge, in a RGRST model to finite many discrete states by partitioning the product space, $\mathbb{R}_+ \times \mathbb{R}_+$ (representing charge and time, respectively), into a number of cells such that each cell corresponds to a phase in a CPH model, while the evolution of the probability of staying in those cells is exactly determined by the given CPH model. More precisely, we have the following theorem.

Theorem 1. *Fix a RGRST process $\{Y(t)\}$ represented as a triple $(p(y,0), q, \rho)$ with $p(y,0)$ being the pdf of initial charge Y_0 and q, ρ as defined in (2). Suppose functions q, ρ, and $p(y,0)$ are smooth and q, ρ satisfy*

$$\frac{\partial \log(\rho)}{\partial y}\cdot q + \frac{\partial \log(\rho)}{\partial t} \equiv -c \quad \rho > 0 \tag{6}$$

for some constant $c > 0$. Then, for any fixed positive integer n, an n-dimensional vector $\alpha > 0$ with $\sum_{i=1}^{n} \alpha_i = 1$, and an $n-1$-dim vector $\lambda > 0$, there exists an n–partition of the space $[0,\infty)^2$ denoted as $\mathcal{P}$ such that the following time-dependent probability mass function $P(t)$ defined on the $n+1$ tuple $\{1,\ldots,n+1\}$:

$$\begin{aligned} P_i(t) &= Prob\left(Y(t) \in \mathcal{P}_i \cap [0,\infty) \times \{t\}, I(T > t) = 1\right), \quad i \in \{1,\ldots,n\} \\ P_{n+1}(t) &= Prob\left(I(T > t) = 0\right), \end{aligned} \tag{7}$$

```
Require: λ = (λ_1, ..., λ_{n-1}),  c = (c_1, ..., c_n),  α = (α_1, ..., α_n);
  Set C_0 ≡ 0, b = [0,∞) × {0} ∪ {0} × [0,∞), ρ_b ≡ 1;
  for i = 1 to n do
    if i < n then
      Set C_i(0) by Eq. (A.8) and α_i;
      Set PDE_i by Eq. (6) subject to boundary condition ρ_b on b
      with c in Eq. (6) replaced by c_i;
      Set ρ_i = exp(solve(PDE_i));
      Set IVP_i by replacing ρ in Eq. (A.9) with ρ_i;
      Set C_i = solve(IVP_i);
      ReSet b = {0} × [C_i(0),∞) ∪ {C_i(t) : t ∈ [0,∞)};
      ReSet ρ_b(y,t) = { 1            (y,t) ∈ {0} × [C_i(0),∞)
                       { ρ_{i-1}(y,t)  (y,t) ∈ {(C_i(t),t) : t ∈ [0,∞)} ;
    else
      Set PDE_n by Eq. (6) subject to boundary condition ρ_b on b
      with c in Eq. (6) replaced by c_n;
      Set ρ_n = exp(solve(PDE_n));
    end if
  end for
  Set C_n ≡ ∞;
  Set ρ = Σ_{i=1}^{n} 1_{C_{i-1}(t) ≤ y ≤ C_i(t)} · ρ_i
  return ρ
```

ALGORITHM 1: Construct_ρ.

is generated by a CPH model with the initial mass α and its transition matrix is given as in (4) with $c_i \equiv c$ for $i = 1, \ldots, n$.

The proof of Theorem 1 is presented in the Appendix. From the proof, it is clear that the connection between RGRST models and CPH models is equivalent to a constraint put on the conditional probability function ρ in (2) of the underlying RGRST model by the condition (6). In fact, the functional form of ρ is completely determined by (6) and the function q, which gives a first-order partial differential equation (PDE) of ρ. This equation turns out to be solvable and has a unique solution for a given boundary condition. Therefore, using the characteristic method, Evans [21], we can solve (6) and express the function ρ as follows:

$$\rho(y,t) = \rho_b\left(g\left(y,t,s^*(y,t)\right), s^*(y,t)\right) \cdot \exp(-c \cdot t), \quad (8)$$

where ρ evaluated at $t = 0$ is constantly 1 which means that all patients have to stay in hospital for a positive time before discharge; the form of the boundary b and the value of the function ρ on b (denoted as ρ_b) are constructed by iteratively solving the Initial Value Problem (IVP) (A.11) in the proof; the details of the iteration are presented in Algorithm 1 of Corollary 2. s^* is the first time when the solution trajectory (g) of IVP (A.11) (starting from (y,t)) touches the boundary curve b. Equation (8) is crucial to determining the parametric form of the joint pdf (3) and the likelihood function used for estimation.

The next corollary is a direct result of Theorem 1. It extends the construction in Theorem 1 to a more general situation where the transition intensity from different transient states to the absorbing state does not have to be identical; i.e., c_i does not have to be equal to c_j for different i, j. Therefore, it is always possible to achieve an arbitrary CPH model from a RGRST model satisfying a generalized version of condition (6) with c replaced by c_i for different i.

Corollary 2. *The smooth requirement on the function ρ in Theorem 1 can be replaced by the following weaker condition.*

Condition 3. The function ρ is continuous and almost everywhere differentiable under the standard Lebesgue measure on $[0,\infty)^2$ and has integrable partial derivatives.

Under the Condition 3, for an arbitrary given CPH model represented by the transition matrix (4) and the initial probability mass vector $\alpha = (\alpha_1, \ldots, \alpha_n)$, there always exists a RGRST model together with a set of partition curves $\{C_0 \equiv 0 < C_1 < \cdots < C_n \equiv \infty\}$ such that the mapping

$$\{(y,t) : C_{i-1}(t) \le y \le C_i(t)\} \mapsto S_i, \quad i \in \{1, \ldots, n\} \quad (9)$$

converts the RGRST model to the given CPH model, where S_i is the ith phase in the CPH model.

Moreover, the desired RGRST model and the partition curves can be inductively constructed through Algorithm 1, where "solve(·)" represents the operation to solve the equation "·".

Notice that given the partition curves $\{C_0 \equiv 0 < C_1 < \cdots < C_{n-1}, C_n \equiv \infty\}$ and the joint pdf (3), deriving the conditional probability density of the cumulative charge $G(t)$

is very simple given that at time t patients stay in the ith-stage, S_i:

$$\text{Prob}(G(t) = y \mid S_i) = \frac{p(y_i,t)\cdot\rho(y_i,t)}{\int_{C_{i-1}(t)}^{C_i(t)} p(x,t)\cdot\rho(x,t)\,dx} \cdot I(C_{i-1}(t) \le y \le C_i(t)). \quad (10)$$

With the help of the conditional density (10), we can define a variety of measures of the "cost" of staying in a stage. For instance, fixing a stage and a time t, we can think of the price as the amount that has been charged since patients arrived in that stage for the first time, the daily price as the amount being charged per day within that stage, and the time cost as the length of time that patients have spent in that stage by t. Formally, the price ($Pr_i(t)$), daily price ($\overline{Pr}_i(t)$), and the time cost ($Ct_i(t)$) for every stage and every time are defined as:

$$Pr_i(t) = \frac{\int_{C_{i-1}(t)}^{C_i(t)} (y - TY_i(y,t))\cdot p(y,t)\cdot\rho(y,t)\,dy}{\int_{C_{i-1}(t)}^{C_i(t)} p(y,t)\cdot\rho(y,t)\,dy}$$

$$\overline{Pr}_i(t) = \frac{\int_{C_{i-1}(t)}^{C_i(t)} ((y - TY_i(y,t))/(t - TT_i(y,t)))\cdot p(y,t)\cdot\rho(y,t)\,dy}{\int_{C_{i-1}(t)}^{C_i(t)} p(y,t)\cdot\rho(y,t)\,dy} \quad (11)$$

$$Ct_i(t) = \frac{\int_{C_{i-1}(t)}^{C_i(t)} (t - TT_i(y,t))\cdot p(y,t)\cdot\rho(y,t)\,dy}{\int_{C_{i-1}(t)}^{C_i(t)} p(y,t)\cdot\rho(y,t)\,dy},$$

where TT_i is the conditional mean of the first arrival time into the stage $i-1$ given the charge level y and current time t, and similarly, TY_i represents the conditional mean of the charge at the first arrival time to the stage $i-1$ given y and t.

Although the price, daily price, and the time cost are defined through the first-order moment, the availability of the conditional probability (10) enables us to define the quantile version of (11). When there are large parts of outliers, a quantile version of those "cost" measures turns out to be more useful.

The information regarding the price and time spent in every such stage, as defined above, is helpful in rationalising the care process, thus reducing waste, in terms of unnecessary or inappropriate treatment, and avoiding delay, often the result of batch and queue processes, in a similar fashion to that adopted for industrial processes (McClean et al. [10]).

2.3. A Two-Stage Algorithm. Corollary 2 implies a two-step algorithm that uses the real hospital charge and LOS data as input to estimate the underlying CPH model and the RGRST model from which the CPH model is derived.

Step 1. Apply the full information maximum likelihood method (FML) and the marginal LOS data to estimate the transition matrix and the initial probability mass that determines the marginal CPH distribution of LOS. The resulting estimators are denoted as $\hat{\lambda} = (\hat{\lambda}_1,\ldots,\hat{\lambda}_{n-1})$, $\hat{c} = (\hat{c}_1,\ldots,\hat{c}_n)$, and $\hat{\alpha} = (\hat{\alpha}_1,\ldots,\hat{\alpha}_n)$.

Step 2. Apply Algorithm 1 to construct the function ρ from the estimators $\hat{\lambda} = (\hat{\lambda}_1,\ldots,\hat{\lambda}_{n-1})$, $\hat{c} = (\hat{c}_1,\ldots,\hat{c}_n)$, and $\hat{\alpha} = (\hat{\alpha}_1,\ldots,\hat{\alpha}_n)$, and construct the joint pdf of charge and LOS by formula (3). With the joint pdf, construct the likelihood function and apply FML to estimate the remaining parameters, which are used to characterize the function q and the initial density $p(\cdot,0)$ (denoted by $\widehat{params}$).

The use of FML guarantees that all estimators obtained from the two-stage algorithm are consistent and asymptotically normal-distributed.

3. Numerical Studies

In this section, we conduct the numerical studies to show the validity of our two-stage estimation procedure. We will apply our procedure to both of the real data and simulation sample.

Our data source is the medical outcome database, New York State's Statewide Planning and Research Cooperative System 2013 (SPARCS 2013). The histogram of the entire SPARCS 2013 indicates that the total charge approximately follows a log-normal distribution; therefore, we will take the following parametric form for the function q:

$$q(y,t) = y, \quad (12)$$

and the initial Y_0 is assumed to satisfy

$$\log Y_0 \sim N(\mu,\sigma). \quad (13)$$

It turns out that under (12), (13), and (6), the resulting marginal distribution of total charge is close to a log-normal distribution.

When covariates exist (denoted by X), we assume that the random vector $(\varepsilon_Y,\varepsilon_T)$ is independent from the covariate vector, and $(\exp(\varepsilon_Y),\exp(\varepsilon_T))$ follows the joint pdf given by (3) with the initial pdf, q, and ρ specified as in (13), (12), and (6), respectively. The covariates are linked with the total charge, Y_T, and LOS, T, through the following regression equations:

$$\log Y_T = \theta_0 + \theta\cdot X + \varepsilon_Y$$
$$\log T = \beta_0 + \beta\cdot X + \varepsilon_T. \quad (14)$$

$\theta^+ = (\theta_0;\theta)$, $\beta^+ = (\beta_0;\beta)$ are the regression coefficient vectors.

As for the dimension of the underlying CPH model, we follow the convention in the previous studies of Faddy et al. [5]; Tang [4]; McClean et al. [10] and only consider the two cases where the number of nonabsorbing phases is 3 and 4. After a preliminary study, we select the 4-Phase CPH model as it can generate better fitting to the SPARCS data.

Under the specification above, there are three classes of parameters to estimate. They are (1) the parameter vectors α, c and λ involved in the CPH model, (2) the parameter (μ,σ) involved in the initial pdf, and (3) the regression coefficients (θ^+,β^+). We call the parameters of types (1) and (2) as the dynamic parameters because they specify the joint model that generates the distribution of charge and LOS.

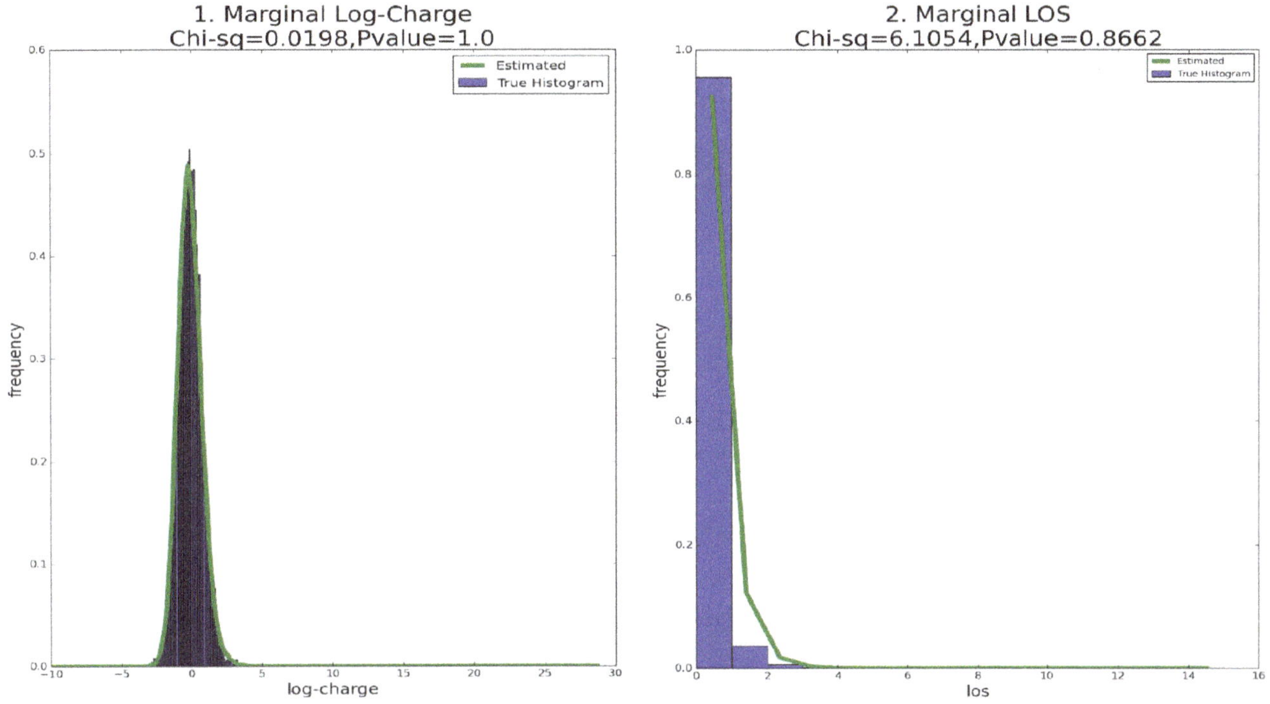

FIGURE 1: Goodness of Fit. Plots 1 and 2 are the fitted marginal CPH-RGRST distribution versus empirical histogram for log-charge and LOS.

In the real data study, we draw 5000 subsamples from SPARCS 2013 with the covariates consisting of the Severity of Illness, Mortality Risk of Illness (In SPARCS 2013, both of the two variables, Severity and Mortality, are quantified through a grading score, which is a number in the set $\{1, 2, 3, 4\}$.), and 24 categorical variables which represent 25 Major Diagnosis Codes (MDC), each of which associates with a class of illness. The summary statistics of our subsample verses the entire SPARCS 2013 with respect to the covariates are described in Table 1.

In the simulation study, we generate 5000 samples from a joint model without covariates and the true value of the dynamic parameters is taken as the estimated value from the real data study, which is given as in Table 2.

In both of the real data and simulation studies, the computer code is written in the language of Python 2.7 with python-scipy, python-numpy libraries being used.

3.1. Simulation Study. The goodness of fit is measured through comparing the fitted curves and the empirical histogram (drawn from the simulation sample) for both of the marginal charge and LOS, as shown in first line of Figure 1. We conduct Pearson's χ^2 test; the value of the χ^2 statistics and the associated P values are (0.0171, 1.0) for the marginal charge and (6.1054, 0.8662) for the marginal LOS. From both of the fitting plots and the results of χ^2 test, our fitting is fairly good.

We also evaluate the goodness of fit in terms of the joint distribution through Pearson's χ^2 test; the χ^2 statistics and its P value are (0.1911, 1.0), which is consistent with Figure 1. Therefore, the simulation study verifies the effectiveness of our two-step estimation procedure.

3.2. Real Example Study

3.2.1. Regression Coefficients. The estimated regression coefficients are reported in Table 3, from which both of the severity and mortality of illness have significantly positive effect on both of the total charge and LOS that is consistent with the intuition.

On the other hand, among all the MDC groups, the Newborn And Other Neonates (MDC_15) and the Diseases and Disorders of the Musculoskeletal System And Connective Tissue (MDC_8) has the greatest negative and positive effects on the total charge, respectively, which is also consistent with the intuition. In contrast, the MDC groups with greatest negative and positive effect on LOS are the Diseases and Disorders of the Ear, Nose, Mouth and Throat (MDC_3) and the Mental Diseases and Disorders (MDC_19), respectively.

In addition, it turns out that the effects of different illnesses on the charge and LOS are not always homogeneous. There are a couple of MDC groups which affect the total charge and LOS in distinct direction. They are the Diseases and Disorders of the Nervous System (MDC_1), Diseases and Disorders of the Circulatory System (MDC_5), Diseases and Disorders of the Male Reproductive System (MDC_12), Diseases and Disorders of the Female Reproductive System (MDC_13), and Alcohol/Drug Use or Induced Mental Disorders (MDC_20). Among them, except the MDC_20 group, all the other groups have a more expensive bill but shorter hospital stay, and therefore a higher daily charge. In contrast, patients with alcohol/drug abuse tend to pay less but stay in hospital longer.

Combining the estimated coefficients in Table 3 and dynamic parameter in Table 2, we can even identify the stage

Table 1: Descriptive statistics of SPARCS 2013.

Characteristics	Group	N (%)	Sample_N (%)	LOS (SD)	Sample_LOS (SD)	Charge (SD)	Sample_Charge (SD)
All Patients		2418874 (100)	5000 (100)	5.46 (8.11)	5.51 (8.16)	36931.77 (68973.47)	36861.8 (67053.64)
MDC	0.0	17.0 (0.0)		11.0 (24.69)		102910.82 (280754.64)	
	1.0	142651.0 (5.9)	298.0 (5.96)	5.7 (8.69)	5.01 (6.14)	46962.08 (83724.59)	41911.53 (50501.65)
	2.0	4138.0 (0.17)	13.0 (0.26)	3.62 (5.18)	3.38 (1.89)	27185.04 (37576.18)	28478.72 (22611.85)
	3.0	32743.0 (1.35)	72.0 (1.44)	3.59 (5.59)	2.81 (2.72)	29468.92 (50592.3)	22093.15 (20516.67)
	4.0	206374.0 (8.53)	425.0 (8.5)	5.81 (7.64)	5.42 (6.99)	37165.6 (64478.26)	35254.34 (48416.02)
	5.0	320765.0 (13.26)	655.0 (13.1)	4.78 (6.58)	4.68 (5.4)	50065.14 (84839.8)	48514.49 (67896.89)
	6.0	211325.0 (8.74)	461.0 (9.22)	5.11 (6.63)	5.56 (7.16)	35785.32 (54820.39)	37176.32 (45615.65)
	7.0	65928.0 (2.73)	116.0 (2.32)	5.6 (6.96)	4.91 (4.31)	42718.49 (78816.64)	34176.78 (38341.19)
	8.0	201134.0 (8.32)	419.0 (8.38)	4.91 (5.95)	5.0 (5.35)	50655.45 (55819.15)	50609.01 (45334.44)
	9.0	66120.0 (2.73)	136.0 (2.72)	4.6 (5.95)	5.07 (8.42)	28073.74 (37308.49)	28829.12 (29869.57)
	10.0	74993.0 (3.1)	171.0 (3.42)	3.97 (5.83)	4.05 (4.72)	28568.47 (43837.41)	27236.6 (30456.03)
	11.0	103597.0 (4.28)	221.0 (4.42)	5.43 (6.75)	5.09 (5.1)	36812.91 (53368.81)	33884.47 (38131.54)
	12.0	11181.0 (0.46)	21.0 (0.42)	3.44 (6.27)	4.81 (10.56)	30593.31 (30945.72)	39233.29 (46533.28)
	13.0	31682.0 (1.31)	57.0 (1.14)	3.13 (5.23)	2.47 (2.03)	28998.31 (33592.18)	31389.63 (20325.52)
	14.0	257203.0 (10.63)	504.0 (10.08)	2.91 (2.54)	2.88 (2.47)	16435.92 (17226.17)	16714.7 (18104.7)
	15.0	236599.0 (9.78)	439.0 (8.78)	3.78 (7.99)	4.06 (7.8)	17912.83 (85865.5)	18682.72 (72830.49)
	16.0	37899.0 (1.57)	92.0 (1.84)	5.01 (6.87)	4.77 (3.79)	37100.38 (83604.25)	36537.56 (52336.47)
	17.0	22289.0 (0.92)	55.0 (1.1)	9.57 (12.73)	9.38 (11.59)	87130.44 (139632.35)	81519.0 (128268.96)
	18.0	108416.0 (4.48)	224.0 (4.48)	9.09 (10.7)	10.24 (15.07)	63423.77 (99592.33)	80804.11 (200106.77)
	19.0	116683.0 (4.82)	245.0 (4.9)	12.94 (16.11)	12.62 (17.7)	34162.28 (57058.45)	32507.77 (49653.33)
	20.0	75432.0 (3.12)	170.0 (3.4)	6.34 (7.45)	6.6 (7.65)	17400.15 (23797.61)	17228.44 (20575.0)
	21.0	30203.0 (1.25)	71.0 (1.42)	4.29 (7.18)	4.77 (10.44)	31248.52 (64435.64)	33845.59 (75320.46)
	22.0	1929.0 (0.08)	2.0 (0.04)	9.06 (13.5)	8.0 (2.83)	79337.2 (184652.6)	51080.31 (29187.33)
	23.0	46924.0 (1.94)	106.0 (2.12)	10.87 (10.27)	11.18 (8.88)	46721.27 (52350.27)	45356.56 (37999.3)
	24.0	8733.0 (0.36)	20.0 (0.4)	8.6 (11.36)	8.55 (8.81)	57383.57 (105543.15)	40839.06 (39649.57)
	25.0	3916.0 (0.16)	7.0 (0.14)	10.77 (12.01)	11.0 (7.44)	103841.73 (118285.21)	73790.14 (54114.8)
Severity	0.0	40.0 (0.0)		6.35 (16.4)		47710.78 (186214.68)	
	1.0	881300.0 (36.43)	1760.0 (35.2)	3.09 (3.97)	3.02 (3.37)	20164.74 (25917.49)	20249.04 (23995.3)
	2.0	929347.0 (38.42)	1939.0 (38.78)	4.96 (6.89)	5.16 (7.76)	30512.25 (37884.57)	30602.25 (38507.07)
	3.0	479712.0 (19.83)	1048.0 (20.96)	7.73 (8.46)	7.57 (7.68)	51935.05 (65352.31)	51307.28 (61645.27)
	4.0	128475.0 (5.31)	253.0 (5.06)	16.83 (18.2)	17.06 (18.36)	142361.38 (210806.88)	140564.83 (210012.56)
Mortality	Extreme	106154.0 (4.39)	210 (4.2)	14.96 (16.66)	13.81 (15.11)	129939.83 (200746.65)	114408.34 (172257.11)
	Major	311482.0 (12.88)	692 (13.84)	8.69 (10.14)	8.51 (9.96)	61247.22 (92604.92)	64073.56 (108815.34)
	Minor	1482115.0 (61.27)	3007 (60.14)	4.03 (6.16)	4.02 (6.31)	24133.09 (33016.21)	23905.06 (31377.21)
	Moderate	519083.0 (21.46)	1091 (21.82)	5.67 (7.03)	6.12 (7.96)	39863.27 (55375.06)	40386.64 (51083.0)

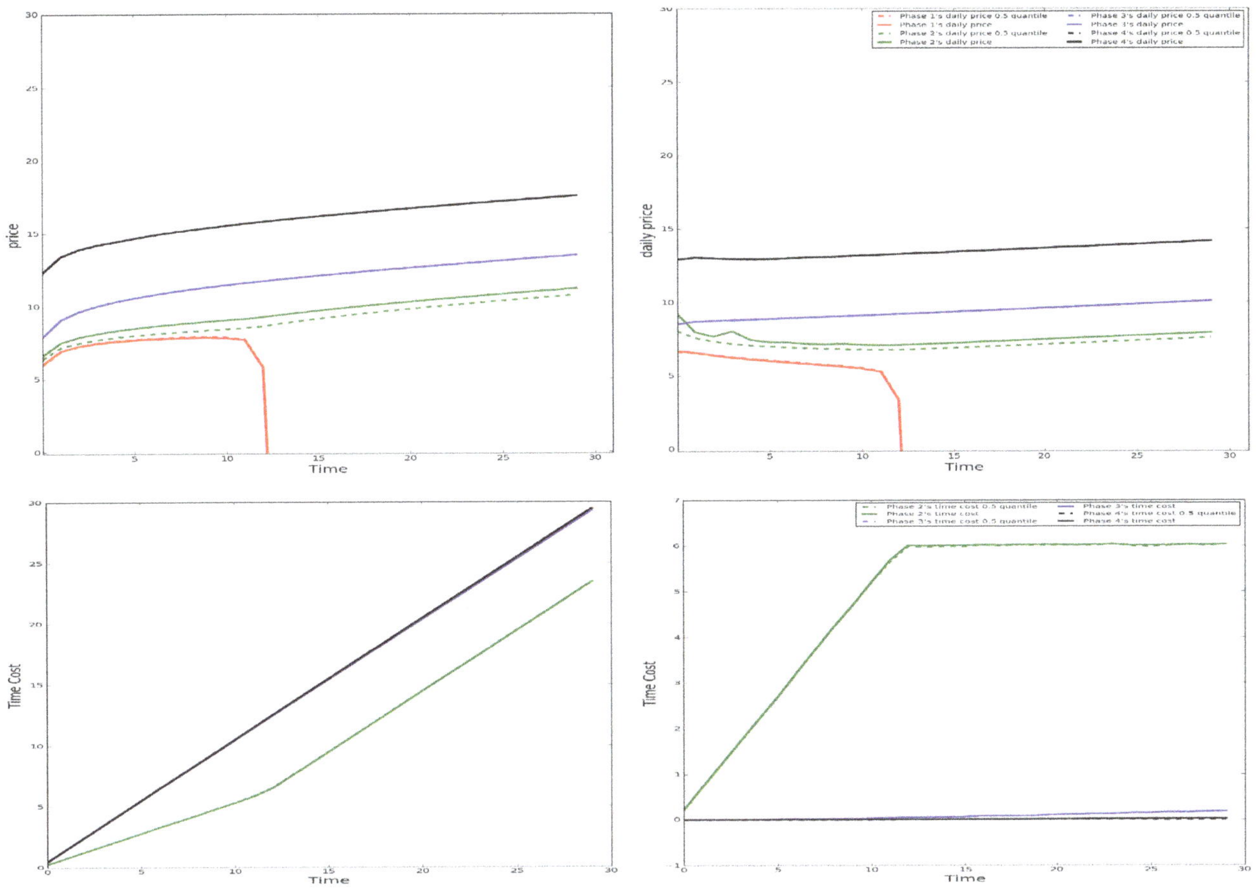

FIGURE 2: Cost of Stages. Plots 1, 2, and 3 sketch the log of the price, daily price, and the time cost (as defined in (11)) versus their quantile version, respectively. Plot 4 shows the other version of the time cost (= $s - Ct_i(s)$ with $s > 0$) versus its quantile version.

TABLE 2: Estimated dynamic parameters.

Dynamic Parameters	Values
(μ, σ)	(−0.5715 , 0.7149)
α	(0.9922, ≈0.0, 0.0001, 0.0077)
c	(≈0.0, 4.4796, ≈0.0, 0.9934)
λ	(4.4905, ≈0.0, 0.029)

from which a patient exits to discharge. The discharge stage encodes critical information of the treatment pathways and is important for management purpose. Table 4 reports the estimated conditional mean (log-)charge, LOS, severity, and mortality risk for patients who exit from every stage. It is clear that the value of all the four variables monotonically increases as patients get discharged from later stages. Especially for severity and LOS, there are clear jumps from stages 1 and 2 to stages 3 and 4. The mean severity is doubled when transiting from stage 2 to stage 3 while the mean LOS almost gets tripled. This gap suggests that patients who are diagnosed with more severe conditions during admission are more likely to go over the treatment in stage 3 or 4, while their rehabilitation usually takes more time and more medical resources (McClean et al. [10]). This observation is consistent with the intuition and, to some extent, verifies the viewpoint that interprets the entire treatment process as a series of transitions among multiple medical stages.

3.2.2. Cost. As discussed in the end of Section 2.1, the CPH-RGRST model enables us to evaluate the "cost" of each medical stage in different manners. Using the estimation results provided in the previous section, we can numerically compute the "cost" for our SPARCS sample.

In Figure 2, we plot the estimated mean price, mean daily price, and mean time of staying for each of the four stages of the CPH model, where the "mean" refers to the CPH-RGRST process that generates the mean charge and LOS, $\overline{Y}_T = \exp(\varepsilon_Y)\exp(E_X(\widehat{\theta_0}+\widehat{\theta}X))$, and $\overline{T} = \exp(\varepsilon_T)\exp(E_X(\widehat{\beta_0}+\widehat{\beta}X))$. In Figure 3, the probability of staying in every nonabsorbing stage is plotted against the time. There are the following three major findings.

(i) From the plot 2 in Figure 2, the daily price for stage 1 declines over time, which is caused by the fact that, for those long-stay patients, they must have already switched into the higher stage treatments after the preexam period (represented by stage 1), which is very well captured in plot 1 of Figure 3. In contrast, for all the stage 2, 3, and 4, the daily price inclines to grow up in long run, which rejects the piece-wise linear assumption claimed in McClean et al. [11]. In fact, in contrast to the constant growth rate of charge within each

Table 3: Estimated regression coefficients.

Groups	Log-Charge (P values)	Log-LOS (P values)
Intercept	9.3245 (<0.0001)	1.7512 (<0.0001)
MDC_1	0.0697 (<0.0001)	−0.1008 (<0.0001)
MDC_2	0.2756 (<0.0001)	0.519 (<0.0001)
MDC_3	−0.1522 (<0.0001)	−0.3564 (<0.0001)
MDC_4	−0.2062 (<0.0001)	−0.187 (<0.0001)
MDC_5	0.1018 (<0.0001)	−0.2451 (<0.0001)
MDC_6	−0.0072 (<0.0001)	−0.1214 (<0.0001)
MDC_7	0.0686 (<0.0001)	−0.0432 (<0.0001)
MDC_8	0.5344 (<0.0001)	0.0258 (<0.0001)
MDC_9	−0.1364 (<0.0001)	−0.1597 (<0.0001)
MDC_10	−0.1132 (<0.0001)	−0.2823 (<0.0001)
MDC_11	−0.265 (<0.0001)	−0.2736 (<0.0001)
MDC_12	0.1164 (<0.0001)	−0.3405 (<0.0001)
MDC_13	0.0504 (<0.0001)	−0.2928 (<0.0001)
MDC_14	−0.3242 (<0.0001)	−0.1945 (<0.0001)
MDC_15	−1.0351 (<0.0001)	−0.0311 (<0.0001)
MDC_16	−0.0948 (<0.0001)	−0.1035 (<0.0001)
MDC_17	0.2244 (<0.0001)	0.1522 (<0.0001)
MDC_18	−0.0289 (<0.0001)	−0.06 (<0.0001)
MDC_19	0.0381 (<0.0001)	0.9866 (<0.0001)
MDC_20	−0.5335 (<0.0001)	0.2749 (<0.0001)
MDC_21	−0.2574 (<0.0001)	−0.1887 (<0.0001)
MDC_22	0.3689 (<0.0001)	0.3077 (<0.0001)
MDC_23	0.1332 (<0.0001)	0.51 (<0.0001)
MDC_24	−0.2957 (<0.0001)	−0.2083 (<0.0001)
APR Risk of Mortality	0.1436 (<0.0001)	0.18 (<0.0001)
APR Severity of Illness	0.3605 (<0.0001)	0.3338 (<0.0001)

Table 4: Summary of discharge stages.

	Stage 1	Stage 2	Stage 3	Stage 4
severity	0.099	0.454	1	2.238
mortality	1.524	1.814	3	3.355
charge	8.062	9.842	11.525	11.505
LOS	2.48	5.732	13	14.87

stage, the increasing growth rate tends to be more reasonable, because a longer stay usually implies a worse health condition for a patient, who, therefore, needs better care, including more expensive medicines, more frequent exams, and the like. These items lift up the cost of stay per day. The same reasoning also applies well to the observation that the time cost of all stages is increasing over time as shown in plots 3 and 4 in Figure 2.

(ii) Although the time cost is slightly lower in stage 3 than in stage 4, both of the two stages (by (11), the time cost for stage 1 is trivial and constantly equal to the total time in hospital, so we omitted it in Figure 2) have their time cost almost identical to the total time that patients spent in hospital since they were admitted. In contrast, the time cost of stage 2 displays quite different features, which is not only much lower than that of the other stages, but, within the first 13 days, its growth rate is also slower. The different features of stage 2 are consistent with the estimated dynamic parameters in Table 2 and plot 2 in Figure 3. From Table 2, it is clear that the intensity of switch-in and switch-to-discharge in stage 2 is significantly higher than in the other stages, which means that there are two factors that lower down the time cost at stage 2. (1) There are a large portion of patients switching from stage 1 to stage 2 in the early time (<5 days, see plots 1 and 2 in Figure 3); in contrast there is almost no patient who could switch from lower stage to stage 3 or 4 (see plots 3 and 4 in Figure 3), which implies on average that the first arrival time to stage 2 is later than to stages 3 and 4. (2) The portion of patients switching out of stage 2 (mainly to discharge by plots 3 and 4 in Figure 3) is also high, which is not the case for stages 3 and 4 (reflected as the scale of plots 3 and 4 being much smaller than plots 1 and 2 of Figure 3). Therefore, the switch-out time from stage 2 is earlier than from stage 3 or 4 on average.

Factors (1) and (2) shown in Figure 2 and Table 2 indicate that stage 2 should associate to the major treatment procedures, like the main surgery, that most inpatients have to experience when staying in hospital. In fact, it is usual that patients need a couple of days as the preparation period

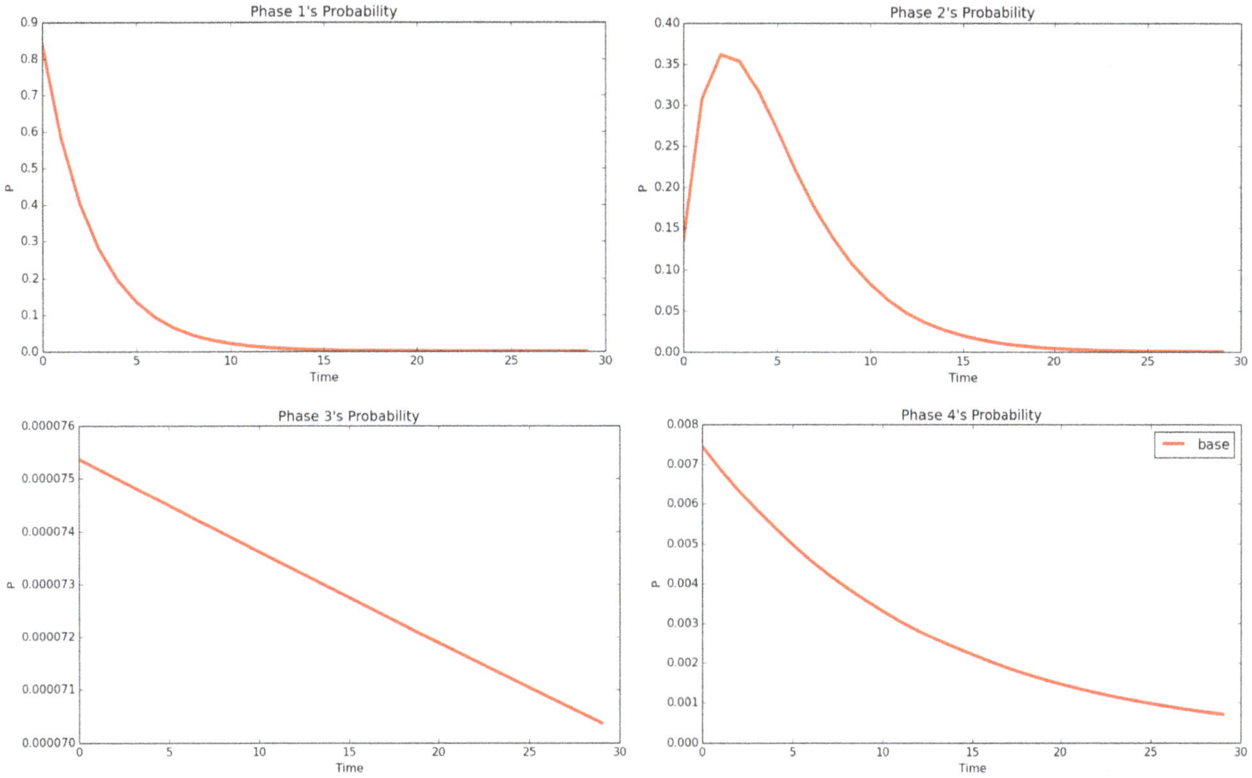

FIGURE 3: Probability of staying in every stage by time.

before the main surgery, such as the period for preexams. This preparation period is exactly captured by factor (1) of stage 2. On the other hand, patients usually recovered soon after the main treatment procedure gets done, and then are discharged, which is reflected by factor (2) of stage 2.

(iii) The third interesting observation from Figure 2 is regarding the median price of stage 2. From plots 1 and 2 in Figure 2, we can see that only at stage 2 there is a clear deviation between the expectation version and the median version of the price. More precisely, at stage 2 the median price is significantly lower than the price defined through the first-order moment, and this fact holds at almost all the time t and also holds for the daily price. It is well known that when the median of a distribution is below its first-order moment, there exists a group of outliers with extremely great value. In the other words, Figure 2 indicates that a portion of patients in stage 2 are charged much higher than the others in that stage and all the time. From the perspective of patient's welfare and the effective allocation of medical resources, it is meaningful to have some further researches in identifying the causes that make some patients in stage 2 being charged more.

Remark 3. By Figure 3, it is clear that the probability of staying in stages 3 and 4 is small over all time. This fact might be induced by model overfitting as pointed out by a referee, but it is not. In contrast, the low probability reflects a deep-level distributional property of SPARCS data. A very large proportion of inpatients recorded in SPARCS only have extremely short hospital stay and 99+ percent of them get discharged by day 10, while no more than 0.01 percent of patients can stay in hospital for more than 25 days. But at the meantime, there do exist a small group of patients who can live in hospital for a couple of months before discharge. The same pattern can be observed for the total charge; the most expensive expenditure can take million dollars while more than 99 percent of patients are charged no more than 100,000 dollars.

Based on the observation above and the nondecreasing design of the CPH-RGRST models that higher stages correspond to longer hospital stay and higher total costs, the low probability of staying in the highest two stages just reflects a fact that both of the charge and LOS data in SPARCS 2013 have a very long and thin tail to the right. This tail property may not be well fitted if a CPH-RGRST model with fewer phases is used, because there will not be enough freedom to distinguish the portion of patients in the tail from those whose charge and LOS stay around the mode.

4. Summary

We introduced a methodology whereby the widely used CPH models and RGRST models can be combined together and a variety of measures of the cost of phases in the CPH model can be defined. A two-step procedure is proposed to estimate the combined CPH-RGRST model and the simulation study is done to verify the effectiveness of the estimation procedure. With the data sampled from SPARCS 2013, we estimated a four-phase CPH-RGRST model and drew the cost curves for every phase. To distinguish the effect of different types of illness on the charge and LOS distribution, we incorporated MDC groups and the severity and mortality risk of illness as covariates into the estimation.

We found that the effect of illness on the total charge and LOS is not always homogeneous. In particular, there are five MDC groups that affect the charge and LOS in different direction. Among them, there is only one MDC group, representing the alcohol/drug abuse, which has the negative effect on the final charge while it lifts up the LOS drastically.

The daily charge for all the stages, 2, 3, and 4, is increasing over time. This fact implies a nonlinear charge accumulation process within every stage and therefore contradicts the piece-wise linear assumption used by the other authors, McClean et al. [11]. We believe that the increasing daily charge is more realistic and reflects dynamic interaction between the health condition of patients and the treatment they accept.

Among all the four stages, stage 2 shows quite different features in both the price measure and the time cost measure. In terms of the time cost, stage 2 is significantly lower than stages 3 and 4 almost all the time. This observation is consistent with the relatively high switch-in and switch-to-discharge intensity that the stage 2 has and associates the stage 2 with the major treatment procedures that most patients need to experience when staying in hospital.

The median is much lower than the mean of both the price and daily price in stage 2, while this kind of deviation does not exist for the other stages, and it implies that there is a portion of outlier patients who are charged much more than the other patients in stage 2. We believe that further studies are needed to find out the causes of those patients being charged more in stage 2, since it matters to the efficiency of the allocation of medical resources.

Appendix

Proof of Theorem 1

The main idea of the proof is to construct the partition $\mathcal{P}$ by induction. Assume, firstly, that the partition $\mathcal{P}$ is formed by n curves in $[0, \infty)$ (denoted as $(t, C_i(t))$ for $i \in \{0, 1, \ldots, n-1\}$) satisfying increasing condition as follows:

$$\begin{gathered} C_{i+1}(t) > C_i(t) \geq 0 \\ C_0(t) \equiv 0 \end{gathered} \tag{A.1}$$

in such a way that $\mathcal{P}_i = \{(y,t) : C_{i-1}(t) \leq y < C_i(t)\}$ for $i \in \{1, \ldots, n\}$ (for simplicity of notation, we assume $C_n(t) :\equiv \infty$.). So, to prove the theorem, it suffices to find out a family of increasing curves $\{C_i : i \in \{0, 1, \ldots, n-1\}\}$ with the induced transition matrix being as stated in the theorem.

Firstly, notice that, by condition (6), we have for $i \in \{0, 1, \ldots, n-1\}$ and any family of n curves $\{C_i : i \in \{0, 1, \ldots, n-1\}\}$ satisfying increasing condition (A.1) the fact that the following holds:

$$\begin{aligned} &\lim_{\delta \downarrow 0} \frac{\operatorname{Prob}\left(I(T > t + \delta) = 0 \mid Y(t) \in \left[C_i(t), C_{i+1}(t)\right), I(T > t) = 1\right)}{\delta} \\ &\quad = \frac{\int_{C_i(t)}^{C_{i+1}(t)} -\left((\partial \rho/\partial y) \cdot q + \partial \rho/\partial t\right)(y,t) \cdot p(y,t)\, dy}{\int_{C_i(t)}^{C_{i+1}(t)} \rho(y,t) \cdot p(y,t)\, dy} \equiv c. \end{aligned} \tag{A.2}$$

Moreover, because

$$\operatorname{Prob}\left(Y(t) \geq C_n(t) = +\infty, I(T > t) = 1\right) = 0, \tag{A.3}$$

we can conclude that no matter the choice of $\{C_i : i \in \{0, 1, \ldots, n-1\}\}$, the transition probability matrix A always has its column $n+1$ of the following form:

$$A_{n+1} = \begin{Bmatrix} c \\ \vdots \\ c \\ 0 \end{Bmatrix} \tag{A.4}$$

On the other hand, the increasing condition (A.1) and the nonincreasing property of the event processes $I(t)$ guarantee that for all $i, j \in \{0, 1, \ldots, n-1\}$ with $j \neq i$ or $i+1$ and small enough δ

$$\begin{aligned} &\operatorname{Prob}\left(Y_{t+\delta} \in \left[C_j(t), C_{j+1}(t)\right) \mid Y(t)\right. \\ &\qquad \left. \in \left[C_i(t), C_{i+1}(t)\right), I(T > t) = 1\right) = 0, \\ &\operatorname{Prob}\left(Y_{t+\delta} \in \left[C_j(t), C_{j+1}(t)\right), I(T > t + \delta)\right. \\ &\qquad \left. = 1 \mid I(T > t) = 0\right) = 0. \end{aligned} \tag{A.5}$$

That is, the induced transition matrix A satisfies

$$\begin{aligned} &A_{i,j} = 0, \quad j \notin \{i, i+1\},\ i, j \in \{1, \ldots, n\}, \\ &A_{n+1,j} = 0, \quad j \in \{1, \ldots, n\} \end{aligned} \tag{A.6}$$

So, to prove the theorem, it suffices to construct a family of increasing curves $\{C_i : i \in \{0, 1, \ldots, n-1\}\}$ guaranteeing that

$$\begin{aligned} A_{i,i+1} &= \lambda_i, \quad i \in \{1, \ldots, n-1\}, \\ P_i(0) &= \alpha_i, \quad i \in \{1, \ldots, n-1\} \end{aligned} \tag{A.7}$$

However, these two conditions are equivalent to finding

(1) a sequence $\{c_i : i \in \{0, 1, \ldots, n\}\}$ with $c_0 = 0$ and $c_n = \infty$ such that

$$\alpha_i = \int_{c_{i-1}}^{c_i} p(y,0)\, dy, \quad i \in \{1, \ldots, n-1\}; \tag{A.8}$$

(2) a sequence of solutions $\{y_i(t) : i \in \{0, 1, \ldots, n-1\}\}$ with $y_0 \equiv 0$ to initial value problems (IVP) for $i \in \{1, \ldots, n-1\}$

$$\begin{aligned} \frac{dy_i}{dt} &= q(y_i,t) - \lambda_i \cdot \frac{\int_{y_{i-1}}^{y_i} p(x,t) \cdot \rho(x,t)\, dx}{p(y_i,t) \cdot \rho(y_i,t)} \\ y_i(0) &= c_i \end{aligned} \tag{A.9}$$

Condition (A.9) arises from the following equality:

$$\begin{aligned} &\lim_{\delta \downarrow 0} \frac{\text{Prob}\left(Y_{t+\delta} \in [C_i(t+\delta), C_{i+1}(t+\delta)), I(T > t+\delta) = 1 \mid Y(t) \in [C_{i-1}(t), C_i(t)), I(T > t) = 1\right)}{\delta} \\ &= \lim_{\delta \downarrow 0} \frac{\text{Prob}\left(Y_{t+\delta} \in [C_i(t+\delta), C_{i+1}(t+\delta)), I(T > t+\delta) = 1, Y(t) \in [C_{i-1}(t), C_i(t)), I(T > t) = 1\right)}{\delta \cdot \text{Prob}\left(Y(t) \in [C_{i-1}(t), C_i(t)), I(T > t) = 1\right)} \\ &= \lim_{\delta \downarrow 0} \frac{\int_{C_i(t+\delta)}^{g^{-1}(C_i(t),t,t+\delta)} p(y,t+\delta) \cdot \rho(y,t+\delta)\, dy}{\delta \cdot \int_{C_{i-1}(t)}^{C_i(t)} p(y,t) \cdot \rho(y,t)\, dy} \\ &= \frac{p(C_i(t),t) \cdot \rho(C_i(t),t) \cdot \left(\lim_{\delta \downarrow 0}\left(\left(g^{-1}(C_i(t),t,t+\delta) - g^{-1}(C_i(t),t,t)\right)/\delta - dC_i(t)/dt\right)\right)}{\int_{C_{i-1}(t)}^{C_i(t)} p(y,t) \cdot \rho(y,t)\, dy} \\ &= \frac{p(C_i(t),t) \cdot \rho(C_i(t),t) \cdot \left(q(C_i(t),t) - dC_i(t)/dt\right)}{\int_{C_{i-1}(t)}^{C_i(t)} p(y,t) \cdot \rho(y,t)\, dy} = \lambda_i, \end{aligned} \tag{A.10}$$

where the time-dependent density function p of the potential charge process $\{G(t)\}$ has the form of $p(y,t) = p(g(y,t,t),0) \cdot \partial g(y,t,t)/\partial y$. The involved function g, viewed as a family of functions in variable s, solves the following family of IVPs:

$$\begin{aligned} \frac{dy}{dt} &= -q(y, t-s) \\ g(y,t,0) &= y \end{aligned} \tag{A.11}$$

and g^{-1} is defined as the inverse to g such that $g^{-1}(y,0,t) = \{x : g(x,t,t) = y\}$.

It is easy to check that condition (1) does always hold. Finally, thanks to the existence and uniqueness theorem of solutions to IVPs, the solution curves

$$\{y_i(t) : i \in \{0, 1, \ldots, n-1\}\} \tag{A.12}$$

do exist to the IVPs in (A.9).

Conflicts of Interest

The authors declare that they have no conflicts of interest.

Acknowledgments

This work was partially supported by the NSFC under Grant no. 11271317 and Zhejiang Provincial Natural Science Foundation under Grant no. LY16A010007, First Class Discipline of Zhejiang A (Zhejiang University of Finance and Economics-Statistics).

References

[1] M. Gold, "Panel on cost-effectiveness in health and medicine," *Medical Care*, vol. 340, no. 12, pp. 197–S199, 1996.

[2] J. Lipscomb, M. Ancukiewicz, G. Parmigiani, V. Hasselblad, G. Samsa, and D. B. Matchar, "Predicting the cost of illness: A comparison of alternative models applied to stroke," *Medical Decision Making*, vol. 18, no. 2, pp. S39–S56, 1998.

[3] D. Y. Lin, E. J. Feuer, R. Etzioni, and Y. Wax, "Estimating medical costs from incomplete follow-up data," *Biometrics*, vol. 53, no. 2, pp. 419–434, 1997.

[4] X. Q. Tang, *Modeling hospital length of stay and cost with heterogeneity [Ph.D. thesis]*, Mechigan State University, Department of Statistics, 2012.

[5] M. Faddy, N. Graves, and A. Pettitt, "Modeling length of stay in hospital and other right skewed data: Comparison of phase-

type, gamma and log-normal distributions," *Value in Health*, vol. 12, no. 2, pp. 309–314, 2009.

[6] A. H. Marshall, B. Shaw, and S. I. McClean, "Estimating the costs for a group of geriatric patients using the Coxian phase-type distribution," *Statistics in Medicine*, vol. 26, no. 13, pp. 2716–2729, 2007.

[7] A. Marshall, C. Vasilakis, and E. El-Darzi, "Length of stay-based patient flow models: Recent developments and future directions," *Health Care Management Science*, vol. 8, no. 3, pp. 213–220, 2005.

[8] A. H. Marshall, S. I. McClean, C. M. Shapcott, and P. H. Millard, "Modelling patient duration of stay to facilitate resource management of geriatric hospitals," *Health Care Management Science*, vol. 5, no. 4, pp. 313–319, 2002.

[9] M. Fackrell, "Modelling healthcare systems with phase-type distributions," *Health Care Management Science*, vol. 12, no. 1, pp. 11–26, 2009.

[10] S. McClean, M. Faddy, and P. Millard, "Markov model-based clustering for efficient patient care," in *Proceedings of the 18th IEEE Symposium on Computer-Based Medical Systems*, pp. 467–472, gbr, June 2005.

[11] S. McClean, J. Gillespie, L. Garg, M. Barton, B. Scotney, and K. Kullerton, "Using phase-type models to cost stroke patient care across health, social and community services," *European Journal of Operational Research*, vol. 236, no. 1, pp. 190–199, 2014.

[12] J. G. Ibrahim, H. Chu, and L. M. Chen, "Basic concepts and methods for joint models of longitudinal and survival data," *Journal of Clinical Oncology*, vol. 28, no. 16, pp. 2796–2801, 2010.

[13] A. A. Tsiatis and M. Davidian, "Joint modeling of longitudinal and time-to-event data: an overview," *Statistica Sinica*, vol. 14, no. 3, pp. 809–834, 2004.

[14] R. Henderson, P. Diggle, and A. Dobson, "Joint modelling of longitudinal measurements and event time data," *Biostatistics*, vol. 1, no. 4, pp. 465–480, 2000.

[15] S. Kim, D. Zeng, Y. Li, and D. Spiegelman, "Joint modeling of longitudinal and cure-survival data," *Journal of Statistical Theory and Practice*, vol. 7, no. 2, pp. 324–344, 2013.

[16] I. Sousa, "A review on joint modelling of longitudinal measurements and time-to-event," *Revstat Statistical Journal*, vol. 9, no. 1, pp. 57–81, 2011.

[17] A. L. Gould, M. E. Boye, M. . Crowther et al., "Joint modeling of survival and longitudinal non-survival data: current methods and issues. Report of the DIA Bayesian joint modeling working group," *Statistics in Medicine*, vol. 34, no. 14, pp. 2181–2195, 2015.

[18] J. C. Gardiner, Z. Luo, C. J. Bradley, E. Polverejan, M. Holmes-Rovner, and D. Rovner, "Longitudinal assessment of cost in health care interventions," *Health Services and Outcomes Research Methodology*, vol. 3, no. 2, pp. 149–168, 2002.

[19] J. C. Gardiner, Z. Luo, C. J. Bradley, C. M. Sirbu, and C. W. Given, "A dynamic model for estimating changes in health status and costs," *Statistics in Medicine*, vol. 25, no. 21, pp. 3648–3667, 2006.

[20] E. Polverejan, J. C. Gardiner, C. J. Bradley, M. Holmes-Rovner, and D. Rovner, "Estimating mean hospital cost as a function of length of stay and patient characteristics," *Health Economics*, vol. 12, no. 11, pp. 935–947, 2003.

[21] L. C. Evans, *Partial Differential Equations*, American Mathematical Society, Providence, RI, USA, 2010.

16

Exploration of Neural Activity under Cognitive Reappraisal using Simultaneous EEG-fMRI Data and Kernel Canonical Correlation Analysis

Biao Yang,[1,2] Jinmeng Cao,[1,2] Tiantong Zhou,[1,2] Li Dong,[3] Ling Zou,[1,2] and Jianbo Xiang[4]

[1]*School of Information Science and Engineering, Changzhou University, Changzhou, Jiangsu 213164, China*
[2]*Changzhou Key Laboratory of Biomedical Information Technology, Changzhou, Jiangsu 213164, China*
[3]*School of Life Science and Technology, University of Electronic Science and Technology of China, Chengdu, Sichuan 610054, China*
[4]*Changzhou No. 2 People's Hospital Affiliated with Nanjing Medical University, Changzhou, Jiangsu 213164, China*

Correspondence should be addressed to Ling Zou; zouling@cczu.edu.cn and Jianbo Xiang; hx_bob@163.com

Academic Editor: Miguel García-Torres

Background. Neural activity under cognitive reappraisal can be more accurately investigated using simultaneous EEG- (electroencephalography) fMRI (functional magnetic resonance imaging) than using EEG or fMRI only. Complementary spatiotemporal information can be found from simultaneous EEG-fMRI data to study brain function. *Method.* An effective EEG-fMRI fusion framework is proposed in this work. EEG-fMRI data is simultaneously sampled on fifteen visually stimulated healthy adult participants. Net-station toolbox and empirical mode decomposition are employed for EEG denoising. Sparse spectral clustering is used to construct fMRI masks that are used to constrain fMRI activated regions. A kernel-based canonical correlation analysis is utilized to fuse nonlinear EEG-fMRI data. *Results.* The experimental results show a distinct late positive potential (LPP, latency 200-700ms) from the correlated EEG components that are reconstructed from nonlinear EEG-fMRI data. Peak value of LPP under reappraisal state is smaller than that under negative state, however, larger than that under neutral state. For correlated fMRI components, obvious activation can be observed in cerebral regions, e.g., the amygdala, temporal lobe, cingulate gyrus, hippocampus, and frontal lobe. Meanwhile, in these regions, activated intensity under reappraisal state is obviously smaller than that under negative state and larger than that under neutral state. *Conclusions.* The proposed EEG-fMRI fusion approach provides an effective way to study the neural activities of cognitive reappraisal with high spatiotemporal resolution. It is also suitable for other neuroimaging technologies using simultaneous EEG-fMRI data.

1. Introduction

Emotional regulation is known as a unique ability of human beings to control experience and expression of their emotions. It has been the focus of many fields (e.g., cognitive neuroscience, clinical medicine, and sociology) due to its importance to human mental health [1, 2]. Two well-established emotional regulation strategies are widely applied to control emotional experiences, including expressive suppression and cognitive reappraisal. The former is a way of response modulation whereby individual voluntarily inhibits emotional expressive behavior [3]. However, according to the catharsis model, emotions are supposed to "pile up" if not expressed [4]. Hence, expressive suppression may enhance emotional experience which harms mental health. Cognitive reappraisal, on the other hand, is an approach to change the way people think about a potentially emotion eliciting condition to decrease the emotional influence [5]. For instance, one's representative reaction to a scene of a person shooting at another one may be decreased by imaging the scene as a film scene. On the contrary, the reaction may be enhanced by imaging the person is shot by his/her close relative. By utilizing cognitive reappraisal, discomfort to events (e.g., sick, horror, and self-abasement) can be alleviated at an early stage. Despite recent studies show that cognitive reappraisal is correlated to facial frown muscle activities [6], heart rate, and skin conductance [3], studying the essence of cognitive reappraisal is still urgent.

Recently, several neuroimaging technologies (e.g., EEG (electroencephalography) and fMRI (functional magnetic resonance imaging)) are utilized to explore the essence of cognitive reappraisal. Submillisecond temporal resolution of EEG makes it suitable to explore the subtle temporal dynamics of neural activity, which is expressed by electric potential fluctuations spread to the scalp. Event Related Potential (ERP) is widely used to study the characteristics of EEG signals under different emotional states due to its high temporal resolution. An essential component of ERP, Late Positive Potential (LPP), is found to indicate the ability of cognitive reappraisal using emotional regulation. The facilitated processing of emotional stimuli is indicated by the LPP as a central-parietal slow positive deflection in the ERP. The amplitude of LPP turns out to be increased for emotionally eliciting compared with neutral stimuli, beginning with approximately 200ms after stimulus onset and continuing several seconds [7]. Meanwhile, it is susceptible to spontaneous emotional regulation. Hence, a decrease of LPP amplitude can be found when participants are asked to distract attention from the pictures which may arouse unpleasant emotion via cognitive reappraisal [8]. Moreover, LPP reduction can also be found from positive emotional regulation by cognitive reappraisal [9, 10]. However, emotional eliciting sources are hard to locate due to the poor spatial resolution of EEG. FMRI is another widely used technology to study the brain function. It can localize both superficial and deep sources of activity with mm-scale spatial resolution via detecting the variations of blood oxygenation level-dependent (BOLD). Cerebral regions which participate in emotional regulation can be found via fMRI due to its high spatial resolution. Recent fMRI researches show that voluntary reappraisal can influence modulated neural activities in the amygdala [11, 12]. It also indicates that the employment of cognitive reappraisal influences the neural activities in the dorsal parts of the anterior cingulate cortex, the ventromedial prefrontal cortex, and the dorsolateral prefrontal cortex [13]. However, the low resolution temporal variations of these regions are not suitable for studying the neural activity under cognitive reappraisal.

To resolve the abovementioned insufficient of monomodality neuroimaging technology, simultaneous EEG-fMRI fusion is utilized to study the neural activity under cognitive reappraisal due to its high spatiotemporal resolution. In general, there are mainly three approaches for simultaneous EEG-fMRI fusion, including fMRI aided EEG analysis, EEG aided fMRI analysis, and symmetric EEG-fMRI analysis. For fMRI aided EEG analysis, fMRI information with high spatial resolution is used to support the inverse issue of EEG source reconstruction. Kyathanahally *et al.* proposed a framework to invest decision-making in the brain using simultaneous EEG-fMRI data [14]. Thinh *et al.* developed a novel multimodal EEG-fMRI fusion approach by employing the most probable fMRI spatial subsets to guide EEG source localization in a time-variant fashion [15]. For EEG informed fMRI analysis, EEG features (e.g., ERP amplitude, the power spectrum, and epileptic) are used to forecast the BOLD changes in fMRI. Liu *et al.* proposed a general linear model (GLM) model for EEG-fMRI fusion. The fusion results indicate that the intraparietal sulcus and frontal executive areas are the primary sources of biasing influences on task-related visual cortex, whereas task-unrelated default mode network and sensorimotor cortex are suppressive during visual attention [16]. Ahmad *et al.* developed a framework to recognize different visual brain activity patterns using simultaneous EEG-fMRI data. A GLM model was utilized for EEG-fMRI fusion and the results were further classified into different patterns by multilayer perceptron [17]. For symmetric EEG-fMRI analysis, both data are jointly processed by a generative model or changed into a common feature/data space. Yu *et al.* developed a framework to construct multimodal brain graphs using EEG-fMRI data which were simultaneously sampled during eyes open and eyes closed resting states [18]. FMRI data were decomposed into independent components with associated time courses by group independent component analysis (ICA) and EEG time series were segmented into spectral power time courses by superposed average of five frequency bands (alpha, theta, beta, delta, and low gamma). However, ICA assumes that all sources are independent. This strong assumption restricts the power of ICA fusion approach in exploring the underlying sources. Canonical correlation analysis (CCA) was employed by Correa *et al.* to fuse simultaneous EEG-fMRI data with weak assumption [19]. Dong *et al.* also proposed a CCA based EEG-fMRI fusion approach to study familial cortical myoclonic tremor and epilepsy [20]. The proposed local multimodal serial analysis was specifically designed to handle the change of hemodynamic response functions (HRFs).

Despite the widely developed approaches to analyze EEG-fMRI data, there is still no method that focuses on two challenging issues of simultaneous EEG-fMRI fusion; one is to handle the mutual interference between EEG and fMRI, and the other is to handle the nonlinearity of EEG-fMRI data. Aiming to resolve these challenges, we propose an effective fusion framework based on CCA. Empirical mode decomposition (EMD) is used to increase SNR of EEG data that is polluted by MR scanning. FMRI masks are constructed and are used to eliminate unwanted fMRI components that are correlated with wanted EEG components. RBF kernel is embedded into the CCA framework to handle the nonlinearity of EEG-fMRI data. Participants are shown with visual stimuli paradigm. Based on previous researches that study EEG and fMRI, respectively [7], we expect (1) the correlated ERP components and fMRI activated regions related to cognitive reappraisal can be simultaneously be extracted from the EEG-fMRI data, and (2) LPPs under three emotional states can be observed from the correlated ERP components and amplitudes of different LPPs coincided with the existed studies, and (3) the correlated fMRI activated regions coincided with the previous found regions (e.g., amygdala, dorsomedial PFC, dorsolateral prefrontal cortex (PFC), anterior cingulate cortex, and orbitofrontal cortex). There are mainly two contributions of our work: (1) providing

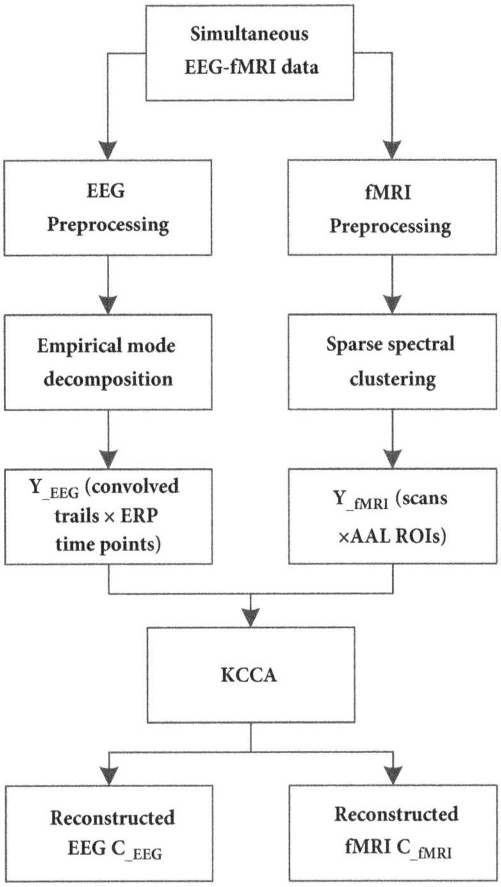

FIGURE 1: Pipeline of the proposed EEG-fMRI fusion approach.

an effective framework for simultaneous EEG-fMRI fusion and (2) exploring the neural activity under cognitive reappraisal in high spatiotemporal resolution.

2. Materials and Methods

2.1. The EEG-fMRI Fusion Framework. The framework of the fusion approach is demonstrated in Figure 1. Simultaneous EEG-fMRI data is preprocessed, respectively. EMD is further used to eliminate noise of EEG data. Sparse spectral clustering (SSC) is employed to construct fMRI masks that indicate the emotion-related cerebral regions. EEG feature to be fused is defined as $Y_{\_EEG}$ (convolved trails × ERP time points), which are obtained by convolving the ERP values at different time points with a standard HRF. On the other hand, fMRI feature to be fused is defined as $Y_{\_fMRI}$ (scans ×AAL ROIs), which are obtained by calculating mean values in anatomical automatic labeling (AAL) cerebral regions under the constraints of fMRI masks. Then, $Y_{\_EEG}$ and $Y_{\_fMRI}$ are fused using a kernel-based CCA (KCCA) framework. EEG and fMRI components ($C_{\_EEG}$ and $C_{\_fMRI}$) are finally reconstructed based on the selected correlated components.

2.2. Subjects. A total of 15 healthy adults, 5 females and 10 males, aged from 19 to 24 years (M (mean value) =23, SD (standard deviation) =1.48), are recruited from Changzhou University to implement the experiments.

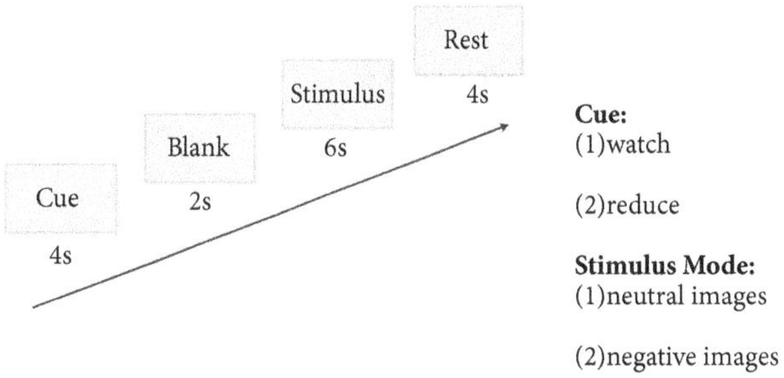

FIGURE 2: Illustration of the visual stimuli paradigm.

Participants have regular or corrected regular vision without history of neurological, medical, or psychiatric disorders. They have been tested for psychological profile to discard some comorbid issues as depression or psychiatric symptoms that can affect emotional evaluation. All participants provide written informed consent to be part of the experiment, which is approved by the local ethics committee (Changzhou University, Changzhou, China). Each subject receives 42-minute fMRI scan (structure: 5 min, resting state: 5 min, and task state: 32 min).

2.3. Paradigm. The visual stimuli paradigm [21] is implemented in a block fMRI design as shown in Figure 2. The entire experiment for one participant contains 120 trials, including 4 circulations in which 30 trials are implemented. Three conditions, including watching neutral images (e.g., buildings, neutral faces, and food), watching negative images (e.g., sadness, disasters, and violence), and watching negative images with cognitive reappraisal, are randomly implemented in 40 trials, respectively. All the images used are chosen from the international affective picture gallery. The arousal for neutral images is M (mean) = 2.91 and SD (standard deviation) = 1.93; meanwhile, for negative images it is M = 5.71 and SD = 2.61. Procedure of a single trial can last at most 16 seconds as proposed in [22]. Initially, cue word "reduce" or "watch" is shown on the screen for 4 seconds in the cue period. After a 2-second blank period, the stimulus period will last for 6 seconds. At this period, neutral and negative images will randomly appear with cue word "watch", while only negative images will appear with cue word "reduce". Notably, cognitive reappraisal will be used if the cue word "reduce" appears. Finally, the rest period will last for 4 seconds.

2.4. Simultaneous EEG-fMRI Acquisition. EEG acquisition system of EGI company (Eugene, the USA) is used in the experiment. EEG is sampled continuously at 1000Hz. An amplifier is placed inside the MR scanner room. Subjects are fitted with an electrode cap containing 64 electrodes with Cz as online reference. Later, the data are referenced to zero by reference electrode standardization technique [23]. It is recently confirmed being close to the idea of zero reference [24, 25]. Impedances are kept low below 50kΩ. The helium pump is turned off during experiments to avoid related artifacts.

Functional imaging data are sampled with 3-Tesla superconducting type nuclear magnetic resonance imaging system

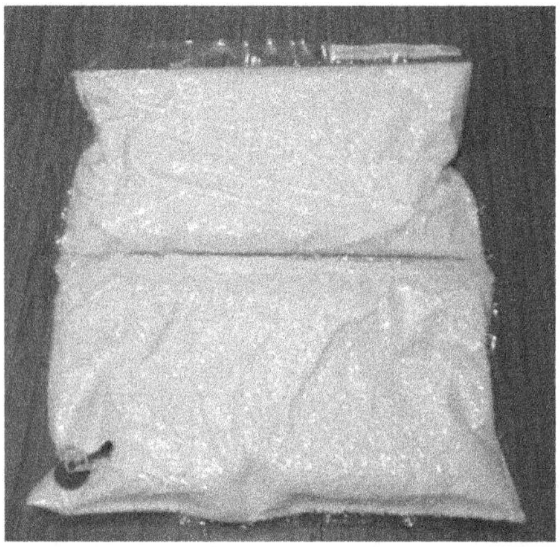

FIGURE 3: The foam pads used to prevent head movement.

of Philips Company. Single excitation gradient echoes planar sequence is utilized to acquire functional images. After a whole paradigm finished, 960 BOLD sensitive echo planar images (EPI) are gathered during four sessions. EPI volumes are aligned with the anterior-posterior commissural line. It contains 24 axial slices with 4mm thickness including flip angle: 90 degree; TR (repetition time): 2s; TE (echo time): 35ms; FOV (field of view): 230mm∗182mm; matrix: 96×74. Subjects are mandated to lie in the MRI scanning room, staying awake, and blinking as little as possible. The foam pads (Figure 3) are used to prevent head movement.

2.5. EEG Data Processing. Processing of EEG data contains two parts, one is denoising and the other is extracting EEG feature. In consideration of the influence caused by MR scanning, denoising is achieved through two steps: traditional denoising using net-station toolbox and further increasing SNR using EMD.

For traditional denosing, noises such as gradient artifact, ECG, and power interference are eliminated as follows: (1) Gradient artifact is removed by template elimination method. The gradient artifact template is constructed in a weighted average mean by labeling the timing that fMRI triggered EEG. Then, an average artifact subtraction method is utilized to eliminate the gradient artifact. (2) Band-pass filtering is employed with the band 0.01-40Hz. (3) Optimal basis set approach is used to eliminate ballistocardiogram artifacts caused by the heartbeat. (4) The EEG data are segmented into different fragments based on the stimulus time point. Each fragment ranges from 200ms before stimulus and 1500ms after it. (5) Artifacts such as head movements and blinking are detected in all fragments of all electrodes. The electrode with artifacts is labeled as bad electrode. (6) The bad electrode is replaced by the average of its 3 surrounding electrodes. (7) The first 200ms of each fragment is used for baseline correction.

After traditional denoising, EMD is employed to further increase SNR of EEG data that is affected by MR scanning [26]. EMD tries to find functions which form a complete and nearly orthogonal basis of the original signal. These functions are termed as Intrinsic Mode Functions (IMFs). Then, increasing SNR can be achieved through removing IMFs that are taken as disturbance. Details of increasing SNR through EMD can be found in our former work [27].

After denoising, emotion-related ERP extracted from EEG is used to study the neural activity under cognitive reappraisal [7]. Amplitudes of ERP (extracted from Poz channel) at different time points are termed as EEG feature. At each time point, the trial-to-trial dynamics are convolved with a standard HRF to coincide with fMRI (5 volumes in each trial) due to the BOLD delay. We restrict the analysis to 900ms (225 uniform and consecutive time points) after stimulus onset because the most emotion-related components in the EEG are considered to appear during the first 200-700ms after stimulus onset. Finally, the dimension of the extracted EEG feature is 600 (convolved trails) × 225 (ERP time points).

2.6. FMRI Data Processing. FMRI data are processed using reference electrode standardization technique and statistical parametric mapping (SPM) to correct slice time and exclude head motion. Then the data are normalized and further registered to the Montreal Neurological Institute (MNI) space. Finally, a Gaussian filter (full-width at half-maximum of 8 mm) is used for smoothing filtering and only five fMRI activation regions (three in stimulus period and two in rest period) after stimulus presentation are selected in each trial. Each fMRI activation region is represented by its mean values in different AAL ROIs [28]. Finally, the dimension of the extracted fMRI feature is 600 (scans) × 90 (AAL ROIs).

Notably, some fMRI regions irrelevant to emotion processing are also activated. These undesired activation regions should be removed to guarantee the accuracy of EEG-fMRI fusion. Otherwise, they may correlate with the wanted EEG components. In this work, an fMRI mask is constructed through spatiotemporal clustering of all fMRI activation. SSC is used to cluster the fMRI activation because SSC is insensitive to the number of features and, thus, can avoid dimension disaster [29]. Then, there is no undesired fMRI activation in the fMRI mask because undesired activation mostly sustain for a short period in certain cerebral regions. Finally, for each row of the fMRI feature, an "and" operation with fMRI mask will be performed to restrain the influence of undesired fMRI activation.

2.7. Simultaneous EEG-fMRI Data Fusion Using KCCA. CCA searches for a pair of linear transformations of the variable set in the manner of one for each. It is commonly used for symmetric EEG-fMRI analysis. Given two data X ($Y_{\_EEG}$) and Y ($Y_{\_fMRI}$), their generative models are given by

$$\begin{aligned} X &= A_X C_X \\ Y &= A_Y C_Y \end{aligned} \tag{1}$$

where A_X and A_Y are canonical variate matrices and C_X and C_Y are associated EEG and fMRI components. Let a_{Xk} and a_{Yk} represent the kth column of A_X and A_Y (the kth pair of canonical variate); then their relational degree is defined as

Table 1: Correlated components of EEG-fMRI with high relational degrees (> 0.55) under three emotional states.

correlated components	relational degrees (KCCA approach / CCA approach)		
	neutral state	negative state	reappraisal state
component 1	**0.951** / 0. 944	**0.971** / 0.966	**0.932** / 0.913
component 2	**0.892** / 0.888	**0.952** / 0.947	**0.834** / 0.801
component 3	0.833 / **0.841**	0.863 / **0.877**	**0.805** / 0.731
component 4	**0.765** / 0.741	**0.821** / 0.816	0.704 / **0.716**
component 5	0.643 / **0.681**	0.753 / **0.765**	**0.613** / 0.606
component 6	**0.586** / N/A	**0.712** / 0.660	**0.551** / 0.537
component 7	N/A / N/A	**0.605** / 0.584	N/A / N/A

$$\rho_k = \frac{a_{Xk}{}^T S_{XY} a_{Yk}}{\sqrt{a_{Xk}{}^T S_{XX} a_{Xk}} \times \sqrt{a_{Yk}{}^T S_{YY} a_{Yk}}} \quad (2)$$

$$S = S(X,Y) = \begin{bmatrix} S_{XX} & S_{XY} \\ S_{YX} & S_{YY} \end{bmatrix} \quad (3)$$

where ρ_k indicates the relational degree of the kth pair of associated components. The total covariance matrix S is represented as a block matrix. The within-sets covariance matrices are S_{XX} and S_{YY}. The between-sets covariance matrices are $S_{XY} = S_{YX}{}^T$. Then, those associated components whose relational degrees are larger than a given threshold (0.55) are used to reconstruct the wanted EEG component $\widehat{C}_X$ and fMRI component $\widehat{C}_Y$, which are defined as follows:

$$\widehat{C}_X = \left(\widehat{A}_X^T \widehat{A}_X\right)^{-1} \widehat{A}_X^T X$$
$$\widehat{C}_Y = \left(\widehat{A}_Y^T \widehat{A}_Y\right)^{-1} \widehat{A}_Y^T Y \quad (4)$$

where $\widehat{A}_X$ and $\widehat{A}_Y$ only contain the selected pairs of canonical variate. Details of solving a CCA problem can be referred to [19].

However, CCA cannot process nonlinear data. Thus, kernel is used to resolve such problem through mapping data into a high dimensional feature space. A kernel κ for all X, Y $\in$ R is defined as follows:

$$\kappa(X,Y) = \langle \varphi(X), \varphi(Y) \rangle \quad (5)$$

where φ is a mapping from the original data space R to a new feature space F (φ: R->F). Great flexibility can be achieved by applying different kernels such as linear kernel, Gaussian kernel, and RBF. Based on kernel, the directions a_{Xk} and a_{Yk} can be represented as follows:

$$a_{Xk} = X\alpha$$
$$a_{Yk} = Y\beta \quad (6)$$

where α and β indicate the transformations from original data to their canonical variate. Then, (2) can be represented as follows:

$$\rho_k = \frac{\alpha' X' XY' Y\beta'}{\sqrt{\alpha' X' XX' X\alpha \bullet \beta' Y' YY' Y\beta}} \quad (7)$$

Notable, linear transformations X'X and Y'Y cannot process nonlinear data very well. Hence, RBF kernel is used to replace the linear transformations due to its superiority in processing nonlinear data. Then, (2) can be rewritten as follows:

$$\rho_k = \frac{\alpha' K_X K_Y \beta}{\sqrt{\alpha' K_X{}^2 \alpha \bullet \beta' K_Y{}^2 \beta}} \quad (8)$$

where K_X and K_Y represent the RBF kernel matrices. Relational degrees calculated using (8) is more suitable to nonlinear EEG-fMRI data than that calculated using (2).

3. Experimental Results

3.1. Comparisons between KCCA and CCA. This work focuses on the highly correlated components between EEG temporal evolution and fMRI spatial activation. Ninety correlated components are obtained using KCCA fusion. Table 1 demonstrates the correlated components whose relational degrees are larger than 0.55. As shown in the table, there are six pairs of correlated components under neutral and reappraisal states, and seven pairs of correlated components under negative state. Our former work using CCA fusion is used as comparison [27]. It is obvious that relational degrees obtained using KCCA is larger than that obtained using CCA.

Figures 4–6 illustrate the fifteen subjects' superposed average results of the correlated EEG-fMRI components. Correlated components whose relational degrees are larger than 0.55 are used for superposed average. For each figure, subfigure (a) indicates the superposed average result of correlated EEG component extracted from Poz electrode. Furthermore, x-axis represents time (ms) and y-axis represents normalized amplitude (dimensionless). Subfigure (b) illustrates the correlated fMRI activation under the same state, while the color-bar indicates the normalized activated intensity. Then, neural activities caused by the same stimuli can be observed in both high temporal (correlated EEG component) and spatial resolutions (correlated fMRI activation).

Aside from the differences in relational degrees, differences in EEG components are also evaluated between CCA [27] and KCCA. Figure 7(a) illustrates the fifteen subjects' superposed average results of reconstructed EEG

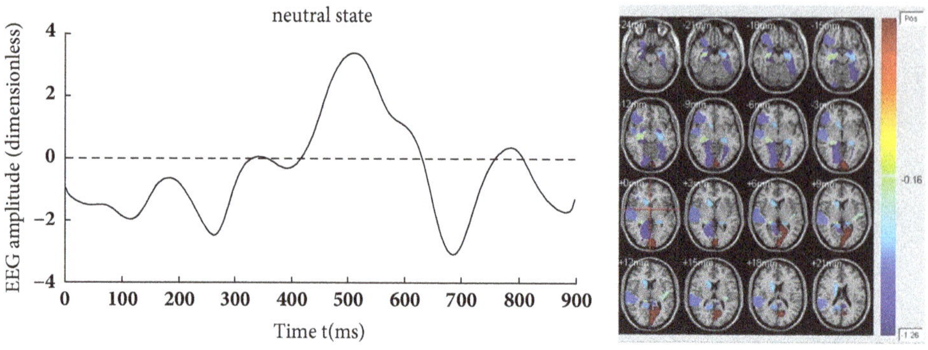

(a) (b)

FIGURE 4: Fifteen subjects' superposed average result of correlated EEG-fMRI under neutral state. (a) Correlated EEG component and (b) correlated fMRI activation.

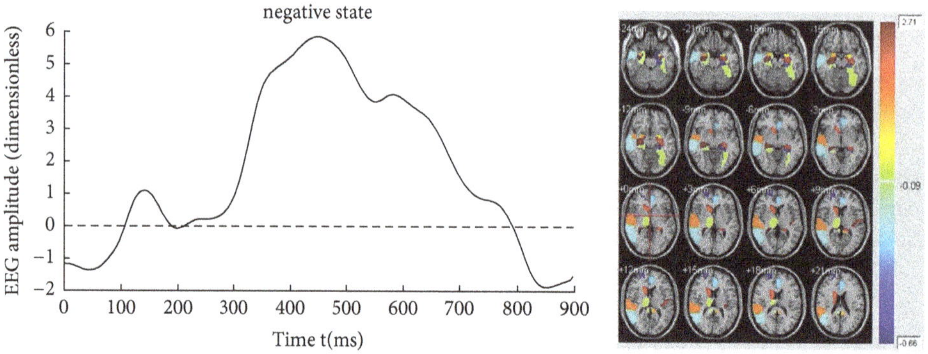

(a) (b)

FIGURE 5: Fifteen subjects' superposed average result of correlated EEG-fMRI under negative state. (a) Correlated EEG component and (b) correlated fMRI activation.

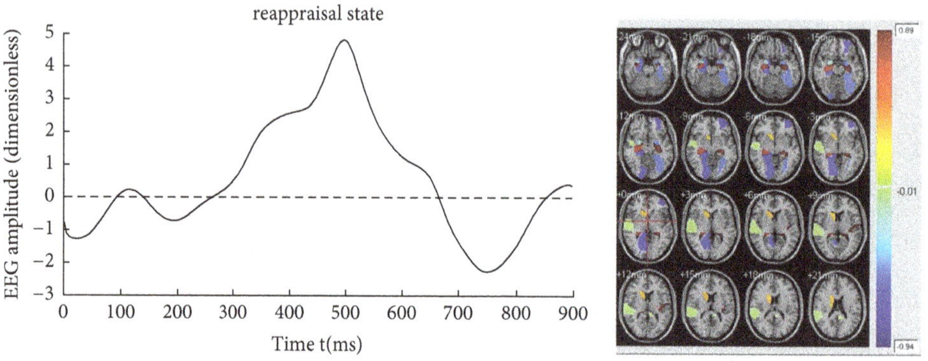

(a) (b)

FIGURE 6: Fifteen subjects' superposed average result of correlated EEG-fMRI under reappraisal state. (a) Correlated EEG component and (b) correlated fMRI activation.

components that are calculated by KCCA fusion. All the EEG components are extracted from Poz electrode. Obvious differences can be observed among their LPP components. The amplitude of LPP component under reappraisal state is smaller than that under negative state and is obviously larger than that under neutral state. Figure 7(b) illustrates the fifteen subjects' superposed average results of reconstructed EEG components that are calculated by CCA fusion. Similar results can be observed. However, amplitudes of LPP component under negative state and that under reappraisal state are more or less intersecting at the reported emotion arousing period (200-700ms by [7]) as illustrated in Figure 7(b). The intersection may be caused by nonlinearity of simultaneous EEG-fMRI data.

TABLE 2: Fifteen subjects' superposed average results of correlated fMRI activations under neutral state, negative state, and reappraisal state (using KCCA).

under neutral state		under negative state		under reappraisal state	
AAL ROIs (No)	Z-score	AAL ROIs (No)	Z-score	AAL ROIs (No)	Z-score
Calcarine_L (43)	0.355	Hippocampus_R (38)	2.711	Heschl_L (79)	0.887
Hippocampus_R (38)	0.208	Heschl_L (79)	2.485	Hippocampus_L (37)	0.870
Heschl_L (79)	0.178	Hippocampus_L (37)	2.317	Hippocampus_R (38)	0.776
Caudate_R (72)	0.068	Caudate_R (72)	1.990	Caudate_R (72)	0.550
N / A	N / A	Temporal_Sup_R (82)	1.383	Amygdala_ R (42)	0.043
N / A	N / A	Cingulum_Post_L (35)	1.249	Temporal_Sup_R (82)	0.038
N / A	N / A	Amygdala_R (42)	1.233	Amygdala_L (41)	0.031
N / A	N / A	Cingulum_Mid_R (34)	0.672	Cingulum_Post_L (35)	0.006
N / A	N / A	Cingulum_Mid_L (33)	0.627	N / A	N / A
N / A	N / A	Amygdala_L (41)	0.567	N / A	N / A
N / A	N / A	Fusiform_L (55)	0.223	N / A	N / A
N / A	N / A	Thalamus_R (78)	0.220	N / A	N / A
N / A	N / A	Cingulum_Post_R (36)	0.121	N / A)	N / A
N / A	N / A	ParaHippocampal_R (40)	0.090	N / A	N / A

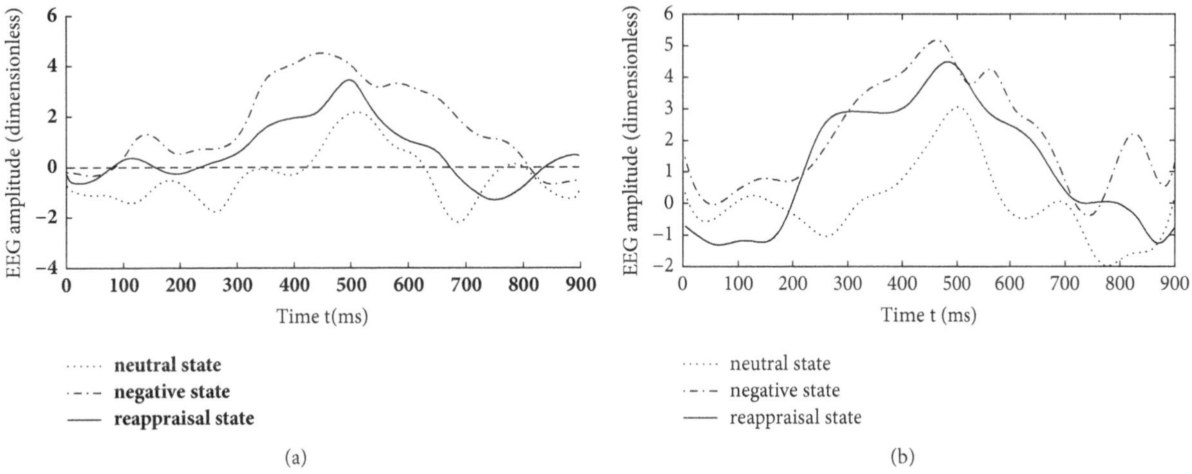

FIGURE 7: Fifteen subjects' superposed average results of EEG correlation components under three emotional states using (a) KCCA fusion and (b) CCA fusion.

A quantitative comparison is performed on the average correlated EEG components of fifteen subjects under three emotional states. 225 samples are uniformly sampled from 700ms EEG component and their amplitudes are used as input. F-test is used for evaluation and different emotional states are used as the factors of ANOVA. The result shows distinct differences in EEG components of different emotional states. The mean of the differences (MOD) between conditions under negative and neutral states is 23, with $F(1, 224) = 262.65 (P < 0.01)$. The MOD between conditions under reappraisal and negative states is 11, with $F(1, 224) = 70.49 (P < 0.01)$. The MOD between conditions under reappraisal and neutral states is 13, when $F(1, 224) = 83.04 (P < 0.01)$. Obviously, the quantitative result is confirmed to the result of Figure 7.

3.2. Comparisons between KCCA and GLM. Comparisons between KCCA and GLM are performed to verify the superiority of symmetric EEG-fMRI analysis in studying the neural activities of cognitive reappraisal. Table 2 demonstrates fifteen subjects' superposed average results of correlated fMRI activation under three emotional states using KCCA. Intensities of fMRI activation are measured by the Z-score values in different AAL ROIs. A big Z-score value indicates a strong fMRI activation. Notably, only AAL ROIs whose

Table 3: Fifteen subjects' superposed average results of correlated fMRI activations under neutral state, negative state, and reappraisal state (using GLM).

under neutral state		under negative state		under reappraisal state	
AAL ROIs (No)	Z-score	AAL ROIs (No)	Z-score	AAL ROIs (No)	Z-score
Parietal_Sup_L (59)	0.516	Heschl_L (79)	1.587	Parietal_Inf_R (62)	0.887
Paracentral_Lobule_R (70)	0.366	Parietal_Sup_L (59)	1.466	Parietal_Sup_L (59)	0.870
Parietal_Sup_R (60)	0.159	Parietal_Sup_R (60)	1.039	Occipital_Mid_R (52)	0.776
Occipital_Mid_L (51)	0.020	Precuneus_L (67)	0.922	ParaHippocampal_L (39)	0.350
N / A	N / A	Paracentral_Lobule_L (69)	0.790	Angular_R (66)	0.006
N / A	N / A	Paracentral_Lobule_R (70)	0.725	N / A	N / A
N / A	N / A	Occipital_Mid_R (52)	0.569	N / A	N / A
N / A	N / A	Occipital_Mid_L (51)	0.507	N / A	N / A
N / A	N / A	Occipital_Sup_R (50)	0.478	N / A	N / A
N / A	N / A	Parietal_Inf_L (61)	0.292	N / A	N / A
N / A	N / A	Temporal_Pole_Mid_L (87)	0.159	N / A	N / A
N / A	N / A	SupraMarginal_L (63)	0.126	N / A	N / A
N / A	N / A	Precuneus_R (68)	0.116	N / A	N / A
N / A	N / A	SupraMarginal_R (64)	0.114	N / A	N / A
N / A	N / A	Heschl_R (80)	0.108	N / A	N / A
N / A	N / A	Cingulum_Mid_L (33)	0.084	N / A	N / A
N / A	N / A	ParaHippocampal_L (39)	0.080	N / A	N / A
N / A	N / A	Cingulum_Ant_L (31)	0.022	N / A	N / A

Z-score values are larger than 0 (a negative Z-score value in certain AAL ROI indicates that this ROI is irrelevant to emotion processing) are preserved in this table. Meanwhile, no EEG component is evaluated because GLM is mainly used for analyzing fMRI activation. Table 3 demonstrates fifteen subjects' superposed average results of correlated fMRI activation under three emotional states using GLM. Differences between KCCA and GLM exist in both activated regions and intensities. Discussions of their differences will be given in Section 4 in detail.

3.3. Evaluation of the fMRI Masks. FMRI masks are used to restrain the activated fMRI regions due to their ability to eliminate the regions uncorrelated to emotion processing. The clustering results of all subjects under three emotional states are illustrated in Figure 8. As shown in the figure, activated regions under neutral state are the smallest while activated regions under negative state are the biggest.

KCCA fusion without fMRI masks is performed to evaluate the effectiveness of fMRI masks. For fMRI, fifteen subjects' superposed average results of correlated fMRI activation obtained through KCCA but without fMRI masks are illustrated in Figure 9. Correlated fMRI activation varies a lot due to whether fMRI masks are used, especially under negative and reappraisal states. For example, there is obvious activation in cerebral regions such as hippocampus, amygdala, and temporal lobe that are directly related to emotion processing in Figure 5(b). However, no activation can be found in these cerebral regions in Figure 9(a). Same phenomena can be observed in Figures 6(b) and 9(b). There is no activation in emotion-related cerebral regions such as hippocampus and temporal lobe in Figure 9(b), while obvious activation can be observed in these regions in Figure 6(b). There is no obvious difference in activated fMRI regions between Figures 4(b) and 9(c) because fMRI masks do not focus on cerebral regions unrelated to emotion processing.

For EEG, fifteen subjects' superposed average results of EEG correlated components under three emotional states but without clustering mask are shown in Figure 10. Compared with the results in Figure 7, no obvious decrease can be observed in ERP amplitude from negative state to reappraisal state. Meanwhile, EEG evolutions under different emotional states are hard to separate.

4. Discussion and Conclusion

The aim of cognitive reappraisal is to regulate human experience under negative emotion such as depression, fear, and disappointment. Simultaneous EEG-fMRI analysis is used to study the neural activity under cognitive reappraisal due to its complementarity in both spatial and temporal domains. In this work, these neural activities are studied using a KCCA fusion framework. Meanwhile, EMD is used to further increase SNR of EEG data that is sampled under MR scanning. FMRI masks are calculated using SSC and are used to eliminate the activation unrelated to emotion processing. With all these processing, both EEG and fMRI components can be reconstructed based on the selected correlated components (Figures 4, 5, and 6). Results of these figures are very important to study the mechanism of cognitive reappraisal that is useful for human to regulate

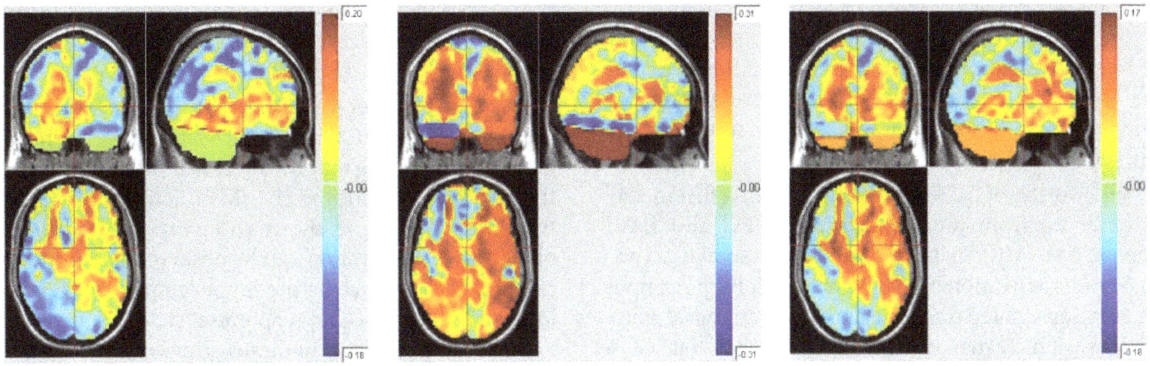

(a) (b) (c)

FIGURE 8: fMRI clustering results of all subjects (a) under neutral state; (b) under negative state; and (c) under reappraisal state (color-bar indicates the activated intensity).

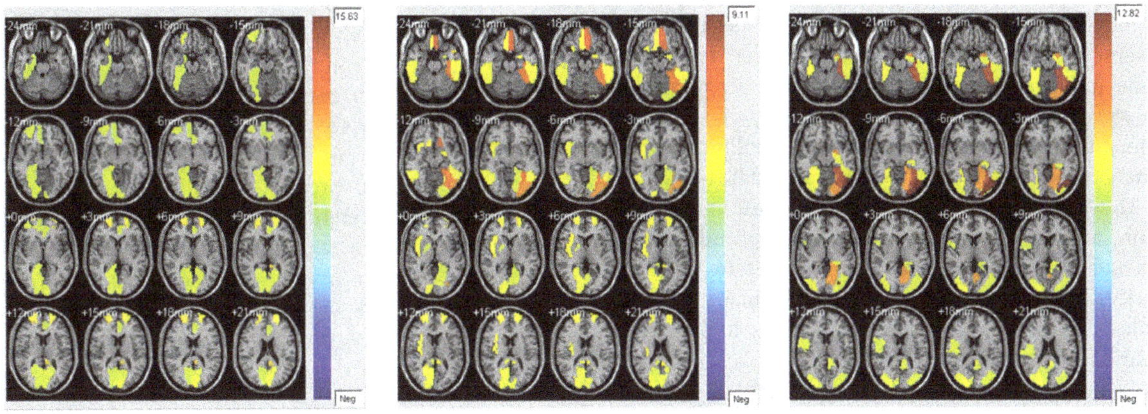

(a) (b) (c)

FIGURE 9: Fifteen subjects' superposed average results of correlated fMRI activation using the proposed method without fMRI masks (a) under negative state, (b) under reappraisal state, and (c) under neutral state.

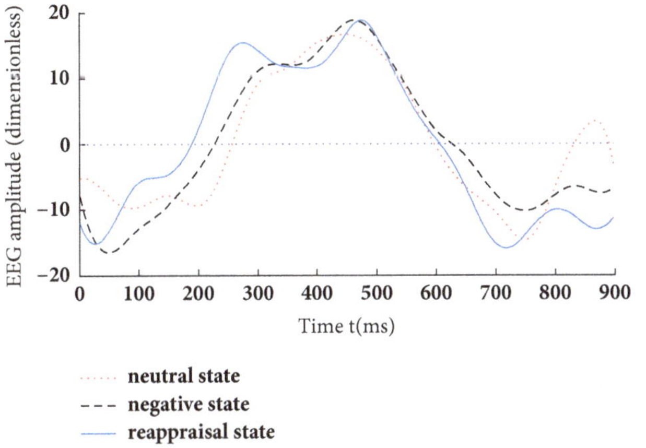

FIGURE 10: Fifteen subjects' superposed average results of EEG correlated components under three emotional states using the proposed method but without clustering mask.

his/her emotion. For spatial analysis, activation in emotion-related cerebral regions (e.g., amygdala, hippocampus, and temporal lobe) under reappraisal state is obviously weaker than that under negative state through introducing the cognitive reappraisal strategy. It reveals that negative emotion can be effectively restricted in emotion-related cerebral regions after applying cognitive reappraisal strategy. For temporal analysis, obvious differences can be observed among different LPP components which are considered to be highly correlated to emotion processing. Peak value of LPP component under reappraisal state is smaller than that under negative state, and obviously larger than that under neutral state. Both the shrunken fMRI activated regions and decreased peak value of LPP component verify the assumptions that negative emotions, e.g., sorrow, fear, and disappointment, can be restrained by using cognitive reappraisal.

Effectiveness of kernel strategy can be observed through the comparisons between KCCA and CCA. CCA fusion is widely used for symmetric EEG-fMRI analysis. However, nonlinearity of the EEG-fMRI data may decrease the fusion accuracy. Thus, we improve the CCA fusion with a kernel strategy. It is not very novel but is effective. KCCA fusion is specially designed to process nonlinear EEG-fMRI data. As shown in Table 1, relational degrees of correlated components derived using KCCA fusion are mainly larger than that derived by CCA fusion. Notably, a larger relational degree indicates a stronger relationship between two components. Thus, the results in Table 1 may indicate the superiority of KCCA fusion to traditional CCA fusion.

The superiority of KCCA fusion to CCA fusion can be also observed from the reconstructed EEG and fMRI components. For fMRI that concentrates on spatial activation, no obvious activation can be observed in hippocampus which is emotion-related under negative or reappraisal states using CCA fusion. It may be caused by the fact that CCA cannot process nonlinear EEG-fMRI data. However, obvious activation can be observed in these regions under the same emotional states using KCCA fusion. It reveals the ability of KCCA in mining effective fMRI activation from nonlinear EEG-fMRI data. For EEG that concentrates on temporal evolutions, amplitude of LPP component under reappraisal state is obviously weaker than that under negative state at the same period using KCCA fusion. The decrease in amplitude indicates the ability of cognitive reappraisal to restrain sorrowful emotion, as pointed out by [4]. However, no obvious decrease can be observed in amplitude of LPP component from negative state to reappraisal state using CCA fusion. Thus, the larger relational degrees, the more fMRI activation, and the obvious decrease in amplitude of LPP component between negative and reappraisal states reveal the superiority of KCCA fusion to CCA fusion. Such superiority is obtained due to the effect of kernel strategy in processing nonlinear EEG-fMRI data.

The superiority of symmetric EEG-fMRI analysis to EEG informed fMRI analysis can be observed through the comparisons between KCCA and GLM (Tables 2 and 3). Only fMRI activation is compared because GLM cannot be used to study the EEG evolutions. Then, for KCCA (Table 2), obvious activation can be observed under negative state in cerebral regions such as the temporal lobe, the hippocampus, the amygdala, and the cingulate gyrus. Meanwhile, activation can be observed under reappraisal state in cerebral regions such as the amygdala, the temporal lobe, the cingulate gyrus, the hippocampus, and the frontal lobe. These activation regions indicate the important role of these cerebral regions in emotional regulation. In the perspective of activated intensity (Z-score), activation in cerebral regions under reappraisal state, especially the regions (e.g., the amygdala, the hippocampus, and the temporal lobe) directly related to emotion processing, is obviously weaker than activation in those regions under negative state through using cognitive reappraisal. Activation in these cerebral regions under neutral state is much weaker than activation in the same regions under the other two states. All these results are basically consistent with the conclusions proposed by [28]. Compared with the fusion results obtained using GLM (Table 3), two results can be concluded: (1) by utilizing KCCA approach, more regions are found to be activated under negative and reappraisal states, and (2) activated intensities of these regions calculated using KCCA fusion are larger than those calculated using GLM fusion. Both results indicate the superiority of KCCA fusion (symmetric EEG-fMRI analysis) in studying the neural activity of cognitive reappraisal.

As a special preprocessing, fMRI masks are useful due to the assumption that strong fMRI activation uncorrelated with emotion processing may be correlated with EEG components, thus leading to omitting the fMRI activation which we are truly interested in. As shown in Figures 4(b), 5(b), and 6(b), obvious fMRI activation can be observed in emotion-related cerebral regions such as the hippocampus and the temporal lobe under negative and reappraisal states. However, no activation can be observed in these regions if fMRI masks are not used as preprocessing. Meanwhile, obvious decrease can be observed in EEG amplitude from negative state to reappraisal state using our fusion approach (Figure 7(a)), while little decrease can be observed under the same condition without fMRI masks (Figure 10).

Based on the above discussions, our fusion approach may provide a fine solution for analyzing simultaneous EEG-fMRI data in high resolution spatiotemporal domains. It can synchronously tell when and where the neural activities related to certain tasks such as cognitive reappraisal occur. It may also provide a useful technological means for fusion-based cerebral area positioning, ERP-induction time determination, and brain imaging feature extraction in the area of brain-human interface. Our fusion approach can be also used in paradigms which can cause LPP with further study on cognitive researches and clinical trials.

There are still some limitations in the proposed fusion approach: (1) for the data to be fused, activation in AAL ROIs is employed instead of original fMRI voxels, aiming at reducing computational complexity. As a result, one cannot study the activation of reconstructed fMRI components at voxel level. (2) Prior knowledge is necessary for our KCCA fusion approach. It is hard to choose suitable parameters that are significant for satisfactory fusion results. There is also no certain criterion in determining the threshold of relational degrees. (3) The number of enrolled subjects is far from enough; thus, the evaluations may lack persuasion. Our future work focuses on implementing EEG-fMRI fusion at voxel level instead of AAL ROIs. Thus, the spatial resolution of reconstructed fMRI components can be greatly boosted.

Conflicts of Interest

The authors declare that they have no conflicts of interest.

Authors' Contributions

Biao Yang and Tiantong Zhou contributed equally to this paper.

Acknowledgments

This work has been partially supported by the National Natural Science Foundation of China (61201096 and 61501060), the Natural Science Foundation of Jiangsu Province (BK20150271), and Qing Lan Project of Jiangsu Province.

References

[1] G. A. Bonanno, A. Papa, K. Lalande, M. Westphal, and K. Coifman, "The importance of being flexible: The ability to both enhance and suppress emotional expression predicts long-term adjustment," *Psychological Science*, vol. 15, no. 7, pp. 482–487, 2004.

[2] R. J. Davidson, K. M. Putnam, and C. L. Larson, "Dysfunction in the neural circuitry of emotion regulation—a possible prelude to violence," *Science*, vol. 289, no. 5479, pp. 591–594, 2000.

[3] D. Driscoll, D. Tranel, and S. W. Anderson, "The effects of voluntary regulation of positive and negative emotion on psychophysiological responsiveness," *International Journal of Psychophysiology*, vol. 72, no. 1, pp. 61–66, 2009.

[4] S. Paul, D. Simon, R. Kniesche, N. Kathmann, and T. Endrass, "Timing effects of antecedent- and response-focused emotion regulation strategies," *Biological Psychology*, vol. 94, no. 1, pp. 136–142, 2013.

[5] J. J. Gross, "Antecedent- and response-focused emotion regulation: divergent consequences for experience, expression, and physiology," *Journal of Personality and Social Psychology*, vol. 74, no. 1, pp. 224–237, 1998.

[6] S. H. Kim and S. Hamann, "The effect of cognitive reappraisal on physiological reactivity and emotional memory," *International Journal of Psychophysiology*, vol. 83, no. 3, pp. 348–356, 2012.

[7] G. Hajcak, A. Macnamara, and D. M. Olvet, "Event-related potentials, emotion, and emotion regulation: an integrative review," *Developmental Neuropsychology*, vol. 35, no. 2, pp. 129–155, 2010.

[8] A. MacNamara, K. N. Ochsner, and G. Hajcak, "Previously reappraised: The lasting effect of description type on picture-elicited electrocortical activity," *Social Cognitive and Affective Neuroscience*, vol. 6, no. 3, pp. 348–358, 2011.

[9] G. Hajcak, J. S. Moser, and R. F. Simons, "Attending to affect: Appraisal strategies modulate the electrocortical response to arousing pictures," *Emotion*, vol. 6, no. 3, pp. 517–522, 2006.

[10] J. W. Krompinger, J. S. Moser, and R. F. Simons, "Modulations of the Electrophysiological Response to Pleasant Stimuli by Cognitive Reappraisal," *Emotion*, vol. 8, no. 1, pp. 132–137, 2008.

[11] S. H. Kim and S. Hamann, "Neutral correlates of positive and negative emotional regulation," *Journal of Cognitive Neuroscience*, vol. 19, pp. 776–798, 2007.

[12] K. N. Ochsner, K. Knierim, D. H. Ludlow et al., "Reflecting upon feelings: An fMRI study of neural systems supporting the attribution of emotion to self and other," *Cognitive Neuroscience*, vol. 16, no. 10, pp. 1746–1772, 2004.

[13] H. L. Urry, "Using Reappraisal To Regulate Unpleasant Emotional Episodes: Goals and Timing Matter," *Emotion*, vol. 9, no. 6, pp. 782–797, 2009.

[14] S. P. Kyathanahally, A. M. Francowatkins, X. Zhang et al., "A realistic framework for investigating decision-making in the brain with high spatio-temporal resolution using simultaneous EEG/fMRI and joint ICA," *IEEE Journal of Biomedical and Health Informatics*, pp. 1-12, 2016.

[15] T. Nguyen, T. Potter, T. Nguyen, C. Karmonik, R. Grossman, and Y. Zhang, "EEG Source Imaging Guided by Spatiotemporal Specific fMRI: Toward an Understanding of Dynamic Cognitive Processes," *Neural Plasticity*, vol. 2016, Article ID 4182483, 10 pages, 2016.

[16] Y. L. Liu, J. Bengson, H. Q. Huang et al., "Top-down modulation of neural activity in anticipatory visual attention: control mechanisms revealed by simultaneous EEG-fMRI," *Neuroscience*, vol. 35, no. 20, pp. 7938–7949, 2015.

[17] R. F. Ahmad, A. S. Malik, N. Kamel, F. Reza, H. U. Amin, and M. Hussain, "Visual brain activity patterns classification with simultaneous EEG-fMRI: A multimodal approach," *Technology and Health Care*, vol. 25, no. 3, pp. 471–485, 2017.

[18] Q. Yu, L. Wu, D. A. Bridwell et al., "Building an EEG-fMRI Multi-Modal Brain Graph: A Concurrent EEG-fMRI Study," *Frontiers in Human Neuroscience*, vol. 10, 2016.

[19] N. M. Correa, T. Eichele, T. Adali, Y.-O. Li, and V. D. Calhoun, "Multi-set canonical correlation analysis for the fusion of concurrent single trial ERP and functional MRI," *NeuroImage*, vol. 50, no. 4, pp. 1438–1445, 2010.

[20] L. Dong, P. Wang, Y. Bin et al., "Local Multimodal Serial Analysis for Fusing EEG-fMRI: A New Method to Study Familial Cortical Myoclonic Tremor and Epilepsy," *IEEE Transactions on Autonomous Mental Development*, vol. 7, no. 4, pp. 311–319, 2015.

[21] L. Yuan, R. Zhou, and S. Hu, "Cognitive reappraisal of facial expressions: Electrophysiological evidence of social anxiety," *Neuroscience Letters*, vol. 577, pp. 45–50, 2014.

[22] J. M. Carlson, D. Foti, L. R. Mujica-Parodi, E. Harmon-Jones, and G. Hajcak, "Ventral striatal and medial prefrontal BOLD activation is correlated with reward-related electrocortical activity: a combined ERP and fMRI study," *NeuroImage*, vol. 57, no. 4, pp. 1608–1616, 2011.

[23] D. Yao, "A method to standardize a reference of scalp EEG recordings to a point at infinity," *Physiological Measurement*, vol. 22, no. 4, pp. 693–711, 2001.

[24] Y. Qin, P. Xu, and D. Yao, "A comparative study of different references for EEG default mode network: The use of the infinity reference," *Clinical Neurophysiology*, vol. 121, no. 12, pp. 1981–1991, 2010.

[25] Y. Tian and D. Yao, "Why do we need to use a zero reference? Reference influences on the ERPs of audiovisual effects," *Psychophysiology*, vol. 50, no. 12, pp. 1282–1290, 2013.

[26] H. J. Dong, "Exotic collections asset pricing: the Lagrangian Optimization," *British Journal of Mathematics & Computer Science*, vol. 5, no. 1, pp. 82–91, 2015.

[27] L. Zou, Y. Yan, and B. Yang, "Feature fusion analysis of simultaneously recorded EEG-fMRI in emotion cognitive reappraisal," *Acat Automatica Sinica*, vol. 42, no. 5, pp. 771–781, 2016.

[28] N. Tzourio-Mazoyer, B. Landeau, D. Papathanassiou et al., "Automated anatomical labeling of activations in SPM using a macroscopic anatomical parcellation of the MNI MRI single-subject brain," *NeuroImage*, vol. 15, no. 1, pp. 273–289, 2002.

[29] L. Zou, Y. Xu, Z. Y. Jiang et al., "Functional connectivity analysis of cognitive reappraisal using sparse spectral clustering method," in *Proceedings of the Fifth International Conference on Cognitive Neurodynamics*, pp. 291–297, 2016.

17

Stochastic Periodic Solution of a Susceptible-Infective Epidemic Model in a Polluted Environment under Environmental Fluctuation

Yu Zhao,[1,2] Jiangping Li,[1] and Xu Ma[2]

[1]School of Public Health and Management, Ningxia Medical University, Ningxia, Yinchuan 750004, China
[2]School of Mathematics and Computer Science, Ningxia Normal University, Ningxia, Guyuan 756000, China

Correspondence should be addressed to Xu Ma; maxu@nxnu.edu.cn

Academic Editor: Chung-Min Liao

It is well known that the pollution and environmental fluctuations may seriously affect the outbreak of infectious diseases (e.g., measles). Therefore, understanding the association between the periodic outbreak of an infectious disease and noise and pollution still needs further development. Here we consider a stochastic susceptible-infective (SI) epidemic model in a polluted environment, which incorporates both environmental fluctuations as well as pollution. First, the existence of the global positive solution is discussed. Thereafter, the sufficient conditions for the nontrivial stochastic periodic solution and the boundary periodic solution of disease extinction are derived, respectively. Numerical simulation is also conducted in order to support the theoretical results. Our study shows that (i) large intensity noise may help the control of periodic outbreak of infectious disease; (ii) pollution may significantly affect the peak level of infective population and cause adverse health effects on the exposed population. These results can help increase the understanding of periodic outbreak patterns of infectious diseases.

1. Introduction

In Northern China, coal fire-power industries and heating systems, as well as vehicle emissions, all conduce to air pollution (airborne fine particulate matter $PM_{2.5}$, PM_{10}, and SO_2, etc.), which has threatened the survival of exposed human population and affected the transmission of infectious diseases [1, 2]. Numerous studies have provided cumulative evidence of the health effects of particulate air pollution on the spread of infectious diseases (e.g., measles) [3, 4]. Therefore, investigating the role of pollution on the outbreak of infectious diseases is one of the most interesting and meaningful issues in the recent past [5].

Dynamic mathematical models have provided a deeper understanding of the transmission process of infectious diseases [6, 7]. There are many interesting results (see, e.g., [8–10]), which show that the simple susceptible-infective (SI) model can fit the transmission process of some diseases (measles, chicken pox, etc.) well. Thus, based on the interaction between the environment and the population (see Figure 1), we incorporate the environmental pollution into the SI epidemic model. Let $S(t)$, $I(t)$, $C_0(t)$, and $C_e(t)$ denote the number of people in the susceptible population, the number of people in the infective population, and the concentration of pollution in the organism and in the environment at time t, respectively. The SI epidemic model in a polluted environment is as follows:

$$\begin{aligned}
\frac{dS(t)}{dt} &= \gamma S(t)\left(1-\frac{S(t)+I(t)}{K}\right)-\beta S(t)I(t) \\
&\quad - r_{10}C_0(t)S(t)-\xi S(t), \\
\frac{dI(t)}{dt} &= \beta S(t)I(t)-r_{20}C_0(t)I(t)-\nu I(t), \\
\frac{dC_0(t)}{dt} &= \alpha C_e(t)-(g+m)C_0(t), \\
\frac{dC_e(t)}{dt} &= u(t)-hC_e(t);
\end{aligned} \tag{1}$$

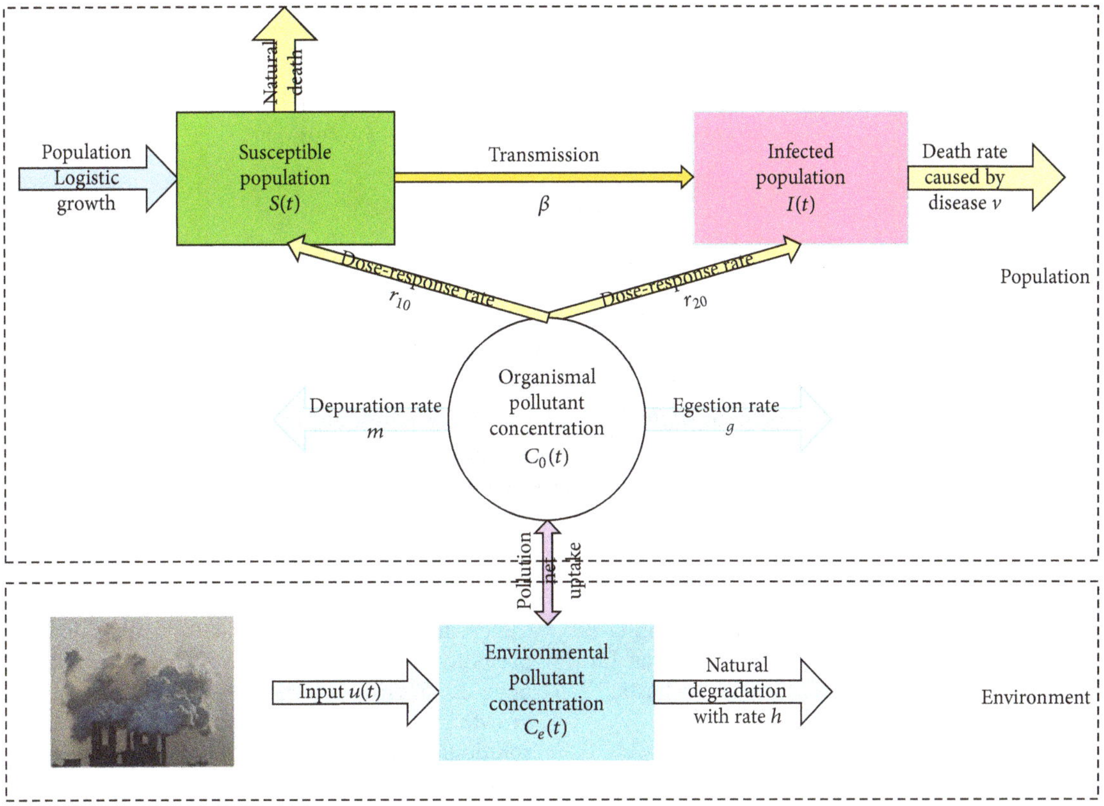

FIGURE 1: Flow chart of the interaction between environmental pollution and population, and the disease transmits from the susceptible subpopulation to infected subpopulation.

all of the parameters are positive constants and the corresponding biological meanings are listed in Table 1. Liu et al. [8] obtained the sufficient conditions of the ultimate boundedness of solutions and the global asymptotical stability of the equilibria.

In real situations, as was pointed by Britton et al. [11], the transmission of infectious diseases is inevitably disrupted by unpredictable environmental conditions (e.g., absolute humidity [12], temperature [13]) making it more appropriate to use a stochastic model for biological parameters. For example, Yang et al. [14] observed the nonlinear effects of temperature and relative humidity on the incidence of measles. Thus, it is reasonable to model the environmental fluctuation as a stochastic transmission coefficient [15, 16]. If the transmission parameter β in the model (1) is subjected to some random environmental effects (temperature, humidity, etc.), then it is natural to consider that the transmission rate β is replaced by a random variable:

$$\widetilde{\beta} = \beta + \sigma\varsigma(t), \qquad (2)$$

where $\varsigma(t)$ is the Gaussian white noise with mean zero and variance one, $\varsigma(t) = dB(t)/dt$, and $B(t)$ is a scalar Wiener Process defined in $(\Omega, \mathcal{F}, \{\mathcal{F}_t\}_{t\geq 0}, P)$, which is a complete probability space with a filtration $\{\mathcal{F}_t\}_{t\geq 0}$ satisfying the usual conditions (i.e., it is right continuous and $\mathcal{F}_0$ contains all P-null sets). σ is the intensity of the white noise. Thus, we can incorporate the environmental white noises into model (3):

$$\begin{aligned}
dS(t) - S(t) & \\
&\cdot \left[\gamma\left(1 - \frac{S(t)+I(t)}{K}\right) - \beta I(t) - r_{10}C_0(t) - \xi\right] dt \\
&- \sigma S(t) I(t) dB(t), \\
dI(t) &= I(t)\left[\beta S(t) - r_{20}C_0(t) - v\right] dt + \sigma S(t) \\
&\cdot I(t) dB(t), \\
\frac{dC_0(t)}{dt} &= \alpha C_e(t) - (g+m) C_0(t), \\
\frac{dC_e(t)}{dt} &= u(t) - hC_e(t).
\end{aligned} \qquad (3)$$

Moreover, outbreaks of infectious diseases always fluctuate over time and exhibit seasonal patterns of incidence [17]. Ferrari et al. [18] pointed out that outbreaks of measles in the tropics have more variable seasonal patterns driven by accumulation and decline of susceptible individuals. Regular oscillatory patterns of measles outbreaks in Baltimore (USA) with an average period of three years have also been reported [19]. To describe the seasonal effect in the model, many

TABLE 1: Biological meanings of the parameters in model (1).

Parameters	Biological meanings	Unit
γ	The intrinsic growth rate in absence of the toxicant	t^{-1}
K	Carrying capacity of the population in absence of the toxicant	Person
β	Probability of infection	-
ξ	The population natural death rate	t^{-1}
v	The death rate caused by disease	t^{-1}
r_{10}	The dose-response rate due to uptake of pollution for the susceptible	t^{-1}
r_{20}	The dose-response rate due to uptake of pollution for the infected	t^{-1}
α	The organisms net uptake rate of pollution from environment	t^{-1}
g	The egestion rate of pollution in the organism (metabolism)	t^{-1}
m	The depuration rate of pollution in the organism	t^{-1}
h	The environmental pollution loss rate due to natural degradation	t^{-1}
$u(t)$	The exogenous rate of pollutant input into the environment	t^{-1}

existing studies [20–23] assume that the system parameters are subjected to a periodic rhythm. Therefore, we can further consider the following nonautonomous stochastic SI epidemic model as follows:

$$\begin{aligned} dS(t) &= S(t)\left[\gamma(t)\left(1-\frac{S(t)+I(t)}{K(t)}\right)-\beta(t)I(t)\right. \\ &\quad \left. - r_{10}(t)C_0(t)-\xi(t)\right]dt-\sigma(t)S(t)I(t)\,dB(t), \\ dI(t) &= I(t)\left[\beta(t)S(t)-r_{20}(t)C_0(t)-v(t)\right]dt \\ &\quad +\sigma(t)S(t)I(t)\,dB(t), \\ \frac{dC_0(t)}{dt} &= \alpha C_e(t)-(g+m)C_0(t), \\ \frac{dC_e(t)}{dt} &= u(t)-hC_e(t), \end{aligned} \tag{4}$$

with initial data

$$\begin{aligned} S(0) &= S_0 \geq 0, \\ I(0) &= I_0 \geq 0, \\ 0 &\leq C_0(0) \leq 1, \\ 0 &\leq C_e(0) \leq 1, \end{aligned} \tag{5}$$

where $\gamma(t)$, $K(t)$, $\beta(t)$, $r_{10}(t)$, $r_{20}(t)$, $\xi(t)$, $\sigma(t)$ are all positive, bounded, continuous θ-periodic functions.

Considering the periodic variation and pollution exposure of epidemic models and exploring the existence of stochastic periodic solutions are meaningful to predict and control the outbreaks of infectious diseases. Such analysis has benefited from the theoretical contributions about the nonautonomous stochastic system [24, 25]. We also see that there has been some research in this respect [20, 21, 26, 27]. For example, Jiang et al. [21] considered a stochastic nonautonomous competitive Lotka-Volterra model in a polluted environment and then derived sufficient criteria for the existence and global attractivity of a nontrivial positive periodic solution. Xie et al. [27] presented a stochastic hepatitis B virus infection model with logistic hepatocyte growth and showed that the model has at least one periodic solution. More related results can be found in [22, 28, 29]. To the best of our knowledge, there are few results about the periodic solution of a stochastic SI epidemic model in a polluted environment. Therefore, the main objective of this paper is to concentrate on the effects of pollution and environmental fluctuation on the existence of the positive periodic solution.

The rest of this paper is organized as follows: in the next Section 2, we present the underlying mathematical analysis: the existence of the global positive solution, the sufficient conditions for the nontrivial stochastic periodic solution, and the boundary periodic solution of disease extinction are derived. The subsequent Section 3 describes the numerical simulation, based on the case of measles, carried out to support the theoretical results. Finally, in the last Section 4, the conclusion is presented.

2. Mathematical Analysis

2.1. Preliminary. Since $C_0(t)$, $C_e(t)$ are the concentrations of the pollution and $0 \leq C_0(t) < 1$ and $0 \leq C_e(t) < 1$ must be satisfied, we assume the following.

Assumption 1 ($0 < \alpha \leq g+m$, $u(t) \leq h$). Notice that $u(t)$ is a positive θ-periodic continuous function, so we can prove the following.

Lemma 2. *For model (4), we have* $\lim_{t\to\infty}|C_0(t)-C_0^*(t)| = 0$; *here*

$$C_0^*(t) = \frac{\int_t^{t+\theta} e^{(g+m)(s-t)}\alpha C_e(s)\,ds}{e^{(g+m)\theta}-1}. \tag{6}$$

The proof of this lemma is provided in Appendix.

From now on, we will only consider the following system:

$$dS(t) = S(t)\left[\gamma(t)\left(1-\frac{S(t)+I(t)}{K(t)}\right)-\beta(t)I(t) - r_{10}(t)C_0^*(t)-\xi(t)\right]dt - \sigma(t)S(t)I(t)dB(t),$$
$$dI(t) = I(t)\left[\beta(t)S(t)-r_{20}(t)C_0^*(t)-v(t)\right]dt + \sigma(t)S(t)I(t)dB(t). \quad (7)$$

For a bounded function on $[0,\infty)$, say, $f(t)$, define

$$f^u = \sup_{t\in[0,\infty)} f(t),$$
$$f^l = \inf_{t\in[0,\infty)} f(t), \quad (8)$$
$$\langle f\rangle_\theta = \frac{1}{\theta}\int_0^\theta f(s)\,ds.$$

Now, we shall give some definitions and Lemmas with respect to the periodic Markov process $X(t)$ as the solution of stochastic system

$$X(t) = X(t_0) + \int_{t_0}^t b(s,X(s))\,ds + \sum_{r=1}^k \int_{t_0}^t \sigma_r(s,X(s))\,dB_r(s), \quad x\in\mathbb{R}^l. \quad (9)$$

Definition 3 (see [24]). A stochastic process $\xi(t) = \xi(t,\omega)$ $(-\infty < t < \infty)$ is said to be periodic with period θ, if for every finite sequence of numbers $t_1, t_2, \ldots, t_n$ the joint distribution of the random variables $\xi(t_1+h),\ldots,\xi(t_n+h)$ is independent of h, where $h = k\theta$, $k = \pm1, \pm2, \ldots$.

Remark 4. It follows from [24] that a stochastic Markov process $X(t)$ is θ-periodic if and only if its transition probability function is θ-periodic and the function $\mathcal{P}_0(t,A) = \mathcal{P}\{X(t)\in A\}$ satisfies

$$\mathcal{P}_0(s,A) = \int_{\mathbb{R}^l} \mathcal{P}_0(s,dx)\,\mathcal{P}(s,x,s+\theta,A) \equiv \mathcal{P}_0(s+\theta,A), \quad (10)$$

for every $A\in\mathfrak{B}$, where $\mathfrak{B}$ denotes the Borel σ-algebra in $\mathbb{R}^l$.

Let $\mathcal{L}$ be a linear operator defined by

$$\mathcal{L} = \frac{\partial}{\partial t} + \sum_{i=1}^n b_i(t,x)\frac{\partial}{\partial x_i} + \frac{1}{2}\sum_{i,j=1}^n a_{ij}\frac{\partial^2}{\partial x_i \partial x_j},$$
$$a_{ij} = \sum_{r=1}^k \sigma_r^i(t,x)\,\sigma_r^j(t,x). \quad (11)$$

Lemma 5 (see [24]). *Suppose that the coefficients of system (13) are θ-periodic in t and satisfy*

$$|b(s,x)-b(s,y)| + \sum_{r=1}^k |\sigma_r(s,x)-\sigma_r(s,x)| \le C|x-y|, \quad (12)$$
$$|b(s,x)| + \sum_{r=1}^k |\sigma_r(s,x)| \le C(1+|x|),$$

in every cylinder $I\times U$, where C is a constant; and suppose further that there exists a function $V(t,x)\in\mathbb{R}^l$ which is θ-periodic in t, satisfying

$$\inf_{|x|>R} V(t,x) \longrightarrow \infty, \quad \text{as } R\longrightarrow\infty, \quad (13)$$

$$\mathcal{L}V(t,x) \le -1, \quad \text{outside some compact set.} \quad (14)$$

Then, there exists a solution of system (9) which is a θ-periodic Markov process.

Remark 6. According to the proof of Lemma 2.1 in [24], condition (14) is only used to guarantee the existence and uniqueness of the solution of system (9).

Next, we have the following theorem.

Theorem 7. *For any given initial value (5), model (7) has a unique positive solution $(S(t), I(t))$ on $t\ge 0$, and the solution will remain in $\mathbb{R}_+^2$ with probability one.*

The proof of this Theorem is provided in Appendix.

2.2. Existence of the Positive Stochastic Periodic Solution. In this section, we shall prove the existence of a positive stochastic periodic solution of models (4) and (7). Firstly, we define

$$\lambda_0 = \frac{1}{\theta}\int_0^\theta \left\{\gamma(s) - \left[r_{10}(s)+r_{20}(s)\right]C_0^*(s) - \frac{1}{2}\left(\frac{\gamma^u K^u}{\gamma^l}\right)^2\sigma^2(s) - \xi(s) - v(s)\right\}ds. \quad (15)$$

Now, we obtain the following result regarding the existence of a positive periodic solution of model (7).

Theorem 8. *If $\lambda_\theta > 0$, then model (7) at least has one positive θ-periodic solution $(S^*(t), I^*(t))$.*

Proof. To prove the existence of a positive θ-periodic solution of model (7), it follows from Lemma 2 and Remark 6 that we need to find a C^2-function $V(t,S,I)$ and a closed set $\Theta\in\mathbb{R}_+^2$ such that (13) and (14) hold. Firstly, we assume that $\gamma^u + \gamma^u/K^l - \beta^l - (r_{10}C_0^* + \xi)^l > 0$ and define a nonnegative function as follows:

$$V(t,S,I) = V_1(t,S) + V_2(t,S,I) + V_3(t), \quad (16)$$

where

$$V_1(t,S) = -M\ln S(t) - M\ln I(t),$$

$$V_2(t,S,I) = \frac{1}{2}(S(t)+I(t))^2 + M(S(t)+I(t)),$$

$$V_3(t) = M\overline{\omega}(t),$$

$$M = \frac{2}{\lambda_\theta}\max\left\{1, \sup_{(S,I)\in\mathbb{R}_+^2}\left\{-\frac{\gamma^l}{K^u}S^3 + \left[\gamma^u - (r_{10}C_0^* + \xi)^l - M\frac{\gamma^l}{K^u} + (\sigma^u)^2 I^2\right]\cdot S^2 + \left[\gamma^u - (r_{20}C_0^* + \nu)^l - (r_{10}C_0^* + \xi)^l - M\frac{\gamma^l}{K^u}\right]SI - (r_{20}C_0^* + \nu)^l I^2 + M\left[\frac{\gamma^u}{K^l} + \gamma^u - \beta^l - (r_{10}C_0^* + \xi)^l\right]S + M\left[\frac{\gamma^u}{K^l} + \beta^u - (r_{20}C_0^* + \nu)^l\right]I\right\}\right\}. \quad (17)$$

It is easy to see that $M\lambda_\theta/2 \geq 1$ and $\overline{\omega}(t)$ satisfies the following:

$$\dot{\overline{\omega}}(t) = -\lambda_\theta + \gamma(t) - [r_{10}(t) + r_{20}(t)]C_0^*(t) - \frac{1}{2}\left(\frac{\gamma^u K^u}{\gamma^l}\right)^2\sigma^2(t) - \xi(t) - \nu(t), \quad (18)$$

$$\overline{\omega}(0) = 0.$$

Integrating (18) from t to $t+\theta$ yields

$$\overline{\omega}(t+\theta) - \overline{\omega}(t) = \int_t^{t+\theta}\dot{\overline{\omega}}(s)\,ds = \int_t^{t+\theta}\left[-\lambda_\theta + \gamma(s) - [r_{10}(s) + r_{20}(s)]C_0^*(s) - \frac{1}{2}\left(\frac{\gamma^u K^u}{\gamma^l}\right)^2\sigma^2(s) - \xi(s) - \nu(s)\right]ds - \int_0^\theta\left[-\lambda_\theta + \gamma(s) - [r_{10}(s) + r_{20}(s)]C_0^*(s) - \frac{1}{2}\left(\frac{\gamma^u K^u}{\gamma^l}\right)^2\sigma^2(s) - \xi(s) - \nu(s)\right]ds = 0. \quad (19)$$

Thus, we can see that $\overline{\omega}(t)$ is a θ-periodic function on $[0,\infty)$ and

$$\liminf_{\epsilon\to 0,(S,I)\in\mathbb{R}_+^2\setminus\Theta_\epsilon} V(t,S,I) = \infty, \quad (20)$$

where $\Theta_\epsilon = \{(S,I) : (S,I) \in (\epsilon, 1/\epsilon)\times(\epsilon, 1/\epsilon)\}$. Thus, $V(t,S,I)$ is θ-periodic with respect to t.

Now, we have the requisite information to verify (14) in Lemma 5. Applying the Itô formula to $V(t,S,I)$, one can obtain

$$\begin{aligned}\mathscr{L}V_1 &= -M\left[\gamma(t) - \frac{\gamma(t)}{k(t)}(S+I) - r_{10}(t)C_0^*(t) - \beta(t)I - \xi(t) - \frac{\sigma^2(t)I^2}{2} + \beta(t)S - r_{20}(t)C_0^*(t) - \nu(t) - \frac{\sigma^2(t)S^2}{2}\right] \leq M\left\{-[\gamma(t) - (r_{10}(t) + r_{20}(t))C_0^*(t) - \xi(t) - \nu(t)] + \frac{\gamma^u}{K^l}S + \left(\frac{\gamma^u}{K^l} + \beta^u\right)I + \left(\frac{\gamma^u K^u}{\gamma^l}\right)^2\sigma^2(t) - \beta^l S\right\}\\ &= M\left\{-\left[\gamma(t) - (r_{10}(t) + r_{20}(t))C_0^*(t) - \frac{1}{2}\left(\frac{\gamma^u K^u}{\gamma^l}\right)^2\sigma^2(t) - \xi(t) - \nu(t)\right] + \frac{\gamma^u}{K^l}S + \left(\frac{\gamma^u}{K^l} + \beta^u\right)I - \beta^l S\right\},\end{aligned}$$

$$\begin{aligned}\mathscr{L}V_2 &= (S+I)\left[\gamma(t)S\left(1 - \frac{S+I}{K(t)}\right) - (r_{10}(t)C_0^*(t) + \xi(t))S - (r_{20}(t)C_0^*(t) + \nu(t))I\right] + M\left[\gamma(t)\cdot S\left(1 - \frac{S+I}{K(t)}\right) - (r_{10}(t)C_0^*(t) + \xi(t))S - (r_{20}(t)C_0^*(t) + \nu(t))I\right] + \sigma^2(t)S^2I^2 \leq \gamma^u S^2\\ &- \frac{\gamma^l}{K^u}S^3 - \frac{\gamma^l}{K^u}S^2 I - (r_{10}C_0^* + \xi)^l S^2 - (r_{20}C_0^* + \nu)^l\cdot SI - \frac{\gamma^l}{K^u}S^2 I - \frac{\gamma^l}{K^u}SI^2 - (r_{10}C_0^* + \xi)^l SI - (r_{20}C_0^* + \nu)^l I^2 + \gamma^u SI + (\sigma^u)^2 S^2 I^2 + M\gamma^u S - M\frac{\gamma^l}{K^u}S^2 - M\frac{\gamma^l}{K^u}IS - M(r_{10}C_0^* + \xi)^l S - M(r_{20}C_0^* + \nu)^l I\\ &\leq \left\{-\frac{\gamma^l}{K^u}S^3 + \left[\gamma^u - (r_{10}C_0^* + \xi)^l - M\frac{\gamma^l}{K^u} + (\sigma^u)^2 I^2\right]S^2 - (r_{20}C_0^* + \nu)^l I^2 + \left[\gamma^u - (r_{20}C_0^* + \nu)^l - (r_{10}C_0^* + \xi)^l - M\frac{\gamma^l}{K^u}\right]SI + M\left[\gamma^u - (r_{10}C_0^* + \xi)^l\right]S - M(r_{20}C_0^* + \nu)^l I\right\}.\end{aligned} \quad (21)$$

From (18) and (21), we can get that

$$\begin{aligned}
\mathscr{L}V &= -M\lambda_\theta + M\left(\frac{\gamma^u}{K^l} - \beta^l\right)S + M\left(\frac{\gamma^u}{K^l} + \beta^u\right)I \\
&- \frac{\gamma^l}{K^u}S^3 \\
&+ \left[\gamma^u - (r_{10}C_0^* + \xi)^l - M\frac{\gamma^l}{K^u} + (\sigma^u)^2 I^2\right]S^2 \\
&- (r_{20}C_0^* + v)^l I^2 \\
&+ \left[\gamma^u - (r_{20}C_0^* + v)^l - (r_{10}C_0^* + \xi)^l - M\frac{\gamma^l}{K^u}\right]SI \\
&+ M\left[\gamma^u - (r_{10}C_0^* + \xi)^l\right]S - M(r_{20}C_0^* + v)^l I.
\end{aligned} \tag{22}$$

Define a closed set

$$\Theta_\epsilon = \left\{(S, I) \in \mathbb{R}_+^2 : \epsilon \le S \le \frac{1}{\epsilon},\ \epsilon \le I \le \frac{1}{\epsilon}\right\}, \tag{23}$$

where $0 < \epsilon < 1$ is a sufficiently small number such that

$$\begin{aligned}
&- M\lambda_\theta + M\left[\frac{\gamma^u}{K^l} + \gamma^u - \beta^l - (r_{10}C_0^* + \xi)^l\right]\epsilon + C_1 \\
&\le -1,
\end{aligned} \tag{24}$$

$$- M\lambda_\theta - M\left[\beta^l + (r_{10}C_0^* + \xi)^l\right]\frac{1}{\epsilon} + C_2 \le -1, \tag{25}$$

$$- M\lambda_\theta - (r_{20}C_0^* + v)^l \frac{1}{\epsilon} + C_3 \le -1, \tag{26}$$

where C_i, $i = 1, 2, 3$ are positive constants defined in (29), (32), and (34) later. Moreover, we denote

$$\begin{aligned}
\Theta_\epsilon^1 &= \left\{(S, I) \in \mathbb{R}_+^2 : 0 < S < \epsilon\right\}, \\
\Theta_\epsilon^2 &= \left\{(S, I) \in \mathbb{R}_+^2 : 0 < I < \epsilon\right\}, \\
\Theta_\epsilon^3 &= \left\{(S, I) \in \mathbb{R}_+^2 : S > \frac{1}{\epsilon}\right\}, \\
\Theta_\epsilon^4 &= \left\{(S, I) \in \mathbb{R}_+^2 : I > \frac{1}{\epsilon}\right\}.
\end{aligned} \tag{27}$$

Then $\Theta_\epsilon^c = \mathbb{R}_+^2 \setminus \Theta_\epsilon = \Theta_\epsilon^1 \cup \Theta_\epsilon^2 \cup \Theta_\epsilon^3 \cup \Theta_\epsilon^4$. Next, we shall prove $\mathscr{L}V(t, S, I) \le -1$ on $[0, \infty] \times \Theta_\epsilon^c$.

Case 1. On Θ_ϵ^1, we have $0 < S < \epsilon$:

$$\begin{aligned}
\mathscr{L}V &= -M\lambda_\theta + M\left[\frac{\gamma^u}{K^l} + \gamma^u - \beta^l - (r_{10}C_0^* + \xi)^l\right]S \\
&- \frac{\gamma^l}{K^u}S^3 \\
&+ \left[\gamma^u - (r_{10}C_0^* + \xi)^l - M\frac{\gamma^l}{K^u} + (\sigma^u)^2 I^2\right]S^2 \\
&- (r_{20}C_0^* + v)^l I^2 \\
&+ \left[\gamma^u - (r_{20}C_0^* + v)^l - (r_{10}C_0^* + \xi)^l - M\frac{\gamma^l}{K^u}\right]SI \\
&+ M\left[\frac{\gamma^u}{K^l} + \beta^u - (r_{20}C_0^* + v)^l\right]I \\
&\le -M\lambda_\theta + M\left[\frac{\gamma^u}{K^l} - \beta^l + \gamma^u - (r_{10}C_0^* + \xi)^l\right]\epsilon \\
&+ C_1,
\end{aligned} \tag{28}$$

where

$$\begin{aligned}
C_1 = \sup_{(S,I)\in\mathbb{R}_+^2} &\left\{-\frac{\gamma^l}{K^u}S^3\right. \\
&+ \left[\gamma^u - (r_{10}C_0^* + \xi)^l - M\frac{\gamma^l}{K^u} + (\sigma^u)^2 I^2\right]S^2 \\
&- (r_{20}C_0^* + v)^l I^2 \\
&+ \left[\gamma^u - (r_{20}C_0^* + v)^l - (r_{10}C_0^* + \xi)^l - M\frac{\gamma^l}{K^u}\right]SI \\
&\left.- M\left[(r_{20}C_0^* + v)^l - \frac{\gamma^u}{K^l} - \beta^u\right]I\right\}.
\end{aligned} \tag{29}$$

Therefore, we can say that $\mathscr{L}V(t, S, I) \le -1$ on $[0, \infty] \times \Theta_\epsilon^1$ in lieu of (24).

Case 2. On Θ_ϵ^2, we have $0 < I < \epsilon$:

$$\begin{aligned}
\mathscr{L}V \le -\frac{M\lambda_\theta}{2} + &\left\{-\frac{M\lambda_\theta}{2} + \sup_{(S,I)\in\mathbb{R}_+^2}\left\{-\frac{\gamma^l}{K^u}S^3\right.\right. \\
&+ \left[\gamma^u - (r_{10}C_0^* + \xi)^l - M\frac{\gamma^l}{K^u} + (\sigma^u)^2 I^2\right]S^2 \\
&- (r_{20}C_0^* + v)^l I^2 \\
&+ \left[\gamma^u - (r_{20}C_0^* + v)^l - (r_{10}C_0^* + \xi)^l - M\frac{\gamma^l}{K^u}\right]SI
\end{aligned}$$

$$+ M\left[\frac{\gamma^u}{K^l} + \gamma^u - \beta^l - \left(r_{10}C_0^* + \xi\right)^l\right] S$$
$$+ M\left[\frac{\gamma^u}{K^l} + \beta^u - \left(r_{20}C_0^* + \nu\right)^l\right] I\bigg\}\bigg\}. \tag{30}$$

It follows from the definition of M that $\mathscr{L}V \le -M\lambda_\theta/2 \le -1$, which implies $\mathscr{L}V(t,S,I) \le -1$ on $[0,\infty] \times \Theta_\epsilon^2$.

Case 3. On Θ_ϵ^3, we have $S > 1/\epsilon$:

$$\begin{aligned}\mathscr{L}V &= -M\lambda_\theta - M\left[\beta^l + \left(r_{10}C_0^* + \xi\right)^l\right] S + \bigg\{-\frac{\gamma^l}{K^u}S^3 \\ &+ \left[\gamma^u - \left(r_{10}C_0^* + \xi\right)^l - M\frac{\gamma^l}{K^u} + \left(\sigma^u\right)^2 I^2\right] S^2 \\ &- \left(r_{20}C_0^* + \nu\right)^l I^2 \\ &+ \left[\gamma^u - \left(r_{20}C_0^* + \nu\right)^l - \left(r_{10}C_0^* + \xi\right)^l - M\frac{\gamma^l}{K^u}\right] SI \\ &+ M\left[\frac{\gamma^u}{K^l} + \beta^u - \left(r_{20}C_0^* + \nu\right)^l\right] I \\ &+ M\left(\frac{\gamma^u}{K^l} + \gamma^u\right) S\bigg\} \le -M\lambda_\theta - M\Big[\beta^l \\ &+ \left(r_{10}C_0^* + \xi\right)^l\Big] \frac{1}{\epsilon} + C_2,\end{aligned} \tag{31}$$

where

$$\begin{aligned}C_2 = \sup_{(S,I)\in\mathbb{R}_+^2} &\bigg\{-\frac{\gamma^l}{K^u}S^3 \\ &+ \left[\gamma^u - \left(r_{10}C_0^* + \xi\right)^l - M\frac{\gamma^l}{K^u} + \left(\sigma^u\right)^2 I^2\right] S^2 \\ &- \left(r_{20}C_0^* + \nu\right)^l I^2 \\ &+ \left[\gamma^u - \left(r_{20}C_0^* + \nu\right)^l - \left(r_{10}C_0^* + \xi\right)^l - M\frac{\gamma^l}{K^u}\right] SI \\ &+ M\left[\frac{\gamma^u}{K^l} + \beta^u - \left(r_{20}C_0^* + \nu\right)^l\right] I \\ &+ M\left(\frac{\gamma^u}{K^l} + \gamma^u\right) S\bigg\}.\end{aligned} \tag{32}$$

According to (25), one can get that $\mathscr{L}V(t,S,I) \le -1$ on $[0,\infty] \times \Theta_\epsilon^3$.

Case 4. On Θ_ϵ^4, we have $I > 1/\epsilon$:

$$\begin{aligned}\mathscr{L}V &= -M\lambda_\theta - \left(r_{20}C_0^* + \nu\right)^l I + \bigg\{-\frac{\gamma^l}{K^u}S^3 \\ &+ \left[\gamma^u - \left(r_{10}C_0^* + \xi\right)^l - M\frac{\gamma^l}{K^u} + \left(\sigma^u\right)^2 I^2\right] S^2 \\ &- \left(r_{20}C_0^* + \nu\right)^l I^2 \\ &+ \left[\gamma^u - \left(r_{20}C_0^* + \nu\right)^l - \left(r_{10}C_0^* + \xi\right)^l - M\frac{\gamma^l}{K^u}\right] SI \\ &+ M\left(\frac{\gamma^u}{K^l} + \beta^u\right) I \\ &+ M\left[\frac{\gamma^u}{K^l} + \gamma^u - \beta^l - \left(r_{10}C_0^* + \xi\right)^l\right] S\bigg\} \le -M\lambda_\theta \\ &- \left(r_{20}C_0^* + \nu\right)^l \frac{1}{\epsilon} + C_3,\end{aligned} \tag{33}$$

where

$$\begin{aligned}C_3 = \sup_{(S,I)\in\mathbb{R}_+^2} &\bigg\{-\frac{\gamma^l}{K^u}S^3 \\ &+ \left[\gamma^u - \left(r_{10}C_0^* + \xi\right)^l - M\frac{\gamma^l}{K^u} + \left(\sigma^u\right)^2 I^2\right] S^2 \\ &- \left(r_{20}C_0^* + \nu\right)^l I^2 \\ &+ \left[\gamma^u - \left(r_{20}C_0^* + \nu\right)^l - \left(r_{10}C_0^* + \xi\right)^l - M\frac{\gamma^l}{K^u}\right] SI \\ &+ M\left(\frac{\gamma^u}{K^l} + \beta^u\right) I \\ &+ M\left[\frac{\gamma^u}{K^l} + \gamma^u - \beta^l - \left(r_{10}C_0^* + \xi\right)^l\right] S\bigg\}.\end{aligned} \tag{34}$$

In view of (26), we can deduce that $\mathscr{L}V(t,S,I) \le -1$ on $[0,\infty] \times \Theta_\epsilon^4$.

In summary, we can draw the conclusion that

$$\mathscr{L}V(t,S,I) \le -1 \quad \text{for every } [0,\infty] \times \Theta_\epsilon^c. \tag{35}$$

Thus, the condition (14) of Lemma 5 is satisfied. Consequently, model (7) at least has one positive stochastic θ-periodic solution. □

Remark 9. Theorem 8 implies that the intrinsic growth rate of population should overcome the extinction risks of infected disease and pollution in order to guarantee the survival of the population. In addition, the condition λ_θ means that the susceptible population evolution dynamic (γ, K), the dose-response rates $(r_{i0}, i = 1, 2)$, and intensity of noise (σ) play an important role in determining the periodic outbreak of infectious disease; that is, reducing the possibility of $\lambda_\theta > 1$ is beneficial to the control of the periodic outbreak of infectious diseases.

Remark 10. In contrast to the authors in [8] assume that the exogenous rate of pollutant input $u(t)$ has constant limit(i.e., $\lim_{t\to\infty} u(t) = u^*$) and derived the stability of equilibria, which ignored the periodicity of model. In this paper, we consider the limit periodic system with attractiveness (i.e., $\lim_{t\to\infty}|C_0(t) - C_0^*(t)| = 0$) and obtain the positive stochastic periodic solution, which extends the results in [8] to a stochastic nonautonomous situation.

Combining Lemma 2 and Theorem 8, we can have the following result on the existence of positive stochastic periodic solution of model (4).

Theorem 11. *Under the conditions of Theorem 8, model (4) at least has one positive stochastic θ-periodic solution $(S^*(t), I^*(t), C_0^*(t), C_e^*(t))$.*

2.3. The Boundary Periodic Solution of Disease Extinction. In this section, we shall obtain the sufficient conditions for disease extinction. Firstly, we define

$$\lambda_\theta^0 = \frac{1}{\theta}\int_0^\theta \left[\frac{\beta^2(s)}{2\sigma^2(s)} - r_{20}(s) C_0^*(s) - v(s)\right] ds. \tag{36}$$

Next, we prove the following theorem.

Theorem 12. *For model (7), if $\lambda_\theta^0 < 0$, then the disease $I(t)$ goes to extinct almost surely.*

Proof. Define $W(I) = \ln I(t)$ for $I \in [0, \gamma^u K^u/\gamma^l]$. Utilizing the Itô formula to model (7) yields

$$dW(I(t)) = LW(I(t))\,dt + \sigma(t) S(t)\,dB(t), \tag{37}$$

where

$$\begin{aligned} LW(I(t)) &= \beta(t) S(t) - r_{20}(t) C_0^*(t) - v(t) \\ &\quad - \frac{\sigma^2(t)}{2} S^2(t) \\ &\le \frac{\beta^2(t)}{2\sigma^2(t)} - r_{20}(t) C_0^*(t) - v(t). \end{aligned} \tag{38}$$

Substituting (38) into (37) and integrating both sides of (37), one can deduce that

$$\begin{aligned} &\frac{1}{t}\int_0^t \ln\frac{I(t)}{I(0)} \\ &\quad \le \frac{1}{t}\int_0^t \left\{\frac{\beta^2(s)}{2\sigma^2(s)} - r_{20}(s) C_0^*(s) - v(s)\right\} ds \\ &\quad + \frac{M(t)}{t}, \end{aligned} \tag{39}$$

where $M(t) = \int_0^t \sigma(s) S(s)\,dB(s)$ is a martingale with the following quadratic variation:

$$\begin{aligned} \langle M(t), M(t)\rangle_t &= \int_0^t [\sigma(u) S(u)]^2 du \\ &\le \sup_{s\ge 0}\left\{\left(\frac{\sigma^u \gamma^u K^u}{\gamma^l}\right)^2\right\}, \quad \text{a.s.} \end{aligned} \tag{40}$$

According to the strong law of large numbers for martingales [32], we can get

$$\lim_{t\to\infty}\frac{M(t)}{t} = 0, \quad \text{a.s.} \tag{41}$$

Combining (39), (41), and the coefficients' periodicity of model (7), we get

$$\begin{aligned} &\lim_{t\to\infty}\frac{1}{t}\int_0^t \ln\frac{I(t)}{I(0)} \\ &\quad \le \lim_{t\to\infty}\frac{1}{t}\int_0^t \left\{\frac{\beta^2(s)}{2\sigma^2(s)} - r_{20}(s) C_0^*(s) - v(s)\right\} ds \\ &\quad + \lim_{t\to\infty}\frac{M(t)}{t} \\ &\quad = \frac{1}{\theta}\int_0^\theta \left\{\frac{\beta^2(s)}{2\sigma^2(s)} - r_{20}(s) C_0^*(s) - v(s)\right\} ds = \lambda_\theta^0 \\ &\quad < 0, \end{aligned} \tag{42}$$

and hence $\lim_{t\to\infty} I(t) = 0$, a.s. □

Note the fact that when $\lim_{t\to\infty} I(t) = 0$, model (7) reduces to the following nonautonomous system:

$$d(S(t)) = S(t)[a(t) - b(t) S(t)], \tag{43}$$

where $a(t) = \gamma(t) - r_{10}(t) C_0^*(t) - \xi(t)$, $b(t) = \gamma(t)/K(t)$ are all θ-periodic functions. Define

$$\lambda_\theta^S = \frac{1}{\theta}\int_0^\theta [\gamma(s) - r_{10}(s) C_0^*(s) - \xi(s)]\, ds. \tag{44}$$

Therefore, we have the following θ-periodic solution result of system (43).

Lemma 13 (see Globalism [33]). *For system (43), if $\lambda_\theta^S > 0$ then it has a stable positive θ-periodic solution $S_\theta^0(t)$ which satisfies*

$$\frac{1}{S_\theta^0(t)} = \frac{\int_t^{t+\theta} \exp\left\{\int_t^s a(\tau)\,d\tau\right\} b(s)\,ds}{\exp\left\{\int_0^\theta a(\tau)\,d\tau\right\} - 1}, \quad t \ge 0. \tag{45}$$

In summary, we obtain the following.

Theorem 14. *For model (7), if $\lambda_\theta^0 < 0$ and $\lambda_\theta^S > 0$, then it has a boundary periodic solution of disease extinction $(S_\theta^0(t), 0)$.*

Remark 15. The transmission coefficient β, intensity of noise σ, and pollution level $r_{20}C_0^*$ may determine the fate of the evolution of infected population.

3. Numerical Simulation

In this section, we shall verify the above theoretical results and illustrate the effects of environmental fluctuation and pollution on the periodic outbreak of infectious disease. With help from MATLAB (Mathworks, Inc., Natick, MA, USA) and Milsteins higher order method [34], which is a powerful tool for solving stochastic differential equations, we consider the following discretized equation of model (7) at $t = (k+1)\Delta t, k = 0, 1, \ldots$:

$$S^{k+1} = S^k + S^k\left[\gamma(k\Delta t)\left(1 - \frac{(S^k + I^k)}{K(k\Delta t)}\right) - \beta(k\Delta t) I^k - r_{10}(k\Delta t) C_0^*(k\Delta t) - \xi(k\Delta t)\right]\Delta t - S^k I^k\left[\sigma(k\Delta t)\sqrt{k\Delta t}\xi_k + \frac{\sigma^2(k\Delta t)}{2}\left(\xi_k^2\Delta t - \Delta t\right)\right], \tag{46}$$
$$I^{k+1} = I^k + I^k\left[\beta(k\Delta t) S^k - r_{20}(k\Delta t) C_0^*(k\Delta t) - v(k\Delta t)\right]\Delta t + S^k I^k\left[\sigma(k\Delta t)\sqrt{k\Delta t}\xi_k + \frac{\sigma^2(k\Delta t)}{2}\left(\xi_k^2\Delta t - \Delta t\right)\right],$$

where ξ_k are the $N(0,1)$-distribution independent Gaussian random variables. Let us assume that

$$\begin{aligned}
\gamma(t) &= 3.5 + 0.5\cos\left(\frac{t}{12}\right),\\
K(t) &= 100 + 5\cos\left(\frac{t}{12}\right),\\
\xi(t) &= 0.34 + 0.05\cos\left(\frac{t}{12}\right),\\
v(t) &= 0.05 + 0.01\cos\left(\frac{t}{12}\right),\\
C_0^*(t) &= 0.5 + 0.05\cos\left(\frac{t}{12}\right),\\
\sigma(t) &= 0.01 + 0.005\cos\left(\frac{t}{12}\right),\\
\beta(t) &= 0.25 + 0.05\cos\left(\frac{t}{12}\right).
\end{aligned} \tag{47}$$

Example 16. To illustrate the effect of pollution on the periodic outbreaks of infectious disease, we look at the following two cases that differ with respect to the average pollution level.

Case (i). Assume that $r_{10}(t) = 0.15 + 0.05\cos(t/12), r_{20}(t) = 0.2 + 0.05\cos(t/12)$. After some simple calculations, we can see that $\gamma^u + \gamma^u/K^l - \beta^l - (r_{10}C_0^* + \xi)^l = 1.8711 > 0$ and

$$\lambda_\theta = 3.3871 > 0. \tag{48}$$

Thus, it follows from Theorem 8 that model (7) has at least one positive 24π-periodic solution. As shown in Figures 2(a) and 2(c), the probability density functions (PDFs) of $(S(t), I(t))$ of model (7) are nearly equal (from the shape of stationary distribution aspect) to each other in different periods, which supports the definition of a periodic Markov process (see Figures 2(b) and 2(d)). Therefore, the solution process of model (7) is a 24π-periodic Markov process. Additionally, in the absence of white noise, model (7) reduces to a deterministic system. Hence, we also plot the trajectories of the corresponding deterministic model (7) in Figures 2(a) and 2(c) (red lines). In summary, it can be observed that the sample trajectories of the stochastic model (7) have regular periodicity under small environmental fluctuations, and fluctuation happens around the periodic solution of the corresponding deterministic counterparts.

Case (ii). Assume that $r_{10}(t) = 0.1 + 0.05\cos(t/12), r_{20}(t) = 0.15 + 0.05\cos(t/12)$. After some simple calculations, we can check that $\gamma^u + \gamma^u/K^l - \beta^l - (r_{10}C_0^* + \xi)^l = 1.9711 > 0$ and $\lambda_\theta = 3.4121 > 0$. According to Theorem 8, model (7) has a stochastic 24π-periodic solution (see Figure 3(a), red lines). We can also observe from Figure 3(a) that due to the decrease in pollution, the peak level of infective population increases. Meanwhile, the corresponding PDF moves to the right position, which implies a higher number for population of $I(t)$ (see Figure 2(b)). Thus, pollution may increase the peak level of infective population.

Next, we shall check the existence of a boundary periodic solution.

Example 17. Let us assume that $r_{10}(t) = 0.15 + 0.05\cos(t/12)$, $r_{20}(t) = 0.2 + 0.05\cos(t/12)$, $\beta(t) = 0.0015 + 0.0005\cos(t/12)$; then we can calculate that

$$\begin{aligned}
\lambda_\theta^0 &= -0.2388 < 0,\\
\lambda_\theta^S &= 3.011 > 0.
\end{aligned} \tag{49}$$

It follows from Theorem 12 that there exists a boundary periodic solution of disease extinction $(S_\theta^0(t), 0)$ of model (7), which is consistent with the simulation results as shown in Figure 4.

Now, we are in a position to see the fit of model (7) for a real-world situation (the case of measles).

Example 18. Measles is a highly contagious airborne infectious disease caused by the measles virus, which spreads easily through coughing and sneezing of infected people. Major epidemics occur approximately every 2-3 years, causing an estimated 2.6 million deaths each year [31]. Recent research has showed that the incidence of measles is related to air pollution in China [1, 3, 35] and has provided cumulative evidence of the adverse health effects of particulate air pollution and dust. Thus, using measles as an example, we have the requisite information to fit a real-world situation such as the outbreak of measles by using model (7). The data source for the cases of measles was from the Chinese center for disease control and prevention (CCDCP) [36]. The parameters of the simulation are listed in Table 2.

It can be seen from Figure 5 that our simulation, based on model (7), is a good fit compared to the data on the

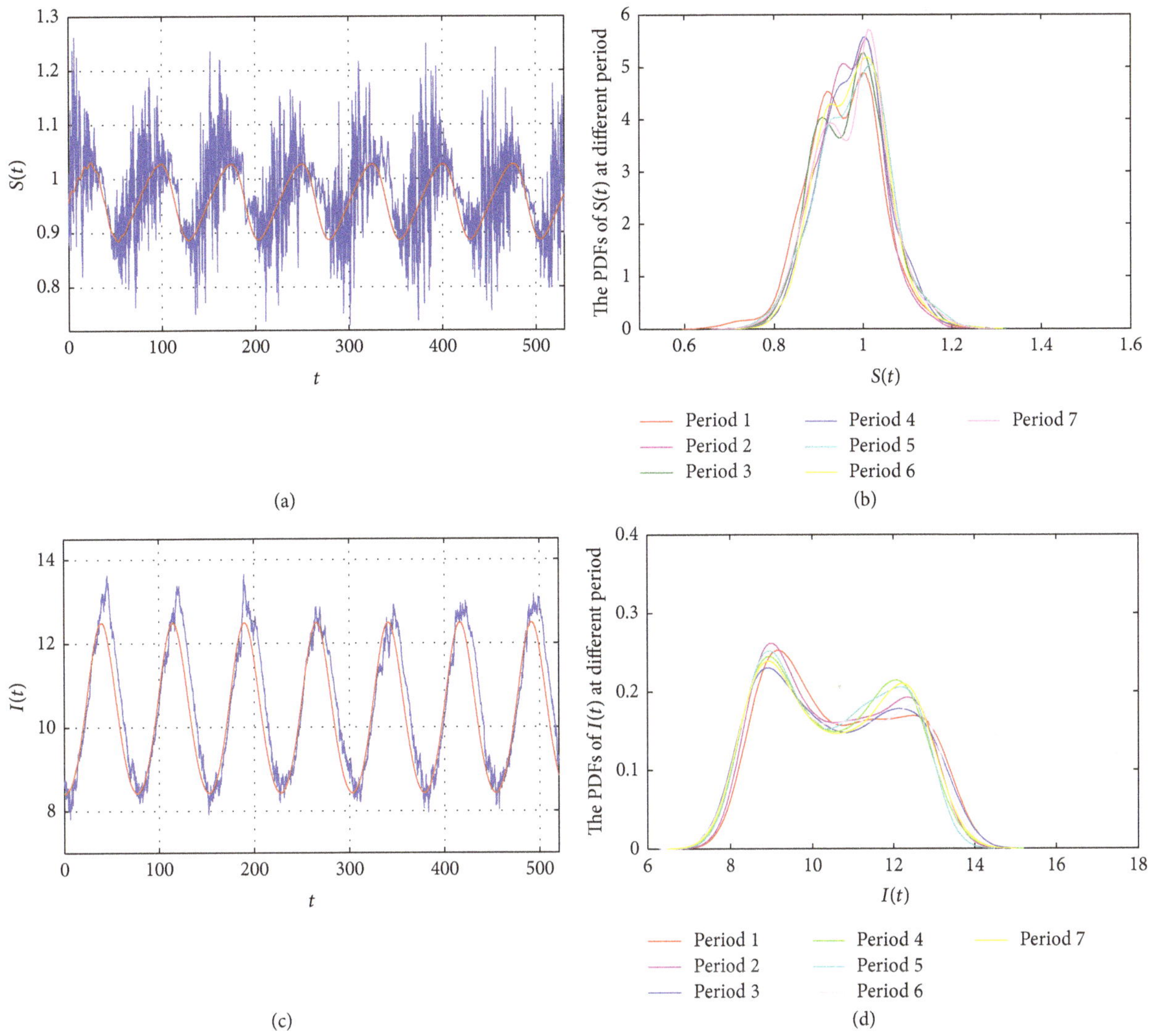

FIGURE 2: (a), (c) The sample trajectory of $S(t)$ and $I(t)$ of model (7) (blue lines) and their corresponding deterministic periodic solution (red lines), respectively. (b), (d) the probability density functions (PDFs) of $S(t)$ and $I(t)$ of model (7) in different periods, respectively. The initial value is $(1, 11)$ and the parameter values are used as in Example 16.

TABLE 2: The values of the parameters in model (46).

Parameters	Mean value	Source
γ	0.01295	[30]
β	0.00495	Estimated
ξ	0.0067	[30]
σ	0.05	[30]
K	1.378×10^9	[30]
ν	0.00175	[31]
$r_{i0}, i = 1, 2$	0.0015	Estimated
C_0^*	1.05	[1]

observed cases of measles in the period from Jan 2014 to Dec 2016. However, the results of fitting the model in the period from Jan 2017 to Dec 2017 are not good; this may be due to the following reasons: (1) by 2016, the government and prevention departments push to improve vaccine coverage may have resulted in the drop in the cases of measles [31]; (2) the Chinese government paid more attention to control the pollution in the environment and enforced strict emission standards, which reduced the negative effect on the population health [35]. Moreover, one interesting finding is that the decrease of susceptible $S(t)$ is beneficial to the decreasing trend of infected cases $I(t)$; that is, if we can reduce the number of the susceptible subpopulation, the cases of measles will show a decreasing trend in the future (see Figure 5, blue lines). Thus, strengthening the coverage of measles vaccination and the environmental quality improvement are advantageous in controlling the outbreak of infectious diseases (e.g., measles).

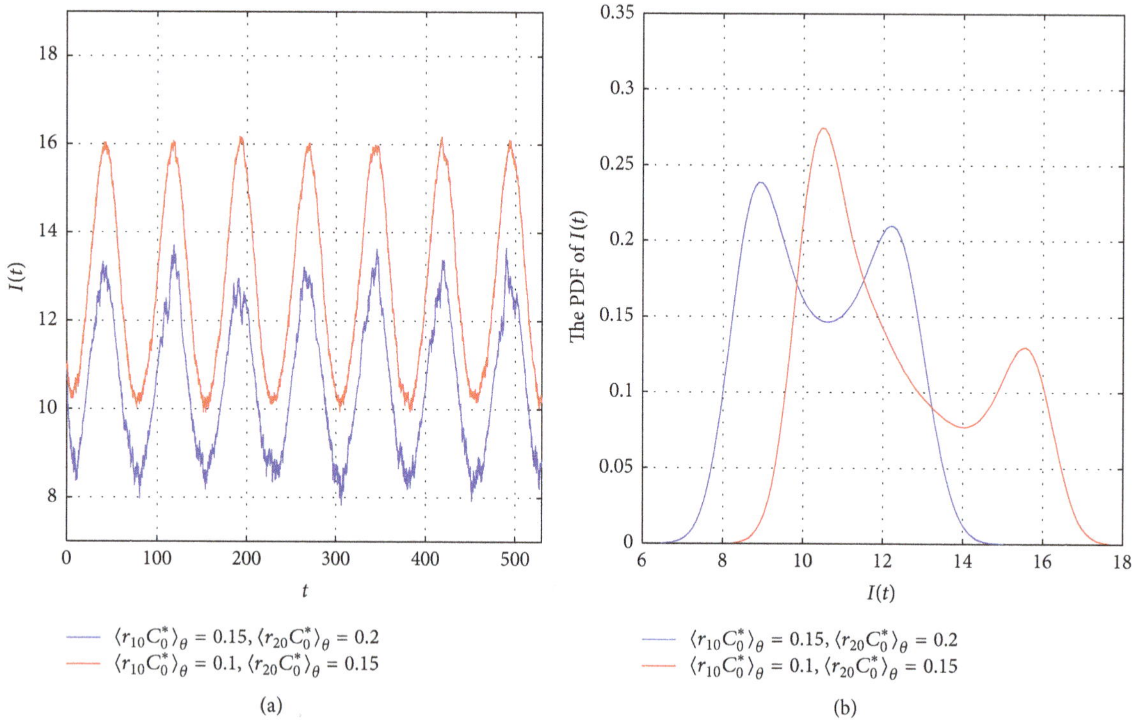

FIGURE 3: (a) The sample trajectory $I(t)$ of model (7) corresponding to different average pollution level $r_{i0}C_0^*$, respectively. (b) the PDFs of $I(t)$ of model (7) in the same period with different average pollution level, respectively.

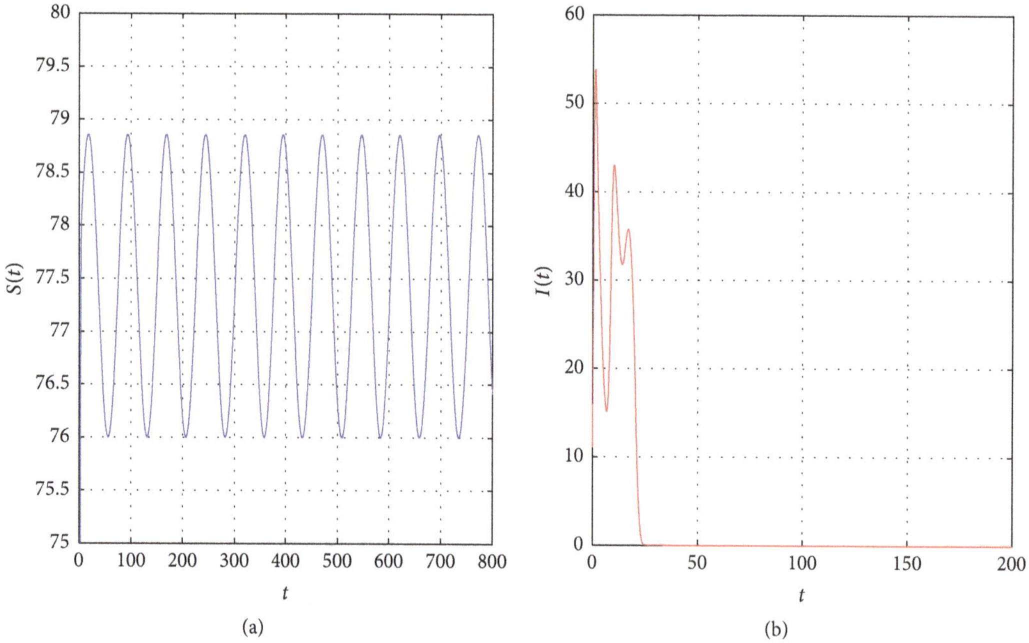

FIGURE 4: The sample trajectory of the boundary periodic solution $(S_\theta^0(t), 0)$ of model (7), with initial values (75, 10).

4. Conclusion

Generally, humans are exposed to some kinds of infectious diseases because the diseases propagate through a polluted environment. Examples include measles spreading through air pollution, snail fever spreading through water pollution, and diarrhea spreading through food pollution. Understanding the transmission of an infectious disease is crucial to predict and prevent major outbreaks of an epidemic [17]. Thus, one of the fundamental questions for the dynamical models of infectious diseases is to find the conditions that identify whether an infectious disease will exhibit a periodic

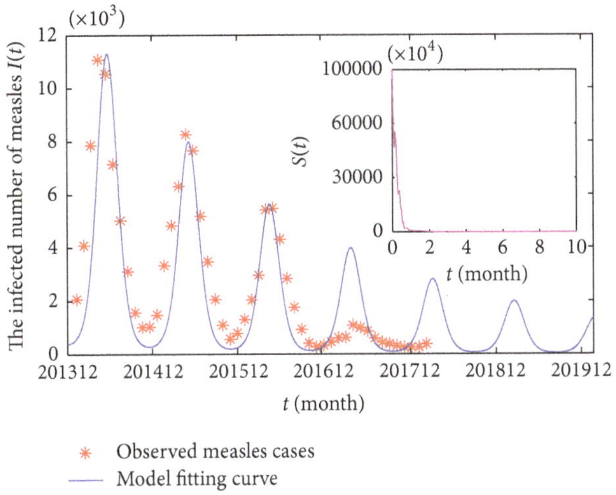

FIGURE 5: Observed (red double cross pattern) of cases of measles $I(t)$ during Jan 2013 to Dec 2016 and model fitted and predicted cases of measles (blue line) from Jan 2013 to Dec 2019. The inner panel is the sample path of $S(t)$.

outbreak or not and determine the risk factors of pollution exposure for such an outbreak in the population. In this paper, we considered a stochastic SI epidemic model in a polluted environment and incorporated the effect of environmental fluctuations as well as pollution. First, we discussed the existence of the global positive solution to the model. The main result of this paper was to obtain the sufficient conditions of the nontrivial stochastic periodic solution (see Figure 2) and the boundary periodic solution of disease extinction (see Figure 4).

Compared to existing research, the main breakthrough of this paper is that we incorporated both environmental white noise as well as pollution into an SI epidemic model, which described two kinds of common phenomena in the transmission process of infectious diseases and explored the effects of environmental fluctuations (noise and pollution) on the dynamical behaviors of an epidemic. The numerical simulations based on the cases of measles showed the following:

(i) The environmental noise σ on β may play an important role in determining the epidemic pattern: (1) it follows from Theorems 8 and 12 that the large intensity of noise σ may adversely affect the existence of the stochastic periodic of model (7) and accelerate the extinction of infectious disease. Thus, the large intensity noise may help the control of periodic outbreak of infectious disease; (2) according to Figure 2, we can see that environmental fluctuations may be responsible for the variations in the seasonal outbreak pattern of a disease in a polluted environment.

(ii) The pollution level ($r_{i0}C_0^*$) plays an important role in susceptible populations, in that it may reduce the number of susceptible population due to the effect of pollution; that is, the pollution causes serious harm to the susceptible population. Therefore, the pollution level may have adverse health effects on the susceptible exposed population, which is also be supported by the measles data (see Figure 5; the decreasing susceptible $S(t)$ may be responsible for the decreasing tendency of $I(t)$.) Moreover, by comparing the peak level of infective population with different average pollution levels $r_{i0}C_0^*$ (see Figure 2), we can see that the peak level of infective population increases with the levels of pollution.

(iii) From an epidemiological viewpoint, our results may provide some theoretical evidence for controlling the infectious disease. For example, in the cases of measles, the strengthening coverage of the measles vaccination and environmental quality improvement are still effective prevention measures in a polluted environment. That is to say, the lesser the population falling within the scope of susceptible subpopulation, the less infected the patients. Therefore, the demographic characteristics of susceptible population may affect the periodic outbreaks of infectious disease. In addition, the pollution control is beneficial to population health, which is consistent with the environmental research results of hemorrhagic fever [37] and influenza [38].

However, this study also has several limitations:

(i) A key assumption of our model is that the pollution affects population dynamics with a linear dose-response function. Since the complicated mechanism of interaction between the pollution and population is still unclear, the dose-response parameter estimation is difficult, since the effect of pollution in vivo is not measurable for human patients. Thus, our model can not accurately describe this interaction, and the numerical simulations do not yet use the polluted data (such as PM2.5 or PM10) to check the effect of the pollution.

(ii) The times series of pollution concentration presents significant variability [39]; however, our model has not included the variability of pollution.

(iii) Some other issues also need to be considered in future, for example, the age-structured modeling [40], the impulse pollution input [41, 42], or the population with partial pollution tolerance [43].

Appendix

Proof of Lemma 2. It follows from the periodicity of $u(t)$ that the solution $C_e^*(t)$ of $dC_e^*(t) = [-hC_e^*(t)+u(t)]dt$ is a positive θ-periodic continuous function, that is,

$$C_e^*(t) = \frac{\int_t^{t+\theta} e^{h(s-t)} u(s)\, ds}{e^{h\theta} - 1}. \tag{A.1}$$

Combining with the third equation of model (4) can result in

$$C_e(t) - C_e^*(t) = (C_e(0) - C_e^*(0)) e^{-ht}, \tag{A.2}$$

which satisfies $d(C_e(t) - C_e^*(t)) = -h(C_e(t) - C_e^*(t))dt$.

Similarly, we can also get that the solution $C_0^*(t)$ of $dC_0^*(t) = [\alpha C_e^*(t) - (g+m)C_0(t)]dt$ is a positive θ-periodic continuous function. According to the variation-of-constants formula, we have

$$\begin{aligned} C_0(t) - C_0^*(t) &= e^{-(g+m)t}\Big[C_0(0) - C_0^*(0) \\ &+ \alpha\int_0^t (C_e(s) - C_e^*(s))\, e^{(g+m)s} ds\Big] = \Big[C_0(0) \\ &- C_0^*(0) - \frac{\alpha(C_e(0) - C_e^*(0))}{g+m-h}\Big] e^{-(g+m)t} \\ &+ \frac{\alpha(C_e(0) - C_e^*(0))}{g+m-h} e^{-ht}, \end{aligned} \tag{A.3}$$

which satisfies $d(C_0(t) - C_0^*(t)) = [\alpha(C_e(t) - C_e^*(t)) - (g+m)(C_0(t) - C_0^*(t))]dt$. Thus, we can obtain

$$\begin{aligned} &\int_0^t |C_0(s) - C_0^*(s)|\, ds \\ &= \frac{1}{g+m}\left|C_0(0) - C_0^*(0) - \frac{\alpha(C_e(0) - C_e^*(0))}{g+m-h}\right| \\ &\cdot \left(1 - e^{-(g+m)t}\right) + \left|\frac{\alpha(C_e(0) - C_e^*(0))}{g+m-h}\right|\left(1 - e^{-ht}\right) \\ &< +\infty. \end{aligned} \tag{A.4}$$

By virtue of the Barbălat Lemma [44] and (A.4), we obtain the required assertion. □

Proof of Theorem 7. Adding the two equations of model (7) yields

$$\begin{aligned} \frac{d(S(t)+I(t))}{dt} &= \gamma(t)S(t)\left(1 - \frac{S(t)+I(t)}{K(t)}\right) \\ &- r_{10}(t)C_0^*(t)S(t) - \xi S(t) \\ &- r_{20}C_0^*(t)I(t) - v(t)I(t) \\ &\le \gamma^u(S(t)+I(t)) \\ &- \frac{\gamma^l(S(t)+I(t))^2}{K^u}, \end{aligned} \tag{A.5}$$

which implies $\limsup_{t\to\infty}(S(t)+I(t)) = \gamma^u K^u/\gamma^l$. Thus, the set

$$\Lambda = \left\{(S,I) \in \mathbb{R}_+^2,\ S+I \le \frac{\gamma^u K^u}{\gamma^l}\right\} \tag{A.6}$$

is a positively invariant set of system (7).

Due to the coefficients of model (7) are local Lipschitz continuous. According to Theorem 3.15 in Mao [32], for any given initial value (5), there is a unique local saturated solution $(S(t), I(t))$ on $t \in [0, \tau_e)$ where τ_e is the explosion time. To show this solution is global, we only need to show that $\tau_e = \infty$ a.s. Since the initial value is positive and bounded, throughout this paper, let m_0 be sufficiently large such that both $S(0)$ and $I(0)$ lie in the interval $[m_0^{-1}, m_0]$. For each integer $m \ge m_0$, define the stopping time

$$\tau_m = \inf\left\{t \in [0,\tau_e) : S(t) \notin \left(\frac{1}{m}, m\right) \text{ or } I(t) \notin \left(\frac{1}{m}, m\right)\right\}, \tag{A.7}$$

and for the empty set define $\inf \varnothing = \infty$. Then, τ_m is an increasing function in terms of m and $\tau_\infty = \lim_{m\to\infty}\tau_m \le \tau_e$ a.s. If we can show that $\tau_\infty = \infty$ a.s. then $\tau_e = \infty$ a.s. and therefore $(S(t), I(t)) \in \mathbb{R}_+^2$ a.s. for all $t \ge 0$. That is to say, to complete the proof all we need to show is that $\tau_\infty = \infty$ a.s. If this statement is false, then for any constant $T > 0$ there is an $\epsilon \in (0,1)$ such that $\mathscr{P}\{\tau_\infty \le T\} > \epsilon$. Hence, there is an integer $m_1 \ge m_0$ such that

$$\mathscr{P}\{\tau_m \le T\} \ge \epsilon, \quad \forall m \ge m_1. \tag{A.8}$$

Define the C^2 functional $U : \mathbb{R}_+^2 \to \mathbb{R}_+$:

$$U(S,I) = -\ln\left(\frac{\gamma^l S(t)}{\gamma^u K^u}\right) + I(t). \tag{A.9}$$

By use of Itô's formula, we have

$$\begin{aligned} dU(S(t),I(t)) &= \Big\{-\gamma(t) + \frac{\gamma(t)}{K(t)}(S+I) + \beta(t)I \\ &+ [r_{10}(t)C_0^*(t) + \xi(t)] + \beta(t)SI \\ &- [r_{20}(t)C_0^*(t) + v(t)]I + \frac{1}{2}\sigma^2(t)I^2\Big\}dt \\ &+ \sigma(t)I(1+S)dB(t) \le \Big[\frac{\gamma^u}{K^l}(S+I) + \beta^u I \\ &+ (r_{10}C_0^* + \xi)^u + \beta^u SI + \frac{1}{2}(\sigma^u)^2 I^2\Big]dt \\ &+ \sigma^u I(1+S)dB(t) \le \Big[\frac{\gamma^u K^u}{K^l} \\ &+ (r_{10}C_0^* + \xi)^u + \beta^u\frac{\gamma^u K^u}{\gamma^l} \\ &+ \left[\beta^u + \frac{1}{2}(\sigma^u)^2\right]\left(\frac{\gamma^u K^u}{\gamma^l}\right)^2\Big]dt + \sigma^u I(1 \\ &+ S)dB(t) = H_1 dt + \sigma^u I(1+S)dB(t), \end{aligned} \tag{A.10}$$

where

$$\begin{aligned} H_1 &= \frac{\gamma^u K^u}{K^l} + (r_{10}C_0^* + \xi)^u + \beta^u\frac{\gamma^u K^u}{\gamma^l} \\ &+ \left[\beta^u + \frac{1}{2}(\sigma^u)^2\right]\left(\frac{\gamma^u K^u}{\gamma^l}\right)^2 < +\infty. \end{aligned} \tag{A.11}$$

Integrating both sides of (A.10) from 0 to $\tau_m \wedge t = \min\{\tau_m, t\}$, and then taking expectations, yields

$$\mathbb{E}U(S(\tau_m \wedge t), I(\tau_m \wedge t)) \le U(S(0), I(0)) + H_1 E(\tau_m \wedge t). \quad (A.12)$$

Set $\Omega_m = \{\tau_m \le T\}$ and it follows from (A.8) that $\mathscr{P}\{\Omega_m\} \ge \epsilon$. Note that, for every $w \in \{\tau_m \le T\}$, there exists one of $S(\tau_m, w)$ and $I(\tau_m, w)$ equals either m or $1/m$, and hence $U(S(\tau_m, w), I(\tau_m, w))$ is no less than

$$C = \min\left\{-\ln\left(\frac{\gamma^l m}{\gamma^u K^u}\right) + m, -\ln\left(\frac{\gamma^l m}{\gamma^u K^u}\right) + \frac{1}{m}, -\ln\left(\frac{\gamma^l}{\gamma^u K^u m}\right) + m, -\ln\left(\frac{\gamma^l}{\gamma^u K^u m}\right) + \frac{1}{m}\right\}. \quad (A.13)$$

Consequently, it follows from (A.12) that

$$\begin{aligned}\mathscr{P}(\tau_m \le T) C &\le \mathbb{E}\left[1_{\tau_m \le T}(w) U(S(\tau_m, w), I(\tau_m, w))\right] \\ &\le U(S(0), I(0)) + H_1 T,\end{aligned} \quad (A.14)$$

where $1_{\{\tau_m \le T\}}$ is the indicator function of $\{\tau_m \le T\}$. Letting $m \to \infty$ gives $\lim_{m\to\infty}\mathscr{P}(\tau_m \le T) = 0$, which contradicts with (A.8). So, $\tau_e = \infty$. Further, notice $T > 0$ is arbitrary. It then follows that $\mathscr{P}(\tau_e = \infty) = 1$. This completes the proof. □

Conflicts of Interest

The authors declare that there are no conflicts of interest regarding the publication of this paper.

Acknowledgments

Research is supported by the University Scientific Research Project of Ningxia (NGY2017086).

References

[1] G. Chen, W. Zhang, S. Li et al., "Is short-term exposure to ambient fine particles associated with measles incidence in China? A multi-city study," *Environmental Research*, vol. 156, pp. 306–311, 2017.

[2] D. W. Dockery, "Health Effects of Particulate Air Pollution," *Annals of Epidemiology*, vol. 19, no. 4, pp. 257–263, 2009.

[3] G. Chen, W. Zhang, S. Li et al., "The impact of ambient fine particles on influenza transmission and the modification effects of temperature in China: A multi-city study," *Environment International*, vol. 98, pp. 82–88, 2017.

[4] X. Wu, Y. Lu, S. Zhou, L. Chen, and B. Xu, "Impact of climate change on human infectious diseases: Empirical evidence and human adaptation," *Environment International*, vol. 86, pp. 14–23, 2016.

[5] F. Wang and Z. Ma, "Persistence and periodic orbits for an SIS model in a polluted environment," *Computers & Mathematics with Applications. An International Journal*, vol. 47, no. 4-5, pp. 779–792, 2004.

[6] C. Viboud, L. Simonsen, and G. Chowell, "A generalized-growth model to characterize the early ascending phase of infectious disease outbreaks," *Epidemics*, vol. 15, pp. 27–37, 2016.

[7] W. Kermack and A. McKendrick, "Contributions to the mathematical theory of epidemics (part I)," in *Proceedings of the Royal Society of London A*, vol. 115, pp. 700–721, 1927.

[8] B. Liu, Y. Duan, and S. Luan, "Dynamics of an SI epidemic model with external effects in a polluted environment," *Nonlinear Analysis: Real World Applications*, vol. 13, no. 1, pp. 27–38, 2012.

[9] S. Usaini, R. Anguelov, and S. M. Garba, "Dynamics of SI epidemic with a demographic Allee effect," *Theoretical Population Biology*, vol. 106, pp. 1–13, 2015.

[10] L. Chen and J. Sun, "Global stability of an SI epidemic model with feedback controls," *Applied Mathematics Letters*, vol. 28, pp. 53–55, 2014.

[11] T. Britton, T. House, A. L. Lloyd, D. Mollison, S. Riley, and P. Trapman, "Five challenges for stochastic epidemic models involving global transmission," *Epidemics*, vol. 10, pp. 54–57, 2015.

[12] J. Shaman and M. Kohn, "Absolute humidity modulates influenza survival, transmission, and seasonality," *Proceedings of the National Acadamy of Sciences of the United States of America*, vol. 106, no. 9, pp. 3243–3248, 2009.

[13] A. C. Lowen, S. Mubareka, J. Steel, and P. Palese, "Influenza virus transmission is dependent on relative humidity and temperature," *PLoS Pathogens*, vol. 3, no. 10, pp. 1470–1476, 2007.

[14] Q. Yang, C. Fu, N. Wang, Z. Dong, W. Hu, and M. Wang, "The effects of weather conditions on measles incidence in Guangzhou, Southern China," *Human Vaccines & Immunotherapeutics*, vol. 10, no. 4, pp. 1104–1110, 2014.

[15] X. Ji, S. Yuan, and J. Li, "Stability of a stochastic SEIS model with saturation incidence and latent period," *Journal of Applied Analysis and Computation*, vol. 7, no. 4, pp. 1652–1673, 2017.

[16] Y. Cai, Y. Kang, and W. Wang, "A stochastic SIRS epidemic model with nonlinear incidence rate," *Applied Mathematics and Computation*, vol. 305, pp. 221–240, 2017.

[17] W. J. Moss, "Measles," *The Lancet*, vol. 390, no. 10111, pp. 2490–2502, 2017.

[18] M. J. Ferrari, R. F. Grais, N. Bharti et al., "The dynamics of measles in sub-Saharan Africa," *Nature*, vol. 451, no. 7179, pp. 679–684, 2008.

[19] H. Emerson, "Measles and Whooping Cough," *American Journal of Public Health*, vol. 27, no. 6_Suppl, pp. 59–83, 1937.

[20] L. Zu, D. Jiang, D. O'Regan, and B. Ge, "Periodic solution for a non-autonomous Lotka-Volterra predator-prey model with random perturbation," *Journal of Mathematical Analysis and Applications*, vol. 430, no. 1, pp. 428–437, 2015.

[21] D. Jiang, Q. Zhang, T. Hayat, and A. Alsaedi, "Periodic solution for a stochastic non-autonomous competitive Lotka-Volterra model in a polluted environment," *Physica A: Statistical Mechanics and its Applications*, vol. 471, pp. 276–287, 2017.

[22] R. Rifhat, L. Wang, and Z. Teng, "Dynamics for a class of stochastic SIS epidemic models with nonlinear incidence and periodic coefficients," *Physica A: Statistical Mechanics and its Applications*, vol. 481, pp. 176–190, 2017.

[23] W. Wang, Y. Cai, J. Li, and Z. Gui, "Periodic behavior in a FIV model with seasonality as well as environment fluctuations," *Journal of The Franklin Institute*, vol. 354, no. 16, pp. 7410–7428, 2017.

[24] R. Khasminskii, *Stochastic Stability of Differential Equations*, vol. 66, Springer, Berlin, Germany, 2nd edition, 2012.

[25] D. Li and D. Xu, "Periodic solutions of stochastic delay differential equations and applications to logistic equation and neural networks," *Journal of the Korean Mathematical Society*, vol. 50, no. 6, pp. 1165–1181, 2013.

[26] Y. Zhao, S. Yuan, and T. Zhang, "Stochastic periodic solution of a non-autonomous toxic-producing phytoplankton allelopathy model with environmental fluctuation," *Communications in Nonlinear Science and Numerical Simulation*, vol. 44, pp. 266–276, 2017.

[27] F. Xie, M. Shan, X. Lian, and W. Wang, "Periodic solution of a stochastic HBV infection model with logistic hepatocyte growth," *Applied Mathematics and Computation*, vol. 293, pp. 630–641, 2017.

[28] X. Zhang, K. Wang, and D. Li, "Stochastic periodic solutions of stochastic differential equations driven by Lévy process," *Journal of Mathematical Analysis and Applications*, vol. 430, no. 1, pp. 231–242, 2015.

[29] Q. Liu, D. Jiang, N. Shi, T. Hayat, and A. Alsaedi, "Nontrivial periodic solution of a stochastic non-autonomous SISV epidemic model," *Physica A: Statistical Mechanics and its Applications*, vol. 462, pp. 837–845, 2016.

[30] "China Population Statistic Yearbook," 2017, http://www.stats.gov.cn/tjsj/ndsj/.

[31] WHO, "Measles," 2017, http://www.who.int/mediacentre/factsheets/fs286/en/.

[32] X. Mao, *Stochastic differential equations and applications*, Horwood Publishing Limited, Chichester, Second edition, 2008.

[33] K. Gopalsamy, *Stability and Oscillations in Delay Differential Equation of Population Dynamics*, vol. 74 of *Mathematics and Its Applications*, Kluwer Academic Publishers, Dordrecht, The Netherlands, 1992.

[34] D. J. Higham, "An algorithmic introduction to numerical simulation of stochastic differential equations," *SIAM Review*, vol. 43, no. 3, pp. 525–546, 2001.

[35] Y. Ma, J. Zhou, S. Yang, Y. Zhao, and X. Zheng, "Assessment for the impact of dust events on measles incidence in western China," *Atmospheric Environment*, vol. 157, pp. 1–9, 2017.

[36] Chinese center for disease control and prevention, 2017, http://www.chinacdc.cn/.

[37] S. S. Han, S. Kim, Y. Choi, S. Kim, and Y. S. Kim, "Air pollution and hemorrhagic fever with renal syndrome in South Korea: An ecological correlation study," *BMC Public Health*, vol. 13, no. 1, article no. 347, 2013.

[38] Y. Liang, L. Fang, H. Pan et al., "PM2.5 in Beijing-temporal pattern and its association with influenza," *Environmental Health: A Global Access Science Source*, vol. 13, no. 1, article no. 102, 2014.

[39] Ministry of environmental protection of the Peoples Republic of China, "China environmental bulletin," 2016, http://www.zhb.gov.cn/.

[40] Y. Zhao, M. Li, and S. Yuan, "Analysis of transmission and control of tuberculosis in Mainland China, 2005-2016, based on the age-structure mathematical model," *International Journal of Environmental Research and Public Health*, vol. 14, no. 10, article no. 1192, 2017.

[41] M. Liu and K. Wang, "Persistence and extinction of a single-species population system in a polluted environment with random perturbations and impulsive toxicant input," *Chaos, Solitons & Fractals*, vol. 45, no. 12, pp. 1541–1550, 2012.

[42] W. Zhao, J. Li, T. Zhang, X. Meng, and T. Zhang, "Persistence and ergodicity of plant disease model with Markov conversion and impulsive toxicant input," *Communications in Nonlinear Science and Numerical Simulation*, vol. 48, pp. 70–84, 2017.

[43] F. Wei, S. A. Geritz, and J. Cai, "A stochastic single-species population model with partial pollution tolerance in a polluted environment," *Applied Mathematics Letters*, vol. 63, pp. 130–136, 2017.

[44] I. Barbălat, "Systems d'equations differentialles d'oscillation nonlinears," *Revue Roumaine des Mathematiques Pures et Appliquees*, vol. 4, no. 2, p. 267, 1959.

18

Mobile Personal Health Monitoring for Automated Classification of Electrocardiogram Signals in Elderly

Luis J. Mena,[1] Vanessa G. Félix,[1] Alberto Ochoa,[2] Rodolfo Ostos,[1] Eduardo González,[1] Javier Aspuru,[2] Pablo Velarde,[3] and Gladys E. Maestre[4]

[1]*Academic Unit of Computing, Master Program in Applied Sciences, Universidad Politecnica de Sinaloa, Mazatlan 82199, Mexico*
[2]*Department of Electronic, Faculty of Mechanical and Electrical Engineering, Universidad de Colima, Colima 28400, Mexico*
[3]*Academic Program of Electronic Engineering, Universidad Autonoma de Nayarit, Tepic 63000, Mexico*
[4]*Department of Biomedical Sciences, Division of Neurosciences and Department of Human Genetics, University of Texas Rio Grande Valley School of Medicine, Brownsville 78520, USA*

Correspondence should be addressed to Luis J. Mena; lmena@upsin.edu.mx

Academic Editor: Masashi Miyashita

Mobile electrocardiogram (ECG) monitoring is an emerging area that has received increasing attention in recent years, but still real-life validation for elderly residing in low and middle-income countries is scarce. We developed a wearable ECG monitor that is integrated with a self-designed wireless sensor for ECG signal acquisition. It is used with a native purposely designed smartphone application, based on machine learning techniques, for automated classification of captured ECG beats from aged people. When tested on 100 older adults, the monitoring system discriminated normal and abnormal ECG signals with a high degree of accuracy (97%), sensitivity (100%), and specificity (96.6%). With further verification, the system could be useful for detecting cardiac abnormalities in the home environment and contribute to prevention, early diagnosis, and effective treatment of cardiovascular diseases, while keeping costs down and increasing access to healthcare services for older persons.

1. Introduction

Cardiovascular diseases (CVD) have remained the leading cause of death globally during the last 15 years. An estimated 17.7 million people died from CVD in 2015, representing 31% of all global mortality. Of these deaths, approximately 6.9 million were in people aged 60 years and older, and over 75% occurred in low and middle-income countries (LMIC) [1, 2]. LMIC are more greatly affected than high-income countries [3–5], largely because people with low socioeconomic status have poor access to healthcare for early diagnosis and treatment of CVD [5]. An increasing urgency exists to tackle CVD in LMIC through effective strategies, guided and monitored by robust estimates of disease prevalence and burden [6]. Thus, technological innovations, including mobile and wireless technologies, are now being developed to improve prevention and control of CVD, and other aspects of healthcare, particularly for older people residing in LMIC [7–9].

The growing application of smartphone technology, due to decreasing costs and increased ease-of-use, combined with parallel advances in sensing technologies, is causing a shift from traditional clinic-based healthcare to real-time monitoring. This shift is supported by the development of mobile personal health monitor (PHM) systems, which are personalized, intelligent, reliable, and noninvasive [10, 11]. PHM systems could improve the quality of care, while reducing costs through timely detection [12–14].

Mobile PHM systems typically consist of a Body Area Network—a set of wearable sensors with wireless data transfer and energy storage capability—integrated by a smartphone as the central processing unit (Figure 1). The physiological signals are processed in real-time by applying machine learning techniques, providing immediate feedback to the

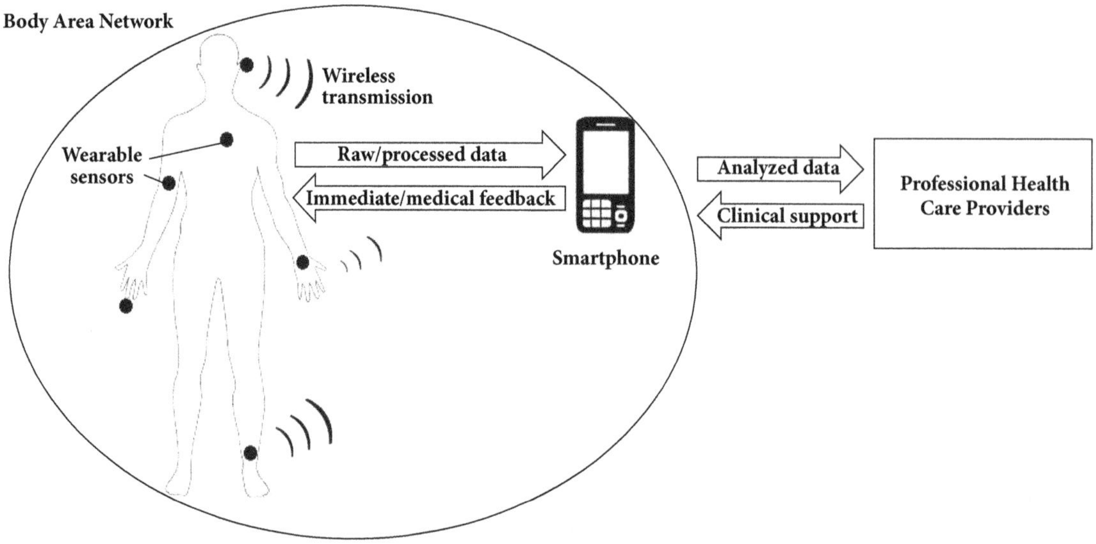

FIGURE 1: General architecture of a mobile personal health monitor system.

user. The data can also be made available to healthcare providers for medical feedback and clinical support [15–17].

PHM systems that offer mobile electrocardiogram (ECG) monitoring have received increasing attention in recent years [18–20]. ECG records are used for screening, diagnosis, and monitoring of several heart conditions from minor to life threatening. Hence, ECG monitoring is a critical and an essential part of healthcare delivery for older adults [17]. Therefore, PHM systems that incorporate ECG data would offer mobile physiological, diagnostic, prognostic, therapeutic, surveillance, and archival capabilities [18, 19] in a wide range of situations, including rural zones, areas lacking cardiologists, and population of solitary elderly, many of whom live alone in their own homes and are restricted physically [21].

However, although a number of PHM systems that collect ECG data have been developed, some of these do not include classification methods for automated detection of arrhythmias or other abnormalities. Among those validated, Kwon et al. proposed a smartphone-integrated ECG monitoring system that works opportunistically during natural smartphone use [22]. The system captured ECG reliably in target situations with a reasonable rate of data drop. Depari et al. developed a single-lead ECG tracing acquisition system based on a smartphone, with a purposely designed application to demodulate the audio signal and extract, plot, and store the ECG tracing [23]. Dinh designed a wearable unit for detecting and sending ECG signals wirelessly to a smartphone [24]. Yu et al. developed a wireless two-lead ECG sensor that transmitted data via Bluetooth and processed and displayed the ECG waveform on a smartphone, all with low power consumption for long-term monitoring [25].

Other PHM systems use commercial monitors or do not provide an intrinsic method for classify ECG signals. Lee et al. designed a wireless system for acquisition and classification of ECG beats integrated with a smartphone. Abnormal beats and other symptoms were diagnosed by cardiologists from results displayed on the screen. Accuracy of beat classification was 97.25% [26]. Miao et al. developed a wearable ECG monitoring system using a smartphone, with automated recognition of abnormal patterns via decision trees in a WEKA environment [27]. The system achieved a 2.6% discrimination ability [28]. Oresko et al. developed a smartphone-based application for real-time CVD detection, using a commercial ECG heart monitor and an adaptive artificial neural network (NN) algorithm for signal preprocessing and classification [29]. The system was trained using the MIT-BIH arrhythmia database [30] and retrained based on real ECG recordings, ultimately demonstrating classification accuracy of 93.32%. None of the aforementioned studies [22–26, 28, 29] reported considerations in software design to address end-user usability and acceptance of mobile PHM systems in older adults.

To improve on previous systems, it would be necessary to enhance the capture as well as the automated classification of ECG signals. We developed a complete mobile PHM system, integrated with a self-designed wireless sensor for ECG signal acquisition, and a native purposely designed smartphone application to be user-friendly to elderly, based on machine learning techniques, for automated classification of captured ECG beats. The signal sensing and transferring process uses a two-lead ECG sensor with Bluetooth technology and an artificial NN approach for identifying abnormal ECG patterns.

The rest of this paper is organized as follows. The methodology of the proposed PHM system is presented in detail in Section 2; the experimental results for ECG signals acquisition, wireless transmission, and assessment of recognition accuracy are shown in Section 3; we conclude our study in Sections 4 and 5, with discussion, limitations, and perspective for further research.

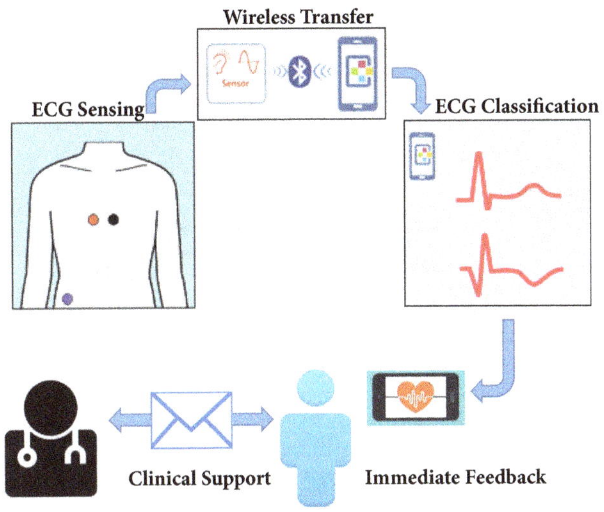

FIGURE 2: Framework of the mobile personal health monitor system.

2. Materials and Methods

The PHM system described in this report operates in five stages: sensing, transferring, classification, immediate feedback, and clinical support (Figure 2). The captured ECG tracings are transmitted and displayed in real-time on a smartphone screen. The presence or absence of arrhythmias, determined using machine learning analysis, is included and is shared via email with healthcare professionals for verification of abnormal ECG patterns.

2.1. ECG Sensor. The sensor design includes acquisition, amplification, filtering, digitalization, and transmission of ECG signals. Three identically sized electrodes and low frequency amplifiers are used to capture the signals and the coupling of impedances. The signal is filtered through low-pass and high-pass filters to improve the signal/noise ratio. The processed signal is then digitized and transmitted by an analog-to-digital converter and Bluetooth module embedded in a microcontroller unit. A 9V primary lithium battery with 1200 mAh capacity powers the ECG sensor.

To acquire reliable ECG signals, two electrodes are attached to the chest as precordial leads V1 and V2 positioned in the fourth intercostal space to the right and left of the sternum, respectively, because incorrect positioning of the precordial electrodes changes the ECG significantly [31], and a reference electrode is placed far from these on the right leg (Figure 3). The reference electrode plays the role of driving the user's body to attenuate the common mode noise caused by external electromagnetic interference [32]. The analog input signal from two lead electrodes was initially amplified through an AD620 differential instrumentation amplifier [33]. Before the next amplifier stage, we coupled the impedance using a TL082 operational amplifier, configured as a voltage follower [34].

The current configuration uses an instrumental amplifier, based on an encapsulation with four LM324 operational amplifiers [35], to amplify the signal with a noninverter amplifier, then filter it, and add voltage (Figure 4). A low power OP97E operational amplifier [36] closes the circuit, protects the user from static charges, and suppresses voltage transients. Two LM324 operational amplifiers act as Butterworth filters, to generate an appropriate low-noise signal that fits within the input range of the analog-to-digital converter [37]. A low-pass active filter with a corner frequency of 40 Hz and a second-order high-pass filter with cutoff frequency of 0.5 Hz remove unnecessary frequency components of the ECG signal. Because the signal obtained consists of positive and negative parts, it was necessary to add a positive carrier signal. To recompose the signal, we used operational LM324 amplifiers as noninverter adders of the two inputs, fed by the ECG signal and a variable power source of 0–9 volts. This increases or decreases the carrier signal, as appropriate. A pair of equal resistances is added, one to the input of the analog signals and another from the inverter input of the operational amplifier to the circuit ground. Thus, the output signal has the same frequency, but with only positive voltage values, and is ready to be read by any microcontroller.

The Blend Micro of Read Bear Labs [38], which combines the Atmega32U4 microcontroller unit with a Bluetooth Low Energy (BLE) module [39, 40], is used for microcontroller processing of the signal. Generic Access Profile (GAP) controls connections and advertising in BLE standard and determines how two devices interact with each other by assigning roles. The ECG sensor and smartphone are defined as peripheral and central devices, respectively. GAP sends advertising out as Advertising Data payload, which can contain up to 31 bytes of data and constantly transmits from the sensor to the smartphone. After a dedicated connection is established, the advertising process stops, and BLE uses Generic Attribute Profile (GATT) services and characteristics to communicate in both directions. This connection is exclusive, because a BLE peripheral only can be connected to one central device at a time.

Communication is established through a generic data protocol, Attribute Protocol, which is used to store services, characteristics, and related data in a simple lookup table. GATT transactions in BLE operate as a server/client relationship. The GATT server is the peripheral that holds the Attribute Protocol, and the GATT client (smartphone) sends requests to this server. All transactions are started by the master device, the smartphone, which receives responses from the slave device, the ECG sensor. A simple Universal Asynchronous Receiver Transmitter type interface [41] defines a custom service containing two specific characteristics for the channels of transmission and reception of the ECG signal.

2.2. Neural Network Approach. We use a three-layered, feed-forward NN approach, built through Matlab NN toolbox [42], for automated classification of acquired ECG tracings. A scaled conjugate gradient back-propagation algorithm with random weights/bias initialization is used for the training stage. The transfer functions are sigmoidal hyperbolic, logarithmic tangential, and lineal. Performance of the NN system was tested with a cross-entropy error function using the mean-squared error parameter, computed for differences between the actual outputs and the outputs obtained in each

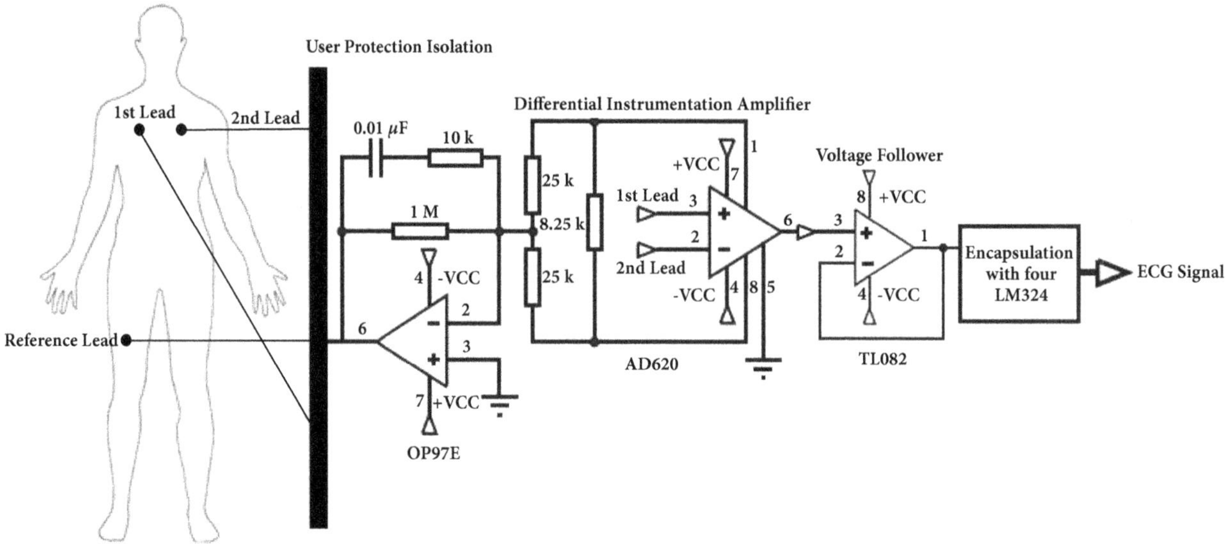

FIGURE 3: Schematic representation of the ECG amplifier circuit and electrode placement on the body.

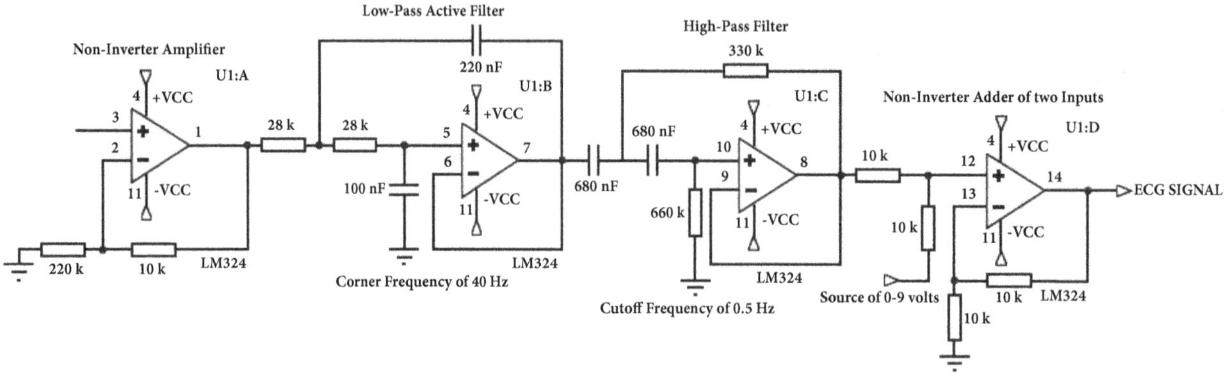

FIGURE 4: Encapsulation with four LM324 operational amplifiers to amplify, filter, and add voltage to the ECG signal.

trained step. The training ended if the total sum of the squared errors was <0.01 or when 3000 epochs were reached. The target outputs for normal and abnormal ECG patterns were (0,1) and (1,0), respectively.

2.3. Data Processing. ECG data for training was obtained from a publicly available source, the Physikalisch-Technische Bundesanstalt Diagnostic ECG Database [43]. This benchmark database contains 549 two-minute digitized ECG records of 290 subjects (mean age 57.2 y; 27.9% women) provided by the National Metrology Institute of Germany. The ECG data includes 15 simultaneously measured signals: the conventional 12 leads, plus 3 Frank Lead ECGs. Each signal is digitized at 1000 samples per second, with 16-bit resolution over a range of ±16 mV and 1 KHz sampling frequency.

We selected data from 268 subjects with clinical summaries available. These included a variety of diagnostic classes: 52 healthy controls, 148 myocardial infarctions, and 68 with other cardiac abnormalities. ECG beats were classified in normal and abnormal heartbeat patterns from ECG records reported as regular and irregular cardiac rhythm. Lead V1 was chosen for the analysis, because it has the highest ratio of atrial to ventricular signal amplitude and, therefore, offers more representative characteristics for identifying the common heart diseases [44, 45]. To avoid overfitting and improve the generalization capability of the NN approach, we added simulated ECG data with artificial corruption, using a Gaussian white-noise model [46], to generate 110 normal and 72 abnormal virtual ECG tracings. The global training dataset contained 8000 beats from all 450 records, for feature extraction of ECG patterns.

The trained NN system was tested on participants of the Maracaibo Aging Study [47], which has 2500 subjects ≥ 55 y of age. One hundred voluntary subjects (mean age 73.5 ± 11.8 y; 74% women) were recruited in the Institute for Biological Research of the University of Zulia, in Maracaibo, Venezuela. All 100 subjects had a previous ECG diagnostic performed by an expert cardiologist, and 13 were diagnosed with some type of cardiac arrhythmia. These ECG records were classified as abnormal and the rest as normal ECG patterns. Recruited participants had reasonable smartphone skills and were assertive about using new technologies. Each volunteer was instructed how to use the smartphone application and underwent 16-second ECG monitoring using the PHM system. ECG acquisitions were performed and supervised by medical staff. The ethical review board of the Institute of Cardiovascular Diseases of the University of Zulia approved the protocol. Informed consent was obtained from each subject or a close family member.

2.4. Software Development. We use Matlab Compiler SDK to save the trained NN as a Matlab function into a shared library for use in an external framework [48]. The smartphone application for plotting the acquired ECG tracing on screen and for return NN output was developed in an Android Studio development environment. The Android Bluetooth serial port profile library [49] establishes the connection with the wearable ECG sensor. Android multithreading [50] allows the smartphone to maintain normal operations, while receiving real-time ECG signals. To make the Android application user-friendly to elderly subjects with reduced vision and manual dexterity, we use a simplified Graphic User Interface with a bright screen, large text and numbers, and simple input buttons with touchscreen technology, all of which have been proven to be efficient for older adults [51]. To provide accurate diagnostic and medical support, application settings include the option to sending screenshots of ECG signal and classification results via email to previously specified healthcare professionals. To assure privacy, reports forwarded to selected recipients lack personal identification, which is already associated with the source email address. The system can be configured to automatically send ECG profiles at the end of each monitoring period or only when abnormal ECG patterns are detected.

3. Results

3.1. Acquisition of ECG Signal. A prototype of the PHM system is shown in Figure 5, and the performance characteristics of the ECG sensor device are given in Table 1. Processing of the ECG tracing, from the first stage of amplification to display on the smartphone, includes (a) amplification by the AD620, (b) coupling of impedance through the TL082, (c) amplification through the LM324, (d) filtering through the low-pass filter, (e) filtering with the high-pass filter, and (f) digitalization and transmission of the positive ECG signal (Figure 6). The analytical process is displayed on the smartphone (Figure 7).

3.2. ECG Classification. When the NN approach was trained on 450 records of the training dataset, the mean-squared error convergence goal (0.0052) was reached in 802 epochs. The best performance was obtained using 10 neurons in the hidden layer of the NN system (Figure 8). Overall classification accuracy in training stage was 97.3%. Correct classification was 92.6% for normal and 100% for abnormal ECG patterns.

When performance of the trained NN approach was tested on real ECG tracings from the test dataset, classification accuracy was 97%. The results are shown in a confusion matrix, where each cell contains the number of ECG records classified for the corresponding combination of estimated and true outputs for normal and abnormal ECG patterns (Table 2).

The total test performance was determined by evaluation metrics (Table 3): accuracy (ratio of the number of correctly classified ECG signals to the total number of ECG signals classified), sensitivity (rate of correctly classified abnormal ECG signals among all abnormal ECG signals), specificity (rate of correctly classified normal ECG signals among all normal ECG signals), and precision (rate of correctly classified abnormal ECG signals among all of detected abnormal

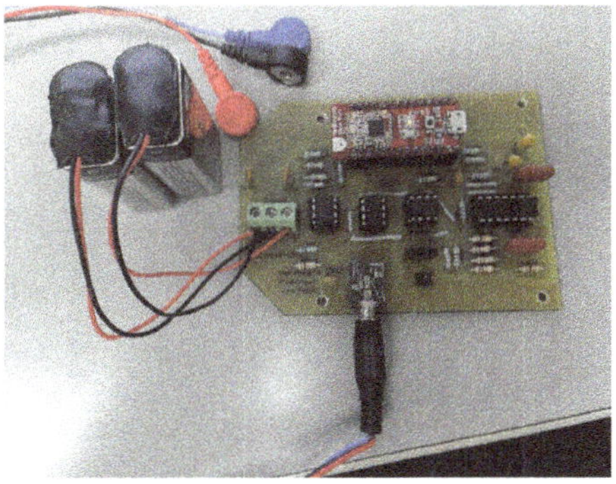

FIGURE 5: Prototype of the self-designed ECG sensor device.

TABLE 1: Performance summary of the ECG sensor device.

Technology	Low-Power Microchip 8-bit AVR RISC-Based Microcontroller
Supply Voltage	3.3 V
Input Impedance	100 MΩ
Frequency Response	Range 0.1Hz and Internal 8MHz Calibrated Oscillator
Common Mode Rejection Ratio	>90dB
Gain	45
Sampling Rate	9.6KHz
Data Bit-Width	8 bits

TABLE 2: Confusion matrix for classification of the test dataset.

	True output	
Estimated output	**Normal**	**Abnormal**
Normal	84	0
Abnormal	3	13

TABLE 3: Total test performance of the mobile PHM system.

Evaluation metrics	**Values** (%)
Sensitivity	100
Specificity	96.6
Accuracy	97
Precision	81.3

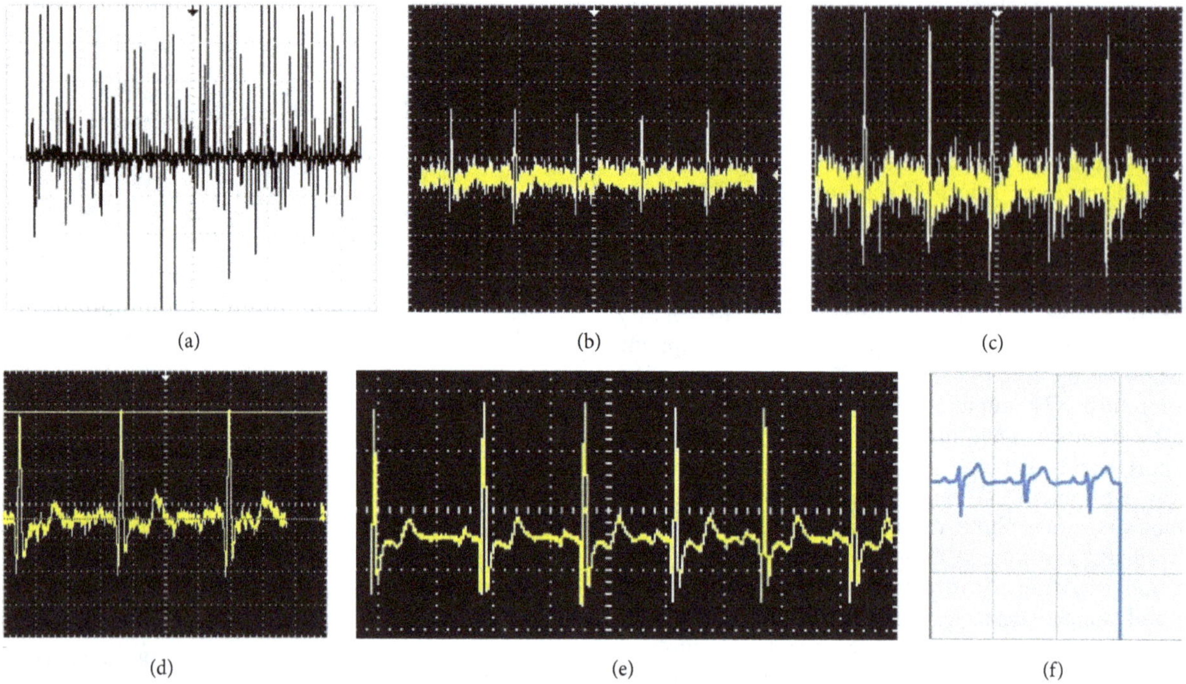

FIGURE 6: ECG signal processing: (a) first stage of amplification; (b) impedance coupling; (c) second stage of amplification; (d) low-pass filtering; (e) high-pass filtering; (f) positive ECG signal on smartphone screen.

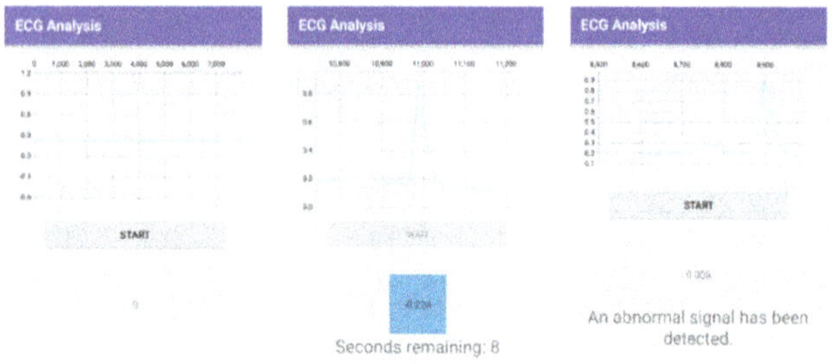

FIGURE 7: Screenshots of ECG analysis process on smartphone.

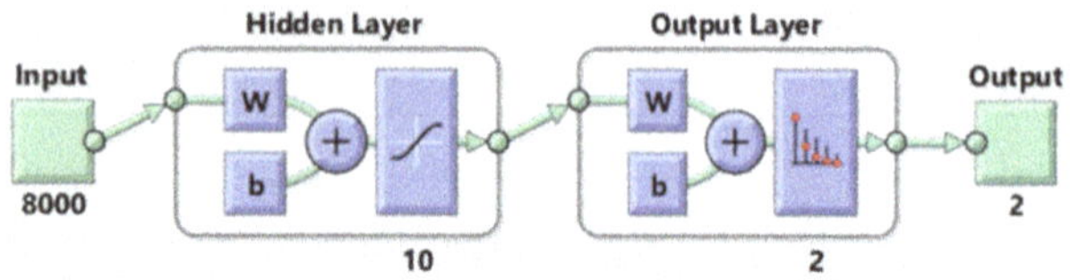

FIGURE 8: Neural network architecture with the best performance.

ECG signals). These metrics are relevant to performance for medical diagnosis applications [52]. Finally, a posterior survey indicated that the majority of the participants found the smartphone application easy to use and considered the time spent learning how to use the mobile ECG monitoring system was reasonable.

4. Discussion

Recent technological advances in integration and miniaturization of physical sensors and increasing computing capability of smartphones have enabled the development of mobile PHM systems as a cost-effective strategy to support healthcare that is focused on the consumer, transparency, convenience, and prevention [53]. Clinical studies reported high sensitivity and specificity at detecting atrial fibrillation [54] and other cardiac abnormalities using wireless mobile ECG devices [55–58]. The ability to provide pervasive heart monitoring to anyone at any time, through natural interactions between smartphone and user, overcomes constraints of place, time, and character and provides personalized information in a transparent form. Users can configure mobile PHM systems to their individual needs and preferences, taking into account age, gender, and ethnicity. Immediate feedback alerts the user of abnormal conditions or abrupt changes in near real-time, potentially improving outcomes. As a final point, clinicians can receive automated updates, providing structured CVD management while minimizing clinical visits.

On the other hand, results of a 2014 consumer survey, performed by PricewaterhouseCoopers Health Research Institute, showed that almost half of respondents were ready to have an ECG device attached to their smartphone, with results wirelessly sent to their physician [59]. Latest evidence from LMIC suggests that mobile PHM systems can improve lifestyle behaviors and healthcare management related to CVD, particularly for aged people and frail users [60].

Elderly should be the primary target of mobile ECG monitoring systems for several reasons. Mainly, because the population aged 65 and older is projected to be about 83.7 million in 2050 [61], worldwide epidemic of chronic diseases is strongly linked to population aging, and the leading contributors to disease burden in older people are CVD [6]. Nevertheless, mobile PHM systems remain in its nascent stages related to behavioral health and older adults [9].

While research in PHM systems have demonstrated feasibility and effectiveness across a variety of populations and health problems, studies generally exclude older adults or do not report significant age differences in responses to the interventions [9]. A possible explanation is the persistence of stereotypes that older adults are afraid, reluctant, and incompetent to use modern technology. Besides, seniors who may believe themselves incapable of learning to use new technologies perpetuate many of these stereotypes [62–64]. Therefore, usability and acceptance of mobile PHM by older adults is not only based on their healthcare requirements, but also on their perspective of technology. Since cognitive performance commonly declines with age, minimizing the complexity of smartphone applications and user-interactions could be key to the adoption of mobile PHM systems by elderly users and should be considered in stages of design and development [65].

In this sense, we developed a mobile PHM system for ECG monitoring and automated classification of heartbeat patterns to identify potential arrhythmias in elderly. The system combines a wearable wireless sensor, mobile technology, and machine learning techniques. Software design included specific characteristics aimed to improve usability and acceptance of older persons. User interface to display and classify ECG signals was simplified at one dedicated button to minimize the amount of steps to be memorized (Figure 7). Additionally, security mechanisms such as user identification and password were omitted to access smartphone application.

Our system has a number of advantages over previously developed mobile PHM systems for monitoring ECG signals, which do not report software design concept to address the user acceptability and acceptance issue in elderly [22–26, 28, 29], do not include automated classification [22–25], operate with commercial sensors [29], or do not provide internal methods for classifying arrhythmias [26, 28]. The prototype detected normal and abnormal ECG patterns in a group of older adults residing in a LMIC with a high degree of accuracy (97%), sensitivity (100%), and specificity (96.6%). Thus, our mobile ECG monitoring approach could be useful for detecting cardiac abnormalities in the home environment and contribute to prevention, early diagnosis, and effective treatment of CVD, while keeping costs down and increasing access to healthcare services for older persons.

However, the ECG monitoring and classification system described herein has several potential limitations. First, our system and most other mobile ECG monitors record a single-channel ECG signal, which provides more limited information than 12-lead ECG devices. Nevertheless, a recent study found good correlation between smartphone ECG and 12-lead ECG data, before and after antiarrhythmic drug therapy [66]. Second, despite high overall recognition, the precision of the NN classifier is only 81.3%, although false positive signals would be recognized by physician evaluation. Third, the system provides timely detection of abnormal ECG patterns for further diagnosis by healthcare professionals but does not identify specific types of cardiac disorders. Finally, the system was tested using a relatively small sample (n = 100) at a single center and primarily included Venezuelan females; thus, the system performance characteristics might not be generalizable to other user populations. Therefore, further studies are necessary to extend use of mobile ECG monitoring to other geographically diverse elderly populations as well as provide a better characterization of heart rhythm abnormalities.

5. Conclusions

The mobile ECG monitoring system described in this report provides near real-time data and automated classification of ECG signals from older adults. The machine learning classifier discriminates between normal and abnormal cardiac rhythms with high accuracy. With further development and verification, the system could provide a cost-effective strategy for primary diagnosis of potential arrhythmias and improve preventive healthcare, particularly in population of solitary elderly.

Conflicts of Interest

The authors declare that there are no conflicts of interest regarding the publication of this paper.

Acknowledgments

This research is financially supported by Grants DSA/103.5/15/11115 and PFCE/1585/17 from Secretaria de Educación Pública, México, and Grants 1R01AG036469-01A1 and R03AG054186 from the National Institute on Aging and Fogarty International Center.

References

[1] *World health statistics 2017: Monitoring health for the SDGs, Sustainable Development Goals*, World Health Organization, Geneva, Switzerland, 2017.

[2] *Global Health Estimates 2015: Deaths by Cause, Age, Sex, by Country And by Region, 2000–2015*, World Health Organization, Geneva, Switzerland, 2016.

[3] V. J. Wirtz, W. A. Kaplan, G. F. Kwan, and R. O. Laing, "Access to medications for cardiovascular diseases in low- and middle-income countries," *Circulation*, vol. 133, no. 21, pp. 2076–2085, 2016.

[4] L. Allen, J. Williams, N. Townsend et al., "Socioeconomic status and non-communicable disease behavioural risk factors in low-income and lower-middle-income countries: a systematic

review," *The Lancet Global Health*, vol. 5, no. 3, pp. e277–e289, 2017.

[5] M. Di Cesare, Y.-H. Khang, P. Asaria et al., "Inequalities in non-communicable diseases and effective responses," *The Lancet*, vol. 381, no. 9866, pp. 585–597, 2013.

[6] M. J. Prince, F. Wu, Y. Guo et al., "The burden of disease in older people and implications for health policy and practice," *The Lancet*, vol. 385, no. 9967, pp. 549–562, 2015.

[7] C. Free, G. Phillips, L. Watson et al., "The Effectiveness of Mobile-Health Technologies to Improve Health Care Service Delivery Processes: A Systematic Review and Meta-Analysis," *PLoS Medicine*, vol. 10, no. 1, Article ID e1001363, 2013.

[8] *Monitoring and Evaluating Digital Health Interventions: A Practical Guide to Conducting Research And Assessment*, World Health Organization, Geneva, Switzerland, 2016.

[9] A. Kuerbis, A. Mulliken, F. Muench, A. A. Moore, and D. Gardner, "Older adults and mobile technology: Factors that enhance and inhibit utilization in the context of behavioral health," *Mental Health and Addiction Research*, vol. 2, no. 2, pp. 1–11, 2017.

[10] M. B. del Rosario, S. J. Redmond, and N. H. Lovell, "Tracking the evolution of smartphone sensing for monitoring human movement," *Sensors*, vol. 15, no. 8, pp. 18901–18933, 2015.

[11] L. J. Mena, V. G. Felix, R. Ostos et al., "Mobile personal health system for ambulatory blood pressure monitoring," *Computational and Mathematical Methods in Medicine*, vol. 2013, Article ID 598196, pp. 1–13, 2013.

[12] Y.-L. Zheng, X.-R. Ding, C. C. Y. Poon et al., "Unobtrusive sensing and wearable devices for health informatics," *IEEE Transactions on Biomedical Engineering*, vol. 61, no. 5, pp. 1538–1554, 2014.

[13] M. Singh and N. Jain, "A Survey on Integrated Wireless Healthcare Framework for Continuous Physiological Monitoring," *International Journal of Computer Applications*, vol. 86, no. 13, pp. 37–41, 2014.

[14] E. Agu, P. Pedersen, D. Strong et al., "The smartphone as a medical device: Assessing enablers, benefits and challenges," in *Proceedings of the 2013 10th Annual IEEE Communications Society Conference on Sensing and Communication in Wireless Networks (SECON)*, pp. 76–80, New Orleans, LA, USA, June 2013.

[15] W. Z. Khan, Y. Xiang, M. Y. Aalsalem, and Q. Arshad, "Mobile phone sensing systems: a survey," *IEEE Communications Surveys & Tutorials*, vol. 15, no. 1, pp. 402–427, 2013.

[16] K. Wac, "Smartphone as a personal, pervasive health informatics services platform: literature review," *Yearbook of Medical Informatics*, vol. 7, pp. 83–93, 2012.

[17] M. M. Baig, H. Gholamhosseini, and M. J. Connolly, "A comprehensive survey of wearable and wireless ECG monitoring systems for older adults," *Medical & Biological Engineering & Computing*, vol. 51, no. 5, pp. 485–495, 2013.

[18] H. L. Kennedy, "The evolution of ambulatory ECG monitoring," *Progress in Cardiovascular Diseases*, vol. 56, no. 2, pp. 127–132, 2013.

[19] P. K. Jain and A. K. Tiwari, "Heart monitoring systems-A review," *Computers in Biology and Medicine*, vol. 54, pp. 1–13, 2014.

[20] S. L. Guo, H. W. Liu, Q. J. Si, D. F. Kong, and F. S. Guo, "The future of remote ECG monitoring systems," *Journal of Geriatric Cardiology*, vol. 13, no. 6, pp. 528–530, 2016.

[21] T. Tsukiyama, "In-home health monitoring system for solitary elderly," *Procedia Computer Science*, vol. 63, pp. 229–235, 2015.

[22] S. Kwon, D. Lee, J. Kim et al., "Sinabro: A smartphone-integrated opportunistic electrocardiogram monitoring system," *Sensors*, vol. 16, no. 3, article no. 361, 2016.

[23] A. Depari, A. Flammini, E. Sisinni, and A. Vezzoli, "A wearable smartphone-based system for electrocardiogram acquisition," in *Proceedings of the 9th IEEE International Symposium on Medical Measurements and Applications, IEEE MeMeA 2014*, IEEE, Lisboa, Portugal, June 2014.

[24] A. Dinh, "Heart activity monitoring on smartphone," in *Proceedings of International Conference on Biomedical Engineering and Technology, ICBET 2011*, pp. 45–49, June 2011.

[25] B. Yu, L. Xu, and Y. Li, "Bluetooth Low Energy (BLE) based mobile electrocardiogram monitoring system," in *Proceedings of the IEEE International Conference on Information and Automation, ICIA 2012*, pp. 763–767, Shenyang, China, June 2012.

[26] S.-Y. Lee, J.-H. Hong, C.-H. Hsieh, M.-C. Liang, S.-Y. C. Chien, and K.-H. Lin, "Low-power wireless ECG acquisition and classification system for body sensor networks," *IEEE Journal of Biomedical and Health Informatics*, vol. 19, no. 1, pp. 236–246, 2015.

[27] F. Miao, Y. Cheng, Y. He, Q. He, and Y. Li, "A wearable context-aware ECG monitoring system integrated with built-in kinematic sensors of the smartphone," *Sensors*, vol. 15, no. 5, pp. 11465–11484, 2015.

[28] M. Hall, E. Frank, G. Holmes, B. Pfahringer, P. Reutemann, and I. H. Witten, "The WEKA data mining software: an update," *ACM SIGKDD Explorations Newsletter*, vol. 11, no. 1, pp. 10–18, 2009.

[29] J. J. Oresko, Z. Jin, J. Cheng et al., "A wearable smartphone-based platform for real-time cardiovascular disease detection via electrocardiogram processing," *IEEE Transactions on Information Technology in Biomedicine*, vol. 14, no. 3, pp. 734–740, 2010.

[30] A. L. Goldberger, L. A. Amaral, L. Glass et al., "PhysioBank, PhysioToolkit, and PhysioNet: components of a new research resource for complex physiologic signals.," *Circulation*, vol. 101, no. 23, pp. E215–E220, 2000.

[31] R. Rajaganeshan, C. L. Ludlam, D. P. Francis, S. V. Parasramka, and R. Sutton, "Accuracy in ECG lead placement among technicians, nurses, general physicians and cardiologists," *International Journal of Clinical Practice*, vol. 62, no. 1, pp. 65–70, 2008.

[32] M. Noro, D. Anzai, and J. Wang, "Common-mode noise cancellation circuit for wearable ECG," *Healthcare Technology Letters*, vol. 4, no. 2, pp. 64–67, 2017.

[33] S. Z. Wang, W. Shan, and L. L. Song, "Principle and application of AD620 instrumentation amplifier," *Microprocessors*, vol. 4, no. 4, pp. 38–40, 2008.

[34] A. M. Soliman, "Novel oscillators using current and voltage followers," *Journal of The Franklin Institute*, vol. 335, no. 6, pp. 997–1007, 1998.

[35] O. Postolache, J. D. Pereira, and P. S. Girão, "Wireless sensor network-based solution for environmental monitoring: Water quality assessment case study," *IET Science, Measurement & Technology*, vol. 8, no. 6, pp. 610–616, 2014.

[36] N. D. A. Ghafur, *Low cost electrocardiogram heart monitor kit [Ph.D. thesis]*, Universiti Teknologi Malaysia, Johor Bahru, Malaysia, 2008.

[37] D. G. E. Robertson and J. J. Dowling, "Design and responses of Butterworth and critically damped digital filters," *Journal*

of Electromyography & Kinesiology, vol. 13, no. 6, pp. 569–573, 2003.

[38] M. Ang, "Combining the Blend micro with the Bluetooth low-energy module," https://www.packtpub.com/books/content/bluetooth-low-energy-blend-micro.

[39] C. Gomez, J. Oller, and J. Paradells, "Overview and evaluation of bluetooth low energy: an emerging low-power wireless technology," *Sensors*, vol. 12, no. 9, pp. 11734–11753, 2012.

[40] K. Townsend, "Introduction to Bluetooth Low Energy," https://cdn-learn.adafruit.com/downloads/pdf/introduction-to-bluetooth-low-energy.pdf.

[41] H. Chun-Zhi, X. Yin-shui, and W. Lun-yao, "A universal asynchronous receiver transmitter design," in *Proceedings of the IEEE International Conference on Electronics, Communications and Control, ICECC 2011*, pp. 691–694, IEEE, September 2011.

[42] H. B. Demuth, M. H. Beale, O. De Jess, and M. T. Hagan, *Neural Network Design*, Martin Hagan, USA, 2014.

[43] R. Bousseljot, D. Kreiseler, and A. Schnabel, "Nutzung der EKG-Signaldatenbank CARDIODAT der PTB über das Internet," *Biomedizinische Technik/Biomedical Engineering*, vol. 40, no. s1, pp. 317-318, 2009.

[44] L. Mainardi, L. Sornmo, and S. Cerutti, *Understanding atrial fibrillation: The signal processing contribution*, Morgan Claypool Publishers, San Rafael, CA, USA, 2008.

[45] A. B. Ramli and P. A. Ahmad, "Correlation analysis for abnormal ECG signal features extraction," in *Proceedings of the 4th National Conference on Telecommunication Technology, NCTT 2003*, pp. 232–237, IEEE, Shah Alam, Malaysia, January 2003.

[46] B. T. Szabó, A. W. van der Vaart, and J. H. van Zanten, "Empirical Bayes scaling of Gaussian priors in the white noise model," *Electronic Journal of Statistics*, vol. 7, pp. 991–1018, 2013.

[47] G. E. Maestre, G. Pino-Ramírez, A. E. Molero et al., "The Maracaibo Aging Study: Population and methodological issues," *Neuroepidemiology*, vol. 21, no. 4, pp. 194–201, 2002.

[48] MathWorks, Compile MATLAB Functions, https://www.mathworks.com/help/compiler_sdk/matlab_code.html.

[49] M. Yan and H. Shi, "Smart living using Bluetooth-based Android smartphone," *International Journal of Wireless & Mobile Networks*, vol. 5, no. 1, pp. 65–72, 2013.

[50] P. Maiya, A. Kanade, and R. Majumdar, "Race detection for android applications," in *Proceedings of the 35th ACM SIGPLAN Conference on Programming Language Design and Implementation, PLDI 2014*, pp. 316–325, Edinburgh, UK, June 2014.

[51] A. Holzinger, "User-Centered Interface Design for Disabled and Elderly People: First Experiences with Designing a Patient Communication System (PACOSY)," in *Lecture Notes in Computer Science*, K. Miesenberger, J Klaus, and W. Zagler, Eds., vol. 2398 of *Lecture Notes in Computer Science*, pp. 34–41, Springer, Berlin, Germany, 2002.

[52] S. Kiranyaz, T. Ince, and M. Gabbouj, "Real-time patient-specific ECG classification by 1-D convolutional neural networks," *IEEE Transactions on Biomedical Engineering*, vol. 63, no. 3, pp. 664–675, 2016.

[53] N. Bruining, E. Caiani, C. Chronaki, P. Guzik, and E. Van Der Velde, "Acquisition and analysis of cardiovascular signals on smartphones: Potential, pitfalls and perspectives: By the Task Force of the e-Cardiology Working Group of European Society of Cardiology," *European Journal of Preventive Cardiology*, vol. 21, no. 2s, pp. 4–13, 2014.

[54] P. A. Wolf, R. D. Abbott, and W. B. Kannel, "Atrial fibrillation as an independent risk factor for stroke: the Framingham study," *Stroke*, vol. 22, no. 8, pp. 983–988, 1991.

[55] J. K. Lau, N. Lowres, L. Neubeck et al., "IPhone ECG application for community screening to detect silent atrial fibrillation: A novel technology to prevent stroke," *International Journal of Cardiology*, vol. 165, no. 1, pp. 193-194, 2013.

[56] N. Lowres, L. Neubeck, G. Salkeld et al., "Feasibility and cost-effectiveness of stroke prevention through community screening for atrial fibrillation using iPhone ECG in pharmacies: The SEARCH-AF study," *Thrombosis and Haemostasis*, vol. 111, no. 6, pp. 1167–1176, 2014.

[57] Z. C. Haberman, R. T. Jahn, R. Bose et al., "Wireless smartphone ECG enables large-scale screening in diverse populations," *Journal of Cardiovascular Electrophysiology*, vol. 26, no. 5, pp. 520–526, 2015.

[58] J. Orchard, N. Lowres, S. B. Freedman et al., "Screening for atrial fibrillation during influenza vaccinations by primary care nurses using a smartphone electrocardiograph (iECG): A feasibility study," *European Journal of Preventive Cardiology*, vol. 23, no. 2, pp. 13–20, 2016.

[59] *New Health Economy Healthcare's new entrants: Who will be the industry's Amazon.com?* PwC Health Research Institute, USA, 2014.

[60] J. D. Piette, J. List, G. K. Rana, W. Townsend, D. Striplin, and M. Heisler, "Mobile health devices as tools for worldwide cardiovascular risk reduction and disease management," *Circulation*, vol. 132, no. 21, pp. 2012–2027, 2015.

[61] J. M. Ortman, V. A. Velkoff, H. Hogan, and H. An aging, *An Aging Nation: The Older Population in The United States*, United States Census Bureau, Suitland, MD, USA, 2014.

[62] J. Durick, T. Robertson, M. Brereton, F. Vetere, and B. Nansen, "Dispelling ageing myths in technology design," in *Proceedings of the 25th Australian Computer-Human Interaction Conference: Augmentation, Application, Innovation, Collaboration, OzCHI 2013*, pp. 467–476, Adelaide, Australia, November 2013.

[63] R. M. McCann and S. A. Keaton, "A Cross Cultural Investigation of Age Stereotypes and Communication Perceptions of Older and Younger Workers in the USA and Thailand," *Educational Gerontology*, vol. 39, no. 5, pp. 326-341, 2013.

[64] Y. Barnard, M. D. Bradley, F. Hodgson, and A. D. Lloyd, "Learning to use new technologies by older adults: perceived difficulties, experimentation behaviour and usability," *Computers in Human Behavior*, vol. 29, no. 4, pp. 1715–1724, 2013.

[65] Z. Lv, F. Xia, G. Wu, L. Yao, and Z. Chen, "iCare: A Mobile Health Monitoring System for the Elderly," in *Proceedings of the 2010 IEEE International Conference on Green Computing and Communications*, pp. 699–705, Hangzhou, China, December 2010.

[66] E. H. Chung and K. D. Guise, "QTC intervals can be assessed with the AliveCor heart monitor in patients on dofetilide for atrial fibrillation," *Journal of Electrocardiology*, vol. 48, no. 1, pp. 8-9, 2015.

19

Numerical and Experimental Investigation of Novel Blended Bifurcated Stent Grafts with Taper to Improve Hemodynamic Performance

Ming Liu,[1] **Zhenze Wang**,[2] **Anqiang Sun**,[1,3] **and Xiaoyan Deng**[1,3]

[1]*Key Laboratory for Biomechanics and Mechanobiology of Ministry of Education, School of Biological Science and Medical Engineering, Beihang University, Beijing 100083, China*
[2]*National Research Center for Rehabilitation Technical Aids, Beijing Key Laboratory of Rehabilitation Technical Aids for Old-Age Disability, Key Laboratory of Rehabilitation Technical Aids Technology and System of the Ministry of Civil Affairs, No. 1 Ronghuazhong Road, Beijing BDA, Beijing 100176, China*
[3]*Beijing Advanced Innovation Centre for Biomedical Engineering, Beihang University, Beijing 100083, China*

Correspondence should be addressed to Xiaoyan Deng; dengxy1953@buaa.edu.cn

Academic Editor: Michele Migliore

The typical helical flow within the human arterial system is widely used when designing cardiovascular devices, as this helical flow can be generated using the "crossed limbs" strategy of the bifurcated stent graft (BSG) and enhanced by the tapered structure of arteries. Here, we propose the use of a deflected blended bifurcated stent graft (BBSG) with various tapers, using conventional blended BSGs with the same degree of taper as a comparison. Hemodynamic performances, including helical strength and wall shear stress- (WSS-) based indicators, were assessed. Displacement forces that may induce stent-graft migration were assessed using numerical simulations and in vitro experiments. The results showed that as the taper increased, the displacement force, helicity strength, and time-averaged wall shear stress (TAWSS) within the iliac grafts increased, whereas the oscillating shear index (OSI) and relative residence time (RRT) gradually decreased for both types of BBSGs. With identical tapers, deflected BBSGs, compared to conventional BBSGs, exhibited a wider helical structure and lower RRT on the iliac graft and lower displacement force; however, there were no differences in hemodynamic indicators. In summary, the presence of tapering facilitated helical flow and produced better hemodynamic performance but posed a higher risk of graft migration. Conventional and deflected BBSGs with taper might be the two optimal configurations for endovascular aneurysm repair, given the helical flow. The deflected BBSG provides a better configuration, compared to the conventional BBSG, when considering the reduction of migration risk.

1. Introduction

Bifurcated stent grafts (BSG) have been widely used in endovascular aneurysm repair (EVAR) for treating patients with abdominal aortic aneurysms (AAAs) [1]. During the EVAR procedure, BSG deployment becomes even more complicated and time-consuming if patients have abnormal AAA features; for example, the aneurysm neck is unfavorable, or the common iliac arteries are highly splayed [2]. To resolve these problems, the deployment technique of intentionally crossing the limbs of the BSG is regularly used [2–4]. With this deployment strategy, the cannulation time and postoperative complication rate in the face of atypical anatomy could be reduced significantly [2, 4, 5].

The typical helical flow observed within the human arterial system has significant physiological effects. The helical flow protects the arterial wall against atherosclerosis and thrombosis formation by affecting the transport of atherogenic lipids [6, 7] and reducing platelet adhesion on the arterial walls [8]. Because of these hemodynamic benefits of helical flow, it has been applied by researchers to design vascular devices to avoid intimal hyperplasia and thrombus formation, which are often caused by an unfavorable hemodynamic environment [9]. In clinical applications, the "crossed limbs" strategy might generate helical flows within the limb of crossed stent grafts [3, 5], which is believed to be advantageous in AAA treatment. One significant feature of the arterial system that needs to be addressed is its taper, or the decreasing diameter of an artery as it becomes an arteriole. Our previous studies revealed that the aortic taper was capable of stabilizing blood flow and maintaining helical flow strength, which evidently reduced the accumulation of low-density lipoproteins on the aortic luminal surface [7]. Accordingly, the taper is of great significance for designing vascular devices.

Optimal design of the stent graft is important for improving its hemodynamic performance. For instance, the blended bifurcated stent graft (BBSG) was proposed by Morris et al.; this graft eliminates the sudden decrease in cross-sectional area at the bifurcation [10]. This type of BBSG is believed to improve hemodynamic performance and provide better long-term outcomes. In this study, the deflected BBSG was proposed based on the specific configuration, including the "crossed limbs" strategy and the BBSG, proposed by Morris et al. [5, 10]. Furthermore, the taper configuration was added to both the conventional and deflected types of BBSGs to obtain the desired high helical flow. In order to assess these new conceptual designs, we analyzed their hemodynamic performance by analyzing numerical simulations. To analyze the displacement force that may induce stent-graft migration, numerical simulation and in vitro experiments were performed to evaluate the migration risk.

2. Methods and Materials

2.1. Geometry. As depicted in Figure 1(a), referring to the BBSG parameters described in the previous literature [11, 12], two series of geometrical models with taper features, in terms of conventional and deflected BBSGs, were generated using SolidWorks (SolidWorks Corp, Concord, MA, USA). The conventional BBSG was designed based on the common BSG with blended features in the bifurcated region, which eliminates the sudden decrease in cross-sectional area at the bifurcation, as proposed by Morris et al. [10]. The deflected BBSG was designed based on the "crossed limbs" deployment strategy. When using the "crossed limbs" strategy in EVAR, the iliac grafts usually get crossed, which generates the helical flow [2, 5]. The differences between the conventional and novel designed deflected BBSGs are that the division surface of the bilateral iliac grafts for conventional BBSG is located in the symmetry plane of the iliac grafts, whereas the division surface of the bilateral iliac grafts for deflected BBSG is located in the base plane of the iliac grafts. The trunk body of all BBSG configurations was kept identical. The overall length (s) was 154.64 mm in the axis direction, and the trunk BSG (t) was 71 mm. The side length (m) was 82 mm. The trunk of the BBSG was 17 mm in diameter (n). Regarding the taper feature, it was set as the internal diameter, and it decreased progressively from the bifurcation region (n) to the outlet (i). For conventional and deflected types of BBSG, three grafts with differing tapers were constructed. Therefore, six models were constructed in total; among these models, conventional BBSGs were denoted as (a1) tapered 17–10 mm BBSG, (a2) tapered 17–9 mm BBSG, and (a3) tapered 17–8 mm BBSG, whereas deflected BBSGs were denoted as (b1) tapered 17–10 mm BBSG, (b2) tapered 17–9 mm BBSG, and (b3) tapered 17–8 mm BBSG. For instance, the tapered 17–10 mm graft had a bifurcation region diameter of 17 mm and an outlet diameter of 10 mm.

2.2. Governing Equations. Numerical simulations were created on the basis of the three-dimensional (3D), incompressible Navier–Stokes in Equation (1) and continuity equations in Equation (2) as expressed below:

$$\rho\left(\frac{\partial \vec{v}}{\partial t} + (\vec{v} \cdot \nabla)\vec{v}\right) = -\nabla p + \nabla \tau, \tag{1}$$

$$\nabla \cdot \vec{v} = 0, \tag{2}$$

where $\vec{v}$ denotes the fluid velocity vector and p refers to the pressure. ρ denotes the blood density ($\rho = 1050\,\text{kg/m}^3$), and τ denotes the stress tensor:

$$\tau = 2\eta(\dot{\gamma})\mathbf{D}, \tag{3}$$

where $\mathbf{D}$ denotes the respective deformation tensor, $\dot{\gamma}$ refers to the shear rate, and η indicates the blood viscosity as a function of the shear rate. $\mathbf{D}(\mathbf{u}) = (1/2)(\nabla\mathbf{u} + \nabla\mathbf{u}^T)$ represents the strain rate tensor, and $\dot{\gamma} = \sqrt{2\mathbf{D} : \mathbf{D}}$ is the strain rate tensor modulus.

The non-Newtonian characteristic of the blood flow was factored in with the Carreau model expressed as follows [13]:

$$\eta(\dot{\gamma}) = \eta_\infty + (\eta_0 - \eta_\infty)\left[1 + (\lambda\dot{\gamma})^2\right]^{((n-1)/2)}, \tag{4}$$

where η_0 denotes the zero shear rate viscosity, η_∞ denotes the infinite shear rate viscosity, and λ refers to the relaxation time constant. The Carreau model was well matched with the experimental data [14], as found, where $\eta_\infty = 3.45\times10^{-3}$ Pa·s, $\eta_0 = 5.6\times10^{-2}$ Pa·s, $n = 0.3568$, and $\lambda = 3.313$ s.

2.3. Boundary Conditions and Meshing. Steady flow was first simulated; subsequently, the solution of steady simulation was employed as the initial condition to further simulate the pulsatile flow. An average velocity of 0.044 m/s was extracted from the velocity waveform in Figure 1(b), and a constant of 13300 Pa was adopted at the inlet and outlets to simulate steady flow. The inlet of the BBSG corresponded to the suprarenal aorta entrance, and the outlets corresponded to the iliac arteries outflow tracts. The Reynolds number used for the steady condition was 204, and the convergence threshold value was 1×10^{-5}. The waveform of time-dependent flat flow velocity presented in Figure 1(b) was set at the inlet, and the waveform of time-dependent pressure boundary was assigned at the outlets to simulate pulsatile flow [15]. The BBSG wall was regarded as rigid and nonslippery [16].

Using ANSYS (ANSYS Inc., Canonsburg, PA), tetrahedral volume meshes were generated for these models. To

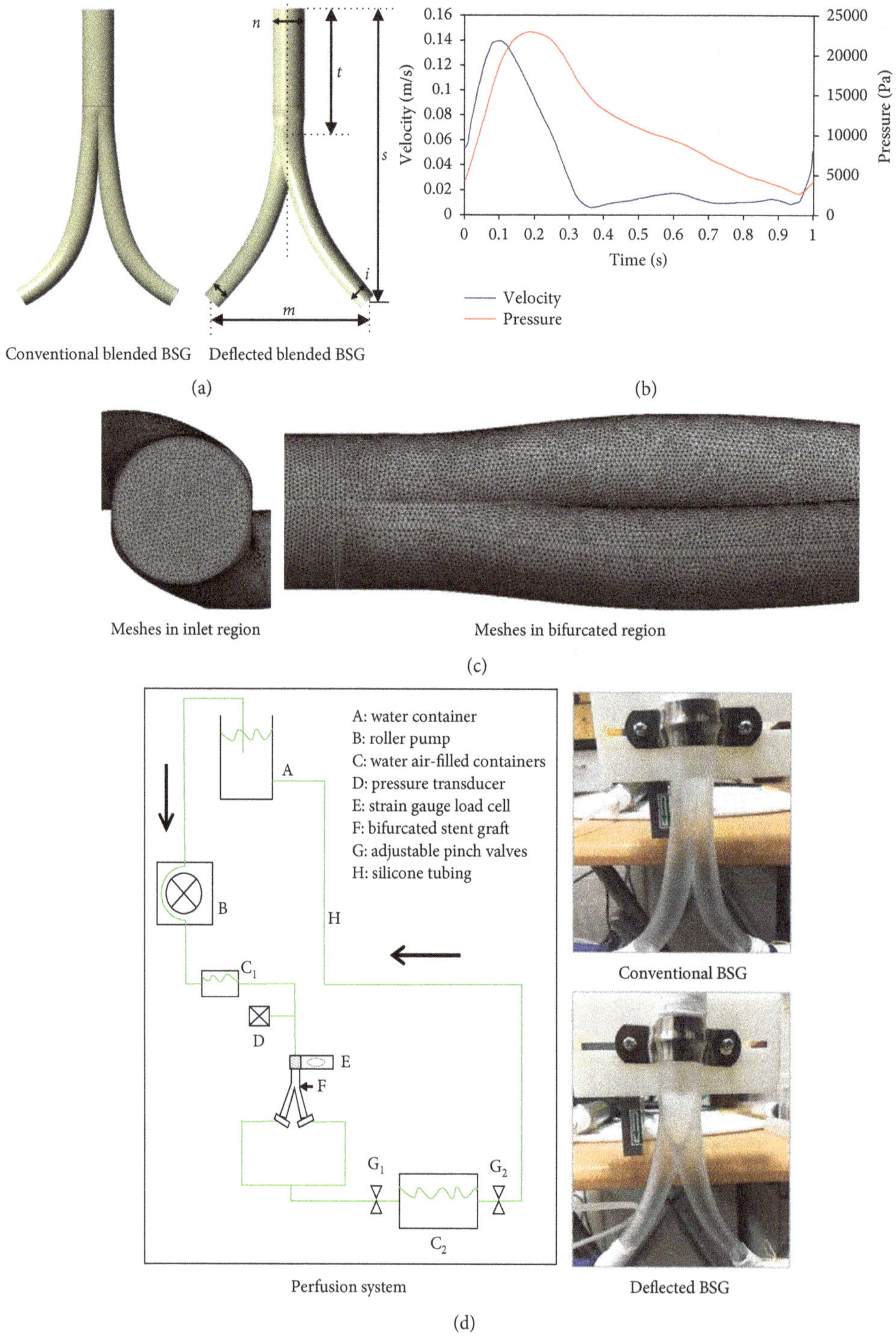

FIGURE 1: (a) Geometrical models of the ideal conventional and deflected types of blended bifurcated stent grafts (BBSGs) with taper to different degrees. (b) Imposed inlet velocity and outlet pressure waveforms. (c) Mesh presentation in the inlet and bifurcated regions. (d) Schematic presentation of the perfusion system and two types of BBSGs made of semitransparent photosensitive resin created with laser rapid prototyping technology.

ensure that our results were mesh independent, three additional mesh sizes were generated and employed to perform the calculations. When the averaged difference in the velocity and pressure of the left outlet between two successive simulations was less than 1% under steady flow (Table 1), mesh independence was considered to be achieved. The meshes that met the standard were directly used to perform the pulsatile simulations. The final volume of the meshes was nearly 1.7 million cells for each model, as shown in Figure 1(b). Details of the mesh-independent study are provided in Table 1, which shows the velocity and pressure differences between consecutive meshes.

Table 1: Mesh-independent study results.

Mesh cells	Mesh nodes	Outlet velocity difference (%)	Outlet pressure difference (%)
973,257	267,382		
1,242,534	332,187	0.05	0.05
1,457,826	397,248	0.03	0.04
1,723,820	462,861	0.01	0.01

2.4. Numerical Scheme. By employing ANSYS Fluent, the numerical simulations were performed by adopting 200 steps per cycle, with step times of 0.005 s [11]. A pressure-based solver was employed with a second-order upwind scheme to spatially discretize the momentum. The residual values for continuity and velocity were set as 1.0×10^{-5} [17]. In total, five periods were computed to ensure that the solutions were periodic. The solutions of the final period were extracted and analyzed using the MATLAB and Tecplot software.

2.5. Quantities of Interest. To better understand the diagnostic and therapeutic aspects of blood flow for treating arterial diseases, numerical simulation studies on hemodynamic effect of blood flow have been widely performed [18, 19]. By simplifying the blood characteristics, several WSS-based descriptors including WSS, time-averaged wall shear stress (TAWSS), oscillating shear index (OSI), and the relative residence time (RRT) could be calculated from the solutions of the simulations. These WSS-based descriptors might represent different hemodynamic disturbances and would present different impacts on endothelial cell homeostasis and platelet activation/aggregation. Therefore, they could potentially be used to predict the representative regions that have a high occurrence risk of stenosis and aneurysm in arteries such as the coronary artery, renal artery, or aorta or occlusion of bypass graft [9, 20].

The helicity can be employed to measure the alignment or misalignment of the local velocity and vorticity vectors, and the rotating direction of the helical structures was indicated by the sign of helicity [21]. The helicity density H_d was defined using the following equation[19, 22]:

$$H_{\mathrm{d}} = \vec{v} \cdot (\nabla \times \vec{v}) = \vec{v} \cdot \omega, \tag{5}$$

By adopting the TAWSS, the WSS on the BSG during the whole cardiac cycle was assessed:

$$TAWSS = \frac{1}{T}\int_0^T |\mathrm{WSS}(s,t)|\, dt, \tag{6}$$

where T denotes the time and s refers to the position on the stent-graft wall.

The OSI was employed to uncover the directional variation of the WSS vector in a pulsatile cycle; a higher value occurred particularly in regions characterized by disturbed flow. This was expressed as follows [23]:

$$\mathrm{OSI} = \frac{1}{2}\left[1 - \left(\frac{\left|\int_0^T \mathrm{WSS}(s,t)\,dt\right|}{\int_0^T |\mathrm{WSS}(s,t)|dt}\right)\right]. \tag{7}$$

RRT is employed for assessing the resident time of blood flow [24] and defined as

$$\mathrm{RRT} = \frac{1}{(1 - 2 \times \mathrm{OSI}) \times \mathrm{TAWSS}}. \tag{8}$$

3. Results

3.1. Flow Pattern. The helicity isosurfaces of $-0.5/0.5\,\mathrm{m \cdot s^{-2}}$ are presented in Figure 2(a). As shown in Figure 2(a), two helical flow structures widely exist along the iliac grafts from the bifurcation region. When the conventional BBSG was observed, the helical flow structures were initially generated form the middle portion of the iliac graft and developed until the outlets. In comparison, the helical flow structures in the deflected BBSG were initially generated from the bifurcated region and developed along the iliac graft until the outlets. The helical flow structures within the deflected BBSG were much more obvious than that in the conventional BBSG. As depicted in Figure 2(b), double-helical flows can be observed at the left iliac graft outlet. As the taper increases, these helical flows become even more apparent. The absolute helicity at the iliac outlet gradually increased from 0.11 to $0.51\,\mathrm{m \cdot s^{-2}}$, until it finally reached $0.63\,\mathrm{m \cdot s^{-2}}$ as the taper for the conventional BBSG increases. The absolute helicity at the left iliac outlet gradually increased from 0.05, to 0.04, to $0.21\,\mathrm{m \cdot s^{-2}}$ for the deflected BBSG with the increasing taper.

The varying trends of absolute area-averaged helicity for the left outlet during the pulsatile calculations are plotted and compared in Figure 3. The absolute helicity in systole evidently surmounts the rest of the cycle. In diastole, helicity remains basically the same and approaches zero. As the taper increased, the peak absolute area-averaged helicity progressively increased from $0.8\,\mathrm{m \cdot s^{-2}}$ (a1) to $2.2\,\mathrm{m \cdot s^{-2}}$ (a3) for the conventional BBSG. Yet the peak absolute area-averaged helicity increases from $0.14\,\mathrm{m \cdot s^{-2}}$ (b1) to $1.05\,\mathrm{m \cdot s^{-2}}$ (b3) for the deflected BBSG as the taper increases.

3.2. Hemodynamic Indicators. As observed in Figure 4(a), the comparatively high WSS areas were observed in iliac grafts, especially in the distal parts of the iliac grafts. The comparatively high WSS areas become progressively apparent as the taper increased. The area-averaged weighted WSS distribution of the iliac grafts was compared using a histogram (Figure 5(a)). As the taper increased, the WSS gradually increased from 0.11 to 0.14 Pa for the conventional BBSG, and from 0.12 to 0.15 Pa, for the deflected BBSG.

As observed in Figure 4(b), the relatively high TAWSS areas could be observed in the distal parts of the iliac grafts. As the taper increased, the relatively high TAWSS areas become even more obvious. The area-averaged weighted TAWSS distribution of the iliac grafts was compared using a histogram (Figure 5(b)). As the taper increased, the TAWSS in the iliac grafts increased from 0.11 to 0.13 Pa for the conventional BBSG and increased from 0.11 to 0.13 Pa for the deflected BBSG. TAWSS on the iliac grafts showed no major differences between the conventional and deflected BBSG.

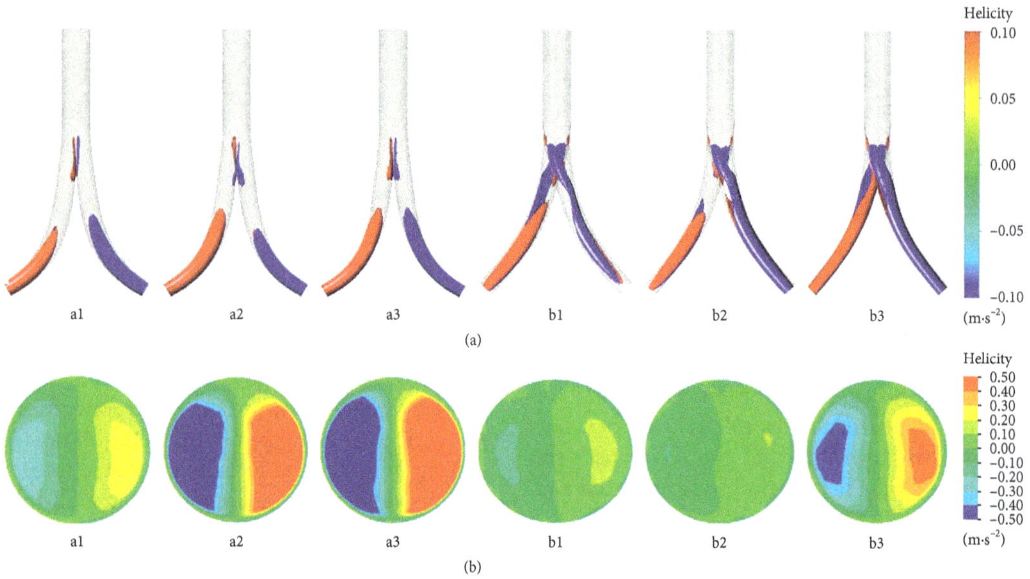

FIGURE 2: (a) Helicity isosurfaces of −0.5/0.5 ms^{-2} under steady-state simulation. (b) Surface contours of helicity at the left iliac graft outlet steady-state simulation. The right-handed helical structure with positive value was colored red, while the left-handed helical structure with negative value was colored blue.

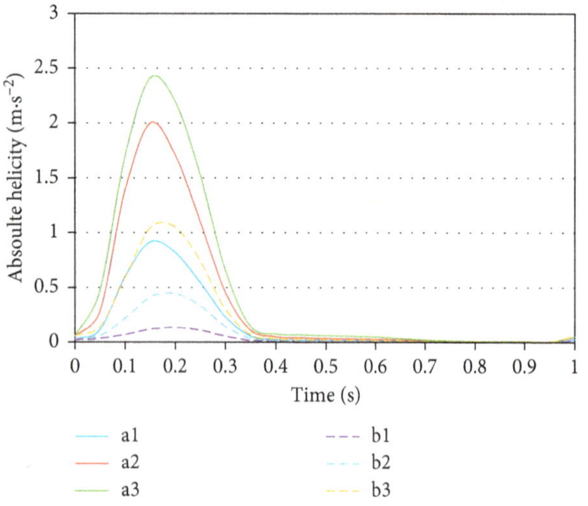

FIGURE 3: Absolute helicity of the left outlet in the pulse cycle during the pulsatile calculations.

The scattered high OSI areas are observed in the bifurcation region, as presented in Figure 4(c). The low OSI area in the inner surface can be observed distributed on the distal parts of BBSG for the conventional BBSG, and the same phenomenon occurs in the deflected BBSG. Figure 5(c) depicts the OSI on the iliac grafts in the form of a histogram. As the taper increases, the area-averaged weighted OSI in the iliac grafts gradually decreases from 0.14 to 0.10 for the conventional BBSG and decreases from 0.14 to 0.11 for the deflected BBSG.

The scattered high RRT areas can be observed in the bifurcation region, as observed in Figure 4(d). The distal parts of BBSG have an apparent low RRT area for the conventional BSG, while the deflected BBSG also presents a low RRT area in the inner face of the distal parts. As shown in Figure 5(d), the area-averaged weighted RRT in the iliac grafts gradually decreases from 13.1 to 10.91 Pa^{-1} for the conventional BBSG with increasing taper, and from 12.92 to 10.72 Pa^{-1}, for the deflected BBSG as with increasing taper.

3.3. Displacement Force. The displacement force likely to induce BSG migration was extracted and compared as variation trends. The displacement force peaked under the maximum pressure, as indicated in Figure 6. The displacement force progressively increased for both types of BBSGs as the degree of the taper increased. The peak displacement force for conventional BBSGs ranged from 3.25 N to 3.9 N and ranged from 2.5 N to 3.5 N for deflected BBSGs. The deflected BBSG clearly had a lower magnitude of displacement force in contrast to the conventional BBSG under the same taper. The peak displacement forces during the pulsatile cycle in both types of BBSG were extracted and compared. It was seen that the peak force in the deflected BBSG was significantly lower than that in the conventional BBSG ($p < 0.05$, t-test), showing that the deflected BBSG posed a lower risk of migration.

3.3.1. In Vitro Experiment. To evaluate the migration risk of the newly designed BSG, we designed an experimental aortic perfusion system to measure the displacement force. As shown in Figure 1(d), the steady flow and aortic pressure within the BSG were provided by the perfusion system. A fluid mixture consisting of 33.3% by volume of glycerol in water was used to mimic blood. The mixed fluid used in the in vitro experiments has characteristics similar to those of blood, with a density of approximately 1050 kg/m^3, and a dynamic viscosity of approximately 0.0035 Pa·s. A roller pump and silicon tubes were used to construct the fluid circuit. The fluid was perfused into the circuit at room

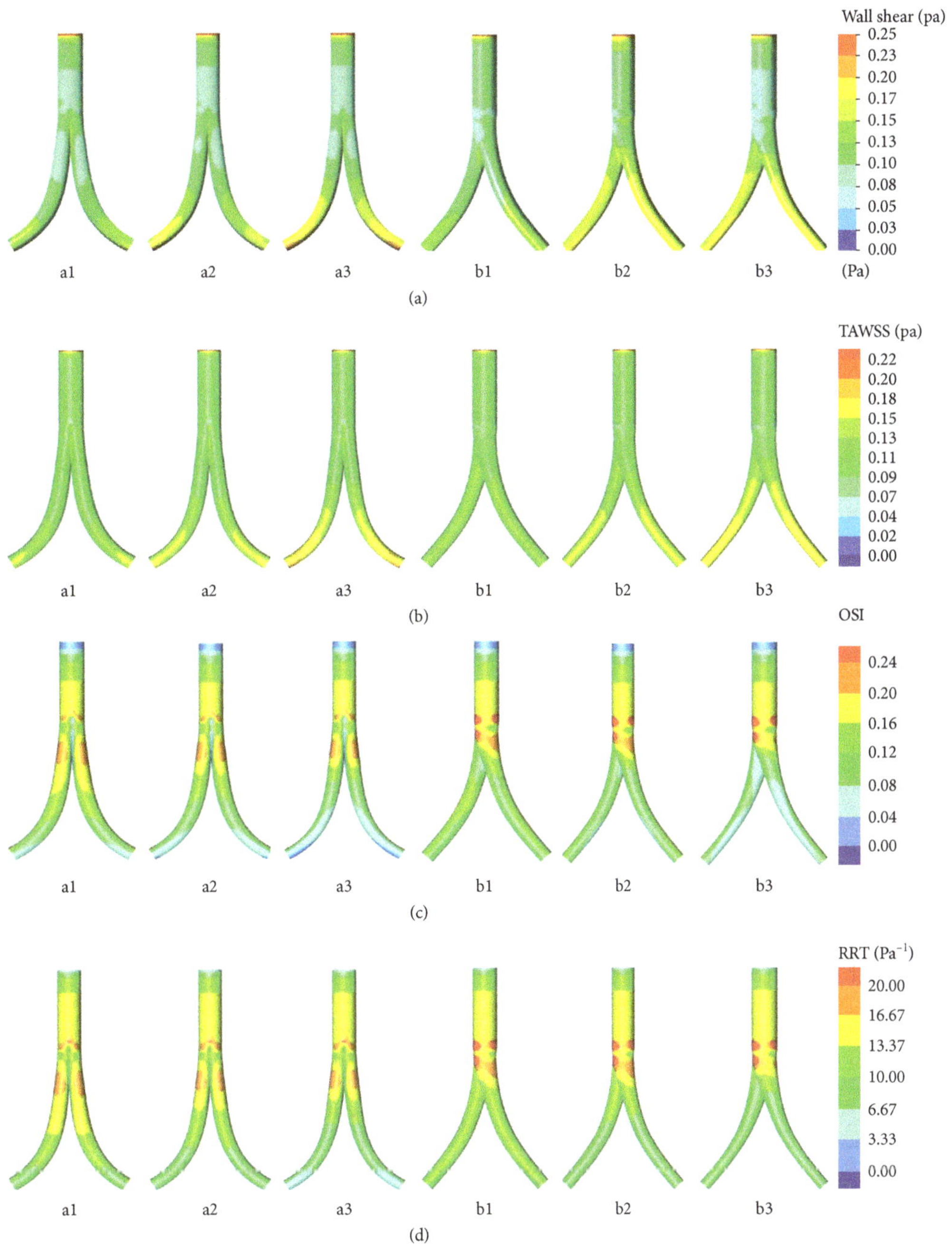

FIGURE 4: Distributions of hemodynamic indicators on the six models. (a) WSS contour; (b) TAWSS contour; (c) OSI contour; (d) RRT contour.

temperature to resemble aortic perfusion. Peripheral resistance was achieved with a container and pinch valves. The pressure was regulated by adjusting the pinch valves and water level in the water/air-filled containers, which were located at the distal part of the circuit. The water/air-filled containers were placed after the roller pump to minimize the flow disturbances.

As depicted in Figure 1(d), all BBSG models used in the experiments were made of photosensitive resin created with laser rapid prototyping technology. The geometrical size of the cavity within the experimental models was exactly the same as that of the geometry model in the computational simulations. The wall thickness of the semitransparent model used in the in vitro experiment was 1 mm. These resin-transparent BBSG models were inserted into the circuit. The proximal part of the BBSG was anchored rigidly to the strain gauge load cells using connectors. The load cell was fixed strongly to ensure that it could sense the displacement changes of the BBSG. The load cell is one type of the weighing sensor that can be used to measure the force along the tension and compression directions. The rated load ranged from 0 to 10 N. The BBSG model was placed on the

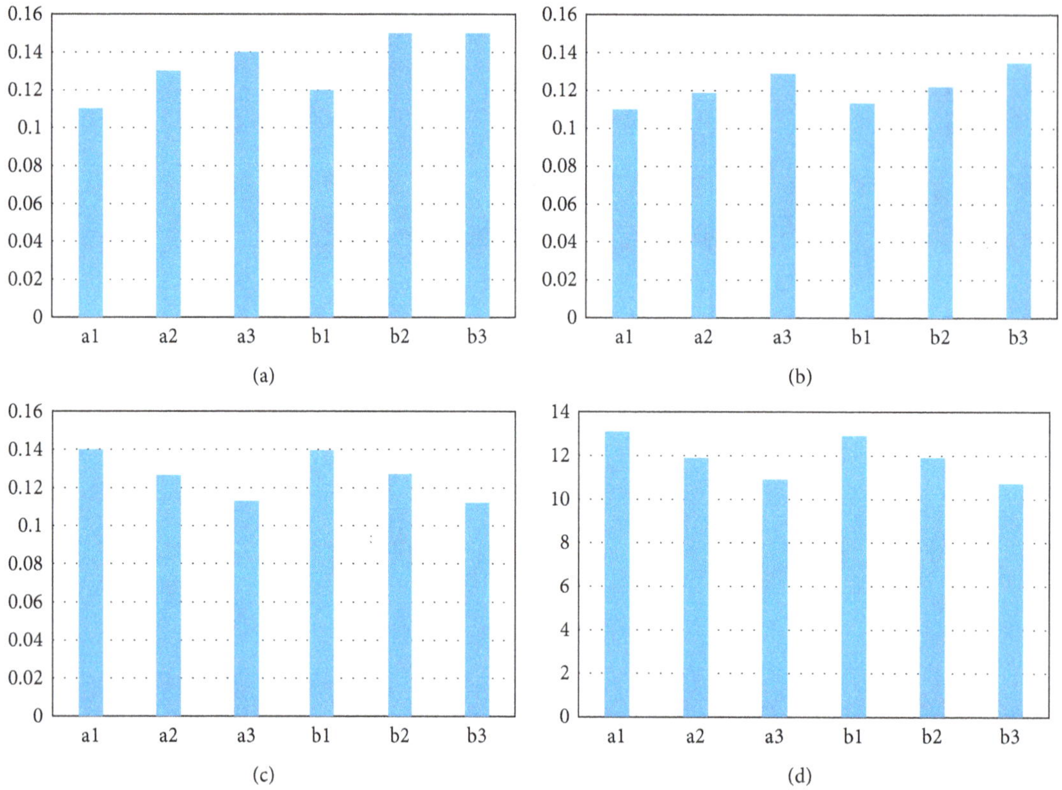

Figure 5: Area-weighted averages of hemodynamic indices in the iliac grafts of the six models. (a) WSS (Pa); (b) TAWSS (Pa); (c) OSI; (d) RRT (Pa^{-1}).

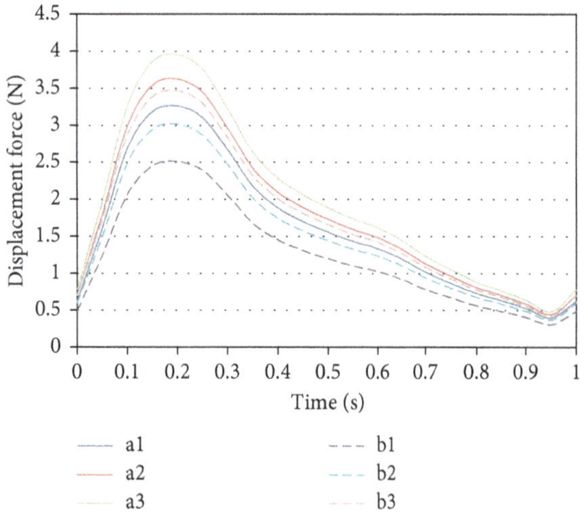

Figure 6: Variation trends of displacement force acting on the BBSG in the pulse cycle.

outside surface of the connectors to ensure that the load cell could fully receive the displacement force induced by the flow. The calibration was performed with weights. The proximal and distal parts of the BBSG were connected to the silicon tube with highly elastic soft rubber tubes to ensure that the measurements would not be influenced. For monitoring the perfusion in the iliac graft, the pressure transducer was deployed and inserted into the circuit. To record the displacement force values, the load cell was linked with a force monitor.

Measurements with both types of BBSG at various degrees of the taper were recorded at the perfusion pressures of 60, 80, and 100 mmHg. Before measurement, we conducted zero leveling and in situ calibration of perfusion pressure. When the flow remained stable, we started to perform the measurements every 20 seconds, after which the force value depicted was recorded 10 times in total. All measurements were performed under conditions of steady flow. The data of displacement force are presented in Table 2 in the format of mean ± SD (standard deviation)

As shown in Table 2, the displacement force gradually increases with the increasing pressure and the increasing degree of the taper. For the deflected BBSG, the displacement forces were smaller than those for the conventional BBSG under identical pressure. Compared with conventional BBSG, deflected BBSG showed a decrease in the displacement force between 0.07 N and 0.11 N in the cases of the three levels of perfusion pressure.

4. Discussion

Optimized design of a BSG is critical for improving its hemodynamic performance and preventing postoperative complications [10, 15, 25]. In this study, we proposed two series of conventional and deflected BBSG models with various degrees of the taper. The hemodynamic performance was assessed and compared by analyzing numerical simulations. The displacement force, which would influence the migration risk, was evaluated by conducting in vitro experiments.

TABLE 2: Displacement forces (N) acting on two types of blended bifurcated stent graft (BBSG) under various degrees of the taper.

	Conventional BBSG			Deflected BBSG		
Taper (mm)	17–10	17–9	17–8	17–10	17–9	17–8
60 (mmHg)	0.78 ± 0.01	0.82 ± 0.01	0.87 ± 0.01	0.71 ± 0.01	0.74 ± 0.01	0.78 ± 0.01
80 (mmHg)	0.93 ± 0.01	0.96 ± 0.01	1.01 ± 0.01	0.89 ± 0.01	0.92 ± 0.01	0.96 ± 0.01
100 (mmHg)	1.12 ± 0.03	1.17 ± 0.01	1.24 ± 0.01	1.03 ± 0.01	1.07 ± 0.01	1.13 ± 0.01

Helicity density was used to qualify the helical flow within the BSG; the sign of helicity density represented the rotating direction of helical structures [19, 26]. As indicated by the simulation results, two dominant helical flows were observed in both the conventional and deflected BBSGs with higher tapers, and the helicity strength increased with an increase in the taper. Helical blood flows are believed to have physiological functions that protect the arteries by suppressing the accumulation of atherogenic low-density lipoproteins within the arterial wall [7], enhancing O_2 supply to the artery [27], and reducing platelet and monocyte adhesions [8, 28]. Liu et al. investigated the hemodynamic performance within the helical graft by adding the taper feature [9]; their findings revealed that the taper feature enhanced the helical flow in the helical grafts, thus reducing the possibility of thrombus formation in the graft and improving the graft patency. The taper feature in our models had a similar effect. Therefore, the proposed blended grafts with taper involving conventional and deflected blended BSGs may decrease the possibility of thrombus formation within the stent grafts and prevent stent-graft failure in the long term. Especially, the helical structure within the deflected BBSG was continually maintained from the bifurcated region till the outlets, which is much wider than that seen in the conventional BBSG. Therefore, the deflected BBSG may provide a stronger preventive effect against the thrombosis formation within the iliac graft and reduce the occlusion risk of the stent graft.

The presence of the taper would increase both helicity and hemodynamic performance by elevating WSS and alleviating OSI and RRT in the iliac grafts for both types of BBSGs proposed in this work. It has been well established that low WSS and high OSI are of great significance for intimal hyperplasia, on the basis of their effects on the function of endothelial cells [29]. High OSI and RRT can result in thrombus formation in the way of stimulating platelet aggregation, enhancing the collision of activated platelets and increasing the residence time of procoagulant microparticles [30]. In this regard, the existence of the taper may decrease the risk of thrombus formation in the grafts. Our results indicated the taper would improve the hemodynamic in both conventional and deflected BBSGs. The BBSG showed a higher WSS and lower RRT on the iliac graft. Therefore, the deflected BBSG might provide a better hemodynamic performance than the conventional BBSG.

BSG migration remains a common complication after EVAR and could be impacted by various factors (e.g., the blood condition and configuration of BSG), as demonstrated by numerous researchers [11, 31]. When compared with the displacement force calculated from the simulation and the in vitro experiments, it was found that the variation trends of displacement force following the perfusion pressure consistently increased as the perfusion pressure increased. The changing trends of displacement force following the perfusion pressure were consistent with the results of the study by Li and Kleinstreuer [11]. Our results also showed that the displacement force would increase as the taper degree increased, when considering the taper feature. Roos et al. also investigated the effects of perfusion pressure and the taper feature on displacement force through in vitro experiments [32]. The displacement force waveforms were seen to have similar temporal behavior to those of the perfusion pressure waveform. They also found that the displacement force increased significantly for the tapered stent graft when compared with the nontapered stent graft. Our results obtained via computational simulations and in vitro experiments revealed that the displacement force would increase with the increase of the taper. Accordingly, the taper could also count as one factor that primarily affects the migration behavior of BBSGs as proposed in this paper. Our results also revealed that the displacement force was smaller in the deflected BBSG when compared with that in the conventional BBSG under identical taper conditions. In this regard, the migration risk assumed by the deflected BSG is smaller than that by the conventional BBSG. Thus, the deflected BBSG with taper might be the better optimized design for BBSG from the viewpoint of prohibiting the BSG migration.

In this study, idealized models with rigid walls were employed. As the hemodynamic effect was the main point, we intended to illustrate the characteristics of stent graft were not considered in our study. This could be one limitation of our study. These simplifications have been proposed as reasonable [9, 33] and provide clear comparisons, enabling a distinct conclusion; meanwhile, these simplified settings could be verified by conducting in vitro experiments. The biological response of platelets to the shear stress is not considered in the BBSG. The formation of thrombosis within the stent graft and the migration behavior of stent graft remain a gradual process. Therefore, a larger observational period is needed to detect the outcomes of endovascular aneurysm repair. Although potential risk of endograft migration and thrombosis can be evaluated using computational simulation and in vitro experiment, the conclusion is a preliminary conclusion and needs further study.

5. Conclusion

In summary, the present study revealed that novel BBSGs with taper, including conventional and deflected types, would generate helical flow and that the existence of the taper feature could enhance helical flow and hemodynamic performance. Therefore, the taper feature might serve as one optimal configuration for designing the BSG when considering the benefits of the helical flow mechanism. As the hemodynamic performance and migration risk must also be considered when optimizing the design of the BBSG, the risk of the deflected BBSG may be the better choice (when compared with the conventional BBSG) as it can provide better hemodynamic performance and poses a reduced risk of migration.

Conflicts of Interest

The authors declare that they have no conflicts of interest.

Authors' Contributions

Ming Liu and Anqiang Sun designed the study and drafted the manuscript; Anqiang Sun and Xiaoyan Deng performed the study; Zhenze Wang also helped in drafting the manuscript. All the authors approved the manuscript for publication.

Acknowledgments

The authors gratefully acknowledge the financial supports by the National Natural Science Foundation of China (nos. 11472031 and 11572028), National Key Research and Development Plan of China (2017YFB0702501) and the Natural Science Foundation of Jiangsu Province (BK20161366).

References

[1] P. M. De Marino, I. M. Lopez, F. P. Sanchez et al., "Endovascular treatment of abdominal aortic aneurysms with narrow aortic bifurcation using excluder bifurcated stent-grafts," *Journal of Vascular Surgery*, vol. 67, no. 1, pp. 113–118, 2018.

[2] V. G. Ramaiah, C. S. Thompson, S. Shafique et al., "Crossing the limbs: a useful adjunct for successful deployment of the Aneurx stent-graft," *Journal of Endovascular Therapy*, vol. 9, no. 5, pp. 583–586, 2002.

[3] F. Stefanov, T. McGloughlin, and L. Morris, "A computational assessment of the hemodynamic effects of crossed and non-crossed bifurcated stent-graft devices for the treatment of abdominal aortic aneurysms," *Medical Engineering and Physics*, vol. 38, no. 12, pp. 1458–1473, 2016.

[4] J. P. Henretta, L. A. Karch, K. J. Hodgson et al., "Special iliac artery considerations during aneurysm endografting," *American Journal of Surgery*, vol. 178, no. 3, pp. 212–218, 1999.

[5] T. L. Shek, L. W. Tse, A. Nabovati et al., "Computational fluid dynamics evaluation of the cross-limb stent-graft configuration for endovascular aneurysm repair," *Journal of Biomechanical Engineering*, vol. 134, no. 12, article 121002, 2012.

[6] X. Liu, Z. Wang, P. Zhao et al., "Nitric oxide transport in normal human thoracic aorta: effects of hemodynamics and nitric oxide scavengers," *PLoS One*, vol. 9, no. 11, Article ID e112395, 2014.

[7] X. Liu, F. Pu, Y. Fan, X. Deng, D. Li, and S. Li, "A numerical study on the flow of blood and the transport of LDL in the human aorta: the physiological significance of the helical flow in the aortic arch," *American Journal of Physiology Heart and Circulatory Physiology*, vol. 297, no. 1, pp. H163–H170, 2009.

[8] F. Zhan, Y. Fan, X. Deng, and Z. Xu, "The beneficial effect of swirling flow on platelet adhesion to the surface of a sudden tubular expansion tube: its potential application in end-to-end arterial anastomosis," *ASAIO Journal*, vol. 56, no. 3, pp. 172–179, 2010.

[9] X. Liu, L. Wang, Z. Wang et al., "Bioinspired helical graft with taper to enhance helical flow," *Journal of Biomechanics*, vol. 49, no. 15, pp. 3643–3650, 2016.

[10] L. Morris, F. Stefanov, and T. McGloughlin, "Stent-graft performance in the treatment of abdominal aortic aneurysms: the influence of compliance and geometry," *Journal of Biomechanics*, vol. 46, no. 2, pp. 383–395, 2013.

[11] Z. Li and C. Kleinstreuer, "Analysis of biomechanical factors affecting stent-graft migration in an abdominal aortic aneurysm model," *Journal of Biomechanics*, vol. 39, no. 12, pp. 2264–2273, 2006.

[12] Z. Li and C. Kleinstreuer, "Blood flow and structure interactions in a stented abdominal aortic aneurysm model," *Medical Engineering and Physics*, vol. 27, no. 5, pp. 369–382, 2005.

[13] U. Morbiducci, D. Gallo, D. Massai et al., "On the importance of blood rheology for bulk flow in hemodynamic models of the carotid bifurcation," *Journal of Biomechanics*, vol. 44, no. 13, pp. 2427–2438, 2011.

[14] Y. I. Cho and K. R. Kensey, "Effects of the non-Newtonian viscosity of blood on flows in a diseased arterial vessel. Part 1: steady flows," *Biorheology*, vol. 28, no. 3-4, pp. 241–262, 1991.

[15] E. Georgakarakos, A. Xenakis, G. S. Georgiadis et al., "The hemodynamic impact of misalignment of fenestrated endografts: a computational study," *European Journal of Vascular and Endovascular Surgery*, vol. 47, no. 2, pp. 151–159, 2014.

[16] A. A. Owida, H. Do, and Y. S. Morsi, "Numerical analysis of coronary artery bypass grafts: an over view," *Computer Methods and Programs in Biomedicine*, vol. 108, no. 2, pp. 689–705, 2012.

[17] J. Dong, K. K. Wong, and J. Tu, "Hemodynamics analysis of patient-specific carotid bifurcation: a CFD model of downstream peripheral vascular impedance," *International Journal for Numerical Methods in Biomedical Engineering*, vol. 29, no. 4, pp. 476–491, 2013.

[18] E. Kokkalis, N. Aristokleous, and J. G. Houston, "Haemodynamics and flow modification stents for peripheral arterial disease: a review," *Annals of Biomedical Engineering*, vol. 44, no. 2, pp. 466–476, 2016.

[19] D. Gallo, D. A. Steinman, P. B. Bijari et al., "Helical flow in carotid bifurcation as surrogate marker of exposure to disturbed shear," *Journal of Biomechanics*, vol. 45, no. 14, pp. 2398–2404, 2012.

[20] Y. Xue, X. Liu, A. Sun et al., "Hemodynamic performance of a new punched stent strut: a numerical study," *Artificial Organs*, vol. 40, no. 7, pp. 669–677, 2016.

[21] U. Morbiducci, R. Ponzini, M. Grigioni et al., "Helical flow as fluid dynamic signature for atherogenesis risk in aortocoronary bypass. A numeric study," *Journal of biomechanics*, vol. 40, no. 3, pp. 519–534, 2007.

[22] D. Gallo, G. De Santis, F. Negri et al., "On the use of in vivo measured flow rates as boundary conditions for image-based hemodynamic models of the human aorta: implications for

indicators of abnormal flow," *Annals of Biomedical Engineering*, vol. 40, no. 3, pp. 729–741, 2012.

[23] X. He and D. N. Ku, "Pulsatile flow in the human left coronary artery bifurcation: average conditions," *Journal of Biomechanical Engineering*, vol. 118, no. 1, pp. 74–82, 1996.

[24] S. W. Lee, L. Antiga, and D. A. Steinman, "Correlations among indicators of disturbed flow at the normal carotid bifurcation," *Journal of Biomechanical Engineering*, vol. 131, no. 6, article 061013, 2009.

[25] H. Kandail, M. Hamady, and X. Y. Xu, "Patient-specific analysis of displacement forces acting on fenestrated stent-grafts for endovascular aneurysm repair," *Journal of Biomechanics*, vol. 47, no. 14, pp. 3546–3554, 2014.

[26] M. Grigioni, C. Daniele, U. Morbiducci et al., "A mathematical description of blood spiral flow in vessels: application to a numerical study of flow in arterial bending," *Journal of Biomechanics*, vol. 38, no. 7, pp. 1375–1386, 2005.

[27] X. Liu, Y. Fan, and X. Deng, "Effect of spiral flow on the transport of oxygen in the aorta: a numerical study," *Annals of Biomedical Engineering*, vol. 38, no. 3, pp. 917–926, 2010.

[28] F. Zhan, Y. Fan, and X. Deng, "Swirling flow created in a glass tube suppressed platelet adhesion to the surface of the tube: its implication in the design of small-caliber arterial grafts," *Thrombosis Research*, vol. 125, no. 5, pp. 413–418, 2010.

[29] J. J. Chiu and S. Chien, "Effects of disturbed flow on vascular endothelium: pathophysiological basis and clinical perspectives," *Physiological Reviews*, vol. 91, no. 1, pp. 327–387, 2011.

[30] A. J. Reininger, H. F. Heijnen, H. Schumann et al., "Mechanism of platelet adhesion to von Willebrand factor and microparticle formation under high shear stress," *Blood*, vol. 107, no. 9, pp. 3537–3545, 2006.

[31] D. S. Molony, E. G. Kavanagh, P. Madhavan et al., "A computational study of the magnitude and direction of migration forces in patient-specific abdominal aortic aneurysm stent-grafts," *European Journal of Vascular and Endovascular Surgery*, vol. 40, no. 3, pp. 332–339, 2010.

[32] H. Roos, M. Tokarev, V. Chernoray et al., "Displacement forces in stent-grafts: influence of diameter variation and curvature asymmetry," *European Journal of Vascular and Endovascular Surgery*, vol. 52, no. 2, pp. 150–156, 2016.

[33] A. F. Totorean, S. I. Bernad, and R. F. Susan-Resiga, "Fluid dynamics in helical geometries with applications for by-pass grafts," *Applied Mathematics and Computation*, vol. 272, pp. 604–613, 2016.

20

A Practical Guide to Analyzing Time-Varying Associations between Physical Activity and Affect using Multilevel Modeling

Jinhyuk Kim,[1] David Marcusson-Clavertz,[1,2] Fumiharu Togo,[3] and Hyuntae Park[4]

[1]*Department of Biobehavioral Health, The Pennsylvania State University, University Park, PA, USA*
[2]*Department of Psychology, Lund University, Lund, Sweden*
[3]*Educational Physiology Laboratory, Graduate School of Education, The University of Tokyo, Tokyo, Japan*
[4]*Department of Health Care and Science, College of Health Science, Dong-A University, Busan, Republic of Korea*

Correspondence should be addressed to Jinhyuk Kim; juk423@psu.edu and Hyuntae Park; htpark@dau.ac.kr

Academic Editor: Zoran Bursac

There is growing interest in within-person associations of objectively measured physical and physiological variables with psychological states in daily life. Here we provide a practical guide with SAS code of multilevel modeling for analyzing physical activity data obtained by accelerometer and self-report data from intensive and repeated measures using ecological momentary assessments (EMA). We review previous applications of EMA in research and clinical settings and the analytical tools that are useful for EMA research. We exemplify the analyses of EMA data with cases on physical activity data and affect and discuss the future challenges in the field.

1. Introduction

Enabled by technological developments, ecological momentary assessment (EMA) [1] using mobile data collection has become an essential research tool in many fields of social and behavioral sciences and is continuing to spread to other areas of sciences. EMA research covers a wide range of phenomena, including the study of environmental, physical, physiological, psychological, and sociological factors, using repeated or continuous recording. Given the widespread use of EMA methods across the different sciences, various terms have been used to refer to similar procedures. EMA methods focusing on self-report data are frequently referred to as experience-sampling methods (ESM) [2], whereas those focusing on physical, physiological, or biological data are often called ambulatory assessments (AA) [3]. However, we use the term EMA broadly to include all these types of ecological, intensive assessments. To exemplify, EMA studies investigate various behaviors, experiences, and environmental conditions, including depression [4–6], psychological stress [7, 8], self-esteem [9], diet [10], self-reported physical activity [11, 12], smoking [13–15], sexual behavior [16], compulsive buying [17], social interaction [4, 18], work activity and satisfaction [8, 19], diabetes management [18, 20], effects of medication [21, 22], asthma [23, 24], allergies [25, 26], tinnitus [27], and working memory and attention [28]. In addition, technological developments have enabled automated EMA of behaviors (e.g., taking medication [29]) and physical environment (e.g., air sampling [26], sampling in electromagnetic fields [30]). Ambulatory monitoring of cardiovascular function, using portable cardiac monitors, has been used for several decades as a tool for understanding the association between experiences and cardiovascular health [31]. Recent developments have expanded physiological monitoring to other parameters, such as physical activity [32–38], hypothalamic-pituitary-adrenal axis activity [39–42], blood glucose [43], skin temperature [44], pulmonary function [23], and others. Furthermore, these data collections are widely used to evaluate treatment and intervention of crucial health-related behaviors in health psychology and behavioral medicine, such as coping with illness and treatment [45, 46], medication compliance [47, 48], and exercise [49, 50].

Psychiatric (or psychosomatic) disorders studied with EMA include a wide range of psychopathology, such as addictive disorders [51, 52], gastrointestinal disorders [53], sexual dysfunction [54], eating disorders [46, 55, 56], attention deficit hyperactivity disorder (ADHD) [57, 58], mood dysregulation [59], anxiety disorders [60–62], depressive disorders [63–65], bipolar disorder [66], and schizophrenia [67–69].

Why did EMA become frequently used in various areas of researches including clinical settings? One advantage of EMA methods is that they enable us to study a phenomenon in its natural environment. A second advantage is that they allow us to study the time course of target variables. Intensive data collection enables the exploration of development trajectories of psychiatric disorders and physical health conditions and identification of factors that are predictive of these trajectories. For instance, one study used EMA methods to examine if spousal responsiveness to verbal expressions of pain in patients with knee osteoarthritis predicted patients' physical function over time [70]. Such fluctuations in the trajectories cannot be captured by traditional, cross-sectional data collection methods. A third advantage is that EMA enable us to assess related symptoms with other related factors (e.g., physiological states or social and environmental situations) immediately before and just after disorders (e.g., panic attacks [62], binge eating [55]), which give us important insights into pathogenic processes and prevention of psychiatric disorders and poor physical health.

Many EMA studies have examined how a phenomenon covaries with variables that may vary across different levels, including moments (e.g., mood states), days (e.g., work days versus weekends), persons (e.g., unemployed versus employed), or other levels (e.g., organizations, seasons) in various populations, including patients with psychiatric disorders and physical conditions. For example, cardiovascular reactivity [71–74] and cortisol-related reactivity [39–42, 75] were reported to be associated with levels of psychological stress, and changes in pulmonary functions tested by a spirometer were associated with daily positive/negative affect, as well as the symptom of shortness of breath in asthma patients. Health-related behaviors, such as eating [76, 77], smoking [13, 14], and alcohol consumption [78, 79], exhibited associations with variation in physical symptoms and psychological states, e.g., craving, positive/negative affect, and anxiety. Furthermore, associations between physical activity measured by self-report and daily fluctuations in psychological states have been reported [11, 12]. These studies provide strong evidence that biological/physiological measures vary in time with momentary symptoms. Thus, the existence of such objective proxies for subjective symptoms indicates the possibility of the practical use of them for monitoring momentary symptoms in a continuous fashion (i.e., without the need for self-reports). There might also be advantages in simultaneously using self-reported subjective symptoms and objective measures to improve the explanation of health outcomes.

It has been suggested that momentary fluctuations in behavioral data, specifically those on physical activity capturing bodily acceleration, reflect the dynamics of systems organizing human behavior and can be used to examine behavioral disorders, including mental illnesses [32–38]. Indeed, altered physical activity is one of the cardinal signs of psychiatric disorders and included in their diagnostic criteria [80]. For example, major depressive disorders (MDD) are characterized by the presence of symptoms associated with behavioral alterations, including diminished physical activity, psychomotor retardation or agitation, and sleep disturbances [80]. Specifically, several studies using accelerometer have been conducted with patients with depression, showing disruption of the circadian rhythm [32–34]. Research has shown the existence of robust statistical regularities concerning daily life behaviors, specifically how resting and active periods derived from physical activity data are interwoven into daily life [81]. In addition, this research found, in patients with MDD, a significant alteration of a parameter of the robust law representing the distribution of resting periods; compared to healthy subject, these patients exhibited more intermittent behavioral patterns characterized by reduced mean activity levels associated with occasional bursts of physical activity counts [81, 82]. Furthermore, alterations of intermittent properties of physical activity have been reported in schizophrenia and bipolar disorder [83, 84]. Recent studies showed the psychobehavioral correlates of temporal diurnal fluctuations in momentary depressive mood and behavioral dynamics [85, 86]. The results in these studies suggested that an increased intermittency of physical activity (i.e., low mean level and occasional burst of physical activity) appeared concurrently with the worsening of depressive mood in healthy subjects across a wide range of populations (adolescents, undergraduates, and adult office workers) [85], as well as in patients with MDD [86]. Furthermore, the cross validation between healthy subjects and patients with MDD were confirmed, indicating that the same psychobehavioral correlates are shared by both groups [86]. A pilot study suggested that temporal variations in depressive mood are affected by underlying changes in physical activity in older adults. Reduced activity patterns preceded or occurred concurrently with the worsening of depressive mood rather than following (Figures 1(a) and 1(b)) [87]. These findings suggest that physical activity obtained by accelerometer is a useful measure for evaluating behavioral abnormalities associated with psychiatric disorders, and that its characterization is likely to provide an objective measure for these disorders. However, other studies have not found support for associations between some types of mental disorders or psychological states and physical activity. For example, a study reported nonsignificant bidirectional associations between mood (i.e., energetic arousal, valence, and calmness) and physical activity in inactive university students [88]. Another study showed that physical activity contributes to an improvement of positive affect, but not a reduction of negative affect in MDD [89].

In this paper, we describe analytic models that are useful for analyzing EMA data with cases on physical activity data and affect. We also offer Supplementary Materials (available here) with SAS code for how to handle physical activity data obtained by accelerometer and use multilevel modeling techniques on EMA data.

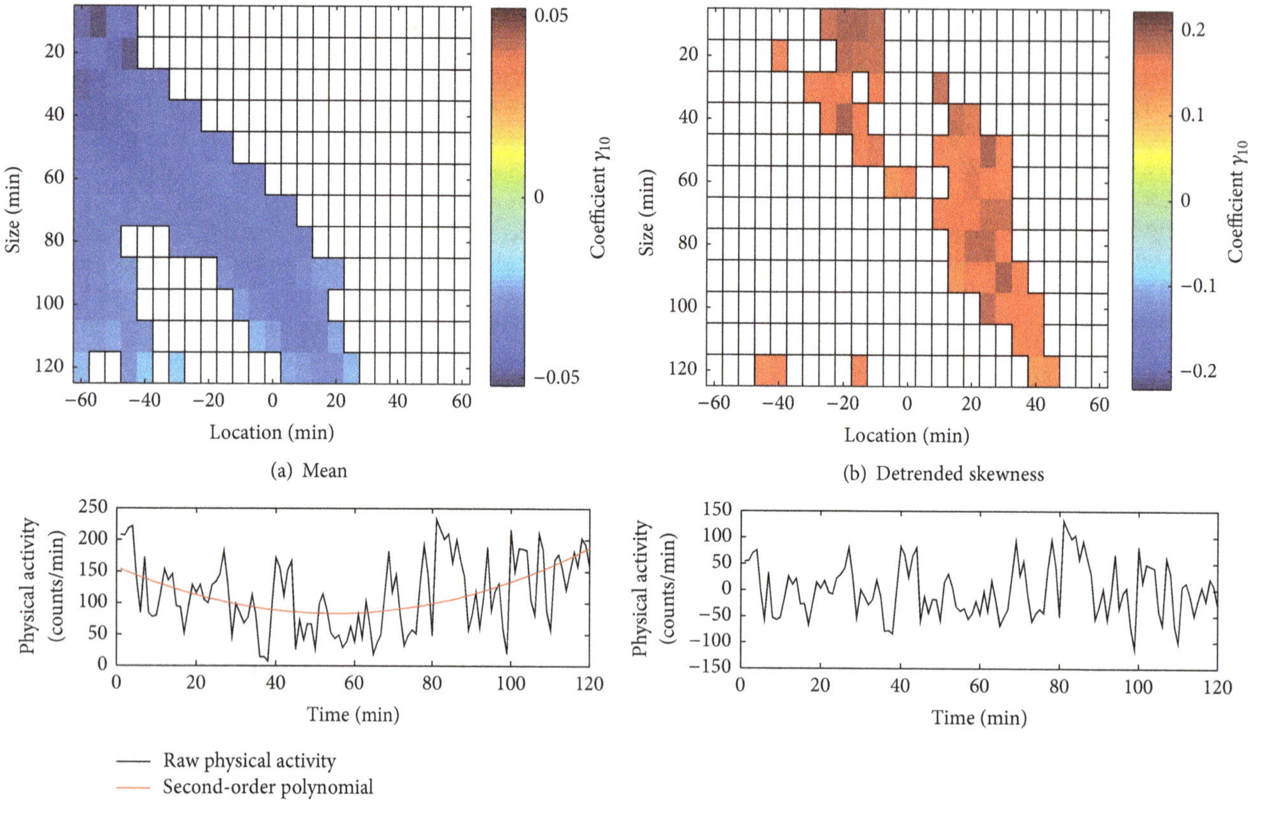

(a) Mean

(b) Detrended skewness

(c) Raw physical activity

(d) Detrended physical activity

FIGURE 1: **Analytic techniques for physical activity.** (a) The temporal associations of depressive mood and local mean of physical activity which evaluates lower/higher mean activity levels. Estimated values of the univariate multilevel model coefficient for the associations are shown in a colored matrix form consisting of 25 columns (different location) and 12 rows (different size) in older adults ($n = 9$). Each grid cell indicates specific location and size of a time frame used for calculating the local mean of physical activity surrounding each EMA recording of depressive mood. A color in each cell represents the value of the model coefficient (γ_{10}) of the predictors. The false discovery rate with the q value of .05 was used as the multiple comparison adjustment. Only the significant cases were shown by colors. Note that the univariate model used for the analysis is as follows. Depressive mood score$_{tj} = \gamma_{00} + \gamma_{10}$ (local statistics of physical activity$_{tj}$) $+ \zeta_{0j} + \varepsilon_{tj}$ [see [85] for details]. (b) The same is shown in panels (a), except for the local mean. Local skewness of physical activity, which evaluates asymmetry of a distribution (i.e., occasional bursts of physical activity in a time window), was used in this panel. (c) A raw physical activity time series for 120 min and the second-order polynomial line (red). (d) The detrended physical activity derived by subtracting the fitted line for the original data.

2. Analytic Tools and Techniques for Evaluating Time-Varying Associations between Physical Activity and Affect

2.1. Multilevel Modeling. Although there are several analytical approaches to examine the association between physical activity and affect in daily life (e.g., correlation, regression, or time series modeling), multilevel modeling is suitable for addressing unbalanced and hierarchical EMA data. In EMA data, multiple observations are typically hierarchically nested within individuals, with the number and timing of observations varying between individuals (see Figure 2 for an example of EMA data structure). In addition, EMA studies usually have missing data due to difficulties in fully complying with the schedule. Traditional techniques such as repeated measures analysis of variance (RM-ANOVA) are not suitable for analyzing these unbalanced data sets [90]. However, such data can be handled by the multilevel modeling approach, which is an extension of traditional regression models and has been recommended for the analysis of data with a hierarchical structure (Figure 2) [90–92].

In multilevel modeling, these within- and between-individual effects can be handled together in the same model by incorporating random effects into model coefficients, i.e., allowing the coefficients to vary across individuals. For example, a researcher might expect that the average level of physical activity and the influence of negative affect on physical activity differ significantly between individuals, and therefore, model these effects as random intercepts and slopes, respectively. Although the multilevel model can be expressed as a single equation, it is easier to understand if it is initially presented as a set of equations separating within- and between-individual levels. In EMA analysis, usually observations are modeled as level 1 (within-individual level)

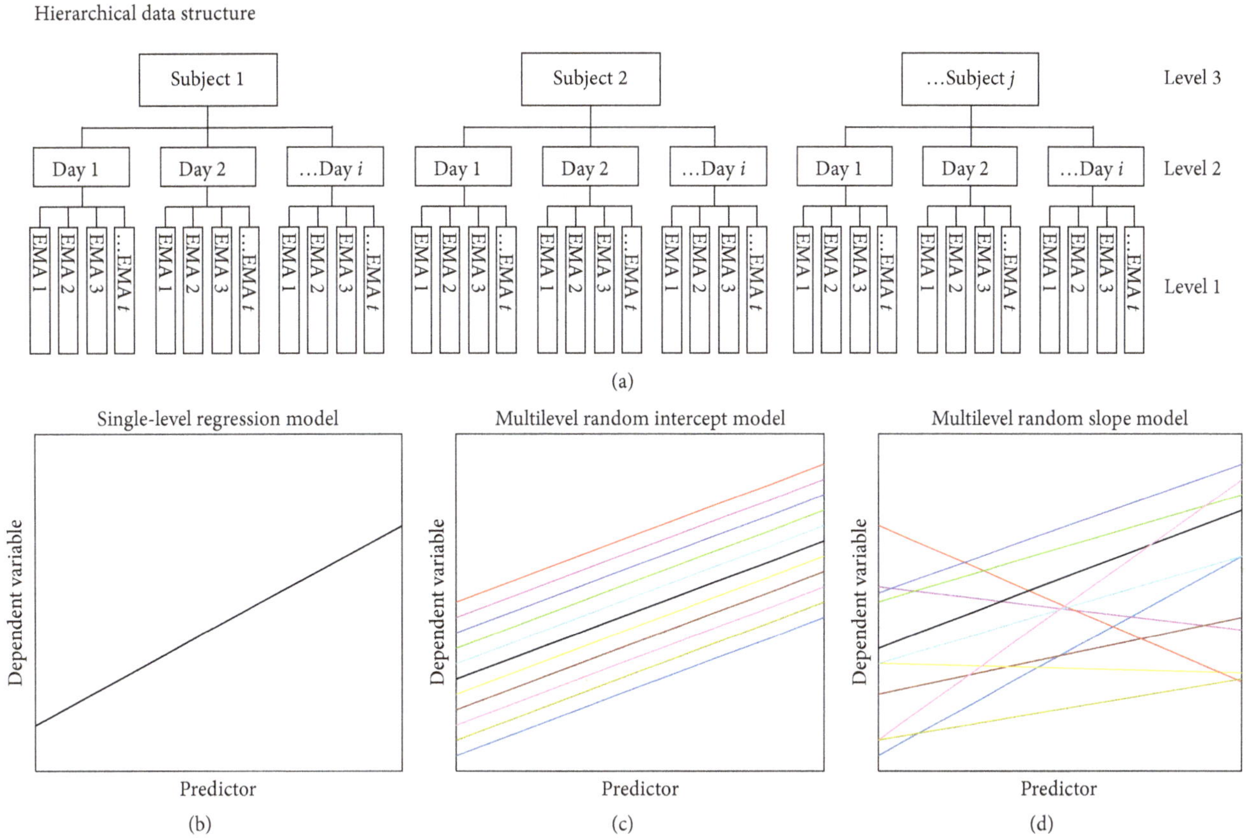

FIGURE 2: **Concept plots illustrate multilevel modeling using hierarchical ecological momentary assessment (EMA) data.** (a) An example of hierarchical data structure in which EMA observations (level 1) nested within days (level 2) nested within subjects (level 3). The number of EMA observations (t) and days (i) can be different in each subject. (b) Traditional regression model with fixed slope and intercept which do not vary across subjects. (c) Multilevel model with random intercepts, which vary across subjects, and fixed slopes. (d) Multilevel model with random intercepts and slopes. The multilevel model can be tested with random slopes and fixed intercepts, but the practical use of the model may be limited.

units nested within individuals who are modeled as level 2 (between-individuals level) units. An example of multilevel models is as follows.

Level 1 Equation (Within-Individual [Observation] Level)

$$Y_{tj} = \pi_{0j} + \sum_{k=1}^{n} \pi_{kj} \left(X_{tj}^{k} - \overline{X}_{j}^{k} \right) + \varepsilon_{tj} \quad (k = 1, \ldots, n) \tag{1}$$

where Y_{tj} indicates the dependent variable (e.g., negative affect or depression) tth momentary observation for the jth subject; X_{tj}^{k} is the kth predictor (e.g., physical activity; k represents the order of predictors) corresponding to the tth momentary observation for the jth subject; $\overline{X}_{j}^{k}$ is the person mean of the kth predictor for centering to estimate the within-person effect of the predictor (physical activity) on the dependent variable of subjective symptoms [93]; n is the total number of predictors; π_{0j} and π_{kj} are the subject j's intercept and coefficient (i.e., slope) of the predictor, respectively; and ε_{tj} is the within-individual residual.

Level 2 Equations (Between-Individual Level)

$$\pi_{0j} = \gamma_{00} + \gamma_{01} Z_j + \zeta_{0j} \tag{2}$$

$$\pi_{kj} = \gamma_{k0} + \gamma_{k1} Z_j + \zeta_{kj} \tag{3}$$

where γ_{00} is the average intercept across all subjects; γ_{k0} is the average slope across all subjects; Z_j is the between-individual level predictor representing, e.g., subject's characteristics; γ_{01} and γ_{k1} are the effect of the variable Z_j; and the random terms ζ_{0j} and ζ_{kj} are the between-individual residuals.

Combined Model

$$Y_{tj} = \gamma_{00} + \gamma_{01} Z_j + \sum_{k=1}^{n} \gamma_{k0} \left(X_{tj}^{k} - \overline{X}_{j}^{k} \right) + \sum_{k=1}^{n} \gamma_{k1} Z_j \left(X_{tj}^{k} - \overline{X}_{j}^{k} \right) + \zeta_{0j} + \sum_{k=1}^{n} \zeta_{kj} \left(X_{tj}^{k} - \overline{X}_{j}^{k} \right) + \varepsilon_{tj} \tag{4}$$

When the groups are nested within additional groups, the data form a 3-level hierarchy and 3-level models can be fitted to account for the additional level, e.g., EMA observations (level 1) nested within days (level 2) nested within individuals (level 3). An example of 3-level multilevel models is as follows (combined model is not shown).

Level 1 Equation (Within-Individual [Observation] Level)

$$Y_{tij} = \pi_{0ij} + \sum_{k=1}^{n} \pi_{kij} \left(X_{tij}^{k} - \overline{X}_{j}^{k} \right) + \varepsilon_{tij} \quad (k = 1, \ldots, n) \quad (5)$$

where Y_{tij} indicates the dependent variable at the tth momentary observation for the jth subject on the ith day; X_{tij}^{k} is the kth predictor corresponding to the tth momentary observations for the jth subject on the ith day; π_{0ij} and π_{kij} are the subject j's intercept and coefficient (i.e., slope) of the predictor on the ith day, respectively; and ε_{tij} is the observation-level residual.

Level 2 Equations (Within-Individual [Day] Level)

$$\pi_{0ij} = \beta_{00j} + \zeta_{0ij} \quad (6)$$

$$\pi_{kij} = \beta_{k0j} + \zeta_{kij} \quad (7)$$

where β_{00j} is the subject j's intercept. β_{k0j} is the subject j's slope; and the random terms ζ_{0ij} and ζ_{kij} are the day-level residuals.

Level 3 Equations (Between-Individual Level)

$$\beta_{00j} = \gamma_{000} + \gamma_{001} Z_j + \delta_{00j} \quad (8)$$

$$\beta_{k0j} = \gamma_{k00} + \gamma_{k01} Z_j + \delta_{k0j} \quad (9)$$

where γ_{000} and γ_{k00} are the average intercept and slope across all subjects, respectively; Z_j is the between-individual level predictor representing, e.g., subject's characteristics; γ_{001} and γ_{k01} are the effect of the variable Z_j; and the random terms δ_{00j} and δ_{k0j} represent the residuals on the between-individual level. See SAS codes in the Supplementary Materials (available here) for the above models.

2.2. Which Statistics Should Be Used to Characterize Physical Activity? Accelerometer is commonly used to objectively measure physical activity and capable of detecting large volumes of small changes in bodily acceleration. A common accelerometer method is to count zero-crossing activities; that is, the number of times that the signal crosses zero within the buffer [94], accumulated to 1-min epochs (we will assume this method in the discussion below, but there are also other ways to assess accelerometer data). The accelerometer enables opportunities to improve the characterization of activity patterns in daily life but also brings new analytic challenges despite expanding efforts to address these issues [95]. A study examined several issues with the use of accelerometer data on algorithms for the time of wearing or taking off the device and activity cut-off points for different intensities of physical activity [96]. The study showed that the choice of epoch length, which refers to the interval of time over which the units of accelerometer measures are aggregated (e.g., 15 seconds or 1 minute), may introduce significant errors when the chosen epoch length mismatches the length originally used for validating the wear time algorithm and activity cut-off points. This indicates that wear time or time spent in different intensities of physical activity cannot be directly compared across studies unless they used the same epoch lengths [96].

In addition to characterizing general activity patterns in daily life, accelerometers are useful tools for estimating the extent of a person's movement over a given period of time, including the intensity, duration, frequency, and the type of movement [95]. There has been growth in research on time spent in different intensities of physical activity (e.g., sedentary behavior [97–100], light, moderate, and vigorous physical activity [101–103]), but a common accelerometer measure is the activity counts per a certain period of time, which represent total volume of physical activity.

Although there are several important issues to consider when analyzing accelerometer data, we focus on how to characterize local (i.e., temporal) physical activity patterns surrounding EMA recordings of affect. To extract and characterize activity patterns in a temporal time window, researchers can analyze local statistics of physical activity data up to the fourth-order moment (i.e., mean, standard deviation [*SD*], skewness, and kurtosis) around EMA recordings (e.g., 60-min local mean of physical activity around the EMA signal). However, a research group focused on mean and skewness because they considered first- and third-order moments to be sufficient to characterize the observed accelerometer data [85, 86]. While *SD* (i.e., the second-order moment) is a standard measure characterizing variability of data, it can be inappropriate when the data do not approximate a normal distribution; the distribution of physical activity has non-negative values, leading to a positively skewed distribution. Intermittency or non-Gaussianity in natural phenomena is known to be successfully captured by the higher-order statistics, such as nonzero skewness or larger kurtosis (flatness) of the probability distribution of the observed data [104, 105], corresponding to the presence of frequent bursts. Indeed, the local *SD* of physical activity did not play a major role in predicting affect (i.e., depressive mood) scores [85, 86]. In contrast, the skewness, as a measure of asymmetry of a distribution, is thought to be more appropriate to characterize the observed asymmetry. Lower or higher mean activity levels quantify the overall states of physical activity. Higher positive skewness quantifies occasional bursts of physical activity [81–83]. Other local statistics of physical activity that can capture the intermittency in physical activity more robustly, such as entropy-type nonlinear statistics, can also be considered.

It is important to consider the effect of time of day on physical activity. A simple way to address this would be by adding a term for time of day (e.g., every 4 hours or morning/afternoon/evening blocks) to (1) or (5) as a controller or moderator [106]. We can also use detrended activity data [85], where a diurnal trend of activity data is subtracted by fitting polynomial functions (e.g., the first-order polynomial to adjust a linear trend) before calculation (Figures 1(c) and 1(d)), which aims at eliminating effects of nonstationarity due to, e.g., daily activities; the effects up the higher-order polynomials can be systematically examined.

2.3. Considering Size and Location of Time Windows for Aggregation of Physical Activity Data. One of the most important questions when examining the association between two (or more) constructs varying over time is how to address the time windows (i.e., location and size) that are used to aggregate each construct. The choice of the size of the time window may be important because it could have a significant impact on the robustness of the statistics and their temporal coincidence with the symptoms. Time windows can be chosen either by using theoretical rationale or by explorative examination. An example of the latter is described below.

One possible attempt is to systematically vary the size and location of the time windows to examine their effects [85]. For example, when the epoch length of physical activity obtained by accelerometer is 1-min, 60-min local mean or *SD* of physical activity is computed from 60 data points, whereas 5-min local statistics are computed from 5 data points. Theoretically, the larger the size of the time window, the greater the stability and reliability of the estimates. However, the choice of larger time windows may obscure more transient fluctuations in the relations between physical activity and self-reported symptoms. Prior studies have used many different sizes of time windows to understand the associations between physical activity and affect states. There are many studies that have focused on very short time windows: 5-30 min [101, 103, 107, 108], which may be useful to check transient associations among target variables or examine health benefits from an even short period of physical activity. One study systematically varied the size of time windows from 5 min (transient) to 2 hours (medium) with a 5-min time interval to test proper time windows predicting depressive mood [85]. Another study used medium (4 hours) time windows of physical activity to compare with affect states assessed every 4 hours [11]. The associations between physical activity and affect on a day level (i.e., relatively long time window) have also been examined [109, 110]. Day-level time windows to aggregate physical activity may be used to examine overall associations with daily affect or event (e.g., sleep), but this examination is sometimes pragmatically made due to the limitation of sparse sampling (i.e., no observations within a day). The size of time windows largely depends upon the research question, but given the large freedom researchers typically have in selecting the size of time windows it is important that future research evaluates the reproducibility of the time-specific effects.

In addition, the choice of the location of the time window plays an important role in the investigation of causal associations, such as whether physical activity precedes or follows changes in momentary symptoms. There is scarcity of research on the bidirectional association between physical activity and momentary symptoms. Some studies showed that physical activity influences mental health benefits [108, 111], whereas others focused on how subjective symptoms predict subsequent physical activity [102, 108, 112]. However, it is a complicated domain and careful consideration of such a trade-off is important, although the optimal choice might be difficult to predict. Figures 1(a) and 1(b) are examples that show an examination of the temporal associations of depressive mood and local mean or detrended skewness of physical activity. Estimated values of the univariate multilevel model coefficient (i.e., slope) for the associations are shown in a colored matrix form consisting of 25 columns (different location) and 12 rows (different size). We considered 25 different locations (−60, −55, −50, . . ., 55, 60 min) and 12 different sizes (120, 110, 100, . . ., 20, 10 min). In total, we considered 300 combinations (25 locations × 12 sizes) for local statistics of physical activity to examine the association with depressive mood assessed by EMA. More specifically, the top left cell in Figure 1(a) represents the model coefficient for the association between depressive mood (EMA) and local mean which calculated from the 10-min size of time window 60 min before EMA (i.e., from −60 to −50 min before EMA). Thus, the colored matrices generally show reduced mean or (detrended) positively skewed activity patterns preceded or occurred concurrently with a higher level of depressive mood rather than following. The false discovery rate with the *q* value of .05 was used as the multiple comparison adjustment [113].

Although we discussed the size and location of time windows which are important when we explore the relationship with self-reported symptoms, the underlying mechanism of sustainability and causality alterations in the levels and patterns of physical activity with affect is uncertain. Further study using the data of high temporal resolution is necessary to clarify this question.

3. Further Challenges

Behavioral patterns characterized by reduced activity and intermittent bursts during low activity periods, as measured by accelerometer, are associated with EMA reports of worse depressive mood in healthy adolescents, older adults, undergraduates, office workers, and patients with MDD. This suggests that behavioral monitoring by the accelerometer may contribute to the identification of changes in subjective symptoms and improved management of these symptoms. While prior studies successfully provided a psychobehavioral measure based on accelerometer data, other types of time-varying changes in daily life should be examined to understand the associations between objective/subjective measures and health-related outcomes.

Many researchers and clinicians these days on the behavioral sciences and other scientific disciplines use mobile data collection incorporating information and communication technologies (ICTs), which enables a more refined understanding of psychiatric disorders including associations among various behavioral/physiological/biological measures. Furthermore, wearable devices (e.g., smartwatch) are increasingly popular to monitor health outcomes such as physical activity, sleep, and heart rate. The abundant information extracted from wearable devices is provided to numerous users often via smartphone applications and have great potential to elicit useful data for health outcomes in academic fields. Another challenge is how to use this information for improved monitoring, management, and intervention of health-related behaviors. For example, the concept of ecological momentary interventions (EMIs), in which real-time interventions are delivered to individuals during their everyday lives in natural settings, is a core elemental technology that is used for novel treatments of diseases including psychiatric disorders [114]. In addition, emerging electronic devices will make "context-sensitive prompting" possible, where questions are automatically triggered based on the subject's behavior, location, physiological states, past responses, and social interactions, which is considered useful for detecting early signs of psychiatric disorders and their pathological transitions [106, 115]. However, actual realization and examination for these novel techniques are necessary in further studies.

4. Conclusion

In this paper, we introduced the multilevel modeling approach, which is useful for analyzing EMA data with observations hierarchically nested within individuals. Although new analytic challenges arise with addressing accelerometer data, it allows for nuanced characterizing of the temporal pattern of physical activity and its correlates. We exemplified different kinds of statistics (e.g., mean and skewness) of physical activity to extract activity patterns in various temporal time windows (i.e., size and location around EMA) which can be widely used according to research questions, but further studies using different types of statistics with a high temporal resolution are necessary to clarify these issues. Detailed SAS codes of multilevel models are shown in the Supplementary Materials.

Conflicts of Interest

The authors declare that there are no conflicts of interest regarding the publication of this paper.

Acknowledgments

This paper was supported by the National Sports Promotion Fund in accordance with the Sports Industry Technology Development Project of the Ministry of Culture, Sports and Tourism in 2017 (S072016032016). The authors would like to thank Drs. H. Shimura and Y. Yamamoto for their contribution to data collection for older adults which are used in Figure 1.

Supplementary Materials

The aim of the Supplementary Materials is to introduce SAS codes for multilevel modeling on the association between local statistics of physical activity based on accelerometer data and self-reported affect based on EMA. It consists of three parts: (a) Aggregating acceleration counts to various time windows (e.g., 60 min). (b) Merging physical activity data with self-reported affect. (c) Reporting the code for multilevel modeling on the association between local statistics of physical activity and affect, as described in Section 2.1. *(Supplementary Materials)*

References

[1] S. Schiffman, A. A. Stone, and M. R. Hufford, "Ecological momentary assessment," *Annual Review of Clinical Psychology*, vol. 4, pp. 1–32, 2008.

[2] J. M. Hektner, J. A. Schmidt, and M. Csikszentmihalyi, *Experience Sampling Method: Measuring The Quality of Everyday Life*, SAGE Publications, Thousand Oaks, Calif, USA, 2007.

[3] T. J. Trull and U. Ebner-Priemer, "Ambulatory assessment," *Annual Review of Clinical Psychology*, vol. 9, pp. 151–176, 2013.

[4] A.-M. Vranceanu, L. C. Gallo, and L. M. Bogart, "Depressive symptoms and momentary affect: The role of social interaction variables," *Depression and Anxiety*, vol. 26, no. 5, pp. 464–470, 2009.

[5] J. Kim, H. Kikuchi, and Y. Yamamoto, "Systematic comparison between ecological momentary assessment and day reconstruction method for fatigue and mood states in healthy adults," *British Journal of Health Psychology*, vol. 18, no. 1, pp. 155–167, 2013.

[6] A. A. Stone, J. M. Smyth, T. Pickering, and J. Schwartz, "Daily mood variability: form of diurnal patterns and determinants of diurnal patterns," *Journal of Applied Social Psychology*, vol. 26, no. 14, pp. 1286–1305, 1996.

[7] A. Steptoe, E. S. Leigh, and M. Kumari, "Positive affect and distressed affect over the day in older people," *Psychology and Aging*, vol. 26, no. 4, pp. 956–965, 2011.

[8] B. Farquharson, C. Bell, D. Johnston et al., "Nursing stress and patient care: Real-time investigation of the effect of nursing tasks and demands on psychological stress, physiological stress, and job performance: Study protocol," *Journal of Advanced Nursing*, vol. 69, no. 10, pp. 2327–2335, 2013.

[9] V. Thewissen, R. P. Bentall, T. Lecomte, J. van Os, and I. Myin-Germeys, "Fluctuations in self-esteem and paranoia in the context of daily life," *Journal of Abnormal Psychology*, vol. 117, no. 1, pp. 143–153, 2008.

[10] R. A. Carels, O. M. Douglass, H. M. Cacciapaglia, and W. H. O'Brien, "An ecological momentary assessment of relapse crises in dieting," *Journal of Consulting and Clinical Psychology*, vol. 72, no. 2, pp. 341–348, 2004.

[11] G. F. Dunton, A. A. Atienza, C. M. Castro, and A. C. King, "Using ecological momentary assessment to examine antecedents and correlates of physical activity bouts in adults age 50+ years: a pilot study," *Annals of Behavioral Medicine*, vol. 38, no. 3, pp. 249–255, 2009.

[12] M. Wichers, F. Peeters, B. P. F. Rutten et al., "A time-lagged momentary assessment study on daily life physical activity and affect," *Health Psychology*, vol. 31, no. 2, pp. 135–144, 2012.

[13] S. Shiffman, M. H. Balabanis, C. J. Gwaltney et al., "Prediction of lapse from associations between smoking and situational antecedents assessed by ecological momentary assessment," *Drug and Alcohol Dependence*, vol. 91, no. 2-3, pp. 159–168, 2007.

[14] S. Chandra, D. Scharf, and S. Shiffman, "Within-day temporal patterns of smoking, withdrawal symptoms, and craving," *Drug and Alcohol Dependence*, vol. 117, no. 2-3, pp. 118–125, 2011.

[15] S. Shiffman and T. R. Kirchner, "Cigarette-by-cigarette satisfaction during ad libitum smoking," *Journal of Abnormal Psychology*, vol. 118, no. 2, pp. 348–359, 2009.

[16] M. Hillbrand and B. M. Waite, "The everyday experience of an institutionalized sex offender: An idiographic application of the experience sampling method," *Archives of Sexual Behavior*, vol. 23, no. 4, pp. 453–463, 1994.

[17] A. Müller, J. E. Mitchell, R. D. Crosby et al., "Mood states preceding and following compulsive buying episodes: An ecological momentary assessment study," *Psychiatry Research*, vol. 200, no. 2-3, pp. 575–580, 2012.

[18] V. S. Helgeson, L. C. Lopez, and T. Kamarck, "Peer relationships and diabetes: retrospective and ecological momentary assessment approaches," *Health Psychology*, vol. 28, no. 3, pp. 273–282, 2009.

[19] T. Rutledge, E. Stucky, A. Dollarhide et al., "A real-time assessment of work stress in physicians and nurses," *Health Psychology*, vol. 28, no. 2, pp. 194–200, 2009.

[20] S. A. Mulvaney, R. L. Rothman, M. S. Dietrich et al., "Using mobile phones to measure adolescent diabetes adherence," *Health Psychology*, vol. 31, no. 1, pp. 43–50, 2012.

[21] D. E. McCarthy, T. M. Piasecki, D. L. Lawrence, D. E. Jorenby, S. Shiffman, and T. B. Baker, "Psychological mediators of bupropion sustained-release treatment for smoking cessation," *Addiction*, vol. 103, no. 9, pp. 1521–1533, 2008.

[22] H. Kikuchi, K. Yoshiuchi, Y. Yamamoto, G. Komaki, and A. Akabayashi, "Diurnal variation of tension-type headache intensity and exacerbation: An investigation using computerized ecological momentary assessment," *BioPsychoSocial Medicine*, vol. 6, article 8, 2012.

[23] T. Ritz, D. Rosenfield, S. DeWilde, and A. Steptoe, "Daily mood, shortness of breath, and lung function in asthma: Concurrent and prospective associations," *Journal of Psychosomatic Research*, vol. 69, no. 4, pp. 341–351, 2010.

[24] R. S. Everhart, J. M. Smyth, A. M. Santuzzi, and B. H. Fiese, "Validation of the asthma quality of life questionnaire with momentary assessments of symptoms and functional limitations in patient daily life," *Respiratory Care*, vol. 55, no. 4, pp. 427–432, 2010.

[25] G. D'Amato and L. Cecchi, "Effects of climate change on environmental factors in respiratory allergic diseases," *Clinical & Experimental Allergy*, vol. 38, no. 8, pp. 1264–1274, 2008.

[26] M. Saito, H. Kumano, K. Yoshiuchi et al., "Symptom profile of multiple chemical sensitivity in actual life," *Psychosomatic Medicine*, vol. 67, no. 2, pp. 318–325, 2005.

[27] J. A. Henry, G. Galvez, M. B. Turbin, E. J. Thielman, G. P. McMillan, and J. A. Istvan, "Pilot study to evaluate ecological momentary assessment of tinnitus," *Ear and Hearing*, vol. 33, no. 2, pp. 179–290, 2012.

[28] R. M. Schuster, R. J. Mermelstein, and D. Hedeker, "Ecological momentary assessment of working memory under conditions of simultaneous marijuana and tobacco use," *Addiction*, vol. 111, no. 8, pp. 1466–1476, 2016.

[29] J. A. Cramer, R. H. Mattson, M. L. Prevey, R. D. Scheyer, and V. L. Ouellette, "How often is medication taken as prescribed?: a novel assessment technique," *Journal of the American Medical Association*, vol. 261, no. 22, pp. 3273–3277, 1989.

[30] L. van Wel, A. Huss, P. Bachmann et al., "Context-sensitive ecological momentary assessments; integrating real-time exposure measurements, data-analytics and health assessment using a smartphone application," *Environment International*, vol. 103, pp. 8–12, 2017.

[31] J. R. Turner, M. M. Ward, M. D. Gellman, D. W. Johnston, K. C. Light, and L. J. P. Van Doornen, "The relationship between laboratory and ambulatory cardiovascular activity: current evidence and future directions," *Annals of Behavioral Medicine*, vol. 16, pp. 12–23, 1994.

[32] B. A. Teicher, S. A. Holden, N. P. Dupuis et al., "Potentiation of cytotoxic therapies by TNP-470 and minocycline in mice bearing EMT-6 mammary carcinoma," *Breast Cancer Research and Treatment*, vol. 36, no. 2, pp. 227–236, 1995.

[33] M. H. Teicher, C. A. Glod, E. Magnus et al., "Circadian rest-activity disturbances in seasonal affective disorder," *Archives of General Psychiatry*, vol. 54, no. 2, pp. 124–130, 1997.

[34] C. Burton, B. McKinstry, A. Szentagotai Tătar, A. Serrano-Blanco, C. Pagliari, and M. Wolters, "Activity monitoring in patients with depression: a systematic review," *Journal of Affective Disorders*, vol. 145, no. 1, pp. 21–28, 2013.

[35] P. Indic, G. Murray, C. Maggini et al., "Multi-scale motility amplitude associated with suicidal thoughts in major depression," *PLoS ONE*, vol. 7, no. 6, Article ID e38761, 2012.

[36] S. Walther, S. Hügli, O. Höfle et al., "Frontal white matter integrity is related to psychomotor retardation in major depression," *Neurobiology of Disease*, vol. 47, no. 1, pp. 13–19, 2012.

[37] A. C. Volkers, J. H. M. Tulen, W. W. Van Den Broek, J. A. Bruijn, J. Passchier, and L. Pepplinkhuizen, "Motor activity and autonomic cardiac functioning in major depressive disorder," *Journal of Affective Disorders*, vol. 76, no. 1-3, pp. 23–30, 2003.

[38] J. O. Berle, E. R. Hauge, K. J. Oedegaard, F. Holsten, and O. B. Fasmer, "Actigraphic registration of motor activity reveals a more structured behavioural pattern in schizophrenia than in major depression," *BMC Research Notes*, vol. 3, article 149, 2010.

[39] T. F. Robles, V. Shetty, C. M. Zigler et al., "The feasibility of ambulatory biosensor measurement of salivary alpha amylase: relationships with self-reported and naturalistic psychological stress," *Biological Psychology*, vol. 86, no. 1, pp. 50–56, 2011.

[40] M. Van Eck, H. Berkhof, N. Nicolson, and J. Sulon, "The effects of perceived stress, traits, mood states, and stressful daily events on salivary cortisol," *Psychosomatic Medicine*, vol. 58, no. 5, pp. 447–458, 1996.

[41] J. Smyth, M. C. Ockenfels, L. Porter, C. Kirschbaum, D. H. Hellhammer, and A. A. Stone, "Stressors and mood measured on a momentary basis are associated with salivary cortisol secretion," *Psychoneuroendocrinology*, vol. 23, no. 4, pp. 353–370, 1998.

[42] A. Steptoe, E. Leigh Gibson, M. Hamer, and J. Wardle, "Neuroendocrine and cardiovascular correlates of positive affect measured by ecological momentary assessment and by questionnaire," *Psychoneuroendocrinology*, vol. 32, no. 1, pp. 56–64, 2007.

[43] E. Boland, T. Monsod, M. Delucia, C. A. Brandt, S. Fernando, and W. V. Tamborlane, "Limitations of conventional methods of self-monitoring of blood glucose: lessons learned from 3 days of continuous glucose sensing in pediatric patients with type 1 diabetes," *Diabetes Care*, vol. 24, no. 11, pp. 1858–1862, 2001.

[44] T. R. Leffingwell, N. J. Cooney, J. G. Murphy et al., "Continuous objective monitoring of alcohol use: twenty-first century measurement using transdermal sensors," *Alcoholism: Clinical and Experimental Research*, vol. 37, no. 1, pp. 16–22, 2013.

[45] M. J. Sorbi, S. B. Mak, J. H. Houtveen, A. M. Kleiboer, and L. J. P. Van Doornen, "Mobile web-based monitoring and coaching: Feasibility in chronic migraine," *Journal of Medical Internet Research*, vol. 9, no. 5, p. e38, 2007.

[46] S. Munsch, A. H. Meyer, N. Milenkovic, B. Schlup, J. Margraf, and F. H. Wilhelm, "Ecological momentary assessment to evaluate cognitive-behavioral treatment for binge eating disorder," *International Journal of Eating Disorders*, vol. 42, no. 7, pp. 648–657, 2009.

[47] G. Jónasson, K.-H. Carlsen, A. Sødal, C. Jonasson, and P. Mowinckel, "Patient compliance in a clinical trial with inhaled

budesonide in children with mild asthma," *European Respiratory Journal*, vol. 14, no. 1, pp. 150–154, 1999.

[48] K. E. MacDonell, S. Naar-King, D. A. Murphy, J. T. Parsons, and H. Huszti, "Situational temptation for HIV medication adherence in high-risk youth," *AIDS Patient Care and STDs*, vol. 25, no. 1, pp. 47–52, 2011.

[49] K. Basen-Engquist, C. L. Carmack, Y. Li et al., "Social-cognitive theory predictors of exercise behavior in endometrial cancer survivors," *Health Psychology*, vol. 32, no. 11, pp. 1137–1148, 2013.

[50] B. C. Focht, V. Ewing, L. Guavin, and W. J. Rejeski, "The unique and transient impact of acute exercise on pain perception in older, overweight, or obese adults with knee osteoarthritis," *Annals of Behavioral Medicine*, vol. 24, no. 3, pp. 201–210, 2002.

[51] D. H. Epstein, G. F. Marrone, S. J. Heishman, J. Schmittner, and K. L. Preston, "Tobacco, cocaine, and heroin: Craving and use during daily life," *Addictive Behaviors*, vol. 35, no. 4, pp. 318–324, 2010.

[52] M. J. Freedman, K. M. Lester, C. McNamara, J. B. Milby, and J. E. Schumacher, "Cell phones for ecological momentary assessment with cocaine-addicted homeless patients in treatment," *Journal of Substance Abuse Treatment*, vol. 30, no. 2, pp. 105–111, 2006.

[53] S. R. Weinland, C. B. Morris, Y. Hu, J. Leserman, S. I. Bangdiwala, and D. A. Drossman, "Characterization of episodes of irritable bowel syndrome using ecological momentary assessment," *American Journal of Gastroenterology*, vol. 106, no. 10, pp. 1813–1820, 2011.

[54] P. Jern, A. Gunst, F. Sandqvist, N. K. Sandnabba, and P. Santtila, "Using ecological momentary assessment to investigate associations between ejaculatory latency and control in partnered and non-partnered sexual activities," *The Journal of Sex Research*, vol. 48, no. 4, pp. 316–324, 2011.

[55] C. Zunker, C. B. Peterson, R. D. Crosby et al., "Ecological momentary assessment of bulimia nervosa: Does dietary restriction predict binge eating?" *Behaviour Research and Therapy*, vol. 49, no. 10, pp. 714–717, 2011.

[56] C. Burd, J. E. Mitchell, R. D. Crosby et al., "An assessment of daily food intake in participants with anorexia nervosa in the natural environment," *International Journal of Eating Disorders*, vol. 42, no. 4, pp. 371–374, 2009.

[57] P. J. Rosen, J. N. Epstein, and G. Van Orden, "I know it when I quantify it: Ecological momentary assessment and recurrence quantification analysis of emotion dysregulation in children with ADHD," *ADHD Attention Deficit and Hyperactivity Disorders*, vol. 5, no. 3, pp. 283–294, 2013.

[58] L. E. Knouse, J. T. Mitchell, L. H. Brown et al., "The expression of adult ADHD symptoms in daily life: An application of experience sampling methodology," *Journal of Attention Disorders*, vol. 11, no. 6, pp. 652–663, 2008.

[59] U. W. Ebner-Priemer, J. Kuo, W. Schlotz et al., "Distress and affective dysregulation in patients with borderline personality disorder: A psychophysiological ambulatory monitoring study," *The Journal of Nervous and Mental Disease*, vol. 196, no. 4, pp. 314–320, 2008.

[60] P. Z. Tan, E. E. Forbes, R. E. Dahl et al., "Emotional reactivity and regulation in anxious and nonanxious youth: A cell-phone ecological momentary assessment study," *Journal of Child Psychology and Psychiatry and Allied Disciplines*, vol. 53, no. 2, pp. 197–206, 2012.

[61] M. C. Pfaltz, T. Michael, P. Grossman, J. Margraf, and F. H. Wilhelm, "Instability of physical anxiety symptoms in daily life of patients with panic disorder and patients with posttraumatic stress disorder," *Journal of Anxiety Disorders*, vol. 24, no. 7, pp. 792–798, 2010.

[62] S. Helbig-Lang, T. Lang, F. Petermann, and J. Hoyer, "Anticipatory anxiety as a function of panic attacks and panic-related self-efficacy: An ambulatory assessment study in panic disorder," *Behavioural and Cognitive Psychotherapy*, vol. 40, no. 5, pp. 590–604, 2012.

[63] E. E. Forbes, A. R. Hariri, S. L. Martin et al., "Altered striatal activation predicting real-world positive affect in adolescent major depressive disorder," *The American Journal of Psychiatry*, vol. 166, no. 1, pp. 64–73, 2009.

[64] L. M. Bylsma, A. Taylor-Clift, and J. Rottenberg, "Emotional reactivity to daily events in major and minor depression," *Journal of Abnormal Psychology*, vol. 120, no. 1, pp. 155–167, 2011.

[65] F. Peeters, N. A. Nicolson, J. Berkhof, P. Delespaul, and M. De Vries, "Effects of daily events on mood states in major depressive disorder," *Journal of Abnormal Psychology*, vol. 112, no. 2, pp. 203–211, 2003.

[66] R. Havermans, N. A. Nicolson, J. Berkhof, and M. W. deVries, "Mood reactivity to daily events in patients with remitted bipolar disorder," *Psychiatry Research*, vol. 179, no. 1, pp. 47–52, 2010.

[67] D. Kimhy, P. Delespaul, C. Corcoran, H. Ahn, S. Yale, and D. Malaspina, "Computerized experience sampling method (ESMc): Assessing feasibility and validity among individuals with schizophrenia," *Journal of Psychiatric Research*, vol. 40, no. 3, pp. 221–230, 2006.

[68] E. Granholm, D. Ben-Zeev, D. Fulford, and J. Swendsen, "Ecological Momentary Assessment of social functioning in schizophrenia: Impact of performance appraisals and affect on social interactions," *Schizophrenia Research*, vol. 145, no. 1-3, pp. 120–124, 2013.

[69] E. Granholm, C. Loh, and J. Swendsen, "Feasibility and validity of computerized ecological momentary assessment in schizophrenia," *Schizophrenia Bulletin*, vol. 34, no. 3, pp. 507–514, 2008.

[70] S. J. Wilson, L. M. Martire, and M. J. Sliwinski, "Daily spousal responsiveness predicts longer-term trajectories of patients' physical function," *Psychological Science*, vol. 28, no. 6, pp. 786–797, 2017.

[71] T. W. Kamarck, J. E. Schwartz, S. Shiffman, M. F. Muldoon, K. Sutton-Tyrrell, and D. L. Janicki, "Psychosocial stress and cardiovascular risk: what is the role of daily experience?" *Journal of Personality*, vol. 73, no. 6, pp. 1749–1774, 2005.

[72] T. W. Kamarck, S. M. Shiffman, L. Smithline et al., "Effects of task strain, social conflict, and emotional activation on ambulatory cardiovascular activity: Daily life consequences of recurring stress in a multiethnic adult sample," *Health Psychology*, vol. 17, no. 1, pp. 17–29, 1998.

[73] T. W. Smith, W. Birmingham, and B. N. Uchino, "Evaluative threat and ambulatory blood pressure: Cardiovascular effects of social stress in daily experience," *Health Psychology*, vol. 31, no. 6, pp. 763–766, 2012.

[74] P. Grossman, G. Deuring, S. N. Garland, T. S. Campbell, and L. E. Carlson, "Patterns of objective physical functioning and perception of mood and fatigue in posttreatment breast cancer patients and healthy controls: An ambulatory psychophysiological investigation," *Psychosomatic Medicine*, vol. 70, no. 7, pp. 819–828, 2008.

[75] V. Bitsika, C. F. Sharpley, N. M. Andronicos, and L. L. Agnew, "Hypothalamus-pituitary-adrenal axis daily fluctuation, anxiety and age interact to predict cortisol concentrations in boys with an autism spectrum disorder," *Physiology & Behavior*, vol. 138, pp. 200–207, 2015.

[76] J. M. Lavender, K. P. De Young, S. A. Wonderlich et al., "Daily patterns of anxiety in anorexia nervosa: Associations with eating disorder behaviors in the natural environment," *Journal of Abnormal Psychology*, vol. 122, no. 3, pp. 672–683, 2013.

[77] R. D. Crosby, S. A. Wonderlich, S. G. Engel, H. Simonich, J. Smyth, and J. E. Mitchell, "Daily mood patterns and bulimic behaviors in the natural environment," *Behaviour Research and Therapy*, vol. 47, no. 3, pp. 181–188, 2009.

[78] M. Muraven, R. L. Collins, S. Shiffman, and J. A. Paty, "Daily fluctuations in self-control demands and alcohol intake," *Psychology of Addictive Behaviors*, vol. 19, no. 2, pp. 140–147, 2005.

[79] S. Jahng, M. B. Solhan, R. L. Tomko, P. K. Wood, T. M. Piasecki, and T. J. Trull, "Affect and alcohol use: An ecological momentary assessment study of outpatients with borderline personality disorder," *Journal of Abnormal Psychology*, vol. 120, no. 3, pp. 572–584, 2011.

[80] American Psychiatric Association, *Diagnostic and Statistical Manual of Mental Disorders*, American Psychiatric Press, Washington, Wash, USA, 4th edition, 2000.

[81] T. Nakamura, K. Kiyono, K. Yoshiuchi, R. Nakahara, Z. R. Struzik, and Y. Yamamoto, "Universal scaling law in human behavioral organization," *Physical Review Letters*, vol. 99, no. 13, Article ID 138103, 2007.

[82] T. Nakamura, T. Takumi, A. Takano et al., "Of mice and men - Universality and breakdown of behavioral organization," *PLoS ONE*, vol. 3, no. 4, Article ID e2050, 2008.

[83] W. Sano, T. Nakamura, K. Yoshiuchi et al., "Enhanced persistency of resting and active periods of locomotor activity in schizophrenia," *PLoS ONE*, vol. 7, no. 8, Article ID e43539, 2012.

[84] T. Nakamura, K. Kiyono, H. Wendt, P. Abry, and Y. Yamamoto, "Multiscale analysis of intensive longitudinal biomedical signals and its clinical applications," *Proceedings of the IEEE*, vol. 104, no. 2, pp. 242–261, 2016.

[85] J. Kim, T. Nakamura, H. Kikuchi, T. Sasaki, and Y. Yamamoto, "Co-variation of depressive mood and locomotor dynamics evaluated by ecological momentary assessment in healthy humans," *PLoS ONE*, vol. 8, no. 9, Article ID e74979, 2013.

[86] J. Kim, T. Nakamura, H. Kikuchi, K. Yoshiuchi, T. Sasaki, and Y. Yamamoto, "Covariation of depressive mood and spontaneous physical activity in major depressive disorder: toward continuous monitoring of depressive mood," *IEEE Journal of Biomedical and Health Informatics*, vol. 19, no. 4, pp. 1347–1355, 2015.

[87] J. Kim, F. Togo, H. Shimura, A. Yasunaga, T. Nakamura et al., "Associations between spontaneous physical activity and mood states in older adults: an ambulatory assessment approach in daily life," in *Proceedings of the The 4th Biennial Conference of Ambulatory Assessment*, State College, Pa, USA, 2015.

[88] B. von Haaren, S. N. Loeffler, S. Haertel et al., "Characteristics of the activity-affect association in inactive people: an ambulatory assessment study in daily life," *Frontiers in Psychology*, vol. 4, article 163, 2013.

[89] J. Mata, R. J. Thompson, S. M. Jaeggi, M. Buschkuehl, J. Jonides, and I. H. Gotlib, "Walk on the bright side: Physical activity and affect in major depressive disorder," *Journal of Abnormal Psychology*, vol. 121, no. 2, pp. 297–308, 2012.

[90] J. E. Schwartz and A. A. Stone, "Strategies for analyzing ecological momentary assessment data," *Health Psychology*, vol. 17, no. 1, pp. 6–16, 1998.

[91] J. J. Hox and J. K. Roberts, *Handbook of Advanced Multilevel Analysis*, Routledge, New York, NY, USA, 2011.

[92] J. D. Singer and J. B. Willett, *Applied Longitudinal Data Analysis: Modeling Change and Event Occurrence*, Oxford University Press, Oxford, UK, 2003.

[93] C. K. Enders and D. Tofighi, "Centering predictor variables in cross-sectional multilevel models: a new look at an old issue," *Psychological Methods*, vol. 12, no. 2, pp. 121–138, 2007.

[94] S. Ancoli-Israel, R. Cole, C. Alessi, M. Chambers, W. Moorcroft, and C. P. Pollak, "The role of actigraphy in the study of sleep and circadian rhythms," *SLEEP*, vol. 26, no. 3, pp. 342–392, 2003.

[95] R. P. Troiano, J. J. McClain, R. J. Brychta, and K. Y. Chen, "Evolution of accelerometer methods for physical activity research," *British Journal of Sports Medicine*, vol. 48, pp. 1019–1023, 2014.

[96] J. A. Banda, K. F. Haydel, T. Davila et al., "Effects of varying epoch lengths, wear time algorithms, and activity cut-points on estimates of child sedentary behavior and physical activity from accelerometer data," *PLoS ONE*, vol. 11, no. 3, Article ID e0150534, 2016.

[97] M. S. Tremblay, S. Aubert, J. D. Barnes et al., "Sedentary Behavior Research Network (SBRN) – Terminology Consensus Project process and outcome," *International Journal of Behavioral Nutrition and Physical Activity*, vol. 14, no. 1, 2017.

[98] N. Owen, G. N. Healy, C. E. Matthews, and D. W. Dunstan, "Too much sitting: the population health science of sedentary behavior," *Exercise and Sport Sciences Reviews*, vol. 38, no. 3, pp. 105–113, 2010.

[99] E. G. Wilmot, C. L. Edwardson, and F. A. Achana, "Sedentary time in adults and the association with diabetes, cardiovascular disease and death: systematic review and meta-analysis," *Diabetologia*, vol. 55, no. 11, pp. 2895–2905, 2012, Erratum in: *Diabetologia*, vol. 56, no. 4, pp. 942–943, 2013.

[100] A. A. Thorp, N. Owen, M. Neuhaus, and D. W. Dunstan, "Sedentary behaviors and subsequent health outcomes in adults: a systematic review of longitudinal studies, 1996–2011," *American Journal of Preventive Medicine*, vol. 41, no. 2, pp. 207–215, 2011.

[101] Y. Liao, C.-P. Chou, J. Huh, A. Leventhal, and G. Dunton, "Examining acute bi-directional relationships between affect, physical feeling states, and physical activity in free-living situations using electronic ecological momentary assessment," *Journal of Behavioral Medicine*, vol. 40, no. 3, pp. 445–457, 2017.

[102] C. Y. Niermann, C. Herrmann, B. von Haaren, D. van Kann, and A. Woll, "Affect and subsequent physical activity: an ambulatory assessment study examining the affect-activity association in a real-life context," *Frontiers in Psychology*, vol. 7, article 677, 2016.

[103] G. F. Dunton, J. Huh, A. M. Leventhal et al., "Momentary assessment of affect, physical feeling states, and physical activity in children," *Health Psychology*, vol. 33, no. 3, pp. 255–263, 2014.

[104] B. Castaing, Y. Gagne, and E. J. Hopfinger, "Velocity probability density functions of high Reynolds number turbulence," *Physica D: Nonlinear Phenomena*, vol. 46, no. 2, pp. 177–200, 1990.

[105] K. Kiyono, "Log-amplitude statistics of intermittent and non-Gaussian time series," *Physical Review E: Statistical, Nonlinear, and Soft Matter Physics*, vol. 79, no. 3, 2009.

[106] A. A. Stone et al., *The Science of Real-Time Data Capture: Self-Reports in Health Research*, Oxford University Press, Oxford, UK, 2007.

[107] T. Bossmann, M. Kanning, S. Koudela-Hamila, S. Hey, and U. Ebner-Priemer, "The association between short periods of everyday life activities and affective states: a replication study using ambulatory assessment," *Frontiers in Psychology*, vol. 4, article 102, 2013.

[108] A. Schwerdtfeger, R. Eberhardt, A. Chmitorz, and E. Schaller, "Momentary affect predicts bodily movement in daily life: An ambulatory monitoring study," *Journal of Sport & Exercise Psychology* , vol. 32, no. 5, pp. 674–693, 2010.

[109] D. Aggio, K. Wallace, N. Boreham, A. Shankar, A. Steptoe, and M. Hamer, "Objectively measured daily physical activity and postural changes as related to positive and negative affect using ambulatory monitoring assessments," *Psychosomatic Medicine*, vol. 79, no. 7, pp. 792–797, 2017.

[110] A. Schöndube, M. Kanning, and R. Fuchs, "The bidirectional effect between momentary affective states and exercise duration on a day level," *Frontiers in Psychology*, vol. 7, article 1414, 2016.

[111] M. Hamer, N. Coombs, and E. Stamatakis, "Associations between objectively assessed and self-reported sedentary time with mental health in adults: An analysis of data from the health survey for England," *BMJ Open*, vol. 4, no. 3, Article ID e004580, 2014.

[112] Y. Liao, E. T. Shonkoff, and G. F. Dunton, "The acute relationships between affect, physical feeling states, and physical activity in daily life: A review of current evidence," *Frontiers in Psychology*, vol. 6, article 1975, 2015.

[113] Y. Benjamini and D. Yekutieli, "The control of the false discovery rate in multiple testing under dependency," *The Annals of Statistics*, vol. 29, no. 4, pp. 1165–1188, 2001.

[114] K. E. Heron and J. M. Smyth, "Ecological momentary interventions: incorporating mobile technology into psychosocial and health behaviour treatments," *British Journal of Health Psychology*, vol. 15, pp. 1–39, 2010.

[115] Z. R. Struzik, K. Yoshiuchi, M. Sone et al., ""Mobile nurse" platform for ubiquitous medicine," *Methods of Information in Medicine*, vol. 46, no. 2, pp. 130–134, 2007.

Permissions

All chapters in this book were first published in CMMM, by Hindawi Publishing Corporation; hereby published with permission under the Creative Commons Attribution License or equivalent. Every chapter published in this book has been scrutinized by our experts. Their significance has been extensively debated. The topics covered herein carry significant findings which will fuel the growth of the discipline. They may even be implemented as practical applications or may be referred to as a beginning point for another development.

The contributors of this book come from diverse backgrounds, making this book a truly international effort. This book will bring forth new frontiers with its revolutionizing research information and detailed analysis of the nascent developments around the world.

We would like to thank all the contributing authors for lending their expertise to make the book truly unique. They have played a crucial role in the development of this book. Without their invaluable contributions this book wouldn't have been possible. They have made vital efforts to compile up to date information on the varied aspects of this subject to make this book a valuable addition to the collection of many professionals and students.

This book was conceptualized with the vision of imparting up-to-date information and advanced data in this field. To ensure the same, a matchless editorial board was set up. Every individual on the board went through rigorous rounds of assessment to prove their worth. After which they invested a large part of their time researching and compiling the most relevant data for our readers.

The editorial board has been involved in producing this book since its inception. They have spent rigorous hours researching and exploring the diverse topics which have resulted in the successful publishing of this book. They have passed on their knowledge of decades through this book. To expedite this challenging task, the publisher supported the team at every step. A small team of assistant editors was also appointed to further simplify the editing procedure and attain best results for the readers.

Apart from the editorial board, the designing team has also invested a significant amount of their time in understanding the subject and creating the most relevant covers. They scrutinized every image to scout for the most suitable representation of the subject and create an appropriate cover for the book.

The publishing team has been an ardent support to the editorial, designing and production team. Their endless efforts to recruit the best for this project, has resulted in the accomplishment of this book. They are a veteran in the field of academics and their pool of knowledge is as vast as their experience in printing. Their expertise and guidance has proved useful at every step. Their uncompromising quality standards have made this book an exceptional effort. Their encouragement from time to time has been an inspiration for everyone.

The publisher and the editorial board hope that this book will prove to be a valuable piece of knowledge for researchers, students, practitioners and scholars across the globe.

List of Contributors

Weifeng Li, Yuxiaotong Shen, Jie Zhang, Xiaolin Huang, Ying Chen and Yun Ge
School of Electronic Science and Engineering, Nanjing University, Nanjing 210023, China

Haochen Zhao, Linai Kuang, Lei Wang and Zhanwei Xuan
College of Information Engineering, Xiangtan University, Xiangtan 411105, China
Key Laboratory of Intelligent Computing and Information Processing, Xiangtan University, Xiangtan 411105, China

Yahui Ji, Wanbiao Ma and Keying Song
Department of Applied Mathematics, School of Mathematics and Physics, University of Science and Technology Beijing, 100083, Beijing, China

Myung Hun Jang
Department of Rehabilitation Medicine, Pusan National University Hospital, Pusan National University School of Medicine, Busan, Republic of Korea

Myung Jun Shin
Department of Rehabilitation Medicine, Pusan National University Hospital, Pusan National University School of Medicine, Busan, Republic of Korea
Biomedical Research Institute, Pusan National University Hospital, Busan, Republic of Korea

Se Jin Ahn
Division of Energy and Electric Engineering, Uiduk University, Gyeongju, Republic of Korea

Jun Woo Lee
School of Mechanical Engineering, Pusan National University, Busan, Republic of Korea

Min-Hyung Rhee
Department of Rehabilitation Medicine, Pusan National University Hospital, Busan, Republic of Korea

Dasom Chae
Biomedical Research Institute, Pusan National University Hospital, Busan, Republic of Korea

Jinmi Kim
Department of Biostatistics, Clinical Trial Center, Biomedical Research Institute, Pusan National University Hospital, Busan, Republic of Korea

Michael J. Paldino
Department of Radiology, Texas Children's Hospital, 6701 Fannin St., Houston, TX, USA

Wei Zhang
Department of Radiology, Texas Children's Hospital, 6701 Fannin St., Houston, TX, USA
Outcomes and Impact Service, Texas Children's Hospital, 6701 Fannin St., Houston, TX, USA

Zili D. Chu
Department of Radiology, Texas Children's Hospital, 6701 Fannin St., Houston, TX, USA
Department of Radiology, Baylor College of Medicine, One Baylor Plaza-BCM360, Houston, TX, USA

Viktoria Muravina and Robert Azencott
Department of Mathematics, University of Houston, 3507 Cullen Blvd, Houston, TX, USA

Eva María Cirugeda-Roldán, Antonio Molina Picó and David Cuesta-Frau
Technological Institute of Informatics, Universitat Politècnica de València, Alcoi Campus, Plaza Ferrándiz y Carbonell 2, Alcoi, Spain

Daniel Novák
Department of Cybernetics, Faculty of Electrical Engineering, Czech Technical University in Prague, Czech Republic

Vaclav Kremen
Czech Institute of Informatics, Robotics and Cybernetics, Czech Technical University in Prague, Czech Republic

Shunxian Zhou
College of Software and Communication Engineering, Xiangnan University, Chenzhou 423000, China
College of Information Engineering, Xiangtan University, Xiangtan 411105, China

Zhanwei Xuan, Lei Wang, Pengyao Ping and Tingrui Pei
College of Information Engineering, Xiangtan University, Xiangtan 411105, China

Aulia K. Heikhmakhtiar and Ki M. Lim
Department of IT Convergence Engineering, Kumoh National Institute of Technology, Gumi 39177, Republic of Korea

Li Yuan, Zhuhuang Zhou, Yanchao Yuan and Shuicai Wu
College of Life Science and Bioengineering, Beijing University of Technology, Beijing, China

Seda Arslan Tuncer
Department of Software Engineering, Faculty of Engineering, Fırat University, 23119 Elazig, Turkey

Turgay Kaya
Department of Electrical-Electronics Engineering, Faculty of Engineering, Fırat University, 23119 Elazig, Turkey

Min Zhao
College of Mathematics, Taiyuan University of Technology, Taiyuan, Shanxi, China

Xiaoyun Wang
College of Mathematics, Taiyuan University of Technology, Taiyuan, Shanxi, China
Department of Scientific C omputing, F lorida State University, Tallahassee, FL, USA

Xiaoqiang Wang
Department of Scientific C omputing, F lorida State University, Tallahassee, FL, USA

Shuping Li
Department of Mathematics, North University of China, Taiyuan, Shanxi, China

Ning Cao and Huirong Liu
Department of Physiology and Pathophysiology, School of Basic Medical Sciences, Capital Medical University, Beijing, China
Beijing Key Laboratory of Metabolic Disorders Related Cardiovascular Diseases, Capital Medical University, Beijing, China

J. Febina
Department of Biomedical Engineering, GRT Institute of Engineering and Technology, Tiruttani, India

Mohamed Yacin Sikkandar
Department of Medical Equipment Technology, College of Applied Medical Sciences, Majmaah University, Al Majmaah 11952, Saudi Arabia

N. M. Sudharsan
Department of Mechanical Engineering, Rajalakshmi Engineering College, Chennai, India

Wenpeng Gao and Yili Fu
School of Life Science and Technology, Harbin Institute of Technology, Harbin, China
State Key Laboratory of Robotics and System, Harbin Institute of Technology, Harbin, China

Xiaoguang Chen
Department of Neurosurgery, TheThird People Hospital of Hainan Province, Sanya 572000, China

Minwei Zhu
Department of Neurosurgery, The First Affiliated Hospital of Harbin Medical University, Harbin 150001, China

Aytuğ Onan
Celal Bayar University, Department of Software Engineering, 45400 Turgutlu, Manisa, Turkey

Yanqiao Zheng and Xiaoqi Zhang
School of Finance, Zhejiang University of Finance and Economics, China

Xiaobing Zhao
School of Data Sciences, Zhejiang University of Finance and Economics, China

Biao Yang, Jinmeng Cao, Tiantong Zhou and Ling Zou
School of Information Science and Engineering, Changzhou University, Changzhou, Jiangsu 213164, China
Changzhou Key Laboratory of Biomedical Information Technology, Changzhou, Jiangsu 213164, China

Li Dong
School of Life Science and Technology, University of Electronic Science and Technology of China, Chengdu, Sichuan 610054, China

Jianbo Xiang
Changzhou No. 2 People's Hospital Affiliated with Nanjing Medical University, Changzhou, Jiangsu 213164, China

Jiangping Li
School of Public Health and Management, Ningxia Medical University, Ningxia, Yinchuan 750004, China

Yu Zhao
School of Public Health and Management, Ningxia Medical University, Ningxia, Yinchuan 750004, China
School of Mathematics and Computer Science, Ningxia Normal University, Ningxia, Guyuan 756000, China

Xu Ma
School of Mathematics and Computer Science, Ningxia Normal University, Ningxia, Guyuan 756000, China

Luis J. Mena, Vanessa G. Félix, Rodolfo Ostos and Eduardo González
Academic Unit of Computing, Master Program in Applied Sciences, Universidad Politecnica de Sinaloa, Mazatlan 82199, Mexico

Alberto Ochoa and Javier Aspuru
Department of Electronic, Faculty of Mechanical and Electrical Engineering, Universidad de Colima, Colima 28400, Mexico

Pablo Velarde
Academic Program of Electronic Engineering, Universidad Autonoma de Nayarit, Tepic 63000, Mexico

Gladys E. Maestre
Department of Biomedical Sciences, Division of Neurosciences and Department of Human Genetics, University of Texas Rio Grande Valley School of Medicine, Brownsville 78520, USA

Ming Liu
Key Laboratory for Biomechanics and Mechanobiology of Ministry of Education, School of Biological Science and Medical Engineering, Beihang University, Beijing 100083, China

Zhenze Wang
National Research Center for Rehabilitation Technical Aids, Beijing Key Laboratory of Rehabilitation Technical Aids for Old-Age Disability, Key Laboratory of Rehabilitation Technical Aids Technology and System of the Ministry of Civil Affairs, No. 1 Ronghuazhong Road, Beijing BDA, Beijing 100176, China

Anqiang Sun and Xiaoyan Deng
Key Laboratory for Biomechanics and Mechanobiology of Ministry of Education, School of Biological Science and Medical Engineering, Beihang University, Beijing 100083, China
Beijing Advanced Innovation Centre for Biomedical Engineering, Beihang University, Beijing 100083, China

Jinhyuk Kim
Department of Biobehavioral Health, The Pennsylvania State University, University Park, PA, USA

David Marcusson-Clavertz
Department of Biobehavioral Health, The Pennsylvania State University, University Park, PA, USA
Department of Psychology, Lund University, Lund, Sweden

Fumiharu Togo
Educational Physiology Laboratory, Graduate School of Education, The University of Tokyo, Tokyo, Japan

Hyuntae Park
Department of Health Care and Science, College of Health Science, Dong-A University, Busan, Republic of Korea

Index

P

R

S

T

W

www.ingramcontent.com/pod-product-compliance
Lightning Source LLC
Chambersburg PA
CBHW080532200326
41458CB00012B/4416
9781632418449